FLESH IN THE AGE OF REASON

FLESH IN THE
AGE OF REASON

ROY PORTER

FOREWORD BY SIMON SCHAMA

W. W. Norton & Company

New York London

Manufacturing by the Maple-Vail Book Manufacturing Group

Library of Congress Cataloging-in-Publication Data
Porter, Roy, 1946–
Flesh in the Age of Reason / Roy Porter; foreword by Simon Schama.
p. cm.
Originally published: London : Allen Lane, 2003.
Includes bibliographical references (p.) and index.
ISBN 0-393-05075-0
1. English Literature—18th century—History and criticism. 2. Body, Human, in
literature. 3. Great Britain—Intellectual life—18th century. 4. Enlightenment—
Great Britain. 5. Mind and body in literature. 6. Rationalism in literature. I. Title.
PR448 B63P67 2004
820.9'3561—dc22   2003070156

ISBN 0-393-32696-8 pbk.

W. W. Norton & Company, Inc.
500 Fifth Avenue, New York, N.Y. 10110
www.wwnorton.com

W. W. Norton & Company Ltd.
Castle House, 75/76 Wells Street, London W1T 3QT

1 2 3 4 5 6 7 8 9 0

To Natsu, the love of my life

For, what was ever understood
By human Kind, but Flesh and Blood?

JONATHAN SWIFT,
'A Receipt to Restore Stella's Youth'

The Corruption of the Senses is the Generation of the
Spirit. JONATHAN SWIFT,
A Discourse Concerning the Mechanical Operation of
the Spirit in a Letter To a Friend. A Fragment

I said, 'we were not stocks and stones' – 'tis very well. I
should have added, nor are we angels, I wish we were,
– but men cloathed with bodies, and governed by our
imaginations. LAURENCE STERNE,
The Life and Opinions of Tristram Shandy

Will this be good for your worships' eyes?

LAURENCE STERNE,
The Life and Opinions of Tristram Shandy

CONTENTS

CONTENTS

PART III. THE FRAILTY OF THE FLESH

PART IV. THE SCIENCE OF MAN
FOR A NEW SOCIETY

FOREWORD

About half way through Roy Porter's intellectual epic, he has his hero Laurence Sterne rail against the 'dirty planet' in which 'strange fatalities' rain down ' "body blows" against the "delicate and fine-spun web" of life, all stage-managed, it seems, by a malignant spirit'. And for those of us who knew, admired and loved Roy Porter, reading *Flesh in the Age of Reason* is necessarily an acutely painful pleasure. For it is mercilessly clear that Roy died at the height of his powers. The book is great Porter, which is to say the best history anyone could ever want to read. Never was the presence of the author so strongly present: deeply serious in the depth of his philosophical inquiry, yet wearing his massive erudition lightly. As always in his work, exacting arguments of intellectual history are made accessible as narrative; the ideas themselves not suspended in some realm of disembodied play, but fleshed out as the title of the work implies and embedded in the lived historical experience of thinkers both mighty and paltry.

The unmistakeably eighteenth-century irony, that the subject of Roy's posthumous masterpiece is itself the long, vexed relationship between the body and the rest of us (soul or mind), would have drawn from the author one of his famously expansive full-body chuckles. But for those of us who bitterly miss his personal as well as his intellectual presence, the exhilaration of reading this shockingly vital and exuberant book is punctuated by the mournfulness of realizing that there will not be another like it. It is, I suppose, some sort of scant consolation that *Flesh in the Age of Reason* actually enacts, in the enduring imprint it leaves on the reader, some of the more optimistic beliefs of its eighteenth-century protagonists, who imagined the mind as the place where identity was built; where consciousness, sentiment and memory dwelled; the lodging-house, in fact, of humanity. But it is, nonetheless, hard for his friends to read Porter's revisitings of the likes of Samuel Johnson, Edward Gibbon, Sterne and Coleridge, all of whose ~~beliefs in the supremacy of vigorous reason were deeply threatened by the fragility of the flesh~~ – and not feel a sharp pang.

For Porter aficionados there are some familiar faces in this volume whom Roy has written about elsewhere – Thomas Beddoes, George Cheyne; Thomas Day; David Hartley; Erasmus Darwin – yet the accounts of what each had to offer to the long debate about the relationship between mind and body never feel stale. (Erasmus Darwin, for example, the founder of the Lunar Society, is made more clearly than ever the progenitor of the theory of evolution consummated by his grandson.) And this is because, in this last work, Porter brought the huge weight of his encyclopedic knowledge to bear on the most demanding questions which have exercised restless minds since Plato: ~~What can we know of ourselves and how would such knowledge be conditioned or compromised by the physical apparatus of its cognition?~~ And, most ambitiously – and for the reader most thrillingly – Porter tackles, through the first hundred or so pages of his book, the history of the idea of the soul. This takes him to places where most eighteenth-century social and cultural historians shrink from trespassing: to the Greeks and the classical Christian philosophers and theologians, and eventually on to René Descartes's dualism. One of the many reasons to be wistful as well as grateful for *Flesh in the Age of Reason* is that one realizes that Porter was warming up to grapple with the torments of the Christian seventeenth century with much the same critical shrewdness and historical sympathy as he had shown for the Enlightenment rationalists of the eighteenth. The readings of Descartes, Milton and Hobbes are as thoughtful and penetrating as those of Hume and Millar for the eighteenth.

As vast as the scale of the undertaking is, the book is never heavy going. It is lightened, not by any relaxation in the sharpness of argument, but by Porter's brief to himself to register the imprint of ideas in social action; and to see, in turn, how such social action might affect the onward discourse of debates about body and mind. So there are, as usual in his work, passages of dazzling description which conjure up whole worlds of freshly agitated self-consciousness. The dawning of the idea that hysteria or hypochondria were physical maladies (rather than purely moral disorders), and were thus susceptible of some sort of corrective regimen, gets vintage Porter analysis, the witty asides always softened by compassionate empathy. And alongside the major figures in the canon Porter makes room for more eccentric figures who nonetheless play their own part in the long, tortured relationship between soul or mind and the body in which it was taken to be imprisoned: Luigi Cornaro, for example, the prophet of a temperate life whose dining habits were so perfectly balanced that he could write 'I feel when I leave the table that I must sing.' Cornaro, Porter tells us, wrote his first book of counsel at 83, his fourth at 95 but then 'passed away prematurely at the disappointing age of 98'. Or at the other end of the scales, George Cheyne, who ballooned to a massive 450 pounds before subjecting himself to the brutal regime of vomits, purges and fasts which entitled the (relatively) skinnier Cheyne to lecture his contemporaries on the perils of gluttony and idleness.

Flesh in the Age of Reason manages, over and again, to spot the moments where a familiar modern preoccupation gets born and circulated in the wider culture, whithout any kind of anachronistic projection. Thus, Porter sees the change in the second half of the eighteenth century, from a culture which celebrated embonpoint and fleshiness as a sign of vitality to Byron's narcissistic regime of diet and exercise, as a genuinely fateful moment: the beginnings of the obsession with youthfulness (especially svelte youth) as a paradigm of beauty. Similarly, he is marvellously illuminating on the first writers, like William Alexander, a whole generation before Mary Wollstonecraft, able to argue that gender was a social construction.

Throughout the whole book flashes Roy Porter's wickedly wonderful way with language; unafraid of importing street talk when it makes sense and delivers his argument with punchy humour. Eighteenth-century England, he writes of the anxieties voiced by Cheyne, was 'becoming a nation of fatties' and 'for certain of Johnson's contemporaries, the blues were a treasured identity badge'. Then, too, Porter allows his almost Johnsonian gift for aphorism full play. The 3rd Earl of Shaftesbury 'was lastingly charmed by the flair and creativity of his genius'. Johnson's 'daily bread was monstrous toil, menial, grinding against the clock; the lexicographer was indeed a drudge'. But these edgy little jabs are just accents in a book where the writing is so exhilarating that it is often difficult to resist smiling at its sheer brio. For Roy Porter, historical prose was never a workaday thing, but in this book, where all of his passions and preoccupations are in overdrive, he lets his feeling for language as a succulent, luscious, toothsome thing, rip. Great writing from the eighteenth century and Romantic masters – Dr Johnson, Gibbon, Hazlitt and Blake – draws from him, as if in irresistible yet admiring emulation, passages worthy of them. The long discussion of the body wars in *Tristram Shandy* may be the single most perceptive and intensely engaged commentary on that book ever written, and, perhaps surprisingly in a book that journeys from Plato to Francis Crick, it is at the very heart of the matter, nowhere more acutely than when Porter writes, movingly as well as wittily:

He was uncommonly sensitive to the conundrum of embodiment. In flesh and blood lay the self and its articulations. With its own elaborate sign-language of gesture and feeling, the body was the inseparable dancing-partner of the mind or soul – now in step, now a tangle of limbs and intentions, mixed emotions. Organism and consciousness, *soma* and psyche, heart and head, the outer and the inner – all merged, and all needed to be minutely observed if the human enigma were ever to be appreciated.

What Porter writes appreciatively of Sterne could also, of course, be written of Porter. And if it is to our everlasting chagrin that such appreciation now comes in the form of an epitaph, this colossal and intellectually thrilling work is at least a vindication of another of its more hopeful, authentically eighteenth-century themes: that though the body may perish, the mind does indeed live on.

writing as legacy

SIMON SCHAMA

PREFACE

Key developments in sixteenth- and seventeenth-century Europe heightened age-old tensions as to the nature of man. In certain respects, the body grew more beset and battered. Endemic warfare, epidemics of bubonic plague, typhus and other urban fevers and the hideous new horrors of syphilis sharpened the woes of this mortal coil. And the prevalent sense of danger and desperation was amplified by the hellfire religious terrorism thundering from Calvinist and Counter-Reformation pulpits and the morbid disgust expressive of extreme Mannerist and Baroque sensibilities.

Yet this was also the age when the humanist revival offered alternatives to the macabre mind-set pervasive since late-medieval times; the body noble, beautiful, orderly, ideal, the dignity of human nature. Vile bodies might still be calumniated, and fleshpots remained siren snares, but the human physique was now equally honoured, thanks to the Renaissance recovery of classical aesthetics, with its veneration ✗ for those macrocosmic–microcosmic harmonies which made the human form the measure and model of all things.

Innovations in medicine, spearheaded by the techniques of dissection developed by Vesalius, further opened the tangible body, the body of the senses, to the probing, penetrative curiosity of the scalpel. Once within the anatomy theatre, the corpse ceased to be inviolable and taboo, and carnal knowledge was no longer forbidden: would not the data gleaned through dissection reveal the glories of Creation and its Divine Artist, and lead to the improvement of medical knowledge and practice? The art and science promoted by the Renaissance and the Scientific Revolution thus promised to metamorphose and resurrect the body in a more secular guise. Meanwhile, however, the Churches continued to elaborate their own teachings about the body:

the Catholic cult of the sacred heart was contemporaneous with William Harvey's *De Motu Cordis*.

Élite drives for the 'reformation of popular culture' aimed to widen the *cordon sanitaire* between bodies superior and inferior. Refined bodily manners would be elevated above coarse flesh via the 'civilizing process'; vile bodies would be firmly consigned to their place; and their subjugation would be reinforced through the pains and penalties of the law (corporal and capital punishment), through training and work discipline (the curse of labour), and through more stringent control of leisure and sexuality.

Not least, intense inquiries – philosophical, medico-scientific, theological – were turning the flesh into a 'body in question'. Down the centuries, it had been the Churches which had arrogated to themselves the authority to pronounce on the riddles of life, from before the cradle to beyond the grave, by way of their canons on the Creation, Fall and Atonement, and specifically on eschatology (study of the four last things: death, judgement, heaven and hell). The state for its part devised doctrines of its own respecting the 'king's two bodies', the 'sacred touch' of the monarch who ruled by Divine Right, and the prince's relation to the 'body politic'. Sacred and temporal, all such tenets were to come under fire from radicals, critics and wits in the free-thinking atmosphere of the Enlightenment. Meanwhile, magical and folklorish beliefs about the flesh (the curative properties of the blood of a hanged man, for instance, or the incorruptibility of the remains of the holy) were being discounted by the élite as 'vulgar errors'.

New metaphysical enigmas loomed. Precisely what were the links between mind and matter, body and soul? Might life be not a divine benefaction after all, but something merely material, a chemical curdling or an electrical spark which triggered vitality? Was the human body, indeed, a machine, pure and simple, of a piece with nature at large as conceived by the new mechanical philosophy? Were the passions to be tamed, or could they be trusted, as part of the wisdom of the body? Was there a *vis medicatrix naturae*, a healing power of Nature, which would preserve life against disease and dissolution? Not least – profanely Promethean thought! – was there any escape from the doom of death? The body Christian, the body pagan; the body medical, the body scientific; the body noble, the body debased; the body free and the body disciplined; the body natural and the body artificial; the body solitary and social; the body sacred and profane – all these were in the melting pot in that great 'crisis' of European thought marking the early Enlightenment, and such questions and attempts to resolve them surface again and again in the body of this book

It will become obvious to readers that certain aspects of this subject receive scant attention. I particularly regret not addressing – for reasons of 'ignorance, Madam, pure ignorance' – changing visualizations of flesh and the self in portraits and caricature in the scholarly tradition pioneered by David Piper and continued by Marcia Pointon, Ludmilla Jordanova and others. I have also made no attempt to explore the problem of personal identity in terms of the preoccupations of contemporary philosophy. The interest in such questions as the 'other minds' debate shown by today's professional philosophers strikes me as 'merely' academic; for those surveyed in this book what was at stake was truly personal, practical and pressing. By way of a final disclaimer, I must make it clear that I engage below almost wholly with the thinking of literate (indeed, literary) élites: a parallel exploration of low and popular culture would be immensely rewarding.

This book follows on from my *Enlightenment: Britain and the Creation of the Modern World* (Allen Lane, 2000). Noting various themes omitted from that book, particularly 'the controversies which raged over mind and body, heaven and hell, the soul, the afterlife, and the *je ne sais quoi* of the self', I announced that 'I plan to address such topics in my next book, which will examine the triangle of the moral, the material and the medical in the anglophone Enlightenment'. This is that. Building upon its broad account of British enlightened thinking, I here present detailed explorations of dilemmas about personal identity in the light of changing beliefs about man's place in nature and human nature. I have not attempted a 'textbook' coverage; rather I present a gallery of contrasting yet interlocking studies meant to be engaging and stimulating rather than encyclopaedic.

ACKNOWLEDGEMENTS

Much of the research for this book was undertaken during the two happy decades I spent at the Wellcome Institute for the History of Medicine in London. Writing began during the first year of its successor, the Wellcome Trust Centre for the History of Medicine at University College London, and it has been completed in the months following my retirement. I am deeply grateful for the facilities generously extended to me since then by Hal Cook, its Director, and its Administrator, Alan Shiel. I am also delighted to acknowledge the unstinting support given to me by members of its staff, notably my former secretary, Emma Ford. Over the years Caroline Overy, Sharon Messenger and Jane Henderson have helped me with research – and Jane has additionally compiled the excellent index. Claire Henderson-Davis also contributed valuable research on folklore. Typing of the seemingly endless proliferation of redrafts has been done by Emma and (as always) by Sheila Lawler. Thanks also to Jed Lawler for coming to the rescue of a computer illiterate. I have been fortunate to have a highly capable copy-editor in Elizabeth Stratford.

PUBLISHER'S NOTE

Roy Porter completed the final draft of this book very shortly before his death. The endnotes were in a half-finished state and these have been dropped. A full bibliography is to be found at the end of the text. Roy often worked from a number of different editions of the same text and without his aid it has proved impossible to construct these references.

The publishers would like to thank Natsu Hattori, Gill Coleridge, David Cannadine and Simon Schama for all their help and comments.

PART I

SOULS AND BODIES

I

INTRODUCTION:
KNOW YOURSELF

Who are we?

Our contemporary Western secular sense of identity stems directly from transformations occurring in the centuries since the Renaissance. These developments are often characterized as the 'death of the soul', but inseparable from such a process, and no less salient, has been the reappraisal of the body. The two have been symbiotic in the refiguring of the self.

The history of the self is commonly told as the rise of modern individualism, the maturing self-consciousness of the self-determining individual. Here lies the fulfilment of the cherished ideals first of 'knowing yourself' – the *gnothi seauton* of the Delphic oracle – and then of 'being yourself': 'this above all, to thine own self be true', as Polonius puts it in *Hamlet*, wearying his son as ever with unwanted advice. In this triumphalist telling, the secret of selfhood is located in authenticity and individuality, and the story presented is one of the surmounting of intractable obstacles in the achievement of autonomy. This great labour of inner character-building typically involves breaking free from religious persecution, political tyranny and the shackles of hidebound convention. Such ideals of self-realization, nobly voiced a century and a half ago in John Stuart Mill's *On Liberty*, still carry a strong appeal, and they square with other values – democracy, freedom of speech, equal opportunities, doing your own thing – which we all hold dear and to which the 'free world' at least pays lip-service.

Received ideas of identity in the West thus presuppose some real and essential 'inner self'. Favoured ways of imagining its realization include the metaphor of a seed maturing into a flower, or

3

the growth-process from birth to adulthood, from dependency to self-sufficiency. These organic metaphors are reflected in popular narratives, or myths, of the historical evolution of the self through the rise of civilization.

It is a tale which begins with the fabled dawn of consciousness. 'Primitive societies' have been deemed to possess a 'tribal' mentality, with all thought-processes being collective and all activities communal. This 'savage mind' was supposedly so gripped by supernatural and magical outlooks, by group rituals and customs, as to preclude any genuine individuality.

It was the golden age of Greece, the story continues, which brought the first stirrings of true individual consciousness, asserted in defiance of clannish taboos and the inexorable decrees of the gods. Socrates and other philosophers began to give expression to ideals of inner goodness, truth and sacred conscience. So threatening to traditional values did such new convictions prove that even the advanced Athenians forced Socrates to drink the hemlock. For their part, Aeschylus, Sophocles and Euripides showed in their dramas how emergent conflicts between the individual and divine and dynastic order were fated to end in tragedy. In later centuries, under imperial despotism in Rome, Stoic philosophers like Seneca valued suicide as the only permitted expression of freedom and autonomy.

The age of faith brought partial advances towards realizing the sovereignty of the inner self. Christianity's core doctrine of a unique, eternal soul inspired those brave acts of personal integrity, modelled on the Crucifixion, which were the making of martyrs; and St Augustine's *Confessions* at the end of the fourth century gave a remarkable self-portrait of the inner trials of the soul of a guilty sinner.

But the Catholic Church had no investment in self-exploration for its own sake. Egoism was anathema. The Church's mission was to teach how mankind's first parents, Adam and Eve, had been punished for disobedience. Did not the early theologian Tertullian insist that 'we have no need for curiosity, after Jesus Christ, nor for investigation after the Gospel'? It was idle curiosity that hankered after forbidden knowledge. The lesson of Original Sin was that the devout must obey the Commandments; self was the wellspring of sin, and Lucifer's fate showed how rebellion (*non serviam*) would be rightly and relentlessly crushed.

Self-denial was the supreme good, as expressed in monastic asceticism and celibacy; saints and mystics transcended their selves in divine love, St John of the Cross seeking the 'annihilation of the self'. All such Christian ideals of self-distrust, of trampling down pride and vanity through submission and selflessly serving in the *Corpus Christi*, the community of the faithful, squared with the medieval feudal principle that everyone had a preordained position in the divine Great Chain of Being, in the hierarchical order of lord and serf, master and man, husband and wife, parent and child; the whole was greater than the part. If the cause of individuality was advanced under medieval Christianity it was largely by those heretics who defied it.

In conventional accounts of the 'ascent of man', it was the age of the Renaissance and Reformation that brought truly decisive breakthroughs. Ever since Jacob Burckhardt, Darwin's contemporary, leading historians and art critics have acclaimed Renaissance Italy as the time and place when 'man' – for which read literate, gifted, élite males – began to break free from the chains of custom, conformity and the Church, taking fearless leaps forward into self-discovery and self-fulfilment at the very time when Columbus was 'discovering' the New World.

As a literary and scholarly movement, humanism rejected the dogma of the miserable sinner required to abase himself before a jealous God, and began to take delight in man himself as the apex of creation, the master of nature, the wonder of the world. New cultural genres – the portrait (above all the *self*-portrait), the diary and the biography (especially the *auto*biography) – reveal heightened perceptions of individuality, the proud ego vaunting and flaunting his own being.

A new sense of personal singularity, and a bold impulse to explore that distinctiveness, radiates from the sixteenth-century French essayist Michel de Montaigne, who posed the fundamental question: *que sçais-je?* (what do I know?), and then humbly tried to answer it through scrupulous introspection. Infinitely curious, that great sceptic proposed that man possessed an *arrière boutique toute nostre* – a room behind the shop all our own: the individual's mind was a unique storeroom of consciousness, a personal new world, ripe for discovery. Montaigne himself retired early from public life, not to commune with God but to scrutinize his own psyche. He might have appreciated Prince Hamlet, for such questions of identity are what Shakespeare's moody, brooding hero soliloquizes upon: who precisely is this 'paragon of animals' who is yet the 'quintessence of dust'? The key role of the soliloquy in Renaissance drama itself marks a new accent on the individual.

Yet, like Socrates and the Christian martyrs, Hamlet too has to die, as do all the other great overreachers portrayed by Renaissance playwrights, such as Marlowe's Dr Faustus and Tamburlaine. Evidently the triumph of the autonomous individual was still a long way off. Highly significant in this respect is the radical ambivalence of Protestantism. Together with other pioneering sociologists of modernization, Max Weber argued in his *The Protestant Ethic and the Spirit of Capitalism* (1904–5) that the Reformation spurred a new individuality, thanks to the reformers' doctrine of the priesthood of all believers: salvation must be a personal pilgrimage, a matter of faith alone (solifidianism); it could not be parcelled out by priests in pardons and other papist bribes. Hence, Protestantism forced believers into soul-searching: Puritans became noted for their breast-beating spiritual diaries. Guilt, sin and submission remained central. Calvin taught predestination and burned heretics, and arguably it was not until Nietzsche proclaimed 'God is dead' late in the nineteenth century that man could fully come into his own as a truly liberated autonomous being.

Ancestor-seeking philosophers have nevertheless identified the seventeenth century as the great divide, the point from which secular rationality served as the foundation of the self-determining individual. According to this reading of Psyche's Progress, it was René Descartes (1596–1650) who staked out a new role for the individual by making the basis of his *Discourse on Method* (1637) the proposition *cogito ergo sum* (I am thinking, therefore I am): my own consciousness is the one thing of which I can be sure, the sole Archimedean point in the human universe. Neither God nor nature, but the ego or consciousness is the spring of human self-understanding.

In medieval thought, as Dante's early fourteenth-century *Divine Comedy* makes clear, the human condition had been conceived through a conspectus of the whole compass of Creation and its macrocosmic–microcosmic correspondences. That cosmological perspective on man's estate was now reversed by an act of self-reflective thought – literally, so Descartes relates, while meditating alone in a small room with a stove, in what seems a licence for solipsism. Indeed, in an astonishingly daring stroke, Cartesian dualism claimed that reason reveals that man is perfectly unique beneath the heavens: he alone, under God, has a conscious mind (*res cogitans*), he alone can *know himself* and so understand the meaning of things. Everything else, the entire animal kingdom included, is mere 'extension' (*res extensa*), that is, inert matter in motion governed by the iron laws of mechanics.

Descartes's dream of the uniqueness of human interiority (self-aware thinking) provoked later introspective philosophers further to probe the mechanisms of the mind. The question *who am I?* was turned into a matter of how our cognitive processes operate: identity resides within the house of intellect. In his highly influential *Essay concerning Human Understanding* (1690), John Locke argued that the mind is not like a furnished flat, prestocked before occupation with innate ideas, but like a home put together piecemeal from mental acquisitions picked up bit by bit. The self is thus the bit-by-bit product of experience and education: we are what we become – or, in Wordsworth's later phrase, the child is father of the man. Particular parents, surroundings and stimuli produce individuated selves. Identity is thus unique because contingent, the cumulative product of ceaseless occurrences. By implication, Locke thus gave his philosophical blessing to change, progress and even diversity, and hence championed freedom of speech and religious toleration.

[margin notes: Dante to Descartes / cosmic to consciousness / Calib Conv- psychol.]

Critics judged this Lockean psychology to be disturbingly relativistic; for supporters, however, it promoted a heroic vision of man making himself – man viewed both as the *producer* but also as the *product* of social development and the civilizing process. Man was no longer to be pictured as an Adam, created by God in His own image, with all his faculties, for good and ill, fully implanted. Rather, the coming myths of the Enlightenment promoted self-made (and God-usurping) man, and thus they made their mark on Marx and the Victorian prophets of progress.

mind = blank slate

Drawing on Francis Bacon's championing of science as the key to human progress, enlightened *philosophes* modelled man as *faber suae fortunae*, the author of his own destiny. Building upon Locke's suggestion that the mind begins as 'white paper, or wax, to be moulded and fashioned as one pleases', attention was now paid to dynamic notions of consciousness-forming. Interaction with nature, and the restless dialectic of needs and wants, latent potential and aspirations, gave man the capacity to progress towards perfectibility, proclaimed the sunny new theories advanced by such thinkers as Condillac, Turgot and Condorcet in France, Priestley, Erasmus Darwin and Godwin in England, and Fichte, Herder and Hegel in Germany.

The story standardly told of the heroic rise of the modern self is not, of course, without its sub-plots, complications and deviations. One centres on that great enigma, Jean-Jacques Rousseau (1712–78), who, like a new Luther, took his stand with painful honesty in his soul-searching autobiographical *Confessions*. 'I know my own heart', the combative solitary proclaimed; and, knowing it, he felt obliged to bare it, good and bad, to all the world – a compulsion for self-exposure that has released, in a great act of homage, a never-ceasing confessional stream, from the poets, artists and geniuses of the Romantic era through to our latter-day drunks, drifters, drug-addicts, drop-outs and depressives. Confession was thereby transformed from an office of the Church into an affirmation of the 'will to truth' of the sacred sovereign self within.

and performance artists

He was quite unlike any other person, Rousseau insisted: he was exceptionally sensitive, he had masochistic leanings, he was addicted to masturbation and other vices, and had abandoned all his infants to an orphanage. In Rousseau, and all the more so in the Marquis de Sade, psychological introspection discovered psycho-pathology – a heart of darkness – and drove the urge to reveal, in the name of truth, what formerly had been judged better left unknown or unsaid and best of all resisted. Formerly a sin, self-centredness was being transformed into the *raison d'être*, the pride and glory, of the modern psyche: thanks to the 'cunning of history', Christian self-denial was thus giving way to the urge – even the 'right' – to self-expression. A century later, patients would 'tell all' on the Freudian couch.

This novel and seemingly inexhaustible fascination with baring the soul reminds us that it was during the eighteenth century that the novel, particularly when cast as first-person narrative, became the prime instrument for the microscopic exploration of fevered inner consciousness. Such classics as Goethe's *Wilhelm Meister's Apprenticeship* (1795–6) took as their very subject the often tortured development (*Bildung*) of the hero's character. 'Sensibility' became essential to goodness and beauty; in the cult of the man and woman of feeling, every sigh, blush and teardrop confirmed the exquisite tuning of the superior soul; and romantic love privileged the boundless questings of the heart. Self-discovery through bitter experience became the dominant Romantic metaphor, with its wanderer protagonist seeking spiritual epiphany through toil and trouble.

The individual moved centre-stage in many other domains of eighteenth-century thinking. Cast as the autonomous bearer of rights, he (women were rarely yet part of the equation) became the basic building-block in a political liberalism which rebutted old Divine Right and absolutist theories with the declaration that the sovereign individual was prior to the state – indeed, was its sole reason for existing. Society was the product of free men coming together to set up a political society to protect fundamental rights to life, liberty and property. Such were the foundations of the new American republic.

In a parallel move, enlightened economic theories also took as their base the private property-holder – the possessive individualist or Robinson Crusoe figure. Finding classic expression in Adam Smith's

Wealth of Nations (1776), political economy imagined the market-place as an arena of independent contractors, each pursuing personal profit through cut-throat competition. Thanks to what Smith called the 'invisible hand', enlightened self-interest, pursued without hindrance, would providentially advantage all – the result would be, in Jeremy Bentham's utilitarian formulation, the greatest happiness of the greatest number, with each individual counting as one unit, no more, no less. What a spectacular reversal of the old moral theology! The Church had rejected selfishness (greed, cupidity) as sin. But such enlightened thinkers as David Hume now contended that the rational hedonism of *homo economicus* was advantageous, both for the individual and for society at large: something scandalously close to 'greed is good'. 'Self-love thus pushed to social, to divine,/Gives thee to make thy neighbour's blessing thine', sang the poet Alexander Pope, while Bernard de Mandeville revelled in the paradox that private vices were public benefits. This new enlightened individualism came to fruition in the American Constitution and in the 'Liberty, Equality and Fraternity' of the French Revolution. Of course, it was not lost on reactionary foes that the Revolution's outcomes – notably the Terror – betrayed those aspirations: sow the wind, and reap the whirlwind.

The revolutionary era moreover inspired the *Sturm und Drang* ('storm and stress') movement in Germany and Romanticism throughout Europe in literature and the arts, thereby pitching individualism onto ever more exalted planes. Rejecting the cash nexus and the insipid despotism of conventional taste, Romanticism idealized the bardic visionary, the Bohemian, the outsider, the Byronic rebel – even victims like Frankenstein's monster, all alone in an unfeeling world.

Romantic social criticism rejected bourgeois respectability: the world is too much with us, complained Wordsworth; urban man was alienated. Communing with Nature was the way to restore harmony with one's true inner self. Life must be a pilgrimage of self-discovery, bitter perhaps – a *Winterreise*. In their distinctive ways, Schiller and Shelley, Coleridge and Chateaubriand, Hölderlin and

Hazlitt each espoused a creed of the sacredness of individual development, in pursuit of what Keats called the 'holiness of the heart's
intentions and the truth of imagination'. Self-development was thus
assuming a sanctified ethos while, in the philosophy of Hegel, the
dialectical strivings of mind or spirit (*Geist*) towards autonomy or full
self-awareness fused personal development with spiritual destiny:
Goethe's *Faust* (first part, 1808; second part, 1832) forms the sublime
instance.

Through the nineteenth century, the Romantic drive to self-
understanding and realization ventured into ever more intense
expression. Schopenhauer, Nietzsche and the novelists and artists of
the *fin de siècle* centred their anguished visions on the solitary individual, solipsistically enduring or enjoying utter isolation from society
and the universe. Often stimulated (or wrecked) by dreams, drugs or
drink, decadent poets dwelt upon their inner experiences. Academic
psychology meanwhile turned subjectivity into an object for scientific
investigation and, through the invention of systematic testing, focused
attention upon individual differences.

Above all, this impassioned quest for the ultimate truth of the self
seemed to make a crucial breakthrough with the 'discovery of the
unconscious'. The upstaging, or rather undermining, of the Cartesian
cogito certainly did not begin with Sigmund Freud – earlier writers
such as Coleridge were fully aware of the 'insensible' and the 'involuntary' aspects of the self, manifest for instance in dreaming – but it
was Freud who theorized the unconscious. Psychoanalysis argued
that the rational understanding proudly cultivated by the Renaissance humanists, and likewise Descartes's prized *cogito*, was not after
all master in its own house, not the real thing. What truly counted was
what had hitherto lurked concealed, an unconscious that was profoundly repressed and hence expressed only obliquely and painfully
through illness and hysteria, nightmare and fantasy.

Freud and his followers thereby opened up new horizons of selfhood, or rather plumbed the psyche's oceanic depths, exposing a
hidden world of secret desires and treacherous drives. Self-discovery
thus became a voyage into inner space, colonization of which was

to have the profoundest implications for twentieth-century psychiatry, art and literature, notably in Surrealism or the stream-of-consciousness novel.

Critically, Freud claimed, too, that he had hit upon a decisive new truth (or one stubbornly silenced): the ultimate secret of the self was sexuality. Depth psychology thus gave a new edge to Polonius's advice. Because the Freudian psyche might not be pleasant to behold – it harboured the incestuous Oedipal libido – ruthless honesty became more essential than ever: nothing should be concealed or rationalized away.

This truth imperative was no less fundamental to one of the key philosophical movements of the twentieth century, existentialism, whose oracle, Jean-Paul Sartre, required the combating of the 'bad faith' of the unexamined life, and all its duplicities. The movement which began with Renaissance autobiography culminated, it thus appears, in existential integrity or angst, the equivocal finest hour of subjective individualism. Meanwhile, on a less exalted plane, the twentieth century spawned scores of creeds and cults, nodding in the direction of Freud and other gurus, which claimed to help people understand and accept themselves, maximize their potential, express themselves and, of course, *be* themselves. The culmination was the post-1960s 'me generation', with its creed of doing your own thing.

Grand narratives of the kind just recounted – of how the West discovered, championed and honed a distinctive self unknown to earlier times, an inner, individualist psyche unfamiliar to the great civilizations of the East – underpin popular attitudes and public platitudes, and continue to carry a huge appeal. Furthermore, they mould familiar stereotypes of 'alternatives': the noble savage, the medieval peasant, the Romantic poet, the free spirit, the lonely crowd, the alienated intellectual, and so on.

Do they not contain a measure of truth? After all, much of our recent artistic and intellectual heritage involves celebration of the exceptional outpourings of mighty, self-absorbed geniuses, such as Beethoven. Yet the tale also has the ring of myth, and an air of soap-box rhetoric, especially when recounted as an epic in which the striving, heroic self scales ridge after ridge until it reaches its peak of perfection in our own times, truly 'authentic' at last – a story flattering to ourselves, when the final twist identifies ours as an age of singular psychic crisis: the self in neurotic torment.

Yet aspects of this meta-narrative must be rejected as self-serving fiction, in particular its Hegelian or teleological assumptions about linear evolution. Belief in an inevitable ascent from some primordial collective psychological soup or swamp to the shining apogee of individual identity now seems a question-begging, self-congratulatory mirage, left over from Herbert Spencer and other Victorians. The horrors of the twentieth century surely demolished the assurance of earlier individualists that the evolution of individuality automatically brought moral improvement.

After all, psychological individualism has a problematic character. In the eighteenth century, Locke's claim that identity is made not given (nurture not nature) served progressive ends – it underwrote political liberation. In the twentieth century, by contrast, the Lockean doctrine of malleability played into the hands of stimulus-response behaviourism, as developed by B. F. Skinner and taken up by totalitarian brainwashing regimes, and of other conservative exponents of social conditioning.

The tensions between self-knowledge and self-possession – the ambiguous implications of science for the psyche – were not lost on Freud. His wholehearted public commitment to pursuing (self-)analysis to the limit required that we be disabused of rose-tinted expectations that such new knowledge would indubitably bring freedom and happiness: in truth, the science of the self would flatten rather than flatter man's self-esteem. 'Humanity has in the course of time had to endure from the hands of science two great outrages upon naive self-love,' Freud explained:

The first was when it realized that our earth was not the centre of the universe, but only a tiny speck in a world-system of a magnitude hardly conceivable; this is associated in our minds with the name of Copernicus, although Alexandrian doctrines taught something very similar. The second was when biological research robbed man of his peculiar privilege of having been specially created, and relegated him to a descent from the animal world, implying an ineradicable animal nature in him: this transvaluation has been accomplished in our own time upon the instigation of Charles Darwin, Wallace and their predecessors, and not without the most violent opposition from their contemporaries. But man's craving for grandiosity is now suffering the third and most bitter blow from present-day psychological research which is endeavouring to prove to the 'ego' of each one of us that he is not even master in his own house, but that he must remain content with the veriest scraps of information about what is going on unconsciously in his own mind. We psycho-analysts were neither the first nor the only ones to propose to mankind that they should look inward; but it appears to be our lot to advocate it most insistently and to support it by empirical evidence which touches every man closely.

Freud thus overturned the Augustinian doctrine of 'forbidden knowledge': pursuit of knowledge about the self did not signal pride, rather it was its antidote.

Yet, for all his innovations and anxieties, Freud was in one crucial respect a traditionalist: he too believed there was indeed an inner core truth of the self – albeit one located in the terrifying subterranean battleground of the id, ego and superego – waiting to be discovered, analysed and even healed. Similarly, the reason why Shakespeare and others had been able to write romantic comedies of 'mistaken identity' was precisely because it was assumed that such confusions could actually be overcome and true identity eventually disclosed: deceptions would end, the masks would come off, all would be revealed. Faced with cases of 'multiple personality', psychoanalysis aimed to expose the false and reinstate the true one.

What has been especially striking in recent decades, however, is the rise of new outlooks challenging the very idea of a nucleated (if evasive) inner personal identity. Gilbert Ryle exposed the myth of the 'ghost in the machine', but crucial here have been the theories of Roland Barthes, Michel Foucault and Jacques Derrida, and more generally of deconstructionists and postmodernists at large. Barthes for his part promoted the notion of the 'death of the author'; in a series of books published over the course of twenty-five years, Foucault challenged liberal belief in individual intention and agency. The conventional humanistic understanding of subjectivity – the individual agent, writer or reader possessing a mind of his or her own and exercising free will through thought and action – was superficial and self-serving. Rather, such anti-humanist iconoclasts argued for the primacy of semantic sign systems, cognitive structures and texts. We don't think our thoughts, they think us; we are but the bearers of discourses, our selves are discursive constructs. Within such frames of analysis, any notion of the ascent of selfhood is but idle teleological myth, a humanist hagiography.

Such a Romantic fallacy had peaked in the nineteenth century (argued Foucault) before collapsing in our own era, partly thanks to the devastating critique mounted by Nietzsche. The death of God, Foucault held, reversing conventional interpretations, entailed the death of man as well: man was decentred or dissolved.

Postmodernism thus maintained that the conventional story of the triumph of the self was no more than an anthropocentric fallacy. Even more scandalously, Foucault and his followers argued that the new individualism heralded in the Enlightenment was in truth – contrary to the claims of its champions and to later apologetics – not an emancipation from social fetters but the very means by which state power cunningly locked subjects into bureaucratic and administrative systems, by stamping them with a clear and distinct identity. Subjectivity was thus a new tool of subjection. Such developments as civil registration required the documenting of names, births and deaths; police mug-shots and fingerprinting were introduced – unique to the individual, and useful mainly as a means of social identification. Continuing controversy in Britain today over the proposed introduction of compulsory identity cards illustrates the point: what has been truly difficult to achieve in modern times is not identity but anonymity.

Traditional tellings of the ascent of man have thus been criticized by those who hold that the prized liberal self is just a rhetorical construct, a trick of language, a ruse or sham. New historicism has thus portrayed Renaissance man as not 'self-discovering' but rather 'self-fashioning', as if – how Jonathan Swift would have loved this – the self were but a suit of clothes. The much-trumpeted Renaissance 'discovery of man' is thereby reduced to yet another stratagem, or at least to a mode of 'social construction'.

Liberal pieties have been further assailed by feminist critiques. The telling of the 'discovery of the self' has been mystificatory, these contend, because it has taken the male sex for granted as normative. Not least, the standard image of the hard, thrusting and self-sufficient ego reflects and has served to legitimate crudely macho stereotypes. The customary saga of the self thus mirrors and reinforces myths of masculinity.

Thus, at the dawn of the twenty-first century, the sense of self needs rethinking. The Lord told Moses: 'I AM THAT I AM', but few of us mortals these days feel so confident about who or what we are. True, right-wing governments in the United States and United Kingdom which champion market-place individualism have the backing of sociobiologists and psychological Darwinians who insist that the selfish gene is Nature's way, and there is no shortage of publicity for a galaxy of styles of self-fulfilment, self-expression and psychotherapy. But such nostrum-mongering is advanced against a backdrop of the erosion of established identities, associated with the disintegration of traditional patterns of family life, employment, gender roles, education and other social institutions. The acceptance of such designer drugs as Prozac, Viagra and Ecstasy heralds a new age in which the chemical modification of the brain calls into question old assumptions about the sovereignty of individual character. Indeed, the explosive controversy in the United States about repressed and recovered memory syndrome – the multiple personality held to follow from childhood sexual abuse – hints at a future in which traditional models of a relatively permanent personality may lose applicability.

Not least, we live in the age of the computer, of artificial intelligence and virtual reality. If robots and androids (in actuality and in science fiction) will think (and feel?) like us, if cyberspace supplants the inner space of personal consciousness, what will happen to the privileged realm of our psyche; indeed, what will happen to the human in us? Will all that be dismissed as 'speciesism'? Will there follow a decisive dissolution of the traditional ego-boundary consciousness, with perhaps a 'reversion' to a 'tribal' – but now electronic or chemical – consciousness?

Bearing in mind these heroic narratives of the odyssey of the self and their recent critiques, this book will concentrate on transformations of the sense of self in Britain in the 'age of reason'. In the 'authorized version' endorsed by the Churches, a person was a familiar paradox: a miserable sinner, promised an eternal destiny beyond the grave. The young Dissenter Isaac Watts could thus, around 1680, insert himself in a scenario familiar ever since St Augustine:

his project

> **I** am a vile polluted lump of earth,
> **S** o I've continued ever since my birth,
> **A** lthough Jehovah grace does daily give me,
> **A** s sure this monster Satan will deceive me,
> **C** ome therefore, Lord, from Satan's claws relieve me.

Watts was a sinner of course, hoping for salvation:

> **W** ash me in Thy blood, O Christ,
> **A** nd grace divine impart,
> **T** hen search and try the corners of my heart,
> **T** hat I in all things may be fit to do
> **S** ervice to thee, and sing thy praises too.

His very name, or self, was inscribed and subsumed in the Christian story of sin and salvation.

Sturdy scriptural fundamentalism steadily lost favour, however, at a time when opinion-shaping élites were ceasing to subscribe to and govern their lives by stern Protestant teachings backed by Bible literalism. New scripts of life were to promote variant readings of a self strutting on a terrestrial, this-worldly stage. Such new concepts of the 'I' were defined less by the transcendental soul than in relation to the body. This book will examine them through exploring how educated élites – opinion-makers – grappled with anxieties as to their nature, individuality and destiny as thinking and feeling humans. In the process they often developed stances at odds with entrenched Christian doctrines, now rejecting, now reinterpreting them.

Christian orthodoxy comprised elements gleaned from the Gospels and given an *imprimatur* by the Churches. The scriptural story of Original Sin, the Fall and the Expulsion from Paradise, and man's subsequent redemption by the Son of God made flesh and crucified at Calvary – these were truths endlessly reiterated not just in *summa* and sermons, but through the liturgy, ceremonials and icons first of the Catholic Church and then of the various Protestant confessions. In England they assumed epic expression in Milton's *Paradise Lost* (1667) and *Paradise Regained* (1671).

A human being, these doctrines explained, was a compound of two distinctive elements, soul and flesh. Composed as it was of spirit, the divine soul by its very nature was immaterial and immortal. Somehow – and this aspect was highly controversial – this soul docked with the quickened foetus in the womb, thereafter cohabiting with the flesh during earthly life. Upon death the soul continued to be sentient, being finally reunited with the resurrected body at the Last Judgement, when it would, for the saved, everlastingly take its place among the heavenly host; otherwise it would end up frying in eternal torment below – the predestined fate, Calvinists taught, of the majority.

Faiths and philosophies the world over have entertained prospects of some existence beyond the grave (perhaps in metempsychosis, the transmigration of souls), and belief in ghosts, shades or the wandering spirits of lost souls has been ubiquitous. Any culture crediting supernatural powers is likely to entertain an afterlife of sorts. But this Christian identification of the self with a 'separate soul' which transcended the flesh was especially indebted to theosophies rooted in the Eastern Mediterranean.

Old Testament Judaism, the immediate seedbed of Christianity, was exceptional in this regard, for it had no developed doctrine of an afterlife in which souls would posthumously participate.* The Promised Land of the children of Israel is emphatically not some post- and extra-terrestrial heaven: and while Jehovah frequently threatens to visit dire punishments upon His Chosen People, they are to fall 'unto the third or fourth generation' of the living rather than upon the shades of the damned in some anticipation of the Christian hell.

While in key ways it was the offshoot of Hebraic monotheism, the theology which became systematized as Christianity, and which established itself, from the fourth century, as the official faith of Imperial Rome, incorporated aspects of Near Eastern Gnostic faiths and Greek metaphysics, including belief (virtually absent from Old Testament Judaism) in a separate, immaterial and immortal soul. Yet while Christ's teachings and Christian theology thus brought this major departure from Judaism, they also absorbed one of its most distinctive features, one repugnant to Asiatic and Hellenistic asceticism: respect for the flesh itself. Levantine Gnostic sects expressed a contempt for the body, regarding it as a dungeon of the spirit and a hothouse of vile appetites. While such leanings clearly left their mark on Christian doctrine (accounting for its teachings on the evils of carnality and the need for the mortification of the flesh), the Church also set a positive value upon the embodied self unknown in matching faiths. After all, did not Scripture teach that man was created by the Father in His own image, and that God Himself became flesh and died upon the Cross? Incarnation was crucial to the Passion – the 'doubting' disciple Thomas needed to finger Jesus's wounds in order to grasp the Resurrection. And, as prefigured by Christ's death and resurrection, in the flesh man would finally rise again.

Far from washing its hands, Christianity thus implicated itself utterly in the dilemmas and dramas of the flesh. Christ performed

---

* This absence of any notion of a disembodied soul, or a heaven or hell, was widely noted by enlightened freethinkers, who exploited it in various ways in their attempts to discredit Judaism, Christianity or religion in general.

over thirty healing miracles, giving sight to the blind, making the lame walk, raising the dead. The faith's popular appeal in the Roman Empire owed much to the fact that, while preaching heavenly salvation, it also, following the parable of the Good Samaritan, tended to bodily needs – for example, by encouraging alms, service and, in due course, the founding of hospitals. Lofty Stoics and wild Cathar heretics might deride such preoccupation with earthly matters as a demeaning bondage to the flesh – hence the Stoic advocacy of noble suicide – but, as Gibbon cynically noted, it was Christianity which successfully appealed to the suffering masses. Through the Eucharist, the doctrine of *Corpus Christi*, the cults of the Virgin, martyrs and holy ascetics, developments in medieval Catholicism further valued and even fetishized the flesh.

The Church's teachings about the mysteries of the flesh and the miracles of saints were wondrous indeed, and controversy was bound to arise once, in less pious times, these truths ceased to be swallowed on faith or authority. The dread of mortality was allayed by the Universal Resurrection at the Last Trump, but how exactly that miracle was to be effected was a true test of faith.

As the following chapters will show, dogma and sedimented popular beliefs were increasingly questioned in the seventeenth and eighteenth centuries by those – be they scholars, scoffers or sceptics – for whom the Christian soul, the Resurrection, and all which hinged upon them were puzzles, wish-fulfilments, sick men's dreams, bizarre blather or pious frauds. Christian teachings about the heavenly hereafter of the rejoined body and soul, cynics eagerly pointed out, especially suited Rome because of the tollbooth the Catholic Church claimed on the stairway to heaven: through indulgences, prayers for the dead and requiem masses, it would ensure that the soul, temporarily detained in purgatory, would ultimately attain its divine destination. All such doctrines of an afterlife might be, as unbelievers avowed, the fabrications of clergy on the make, but they were also fundamental to the hopes of the faithful at large – especially those whose daily life was blighted with poverty, affliction and violence –

those for whom the prospect of eternal bliss was the only redress for this vale of tears: religion, indeed, as the opium of the people.

From Luther onwards, Protestantism had thrown a spanner into the works by repudiating purgatory. While the rejection of purgatory no doubt expressed popular loathing for priestly mercenariness, it must also have been deeply unsettling to those now denied the expected helping hand to heaven. And its erasure from the map of salvation inevitably raised questions about what exactly would happen, after all, to that separate soul when released from the body at death. Where did it go, and tarry? What existence did it enjoy or endure *post mortem*? In lashing the corruptions of the Catholic Church, Protestantism thus prompted the brash questions of rationalists and the later qualms of Victorian honest doubters.

Did the British continue to uphold traditional Christianity as taught by the Anglican catechism and liturgy? Many obviously did: those epics of the biblical narrative, *Paradise Lost* and *Paradise Regained*, lastingly appealed to Protestant tempers, as did the contemporary spiritual autobiography of the redeemed Baptist, John Bunyan's *Grace Abounding* (1666). Gibbon sneeringly depicted his pious maiden aunt Hester swallowing biblical literalism whole, confidently expecting to be translated to a heaven where she would join a angelic choir singing its hallelujahs.

This book will not, however, concentrate on the persistence of orthodoxy, though it will discuss some of those thinkers who, like Samuel Johnson, upheld its tenets, including belief in eternal damnation. Rather, it will address new responses to such pressing questions as 'Who am I?' and 'What will become of me?', that were formulated by liberal Christians and other educated laity.

[margin handwritten note: what he won't and will do]

In part prompted by doubts and criticisms, such new responses were also fanned by winds of cultural change. By consequence of the Glorious Revolution of 1688, the Anglican Church finally lost its quasi-monopoly over the promulgation and policing of religious truth in England. Faith was irrevocably splintered into antagonistic factions – Anglicans both high and low, the Catholic remnant, those Calvinist

Puritans who had been in the driving seat around the time of the Civil War, and the more populist sects which had rooted and shooted since then – Baptists, Congregationalists, Quakers and the motley underground conventicles of Ranters, Fifth Monarchists, Free Spirits, Muggletonians and others who would preach, prophesy and practise as the spirit moved them. Doctrinal controversy – sometimes radical, typically hairsplitting – became endemic: since it bade all to scrutinize the Scriptures, what else could Protestantism expect?

Such developments were spurred, too, by the spread of education, literacy and print, by the temporary breakdown of censorship during the Civil War and Commonwealth, and then by the lapse of the Licensing Act in 1695, after which pre-publication censorship never returned. The Act of Toleration (1689) permitted all to express and practise their faith with a fair prospect of impunity. England thereafter resounded with a cacophony of views about divine providence and human destiny, and God's Englishmen resolutely advanced views of their own on fundamentals rather than docilely taking their cue from the Prayer Book of the Church by law established.

Debate, doubt and difference were fuelled by the print revolution. The explosion of newspapers and magazines, and the emergence of Grub Street around the turn of the eighteenth century inevitably brought, in a free and flourishing country, that proliferation of new-minted truths, discoveries and visions which so incensed Jonathan Swift, who exposed how the novelty of authorship gratified the vain presumption of opinionated egoists and knew it would bring confusion, strife and anguish. The 'Bulk of Mankind', that misanthropic Anglican divine and Tory satirist judged, 'is as well qualified for *flying* as *thinking*'.

great Swiftism

All such new beliefs about man and his fate were also adjustments to socio-cultural change. England was fast urbanizing. Its expanding middle classes were possessed of some learning in their heads and money in their pockets, and its propertied élite was newly basking in civilized refinement. A population was emerging that was no longer submissively inured to the pains and privations of this vale of tears but eager to participate in the pleasures of polite prosperity. If some, like Samuel Johnson, continued to hold that there was more in life to be endured than enjoyed, many were keen to change that, and the quest for social pleasures became a prime mover in the new Georgian order.

Only for a tiny minority did this new worldly milieu and flexible climate of opinion, fostered by print culture and coffee houses, prompt the abandoning of Christianity root and branch; but it certainly kindled questioning and it led the Churches themselves to hearken to their flocks and amend their priorities. There was perhaps less tortured heart-searching now given over to the question: 'What shall I do to be saved?', with its commitment to the prime duty of 'living to die and dying to live'. The ancient priorities of the *ars moriendi* and the *memento mori* retreated in the face of the upcoming assumption that temporal life was meant to be enjoyed – had not a benevolent Deity ordained happiness on earth as an earnest of bliss eternal? Pelagians, Arminians, Latitudinarians and other rational and liberal Christians rejected as unworthy of true religion the notion of a hammer-fisted Almighty meting out woes in this world as a prelude to eternal retribution in the world to come.

As the business, profits and pleasures of temporal existence crowded out the mysteries of eternity, as the big issue turned from 'Shall I be saved?' to 'How shall I be happy?', a further question cast its shadow: 'What is it, then, that I am?' Few educated people explicitly denied that man was, as Christian humanism had taught, the son of Adam, somehow compounded of soul and flesh – incarnated soul or ensouled body – endowed with free will, located a rung beneath the angels on the Great Chain of Being. But exactly what that amounted to was troublingly ambiguous and hotly contested.

In the seventeenth century, as already noted, Descartes signally reiterated the ascendancy of the immaterial by casting it essentially as *res cogitans*, a thinking self. Cartesianism thereby encouraged the naturalistic turn taken by the new rationalism, for this *cogito* stood on its own rational feet, independent of Bible or decretals. Whereas in Christian theology, as in Platonic philosophy, an eternal cosmic order guaranteed the ego within, Descartes's view that our moral resources lie entirely within us inevitably if inadvertently paved the way for modern subjectivity.

Cartesianism, of course, became mired in difficulties of its own, partly because of problems as to precisely how this non-material consciousness was 'earthed' with the body. Descartes's view that the two met at the pineal gland attracted more satire than support. His denigrators, however, put themselves under an obligation to come up with a better alternative, and subsequent philosophical, medical and scientific speculations returned time and again to the nagging difficulty of precisely how soul and body, mind and matter, could mesh and sympathize with each other.

The 'new philosophy' also provoked fresh speculations about the soul, especially, of course, among thinkers who, for varied reasons, were militantly materialist. For some, notably Thomas Hobbes, philosophical materialism served anti-clerical ends; for others, such as Joseph Priestley a century later, materialism was conscripted to reinforce the Christian gospel, however bizarre and heretical that stance seemed to the devout.

Moreover, a materialistic worldliness was to spread in the bubbling commercial atmosphere of the eighteenth century and the birth of 'the consumer society'. With the growth of prosperity and creature comforts, the moneyed became absorbed in the here-and-now, in matters tangible, buyable, disposable; in items of fashion and taste, manufactures, commodities, privacy, domesticity and a new sexualiz-ation of existence. These trends were doubtless, in broad terms, secularizing, but they emphatically did not lead to the deposing of the Christian soul by a new predilection for the flesh as such. For the 'body' remained hardly less puzzling than the soul and, if more concrete, far more objectionable.

Although destined for resurrection, the flesh had, of course, been ceaselessly vilified in medieval preaching and teaching as concupis-cent and corrupt. And it appeared hardly less unsatisfactory, if for different reasons, to the avant-garde of enlightened polite culture. It was, to be sure, indubitably solid and the stuff of science – only the fanciful Bishop Berkeley could dismiss brute matter as some metaphysical chimera. 'Doctor Berkeley, Bishop of Cloyne, a very worthy, ingenious and learned man,' Lord Chesterfield bantered to his son,

has written a book to prove that there is no such thing as matter, and that nothing exists but in idea: that you and I only fancy ourselves eating, drinking, and sleeping; you at Leipsig, and I at London; that we think we have flesh and blood, legs, arms, etc., but that we are only spirit. His arguments are, strictly speaking, unanswerable; but yet I am so far from being convinced by them, that I am determined to go on to eat and drink, and walk and ride, in order to keep that *matter*, which I so mistakenly imagine my body at present to consist of, in as good plight as possible.

Yet the flesh proved deeply problematic, and, as Chesterfield's letters show, if it was a source of pleasure, it was also a thorough nuisance, in constant need of care, attention and apology. To a degree that is hard to imagine nowadays, visible, tangible flesh was all too often experienced as ugly, nasty and decaying, bitten by bugs and beset by sores; it was rank, foul and dysfunctional; for all of medicine's best efforts, it was frequently racked with pain, disability and disease; and death might well be nigh. Letters and diaries – to say nothing of Swift's satires or the cartoons of Hogarth and Gillray – document at length and with passion the intense repugnance people so frequently felt towards their own noisome flesh and that of others. That in part explains why, as Norbert Elias has argued, the period brought such an earnest raising of the thresholds of embarrassment and shame, so as to hide, deodorize, cleanse, purge, exclude and expel those multitudinous aspects of the flesh and of bodily functions experienced as psychosocially threatening, disgusting and dangerous.

The eighteenth century inevitably brought a host of new disciplines of the flesh. Some were personal, – like dieting, deportment, exercise, hygiene and the avoidance of 'self-pollution'. Others were public, finding expression in such corrective and sanitizing institutions as schools, hospitals, workhouses and prisons, culminating, on the drawing-board at least, in Jeremy Bentham's visionary penitentiary, the Panopticon, in which all bodies were permanently under comprehensive all-seeing scrutiny. Meanwhile, élite drives for the reformation of popular culture equated the flesh and the plebs, and hence made the bodily connote all that was vulgar, disorderly, contagious and threatening. Although occasions remained for licensed carnivalesque release, educated opinion reinforced doubts about and revulsion against the flesh.

With the Christian soul problematized but the flesh an object of intensified disquiet and discipline, élite identities associated themselves with the elevation of the mind, that is, with a consciousness which, while distinct from the theological soul of the Churches, was equally distanced from gross corporeality. To speak rather schematically, in crudely reductionist and functionalist terms, opinion-leaders wished to escape the thumb of the beneficed clergy – and hence had to redefine the inherited Christian soul; while they also aimed to lord it over the plebs, which meant that they had to be wary of any uncouth embracing of the body as such. Parading a new mental and cultural authority, progressive thinkers invented a stalking-horse and shibboleth of their own: mind, and eventually the idea of the march of mind. For them, progress became the true, the secular, meaning of salvation, and the doctrine of mind over matter stood for power over the plebs.

structure of chapter briefly

After introductory chapters which offer broad surveys of Christian theology, the philosophical heritage and the doctrines about the body advanced by early science and medicine, this book will proceed, through a series of studies of people and problems, to explore the various innovations, trends and tangents produced by post-Restoration thinking. In coverage it makes no pretence to be definitive or even representative. In an age which brought a striking fragmentation of opinion, what was 'representative' was kaleidoscopic variety, and assurance of adamantine absolute truths was waning, much to the vexation of men like Edmund Burke who saw corrosive questionings as the precondition of the French Revolution, and of Evangelicals insistent that the new self-indulgent narcissism of the age of sensibility flew in the face of Divine Truth. 'The great and high', declared Isaac Milner in 1794, 'have forgotten that they have souls'.

This book explores how, in a manner of speaking, that demise of the soul came about. It investigates how, against the backcloth of the Enlightenment's watchword, *sapere aude* ('dare to know'), individuals reformulated the problems of existence and made sense of the self, with a changing, and waning, reference to the soul. It is a story of the disenchantment of the world, a move from a time when everything was ensouled (animism) towards a present day in which the soul is no longer an object of scientific inquiry, though mind may still just be.

2

RELIGION AND THE SOUL

How my soul, which I look upon to be an immortal Being
in me, that is the Principle of thinking, should extinguish
with my Body I cannot in any reasonable way of thinking
conceive.

THOMAS SYDENHAM

Thy body, when the soule is gone, will be a horrour to all
that behold it, a most loothsome and abhorred spectacle.

ROBERT BOLTON

Western thinking about the human condition long hinged
on the union of two contrasting elements, body and soul. At least
from the time of Plato (*c*.428–*c*.348 BC), models of their relationship
– complementary but conflictual – promoted a dualism which, once
given the blessing of Christianity, proved durable, persuasive and
dominant. A grasp of the emergence of those ideas is essential for
understanding later developments.

The earliest Greek-speaking philosophers, before 500 BC, hoped to
explain the world in terms of a *single* causal entity – water, air and so
on. Their successors and rivals conceptualized it in terms of *multiple*
principles. But with Pythagoras (sixth century BC) and his followers,
and in particular with Plato in fourth-century Athens, these options
('monism', 'pluralism') were challenged by a *dualism*, applied to the
cosmos and man alike, which was to prove astonishingly influential
– indeed, arguably it still rules, or skews, Western outlooks. The
notion that man is a compound of two distinct entities, body and

28

soul, carried with it massive implications, philosophical, moral, scientific and theological. Philosophically, the soul–body pairing presupposed two independent sorts of reality. In natural philosophy, it came to mean the split between an animating principle (First Mover) and a thing moved (matter), while within Christian theology, it would become the hierarchy of Creator and created, Holy Spirit and terrestrial clay.

If the earliest Greek thinkers were primarily interested in 'science' – how the world came to be and how it worked – it was Pythagoras who turned attention to a 'moral' universe, governed by a principle of Truth. For the Pythagoreans, humans were composed of a good (divine) soul and a mutinous body requiring to be mastered. This good–bad split pervaded other domains: in the cosmos, for instance, form, order and light were good; chaos, disorder and darkness, evil. Such macrocosmic–microcosmic correspondences exerted a tenacious hold over later philosophers. The Neoplatonist Plotinus, for instance, described a continuum which extended down from Divine Intellect to brute matter, via angels, man, lower animals, the vegetable kingdom and inanimate matter. As we shall see later, this model of the superiority of the soul in man and the universe alike was still being proclaimed by the Cambridge Platonists as late as the mid-seventeenth century.

The Greeks of the age of Homer (eighth century BC) had thought of *psyche* (breath, or soul; later, *anima* in Latin) not as a moral agent but simply as the breath necessary for life. Filled with *psyche*, the Homeric warrior was all action, defined by deeds more than deliberations, worlds apart from the sophisticated orators and contemplative intellectuals recorded in Plato's dialogues a few hundred years later.

Indeed, the *Iliad* even lacks an abstraction which we could translate as 'person' or 'oneself'. Rather, Homer portrays life and conduct as driven by external, supernatural forces, and his protagonists are puppet-like, often in the grip of terrible powers beyond their control – gods, demons and Furies – which decree their fates and punish, avenge and destroy. The inner life, with its agonizing dilemmas of will, conscience and choice, has not yet become decisive.

A new mental landscape had emerged, however, by Athens's golden age (fifth and fourth centuries BC). The thinking on the psyche that then developed set the mould for mainstream Western reasoning about the mind, as was in effect acknowledged by Freud when he named infantile psycho-sexual conflicts the 'Oedipus Complex', paying tribute to the play by Sophocles. What makes Greek drama so powerful is its combination of elements both of traditional and of newer casts of mind.

The plays of Aeschylus, Sophocles and Euripides dramatize titanic conflicts – the hero or heroine as a plaything of the gods or crushed under destiny, the rival demands of love and honour, of duty and desire, of individual, kin and state. The ineluctable outcome of such conflict is madness and death. Unlike Homer's heroes, the tragedians' protagonists are the *conscious* subjects of reflection, responsibility and guilt, racked by inner conflict, and the agonies of minds divided against themselves are echoed in the contrapuntal utterances of the Chorus. The destructive powers in the tragedies are no longer solely those of external fate, imperious gods and malevolent furies. For ruin is also self-inflicted – their heroes are consumed by *hubris*, by ambition or pride, followed by shame, grief and guilt; they tear themselves apart and heap retribution upon themselves (*nemesis*). The psychic civil war staged by Greek tragedy was then rationalized in the philosophy of Socrates and Plato.

Systematically reasoning about nature, society and mind, the philosophers of Periclean Athens cast the rational individual – that is to say, the well-born and educated male citizen, like themselves – as their ethical and political standard. In thus championing reason, they did not deny the irrational. On the contrary, the credit they granted to the mind affirms the dangerous power they saw in the passions and in the blind destructive force of fate: only the calm pursuit of reason could save humans from catastrophe.

Plato, in particular, condemned appetite as the arch-enemy of freedom and dignity; and the Platonic polarization of the rational and the irrational, enshrining as it did the superiority of mind over matter, became definitive of such later and complementary philosophies as Stoicism, with its celebration of transcendent Order and universal Mind. Through self-knowledge – 'know thyself' – reason could fathom human nature and thereby master the appetites that enslaved man. Terrified by the primordial forces assailing the mind, Platonism, Stoicism and kindred philosophies exposed unreason as a danger and disgrace which mind or soul must combat.

In particular, the soul cast as an immortal intellectual and moral principle was central to Socrates, who memorably deemed the unexamined life not worth living. While indebted to Pythagoras, he did not precisely echo his simple body–soul dualism. For experience showed that wrong was not simply a beast in the body but rather the pursuit of a supposed but mistaken good, due not to evil but to ignorance.

In their struggles to represent the human condition and the good life, Socrates and his pupil Plato tried out various formulations. In Plato's *Phaedo*, for instance, the soul was presented as an elementary entity; but it was not unitary in the *Republic*, the *Phaedrus* or the *Timaeus*. This last work, widely endorsed in medieval and Renaissance psychologies, posited a threefold partition of the soul, each part being mapped onto a specific bodily zone: the rational element in the head, the spirit in the breast and the appetites in the belly. Dividing the rational faculty from the rest, the neck was an isthmus insulating the intellect from contamination.

The same three faculties reappear in a different guise in the *Phaedrus*, in the myth (also popular later) of the charioteer and his pair of horses. This gives a different account of the soul's fate as yoked to the body. The charioteer stands for the rational faculty of the soul, a white horse its spirited element or will (reason's natural ally), and a dark horse its appetites. When the dark horse stumbles, it brings down with it the white horse and the charioteer. In this Platonic allegory of the 'fall', it is thus a principle *within* the soul itself which is responsible for its fate, harnessed as it is to the body.

Socrates and Plato were clearly torn between rival conceptualizations of the driving forces (or ruling classes) within. In the *Timaeus* and the *Phaedrus*, for example, the appetites are envisaged as integral to the soul, and hence it is from the soul that desires emerge. In the *Phaedo*, by contrast, appetites are grossly corporeal and at odds with the soul. When Plato's complex speculations were selectively Christianized, however, what was absorbed was a simplified dualism which pitted fallible flesh against a god-like soul.

Whereas Plato devoted himself to elucidating moral truth, his pupil Aristotle principally sought to explain man and the universe in a naturalistic or scientific way. Furthermore, while Plato maintained that the senses could never deliver certain knowledge of anything – intellect alone could grasp truth – Aristotle looked to them as man's chief source of knowledge, being highly critical of Plato's fanciful postulation of independent, transcendental Forms. Form could not exist apart from matter, pronounced Aristotle, the consummate bio-logical observer – though matter for its part, without form, was simply 'potential'; it was form which provided the immutable principle.

This 'form and content' doctrine underpinned Aristotle's view of soul and body. He proposed a far snugger alliance of the two than Plato: where his mentor saw strife, he emphasized the necessity for their union. The body, for Aristotle, was not the enemy of the soul. Rather, the soul needed to be wedded to the flesh, since only through the body could it function. The two were thus not estranged and competing sovereign entities, but were related as means to ends, potentiality to actualization.

This intimate rapport between body and soul challenged Plato's clear-cut value-judgement distinctions. The Aristotelian soul was neither immured within the body nor the casualty of its cravings, but originated with and within the body, being sexually transmitted through the semen. Moreover, the tripartite soul of the *Timaeus* (reason, spirit, appetite) was simplified to become twofold in Aristotle, rational and irrational – the latter itself being further subdivided into the vegetative and sensitive faculties. These 'lower' souls were also present in plants and animals: nutrition, growth and sense were all attributed to the actions of the respective vegetative and sensitive souls. The Aristotelian viewpoint, which thus stressed continuities rather than polarities between plants and animals on the one hand

and humans on the other, proved lastingly influential in science and medicine, as we shall see in the next chapter.

Beyond this subrational soul lay *nous*, the intellect or rational soul.* The lower part of *nous*, the 'passive intellect', was tied to the body and perished with it – it was, so to speak, the materialization of thought. The active *nous* was, however, divine, immortal, detached from the body and thought of less as a substance than as an activity. This rather elastic account of reason or *nous* eased the assimilation of Aristotelian metaphysics into Christian theology.

Stoicism, too, had a considerable input into Christian formulas. St Paul drew for his notion of the spiritual soul upon the Stoic concept of soul (*pneuma*), viewed by the Apostle as the creative in-breathing of God ('inspiration' in the literal sense). And the Stoic belief that man's end was to live in conformity with the Ruling Principle or Universal Reason, which involved not merely quelling but actually eradicating desires in a positive state of 'apathy' (literally: being without feeling), commended itself to Christian asceticism.

Christianity was an outgrowth from Judaism, and it took the inspiration for its new dispensation for man's salvation from the Old Testament master-narrative which began with Creation as related in Genesis and would end in the New Jerusalem. Christ's prophetic message, as recorded in the Gospels (written up long after His

---

* The fascinating but complex philological issues raised by soul-language cannot here be discussed. But it should be remembered that the soul underpins a whole series of symbols. The chief of these symbols is *breath*, and all its derivatives. The etymology of the Latin word *animus* is in itself related to 'breath' and 'air' as principles of life. *Animus* is the intellectual principle and the seat of desire and the passions, and corresponds to the Greek *anemos* and the Sanskrit *aniti*, meaning 'breath'. Its properties are intellectual and emotional and its range male, while the *anima* is the principle of inhaling and exhaling air and its range is female. Without claiming to teach a complete and coherent system of anthropology, St Paul distinguishes within the individual spirit (*pneuma*), soul (*psyche*) and body (*soma*). If Thessalonians 5: 23 is compared with 1 Corinthians 15: 44, it will be seen that it is the soul-*psyche* which vitalizes the human body while the spirit-*pneuma* is that part of the individual which is exposed to a higher level of life and to the direct influence of the Holy Spirit. It is the latter which is to benefit from salvation and from immortality and the latter which grace makes holy. However, its influence should be radiated by the psyche throughout the body and consequently throughout the individual as a whole, that is, the body which lives and moves in this world and will be resurrected in the life to come.

death), incorporated and enlarged upon Ezekiel, Isaiah and the other prophets; the New Testament is plotted by their apocalyptic expectations, which were further elaborated and reinterpreted down the ages by the Church.

Incorporating earlier biblical texts (especially Genesis, Exodus, the books of the prophets and the apocalyptic visions of Daniel), the book of Revelation, which concludes the New Testament, unveils a succession of events destined to terminate the present wicked world-order, which, through Christ's Second Coming, is to be replaced by the regeneration of mankind. In this sacred chronology, Revelation taught a model of time foreign to the classical world. Unlike Graeco-Roman cyclicalism (Plato's 'great year', the theory of eternal recurrence), the Bible grants earthly history a single storyline, with an opening ('In the beginning': the *fiat* of Creation), a catastrophe (the Fall), a crisis (the Incarnation and Resurrection of Christ), and an imminent end (the Second Coming of Christ as King, followed by 'a new heaven and a new earth'), which will bring the 'tragedy' of man to a happy ending (hence Dante's 'divine *comedy*'). This historical drama, furthermore, had a heavenly Author: 'I am the Alpha and Omega, the beginning and the end, the first and the last.'

Mankind is but a pawn in the blood-curdling chiliastic narrative whose protagonists are the titanic opposing forces of good and evil, light and darkness. Satan, the Beast and the Great Whore – collectively, 'Antichrist' – are ranged against God, Christ and the company of saints. History's consummation will occur only after the annihilation of the forces of evil in this 'war in heaven'.

Early Christians expected 'apocalypse now' to bring about the 'kingdom of God'. This failed to happen. But the Apocalypse, as Milton observed, rises 'to a Prophetick pitch in types, and Allegories', and so it proved easy to adjust apocalyptic symbols to changed circumstances. Over time, the evil empire of the Beast was variously re-identified (and still is) with the Jews, Islam, the Vatican, Communism and so forth. Moreover, a tendency to internalize eschatology via a spiritual reading had begun as early as St Paul's 'behold, the kingdom of God is within you'. Rejecting literal readings of the millennial promise, St Augustine also directed apocalyptic prophecy to the individual soul. His *Confessions* were to form the template for later spiritual autobiographies and allegories like Bunyan's *Pilgrim's Progress*, which depicted the believer wending his spiritual way through the temptations of Satan towards the 'new Jerusalem . . . prepared as a bride adorned for her husband'.

Christianity thus adopted (and universalized) Judaism's providential vision of the destiny of Zion's children unfolding in linear ('real') time. But the soul–body dualism which became equally fundamental to Christian theology was derived not from the Hebrew heritage but from admixtures of Levantine theosophy and Greek philosophy. The Old Testament viewed man primarily as a divinely animated body, not, as in Plato, an immaterial soul, temporarily enfleshed. Admittedly, in Jewish circles around the time of Christ the Pharisees were promoting doctrines of the immortal soul, but this innovation was opposed by powerful Sadducees who upheld the traditional doctrine that the soul perishes with the body.

The Hellenization of Christianity, with its metaphysics of the separate soul, began, perhaps ironically, with Philo the Jew, a first-century Alexandrian deeply sympathetic to Greek thinking. Drawing on the Stoic idea of *pneuma* as the divine substance or soul breathed into man, Philo proposed a radical body–soul dualism that was foreign to Old Testament faith. He also drew on Plato's *Phaedrus* myth of the 'fall' of the soul; dwelling in the body as in a tomb, the soul was condemned to be a 'pilgrim and sojourner' while on earth. In the thinking of the second- and third-century Church Fathers, this model of the polarization of soul and body crystallized, as did the image of the soul trapped in the world – experience of savage persecution evidently made the Neoplatonic body–soul conflict particularly pertinent to early Christians.

For Christians, however, unlike Platonists, certain doctrines integral and singular to Christianity, specifically the Incarnation and Resurrection, precluded wholly negative views of the flesh. Within the Christian eschatology, the immortal life of the soul required the reanimation of the body: had not Christ taught (and St Paul expounded) how His Resurrection after the Crucifixion was the guarantee of a general resurrection? Without that, would not the Saviour have died in vain?

In any case, the need to combat Gnostics, Manichees and members of other ascetic sects and heresies, who execrated the flesh as the Devil's work (tainted by profane earthly powers), also weighed heavily with the Fathers. Countering Gnosticism, Irenaeus (late second century) insisted that it was soul and body melded together which made up a complete person – man was the union of soul, which had received the divine spirit, with flesh, made in God's image. Irenaeus' contemporary, the brow-beating, heretic-hunting Tertullian, demanded respect for God-created flesh.

But other winds were blowing. The third-century theologian Origen gave pride of place to the immateriality of the soul and, in allegorical readings of Scripture, deemed its entry into the material world a 'descent'. The soul of man was pre-existent, he stressed in Neoplatonic manner, and so its embodiment must be punishment for some prior sin. Whereas Tertullian had cast the soul (in a rather Jewish manner) as part and parcel with the flesh, Origen constantly avowed its self-sufficient immateriality. His reputed self-castration squares with such flesh-despising views.

Augustine (354–430) gave Christian thinking yet another twist – one which proved lastingly influential. In his youth he was a Manichee who held, like the Gnostics, that matter was evil and a threat to the soul. Repudiating such views upon becoming a Christian – and putting aside his concubine – he later taught that man's corruptibility and mortality derived not from the flesh *per se* but from the sin of Adam. Without Original Sin, man as a unity – body and soul – would have been immortal: only after the Fall did flesh and spirit descend to civil war. Through the Resurrection, however, the glorified but still physical body, reunited to the soul, would return man to his pristine perfection. Although the corrupt concupiscence of the body in this life – upon which Augustine never failed to dwell – was symptomatic of man's lapsed condition (the spirit is willing but the flesh is weak), the flesh was not in itself base or even (despite the

Christian Platonists) the cause of the Fall, for the first sin came from the soul. When Adam ate of the fruit of the tree of the knowledge of good and evil, it was first and foremost a disobedience of the will.*

While softening the detestation of the flesh characteristic of his Manichee phase (and of Christian Platonists), Augustine thus presented body and soul as the two components of a torn and divided self. The immateriality of the soul was upheld without naïvely elevating it above the body in a way which would have betrayed the specificity of the Christian gospel. Over a thousand years later, in a rather similar manner, that great Augustinian Martin Luther was likewise to insist, against the Platonizers, that the body in itself was not a punishment for Original Sin. Man would have had a bodily presence, flesh and bones, had he never fallen. In a tradition from Augustine to Luther, Christian doctrine thus tried to steer a middle way between the Jewish lack of a separate soul and the Neoplatonic contempt for the flesh.

Throughout medieval and, in due course, Reformation and Counter-Reformation thinking, the human animal continued to be defined as *homo duplex*, the union, incurably discordant, of earthly body and immortal soul – a notion enshrined in the Anglican Prayer Book's reference to 'ourselves, our souls and bodies'. Rival readings of this alliance vied for supremacy. The Aristotelian scholasticism pioneered by Thomas Aquinas in the thirteenth century (and long the staple fare of the universities) portrayed the flesh as the *instrument* of the soul; Christian Platonists by contrast viewed it as the soul's *dungeon*. For some Christian teachers, the body, identified by St Paul with flesh embattled against the spirit (Galatians 5: 17: 'For the flesh lusteth against the Spirit, and the Spirit against the flesh: and these are

---

* Such issues (especially the implication of sex in sin) inevitably posed the question of the propagation and transmission of the soul: when and how did man get his soul? Augustine's insistence on its spiritual nature made it hard for him to uphold, along with Tertullian, the doctrine of physical traducianism. Nevertheless, he did link Original Sin with procreation, which was suggestive of the idea that the infant's soul came in some way from the parents' copulation. His solution to this ever-delicate problem was what he might call spiritual traducianism: the soul of the child came from the soul of the parent. Thus, the transmission of Original Sin was explained, and the spirituality of the soul safeguarded.

contrary the one to the other'), was the inexorable enemy. On the other hand, the divinely created human frame could be depicted as 'the temple of the Holy Ghost' (St Paul again: 1 Corinthians 6: 19), a view sanctified by the Incarnation.

The Church's teachings were further complicated, moreover, because from the earliest Fathers body and soul were not thought of merely as literal objects but metaphorical – in other words, flesh and spirit, denoting degenerate and pure impulses respectively. St Paul's Epistle to the Galatians, just quoted, served as a standard source for this rhetoric of two warring protagonists at large, with its identification of the 'works of the flesh' as 'adultery, fornication, uncleanness, lasciviousness, idolatry, witchcraft, hatred, variance, emulations, wrath, strife, seditions, heresies, envyings, murders, drunkenness, revellings, and such like'. The terms of this rhetorical war provided pulpit orators with limitless ammunition. In his *Of the Combat of the Flesh and Spirit* (1593), the Cambridge Puritan William Perkins explains that 'flesh' and 'spirit' signify contrary impulses within man, the spirit being a 'created quality of holiness' and flesh 'the natural corruption or inclination of the mind, will, and affections'. Both – here Perkins is clearly speaking with a Platonic tongue – are qualities within the soul.

As heathen Europe underwent conversion from the Dark Ages, all such high-theological teachings became intertwined in myriad ways with popular and pagan lore about the supernatural, ghosts and the afterlife. The emergent mission of the Church and the needs of the faithful led to the formulation of much that was barely biblical: the Trinity (with its evident echoes of Plato's tripartite soul), the Eucharist, the Devil (and the Faustian idea of selling one's soul to Satan) and, from the thirteenth century, the doctrines of purgatory and limbo. Superstitions and saints' lives embroidered awesome tales of miraculous bodies and wonder-working souls.

All such teachings were popularized, through the liturgy and sermons, through offices of piety and the frescoes which emblazoned the interiors of churches. A tradition of earthy and sometimes droll body–soul dialogues emerged, dramatizing typically bitter recriminations between a deceased person's body and soul, contesting responsibility for his failings. The Soul blamed sin on the flesh, which it charged with every imaginable carnal enormity. Not so, rejoined the Body: it could not be censured for sin, because it was only passive and subordinate matter acting under orders: evil, as Augustine had argued, began in the mind or will. In any case, should the Soul not have been vigilant in the first place?

Parallel literary genres, like the Dance of Death that was popular after the Black Death, juxtaposed body and soul; and the clichés of the 'body and soul' dialogues – were they not partners in crime? – formed the daily bread of sermons, homilies and devotional tracts. Certain motifs constantly recur in texts and images: *contemptus mundi*, the deathbed with its ever-present devils or the soul escaping from the mouth or nostrils, and gothic visions of souls burning in hell.

Characteristic of these pious and didactic dialogues was the Puritan William Prynne's 'The Soules Complaint against the Bodies Encroachments on Her' (a poem written during his imprisonment in the 1630s and published in 1642), a supplication made by the Soul in which the Body remains duly silent. In its absence, asserts the Soul, the flesh can achieve nothing:

> What is the body, but *a loathsome Masse*
> *Of dust and ashes, brittle as a glasse.*

Along similar lines is an image in Francis Quarles's *Emblems* (1635). Armed with a lengthy spyglass, Spirit can see much farther than Flesh. While the latter heeds objects close at hand which seduce the senses, Spirit descries a vision of the Last Judgement and urges Flesh to renounce its 'present toyes' for 'future joyes'.

Written in the 1650s, Andrew Marvell's 'Dialogue between the Soul and the Body' marks a watershed by departing significantly from traditional religious didacticism. In content it is far removed from the medieval templates, for all references to sin have disappeared, and its tone is philosophical rather than pious. Marvell dramatizes the ceaseless warfare being waged within Everyman. In conventional Christian-Platonic terms, Soul implores:

> O who shall from this Dungeon, raise
> A Soul inslav'd so many wayes?
> With bolts of Bones, that fetter'd stands
> In feet; and manacled in hands.

But the twist is that Soul does not have all the best lines. Body protests at how Soul visits upon the flesh all manner of spiritual ailments which prove terrible torments:

> But Physick yet could never reach
> The Maladies Thou me dost teach;
> Whom first the Cramp of Hope does Tear:
> And then the Palsie Shakes of Fear.
> The Pestilence of Love does heat:
> Or Hatred's hidden Ulcer eat.

Body is indignant at having to take the rap: if the flesh is indeed a tub of troubles, who inflicted them in the first place?

> What but a Soul could have the wit
> To build me up for Sin so fit?

Turning the tables on conventional tropes, and surely echoing the struggles of people against monarch in a Civil War in which Marvell's own sympathies were divided, it is Body no less than Soul which craves release:

> O who shall me deliver whole,
> From bonds of this Tyrannic Soul?
> Which, stretcht upright, impales me so,
> That mine own Precipice I go . . .
> A Body that could never rest,
> Since this ill Spirit it possest.

After several sharp rallies, the contest proves an honourable if bad-tempered draw, or stalemate. Marvell, an MP as well as a poet, was a political trimmer – and his irenical moral is the interdependence, if insurmountable quarrelsomeness, of both elements in man's divided nature, rather as in a stormy marriage. His poem marks a new era which reworked, as much as it reiterated, the old Christian truths.

As a devotional genre, the body–soul *querela* had petered out by the eighteenth century. But, poetically at least, the 'body and soul' pairing remained as pervasive as ever, and its archetypes constituted a powerful way of representing gendered and sexual relations. Love poets had, of course, long distinguished antithetical kinds of love – the one earthbound, the other heavenly, *eros* and *agape*, or *cupiditas* and *caritas*. Other possibilities, too, were explored – indeed, done to death. Of all the metaphorical analogues for the soul–body duo, the most popular and explosive was that of husband and wife. Typically, the body was identified with sensual Eve and the soul, or reason, with Adam. However deployed, body–soul thinking told of the union of opposites, habitually discordant but mutually indispensable.

The finest expressions of the Christian vision in the English-speaking world were *Paradise Lost* and *Paradise Regained*. These works formed the consummation of a tradition while also marking its dissolution.

Milton's God is omnipotent, His moral law inexorable and eternal. But the Lord makes man free (as Milton elsewhere wrote, 'For what obeys reason is free/And reason He made right'), since without freedom of choice there can be no moral order. Lucifer has the liberty to break God's decrees, though the price is expulsion from Heaven. It was God's will to create an earthly Paradise; all He required was that man should live in it according to His law. In Book V, Adam is warned:

> God made thee perfect, not immutable;
> And good he made thee, but to persevere
> He left it in thy power; ordain'd thy will
> By nature free, not over-rul'd by fate
> Inextricable, or strict necessity.

The two epics spell out the consequences of man's disobedience. The original nature of man, glorious in body, lay in Adam and Eve as depicted in the Garden in Book IV:

> Godlike erect, with native honour clad
> In naked majesty seem'd lords of all:
> And worthy seem'd: for in their looks divine
> The image of their glorious Maker shone.

In this divine order, Adam was the superior: 'He for God only, she for God in him'. Yet Eve (body) proved more persuasive, as we see in Book IX:

> She gave him of that fair enticing fruit
> With liberal hand: he scrupl'd not to eat
> Against his better knowledge, not deceiv'd,
> But fondly overcome with Female charm.

Nature was the physical manifestation of God's design for the universe, associated with light and growth. Man was not simply a part of material nature: he was not like the animals, indeed, for he had been given dominion over them. He had a soul, and hence a moral consciousness, and a freedom of choice which set him closer to Heaven than to Earth.

The path of wisdom and goodness was to recognize and obey the will of God. In Book VIII Milton shows the Ptolemaic Adam in conversation with Raphael, questioning the meaning of the universe: could it have been created simply so as to orbit the tiny Earth once in twenty-four hours? The Archangel's answer was also, by implication, Milton's. It was natural that men should speculate ('for Heav'n/Is as the Book of God before thee set'), and from astronomy men could calculate the times and seasons. But further than this man need not go – here lay the lures of forbidden knowledge. Raphael warned against idle speculation:

> Heav'n is for thee too high
> To know what passes there; be lowlie wise:
> Think onely what concernes thee and thy being;
> Dream not of other Worlds.

Though himself a humanist and for many a heretic, what Milton feared was the misuse of reason. In Book IV of *Paradise Regained* the Devil tempts Christ, painting a seductive picture of Greek philosophy and art. From Socrates, Plato and Aristotle, insinuates Satan, Christ can learn the political wisdom he will need to be a real ruler in Heaven. Christ replies:

> But these are false, or little else but dreams,
> Conjectures, fancies, built on nothing firm.

All one needed was divine truth. Philosophers had perplexed themselves and others:

> Ignorant of themselves, of God much more,
> And how the world began, and how men fell
> Degraded by himself, on grace depending.
> Much of the soul they talk, but all awry . . .

Thus Milton put the new science, rationalist philosophy and profane curiosity in their place. Human wickedness took the form of a headstrong conceit and an aversion to submit to God's moral law. The wisdom of salvation was contained in the Scriptures.

Paradise Lost ends with Adam and Eve walking sadly out of Eden:

> The World was all before them, where to choose
> Their place of rest, and Providence their guide:
> They hand in hand with wandering steps and slow,
> Through *Eden* took their solitarie way.

The world was also all before Milton's contemporaries, as they took their hesitant steps away from that closed Christian world of revealed truth and forbidden knowledge towards – they knew not what.

3

MEDICINE AND THE BODY

> We are all like the most of the ladies of Paris: they live
> extremely well without knowing what goes into the stew;
> in the same way we enjoy bodies without knowing what
> they are composed of.
>
> VOLTAIRE

> What then is matter? What is spirit? How does one
> influence the other, and vice versa?
>
> GUSTAVE FLAUBERT

Our sense of self presupposes an understanding of our bodies. But how do we know them? We think we know them instinctively, we speak of 'our bodies, ourselves'; the original meaning of 'autopsy' is to look into one's self.

But here lie problems. It is an elementary fact that we cannot see or, mostly, even feel what is going on inside the skin envelope. Nor do we generally, by act of will, exert much control over our metabolic functions (though this, one of the aims of the yogic and tantric traditions, became, as we shall see in Chapter 23, a hope of the utopian rationalist William Godwin). We may wish and wish, but (most probably) we won't grow a centimetre taller. We cannot command our hair not to fall out, tell our kidneys to secrete or our heart to beat. And we are quite unaware of internal events (digesting food, making cells), unless they are giving us discomfort. The idea of intuitive, internal self-knowledge of bodies (to say nothing of control over them) is thus far more problematic than that of mental introspection. To a large degree our sense of our bodies, and what happens in and to them, is not first-hand but mediated through maps and expectations derived from the culture at large.

Bodies are studied objectively, scientifically, not least by 'autopsies' in the modern sense; and such 'outsider' knowledge shapes and shades our personal ways of thinking the self. Central to those sciences of the body – today the range of natural, human and social sciences is huge – has been medicine: after all, our need to know about our bodies is most pressing when something goes wrong.

Theoretical accounts of what makes up the body, and how it works, in sickness and in health, were first written down in the West by the Greeks and transmitted (through Islam) down the Middle Ages, before being consolidated yet challenged by the spectacular dissections of the Renaissance and the physiological investigations of William Harvey and others in the seventeenth century.

Unlike the medicine of the Mesopotamians and Egyptians, the model of the body championed by Greek-learnt medicine was emphatically, even aggressively, secular. The body was part of a natural order which was law-governed, disease was a regular irregularity. That view was indicative of a bid by a corps of physicians to present themselves as superior to the existing mishmash of soothsayers, magicians, quacks and folk practitioners, those practising what might loosely be called religious, mystical or traditional modes of healing. The ambitious new professional physicians of Greece and Rome insisted that the body functioned within the order of nature, and for that reason was the proper turf of knowledgeable medical men: beware consulting others!

As first recorded in the Hippocratic corpus (fourth century BC: supposedly the thoughts of a distinguished physician from the island of Cos) and codified by the illustrious and amazingly prolific Galen (second century AD), learned medicine repudiated earlier supernatural and magical accounts of health and sickness, which saw them as god-sent. Its explanatory repertoire centred on the 'humours', bodily fluids (generally taken to be four in number) whose equilibrium was adjudged vital for the maintenance of life: the body must not become too hot or too cold, too wet or too dry. Humoral theory voiced the

Greek assumption that healthiness involved a balance of the key fluids in the body and sickness a maladjustment. It was also elaborated to explain much else: sexual and racial differences, character, disposition, psychological traits – in fact, every significant aspect of human life.

What was being kept in equilibrium or upset were bodily fluids or *chymoi* (translated as 'humours'). Sap in plants and blood in animals were viewed as the fount of life. Other and perhaps less salutary bodily fluids appeared mainly in case of illness – for example, the mucus of a cold or the runny faeces of dysentery. Two fluids, bile and phlegm, were particularly associated with illness; though naturally present in the body, both seemed to flow immoderately in sickness. Winter colds were due to phlegm, summer diarrhoea and vomiting to bile, and mania resulted from bile boiling up in the brain. The Hippocratic tract *Airs, Waters, Places* also attributed national characteristics to bile and phlegm: the pasty, phlegmatic peoples of the North were contrasted with the swarthy, hot, dry, bilious Africans – and both were judged inferior to the well-balanced Greeks living in their ideally equable climate.

Bile and phlegm were visible mainly when exuded in sickness, so it made sense to regard them as largely harmful. But what of other fluids? From time immemorial, blood had been associated with life, yet even blood was expelled naturally from the body, as in menstruation or nose-bleeds. Such natural evacuation of the blood suggested the practice of blood-letting, devised by the Hippocratics, systematized by Galen, and serving for centuries as a therapeutic mainstay in case of fevers.

The last of the humours, black bile (melancholy), entered disease theory late, but in the Hippocratic *On the Nature of Man*, it assumed the status of an essential, if mainly deleterious, humour. Visible in vomit and excreta, it was thought of as responsible for the dark hue of dried blood. Indeed, the idea of four humours may have been suggested by observation of clotted blood: the darkest part corresponded to black bile, the serum above the clot was yellow bile, the light matter at the top was phlegm. Black bile completed a coherent, symmetrical grid of four humours in binary oppositions, and the four humours – blood, yellow bile, black bile and phlegm – then proved wonderfully versatile as an explanatory system. They could be correlated to the four primary qualities (hot, dry, cold and wet), to the four seasons, to the four ages of man (infancy, youth, adulthood and old age), to the four elements (fire, air, earth and water), and to the four temperaments (sanguine, bilious, melancholic and phlegmatic). They thus afforded a neat schema with unlimited explanatory scope. On the assumption, for example, that blood predominated in spring and among the young, precautions against excess could be taken, either by eliminating blood-rich foods, like red meat, or by blood-letting (phlebotomy) to purge excess. The scheme – which finds broad parallels in traditional Chinese and Indian medicine – could be made to fit with observations and afforded rationales for disease explanation and treatment within a causal framework.

The Hippocratic medicine developed in Antiquity grounded itself on nature, on physical reality – not in the spiteful whims of the gods, broken taboos, or the spells of malicious sorcerers, all of which were now dismissed as superstitious. It is no accident that the Greek term for nature (*physis*) gives us our words physics and physician. But to say that it was concerned with the physical – with poor diet or the consistency of a sick person's stools – does not mean that it drove a wedge between the material body and the mind. Far from it: Greek medicine was holistic through and through; it presumed the unity of body and behaviour; the physical and the psychological were two sides of the same coin. And its cast of thinking ensured profound and enduring holistic psycho-somatic and somato-psychic strands in the Western tradition.

To explain what activated the flesh, 'animal spirits' were posited, superfine fluids which shuttled between the mind and the vitals, conveying messages and motion. ('Animal' here does not mean pertaining to the beasts but rather relating to the soul or *anima*.) And, following Aristotle, the revered 'father of biology' earlier discussed, classical medicine held that various 'souls' respectively governed specific bodily functions: the 'vegetable soul' directed nourishment and growth (what we would today call autonomic processes and metabolic regulation); the 'animal soul' governed sense, feeling and motion (similar, in our terms, to the sensory/motor system); and the 'intellectual soul' regulated the mental powers, that is, what medieval and Renaissance theorists of human nature were to group as the inner senses of reason, will, memory, imagination and judgement. These 'souls' were corporeal.

In classical medicine, the materiality of the flesh, far from excluding the idea of 'spirit', accommodated and even required it. Responsible for purposive functions and movement, animal spirits were central to Galenic medicine – and thence to subsequent European philosophizings about life for the next millennium and a half. After all, for the soul to act on the flesh, was there not an evident need for bridging media, partaking of the properties of both? Spirits formed precisely those intermediaries. Even when the rational soul was not consciously in charge, spirit represented the vivifying element present, for instance, in the digestive juices or in semen, imparting to them their vigour. Such spirits drew their potency, many thought, from an aerial substance in the atmosphere, the *pneuma*, or divine spirit, breathed into the lungs.

In all such formulations, 'spirit' conveys subtly nuanced shades of meaning: not all 'spirit' was what we would today call 'spiritual'. One meaning pertains to the purely immaterial, as, with the coming of Christianity, the Holy Ghost or Holy Spirit – a spirit which presupposes a difference in kind (the 'spiritual') from things gross, concrete or fleshly. But 'spirit' chiefly conveyed the idea of an exceedingly fine medium, the most ethereal possible, far more delicate than the ponderous substance which 'matter' might routinely suggest. The value of the term 'spirit' in traditional biomedical discourse lay in this very flexibility.

Galenic medicine identified an innate spirit (*spiritus insitus*) which pervaded all parts of the body, approximately the equivalent of 'life' in the most general sense. It found expression in the body's 'innate heat' and 'primitive moisture': without these, there could be no animation. These were what differentiated the living from the inanimate. In addition to this general innate spirit, specific spirits were elaborated – the natural, the vital and the animal. These were superfine in character and relatively localized, being produced in and by specific organs, namely, the liver, the heart and the brain respectively. Each played a special physiological role.

Dominant Galenism also assimilated the Aristotelian doctrine that objects consisted of form and matter. Matter was a potential which could be actualized by form – for instance, wood could be 'in-formed' into a branch or a table. Matter was thus indeterminate, inchoate, rather low-grade stuff, awaiting the form which articulated and enhanced it; but it was also the 'principle of individuation' – what made things particular or unique. Tables were universal in their (Aristotelian) form or (Platonic) Idea – every table had legs and a top, and was for putting things on; but it was the particular type and piece of timber which made this or that table distinctive – which gave it its 'quiddity', its dimensions (or quantity), grain and shade. Qualities or virtues, in other words, were those powers possessed by forms which made them capable of bringing about change in matter. The form of man was the soul, and the soul was the form of the body. In Aristotelian and Galenic thinking, dynamic activity depended on the form; the soul was thus the mover and end (final cause) of all the actions of living bodies (not just humans).

A human being was thus represented in traditional biomedicine as a complex, differentiated but integrated whole (the Platonic or Christian immortal soul, as we have seen, brought additional complications). The humours formed one facet, and their disposition was reflected in the 'complexion' (or outward appearance) and the 'temperament' – or, as we might say, personality. Humours, complexion and temperament constituted an interactive system, equipped with feedback loops.

Within this framework, illness was standardly read not as a random assault from outside, but as a significant life-event, integral to the sufferer's whole being, spiritual, moral and physical, to his or her humoral balance, and to his or her life-course, past, present and future. This view partly stemmed from ingrained beliefs about what caused illness. The explanations offered by doctors regarded good health as a measure of the orderly workings of the individual constitution, and sickness as a sign of its imbalance. To maintain good health, one needed to ensure proper diet, exercise, evacuations, adequate sleep and the like. It was important to reside in a healthy environment, to regulate one's passions, and be moderate and temperate in habits.

Sickness set in when bodily balance was disturbed. If the system grew too hot and dry, this came out in fever; if too cool and wet, it developed a cold. If too little blood were produced, the body lacked nourishment and languished. If excessive blood were generated, for example by drinking too much red wine, one's blood would boil or rush to the head; 'hot-blooded' people were liable to apoplexy or stroke. Thus sickness was largely seen as personal, internal, and brought on by faulty lifestyle. Such 'distempers' (being out of temper) could be treated by restoring the lost equilibrium; hence 'cooling' herbal medicines, blood-letting (phlebotomy) or even cold baths would be good for fevers, while plenty of rich food and red meat would cure 'thin blood'. The enduring popularity, likewise, of purging and blood-letting hinged on the old conviction that sickness followed plethora (excess) or the build-up of 'peccant' (evil) humours in the system, requiring periodic discharge. Better still, attention to all aspects of 'regimen' or lifestyle would prevent or mitigate disease (literally 'dis-ease') in the first place.

This classical framework for understanding the body and the swings of health and sickness, developed in the Hippocratic writings and systematized by Galen, retained its hold throughout the Middle Ages into early modern times. It was rich, inclusive and flexible; it codified common sense and was open to minor alterations. It was first comprehensively challenged by the 'new philosophers' of the seventeenth century. Their mechanical models of nature implied that, precisely like all other inanimate objects, living bodies were machine-like, governed by the universal laws of matter (corpuscles) in motion. 'Mechanical philosophers' thus looked upon the body as a piece of machinery, and, proclaiming that science was a matter of action not words, encouraged hands-on experimental investigation.

The new science launched a war on empty words, on reification. All that old Aristotelian talk (potential and actualization, substance and accidents, qualities and quiddities) and the thinking behind it was now dismissed as futile and fruitless verbiage, mere hot air. As Francis Bacon avowed in his dismissal of Aristotelian final causes (teleology), scholasticism was like a barren virgin which brought forth nothing. Claiming, by contrast, to possess an understanding of matter which was rooted in reality (*res non verba*: things not words), the 'new philosophers' returned to the alternative tradition of atomism, advanced in Antiquity by Epicurus, Democritus and Lucretius but largely sidelined. Ridiculing all the old scholastic blather, they substituted a model of nature composed of matter in motion, and held that matter itself was made up of corpuscles or particles operating in a plenum (according to Descartes, who denied the vacuum) or in void space (as for Newton), whose motions could be given mathematical expression. 'Instead of using only comparative and superlative Words and intellectual Arguments,' explained William Petty, a founder-fellow of the Royal Society, 'I have taken the course . . . to express myself in Terms of *Number*, *Weight*, or *Measure*.' Behind what John Locke called 'secondary qualities' such as colour, smell and so on, which were essentially subjective, lay rock-solid 'primary qualities' – mass, velocity, acceleration.

Through the innovations of Descartes, Gassendi, Boyle, Hooke, Huygens, Newton and many others, the mechanical philosophy transformed physics and astronomy in the seventeenth century; inevitably it also prompted new research programmes in anatomy, physiology and medicine. Investigators were spurred to view living creatures mechanistically, as ingenious contraptions made up of skilfully articulated components (bones, joints, cartilage, muscles, vessels), functioning as levers, pulleys, cogs, pipes and wheels, in line with the laws of mechanics, kinetics, hydrostatics, and so forth. The body became a *machina carnis*, a machine of the flesh.

Faced with the question, 'What makes bodies tick?', the obvious answer given by the mechanical philosophers was that they went by clockwork.

In these developments, William Harvey proved a crucial but transitional and ambiguous figure. The revolutionary anti-Galenic conclusion of his *Exercitatio Anatomica de Motu Cordis et Sanguinis in Animalibus* (An Anatomical Disquisition Concerning the Motion of the Heart and the Blood in Animals: 1628) that the blood continually circulated around the body, driven by a heart which functioned as a pump, became grist to the mill of new philosophers from Descartes onwards. But Harvey himself thought along Aristotelian teleological principles, and it was left to a younger generation to hail his discoveries as evidence in favour of the mechanical philosophy.

One such was Marcello Malpighi. Drawing on the marvellous new invention the microscope, this Professor of Medicine at Pisa conducted a remarkable series of studies into the structure of the liver, skin, lungs, spleen, glands and brain, many of which were published in early numbers of the *Philosophical Transactions* of the Royal Society, chartered by Charles II in 1662. Also in Italy, Giovanni Borelli, among other 'iatrophysicists' (doctors convinced that physics provided the key to the body's operations), studied muscle action, gland secretions, respiration, heart action and neural response. His main contribution was a treatise, *De Motu Animalium* (On Animal Motion: 1680), which set out remarkable observations on birds in flight, fish swimming, muscular contraction, the mechanics of breathing and a host of similar subjects, and attempted, more boldly than any before him, to comprehend bodily functions in terms of mechanics. Investigating what made the body machine work, he postulated the presence of a 'contractile element' in the muscles; their operation was triggered by processes similar to chemical fermentation. Respiration for its part was a purely mechanical process which drove air, via the lungs, into the bloodstream. Familiar with the air-pump experiments conducted by Otto von Giercke in Germany and Robert Boyle in England, in which small creatures expired in 'rarefied' air (that is, a vacuum), Borelli maintained that 'aerated blood' included elements vital to life. Physics and chemistry together, aided by experimentation and the apparatus, both technological and conceptual, provided by the mechanical philosophy, thus promised to lay bare the secrets of life, buried in the flesh and long veiled by scholastic jargon.

Borelli's younger contemporary, Giorgio Baglivi, Professor of Anatomy at the Papal School in Rome, represented the culmination of this 'iatrophysical' programme. His *Praxis medica* (1699) affirmed that 'a human body . . . is truly nothing else but a complex of chymico-mechanical motions, depending upon such principles as are purely mathematical'. Baglivi, however, was only too well aware of the predicament staring champions of scientific medicine in the face: frustratingly, their theories and studies did not seem to yield more effective cures.

A parallel bid to read the body in terms of the new science came from iatrochemistry. Whereas iatrophysics perceived the human frame through mechanics, iatrochemistry thought that chemistry held the secrets. Equally repudiating the humours as vacuous verbiage, its supporters hailed the chemical theories of the Swiss iconoclast Paracelsus (Philippus Aureolus Theophrastus Bombastus von Hohenheim, 1493–1541), who, while widely dismissed as a quackish ignoramus, was respected by others as a towering reformer. Paracelsus had praised the simplicity of Hippocrates, learned from folk medicine, and touted the power of nature and the mind to heal the body. Above all, as his operative principles he replaced the equivocal humours with the three chemical principles of salt, sulphur and mercury.

Devotees of iatrochemistry also revered his Netherlandish follower, Joannes Baptista van Helmont. Modifying Paracelsus's notion of a single 'archeus' (that is, in-dwelling spirit), van Helmont held that each organ possessed its own specific spirit (*blas*) which regulated it. 'Spirit' for him was not mystical or occult but chemical. Indeed, he held all vital processes to be chemical, each being due to the action of a particular ferment or gas. There was, thus, a ferment for converting food into living flesh and blood. Similar transformative processes occurred throughout the body, but particularly in the stomach, liver and heart. Bodily heat was a by-product of chemical fermentations, and the whole system was governed by a 'soul' situated in the pit of the stomach. Chemistry, broadly understood, was thus the key to life. Views like these were unsettling: Gui Patin, leader of Paris's reactionary medical faculty, denounced van Helmont as a 'mad Flemish scoundrel'.

By the close of the seventeenth century, advances in anatomy and physiology had created the promise of a scientific understanding of the body, matching what high-prestige mathematical astrophysics and mechanics had done for the inanimate world. Beliefs about the body were in flux, but one thing was clear: all the new models joined in denouncing Aristotelianism and Galenism as empty and barren – if often in reality recycling their ideas under a different guise, pouring old wine into new bottles.

The new mechanical models elicited pride in the body: what a marvellous machine it was! The Cambridge botanist John Ray extolled 'the admirable Art and Wisdom that discovers itself in the make and constitution, the order and disposition, the ends and uses of all the parts and members of this stately fabrick of Heaven and Earth', praising the body because there was 'nothing in it deficient, nothing superfluous, nothing but hath its End and Use'. A school of physico-theology pointed to the contrivances of the body as the finest proofs of God.

Such mechanical models also called for a rethinking of the nature of life itself. Did it reside in the Christian supernatural soul (*anima*) that was attached to the organism since 'quickening' and animating it? This was essentially the theory of Georg Stahl, Professor of Medicine at Halle (Prussia) in the early eighteenth century. Or was it an external impulse which God had imparted to the bodily machine, like winding up a clock or striking a billiard ball? – the view of the Leiden medical professor, Hermann Boerhaave. Or was life a property inherent in the organism thanks to its high degree of organization? – an interpretation that gained ground in the eighteenth century, especially among materialists and unbelievers. In addition, was *human* life qualitatively different from that of a mush-room, a mouse or a monkey?

The mechanization of the world-picture further required rethinking of the interaction between mind and matter. How did reason govern the body? Did the flesh have a reciprocal capacity to sway the mind? If so, was that – or *should* it be – only in the heat of passion (hot blood), or in sickness, physical or mental?

The crucial catalyst for such speculations was René Descartes. Descartes was a dualist who decried dogmatic materialism; but his writings threw down a challenge to investigators of all convictions to locate where and how consciousness acted within the organism, indeed within the brain. Might such thinking be the slippery slope to reducing the soul to the brain or body altogether? His rationalist philosophy will be discussed in detail in the next chapter, but to see how far the 'new philosophy' had changed expert opinion about the workings of the human animal by the last decades of the seventeenth century, it will be instructive to examine the works of Thomas Willis (1622–75).

Oxford-trained, Anglican by faith and royalist by politics, an associate of Robert Boyle and Robert Hooke, a fellow of the Royal Society and a fashionable London physician besides, Willis represents the cutting edge of respectable scientific thinking. He is remembered for coining 'neurologie', a term for the new discourse of the 'nerves' and 'nervousness' which became so favoured in the eighteenth century, and for his description of the 'Circle of Willis', the arterial circle at the base of the brain. Though a 'modern', his theories of neurological activity continued to draw on much of the baggage of traditional biomedicine, including animal spirits, the intermediaries between body and mind distributed through the nervous system. He too, like Harvey, is thus a fascinating intermediary between old and new.

Harvey's discovery of the circulation of the blood, Willis recognized, called for a rethinking of physiology at large. Building on painstaking anatomical investigations, especially of the nerves, vivi-section experiments and clinical experience, his *Cerebri Anatome* . . .

(Anatomy of the Brain: 1664) put 'neurologie' on the map; his *De Anima Brutorum* (On the Soul of Brutes: 1672) explained the workings of living creatures, while a further study, the *Pathologiae Cerebri et Nervosi Generis Specimen* (Pathology of the Brain, and Specimen of the Nature of the Nerves: 1667), proposed the neurological origins of epilepsy and other convulsive disorders.

Impressed by the mechanical philosophy, Willis rejected not just scholasticism's 'substantial forms' but Paracelsus's 'archeus' doctrine as well. Determining what was unique about living beings, he postulated the 'corporeity' of a soul (*anima* or animating principle), common to beast and man alike. This 'animal soul' depended altogether on the body, being born and dying with it. No medium was needed between the body and this corporeal soul: the various members of the body were all 'organs' of this vivifying principle. It had distinct and extended parts, enabling it to activate the different limbs. This animal soul could be divided, and could continue to exercise its functions of sense and motion even if so divided – as with worms and eels when cut into pieces. Willis's *anima* was roughly what was soon to be called 'irritability' by the Swiss investigator Albrecht von Haller – an organism's capacity to receive and react to stimuli. Responsiveness thus stemmed from the animal soul.

Of what was this 'soul of brutes' (the phrase used by John Pordage, Willis's contemporary translator) composed? Willis likened it to fire, extremely subtle and mobile. As with flame itself, the soul required a twofold food – a sulphurous and a nitrous substance. The animal soul likewise had a double location: in the blood (vital fluid) circulating, as Harvey had shown, through the heart and vessels; and in the 'animal liquor', or nervous fluid, present in the brain and flowing through the nerves, envisaged by Willis as tubes. The aspect of the soul inherent in the blood was comparable to a flame; that within the nerves was like the light rays issuing from such a flame. The soul was not actually constituted of blood and nerve juices but (in Pordage's charmingly flowery and anthropomorphic phraseology) 'inhabits and graces with its presence both these provinces'.

Being corporeal, the animal soul arose 'with the body, out of matter rightly disposed', though, as it was imperceptible to the senses, it could be known only by its effects. Upon the body's decease, the particles of the animal soul were dispersed, without trace, leaving the body subject to rapid corruption. The corporeal soul performed various functions, above all activating the blood (metabolic activity) and the nerve juices (nervous activity). In addition, there was a third aspect, an outgrowth of the 'vital flame', involved in sexual activity and reproduction.

The most subtle agents involved in the operations of the animal soul were the 'animal spirits' which, Willis taught, were vaporized into the brain and cerebellum. They then entered the cortex, flowed down the medulla and spinal marrow and, via the nerve fibres, pervaded the entire body.

Addressing the structure and functioning of the nervous system, Willis distinguished sensory from motor functions. The sensory components, which consisted of images, were transmitted, via the nerve tubes, to the brain where they were represented as on a white sheet – evidently he had in mind a camera obscura. From there they proceeded to the cortex, where they constituted memory. The motor aspects of the nervous system operated through a sequence involving imagination, memory and appetites, with the animal spirits as the vehicle and the nerve ducts as the pathway.

What was the origin of the corporeal soul? Willis held that a 'heap' of subtle atoms or animal spirits – a 'little animal soul, not yet kindled' – lay in the seminal fluid. When, through sexual intercourse, this 'heap' found a suitable berth, a soul was kindled, just as one flame was ignited by another. The animal soul then fashioned the body according to the 'forms' (original types ordained by divine providence). Thereafter, the animal soul served to preserve the body from putrefaction, while the body supported the soul by nourishing it.

Crucial to Willis's thinking was that this *animal* or *corporeal* soul was quite distinct from the *rational* soul of humans, and subordinate to it. Common to mankind and the animal kingdom, the animal soul was material, unlike the superior rational soul (unique to humans), which was immaterial and immortal. The office of the rational soul was the exercise of reason, judgement and will. It presided over the lower soul. Man was thus a bi-souled biped.

Although the brute creation did not possess a rational or immortal soul, animals nevertheless, Willis held, challenging Descartes, enjoyed some measure of inferior reason. To clarify the difference between the minds of animals and of man, he called to mind a pipe organ. The wind makes a rough noise when it passes into a pipe; the fingers of a musician, by contrast, produce wonderfully harmonious and inventive music. A mechanical device, run by water power, may, however, produce tunes on such a pipe organ vaguely comparable to those performed by human fingers. Governing and directing the animal spirits, the rational soul of man is comparable to the musician, playing a pipe; rather, as with a water-powered organ, animals can produce behaviour somewhat comparable to the human.

Animals, Willis happily conceded, exhibit instincts which may dictate operations of great complexity. Brutes also had a certain capacity to learn by experience, example and imitation, thanks to the senses, memory and imagination. They were thus not, as for Descartes, mere automata. Nevertheless, the distinction between the animal and the rational soul was crucial to Willis, biologically, metaphysically and religiously: the corporeal soul of brutes was limited in scope to the objects of the senses, to the material here-and-now, whereas the rational soul had the capacity to embrace abstractions – the immaterial – and also possessed powers of comprehension and discourse.

The 'knowing faculty' (imagination or fantasy) of the corporeal soul was located, Willis held, in mid-brain, where it received sense impressions. Since appearances could obscure or distort the true nature of things, the imagination was prone to being deceived. In man and man alone, however, the intellect presided over the imagination, picking up and correcting its errors. Fed by such sense impressions, it also generated abstract concepts and formulated universals – God, infinity and eternity, and many other ideas far removed from sense and imagination.

Animals were capable of a modicum of reasoning; in man, by

contrast, the intellectual powers were immense. Human reason could make inferences which far transcended mere sense perception; it could formulate axioms, unearth causes, handle mathematics, cultivate the arts, sciences and the 'laws of political society', and build wonderful machines. Above all, the rational mind could grasp the ineffable infinitude of God, and the reality of angels, heaven and hell. The reasoning power of brutes, by contrast, 'will hardly seem greater than the drop of a bucket to the sea'.

The distinction between the animal and the rational soul was thus not just one of degree but of kind – it was qualitative. The animal soul was material, the rational soul immaterial and immortal, divinely implanted. How then – a version of Descartes's dilemma – did Willis envisage the links between the two kinds of soul in man? He endorsed the traditional Christian view of man's tripartite nature: he possessed a body, an animal life shared with the brutes and, lastly, 'spirit, by which is signified the rational soul, at first created by God, which being also immaterial, returns to God'. Man was thus midway between angels and brutes on the Chain of Being.

The relationship between the two souls was complex. The animal soul pervaded the entire body, while the rational soul pertained exclusively to the head, dwelling within the brain as on a throne, just like a king in his palace. Like a monarch, the intellect did not need to attend personally to those functions served by the dutiful corporeal soul.

The rational soul was nevertheless not aloof but plugged into the bodily economy. For its operation, it depended on the imagination, which was itself the end-point of the chain whereby sense impressions were carried to the nerves. Intellects in any case differed – was not one person cleverer than another? This was because of differences in their respective corporeal endowments and brain power. The intellect was thus in certain crucial ways contingent on the brain and hence the body.

This championship of the rational soul shows how Willis, while a staunch advocate of the 'new philosophy', underwrote the Christian orthodoxies of the day: he came up with the physiological rendering of orthodox theological truths. Immaterial and immortal, the rational soul was 'poured' by God into the body. It also enjoyed, nevertheless, a well-defined place in empirical natural philosophy, explaining as it did features that would later be called psychological. Through authors like Willis, science and medicine would gradually replace churchmen as the accredited interpreters of the human.

Just how widely read were Willis's books is unclear, nor is it relevant. What is significant is that thinking such as his was becoming ensconced and diffused. Late-seventeenth-century élites were more or less aware that the old ways of talking about one's body and its experiences – in terms of humours, 'substantial forms' and qualities – were on the way out, being challenged by new models, metaphors and focuses of attention (for instance, the nerves). As the fluids (humours) declined in prominence by contrast to the solids (organs), the guts, belly and bowels (those humoral containers) lost their ancient importance as referents for one's self and its feelings, to be replaced in polite thinking by the head, the brain, and the nervous system. Thereafter, it was vulgar or plebeian to be preoccupied with such 'low' parts. Such shifts may have been reflected in speech. The old customs of declaring that one felt something in one's 'bowels', or of appealing to the 'bowels of Christ', were waning. No longer were the viscera or 'vitals' where the essential self lay. The new centre of symbolic gravity lay up in the head, the brain and the nerves.

Descartes's philosophy certainly met the need for a philosophical vindication of the autonomy and dignity of the soul, reason or self, independent of interdenominational wranglings. But it did so at the cost of reducing to mere 'extension' the whole of the rest of Creation – and that included the human physique. It was a tendentious claim which brought in its wake endless enigmas and created more problems than it solved. English readers found such solutions as Willis's more palatable, with their reassuring sense of man's continued location on a well-defined and traditional Chain of Being, midway between humanoid brutes and the divine – apes and angels.

The mechanical metaphors spun by Willis were both powerful

and attractive, and they carried with them significant implications, not least for free will. Was man just a machine? What did this imply for accountability? It was such problems as these which exploded over the coming century.

4

THE RATIONAL SELF

Self is that conscious thinking thing . . . which is sensible
or conscious of pleasure and pain, capable of happiness
or misery, and so is concerned for itself, as far as that
consciousness extends.

JOHN LOCKE

Know then thyself, presume not God to scan,
The Proper study of mankind is Man.

ALEXANDER POPE

What is Man? *Gnothi seauton*, 'know thyself', spake the
Delphic oracle, *nosce teipsum*, as it came to be Latinized; but that could
seem less a plan of action than an invitation to paradox, as with
Pope's *Essay on Man*.

As just seen, any definition of that 'self' evidently had to include
the mortal coil and what made it tick. But, *pace* Coleridge's dismissal
of the tribe as '*shallow* animals, who having always employed their
minds about Body and Gut . . . imagine that in the whole system of
things there is nothing but Gut and Body',* doctors like Thomas
Willis certainly did not maintain that man was made of flesh alone –
far from it. For its part, Christian divinity taught that the apex of
Creation, made in God's image, was *homo duplex* – if he was the fallen
son of Adam, a pilgrim in this vale of tears, yet he was also a seraphic
soul scripted into an apocalyptic epic. Whether biologically or

---

* Coleridge was derisive because he was a demanding patient and also an erstwhile materialist
himself.

theologically, man was obviously hard to plumb and puzzling – was, as Pope put it, 'the glory, jest and riddle of the world'.

Gaining prominence from the seventeenth century was a further model of man, one which did not so much negate as complement the alternatives already discussed. Philosophers, too, were developing their own visions of the self, principally figured not in terms of the fabric of the flesh or the salvation of the soul but in respect of consciousness. Not just the stuff man was made of ('substantial form', as Aristotelian scholasticism put it) nor his role in the divine comedy, but how he thought and felt – perception, sentience and thinking – also defined who he was, indeed might be truly definitive of it. Such a view was hardly new, of course – its antecedents lay as far back as Socrates and Plato – but what was significant was that, from the rise of Renaissance humanism, such philosophizings increasingly stood on their own two feet, independent of the prop of theology, in what became in time the burgeoning domains of epistemology, cognitive science, ethics and psychology; in short, the core human sciences.

Society too, for official purposes, needed formulations of its own as to what constituted a public person, a legal entity, a bearer of privileges and obligations. Matters of subjecthood and status, judicial and contractual accountability, property ownership, transfer and inheritance, marriage and family law, guardianship and trusteeship, guilt and punishment, the franchise and citizenship – all these required rulings as to who was to count as an independent unit, blessed and burdened with rights and responsibilities.

The humanism of Shakespeare's day prized self-knowledge. 'My self am centre of my circling thought/Only myself I study, learn and know', reflected Sir John Davies in his *Nosce teipsum* (1599), just before Shakespeare's play recorded Polonius's gratuitous advice to his son. For seventeenth-century philosophers, the solution to the riddle of identity would be sought along the road to knowledge. The self which could be known was necessarily the knowing self – the answer to the oracle's *nosce teipsum* would come through exploration of *what* could be known about existence at large and *how*. Rejecting alike the chop-logic *ex cathedra* metaphysics of churchmen and schoolmen, and the sceptical seductions of gentlemanly Pyrrhonism (Montaigne's diffident *'que sçais-je?'*), philosophers intrepidly armed themselves with reason.

First outlined in *The Advancement of Learning* (1605), the empiricism of Francis Bacon – that aristocrat among English intellectuals – boldly claimed (*contra* the sceptics) that sufficiently reliable knowledge could be achieved by disciplined recourse to experience: man had the capacity, right and duty to know the world, the human epitome included, through the five senses. To parry any clerical jealousy over what might be taken as prying into God's secrets – forbidden knowledge – the philosophical Lord Chancellor made a discreet and dutiful concession: investigation 'must be bounded by religion, or else it will be subject to deceit and delusion'. But man was charged to read the Book of God's Works no less than the Book of His Words: Nature as well as Scripture was a God-given fount of truth.

Abstract reason was unsatisfactory because arrogant, and so science had to be grounded in modest experience – modelled not on the solipsistic spider spinning her web from within herself but on the busy bee gathering nectar from the flowers. Empirical knowledge, too, had its weaknesses, and Bacon warned of the distortions, both individual and collective, inherent in the senses, highlighting the four 'idols' (or illusions) which warped perception: those of the cave, herd, theatre and market-place. (The philosophical anti-idolatry that so animated Bacon clearly mirrored its Protestant iconoclastic twin.) This did not mean that the testimony of the senses was to be rejected; rather, it had to be kept on the straight-and-narrow by methodical fact-gathering, recourse to the supports of instrumentation, crucial experiments and submission to collective judgement.

Bacon's programme for the advancement of learning thus side-stepped the uniquely divine soul and occupied itself with the role of the 'sensitive' soul, the operation of the senses. Indeed, that wily statesman ceded the soul to the divines: 'true knowledge of the nature and state of the soul', he shrewdly allowed, 'must come by the same inspiration that gave the substance.'

*

More concerned than the utilitarian Bacon with theorizing as an end in itself was René Descartes. Educated by Jesuits who introduced him to natural philosophy, including the Galilean astronomy, he initially enlisted as a gentleman-soldier before settling to the scholarly life, taking up mathematics and the physical sciences. By his mid-twenties his brilliant mind had glimpsed the possibility of combining algebra and geometry into analytical geometry; and on 10 November 1619, in a quasi-mystical experience recounted in his *Discours de la méthode* (Discourse on Method: 1637), he solemnly dedicated himself to the pursuit of truth, determining to doubt all conventional beliefs root and branch, and to build philosophy afresh on the basis of indubitable first principles. Beginning with the one thing so self-evidently true it could not possibly be questioned, his own consciousness – *cogito ergo sum*: I am thinking, therefore I exist – he aimed, through the rigorous logic of introspection, to establish principles so 'clear and distinct' that the mind of man 'cannot doubt their truth'.

In developing his method of universal doubt and his remarkable claims for the power of reason, Descartes tried to avoid treading on ecclesiastical toes – not for him Galileo's fate. He thus avowedly restricted his account to the rational soul, not meddling with its theological and heavenly twin; the two were complementary, not rivals.

Unlike Bacon, Descartes deprecated sensory knowledge, which could not shake off the uncertainty of subjectivity. Because 'the notion of thought precedes that of all corporeal things and is the most certain', it must be the conscious mind (*res cogitans*) which formed the essential 'I'. This Platonizing ennobling of reason above the senses meant that the two were effectively treated by Descartes as ontologically distinct. Since the senses were unambiguously of the body, there yawned a radical chasm: the flesh was divisible, the rational soul, like that of the Christian, was indivisible; the essence of the bodily was extension (*res extensa*: matter, what filled space), that of the mind, consciousness. In a single intrepid stroke of thought, Descartes had disinherited almost the whole of Creation – all, that is, except the human mind – of the attributes of life, soul and purpose which had infused it since the speculations of Pythagoras and Plato, Aristotle and Galen.

While discounting it as the source of definitive truth, Descartes did not neglect the corporeal; far from it. It was man's duty to study it; and, since it was quite inert, what objection could be raised against it? While living close by the butchers' quarter in Amsterdam he often dissected carcases, and he produced three works devoted to the study of living things: *Tractatus de Formatione Foetus* (Treatise on the Formation of the Foetus: posthumous, 1662), *La Description du corps humain* (Description of the Human Body: 1648), and *Traité de l'homme* (Treatise of Man: 1648). This last outlined a mechanical model of the human animal: drawing analogies with clocks and automata, he proposed, in a tactfully expressed thought-experiment, how an 'artificial' man could be conceived with physiological operations identical to those of humans, fully explicable in terms of matter in motion. Animals for their part did not possess souls (incapable of speech, did they not evidently lack consciousness?) and so were indeed such mechanical automata pure and simple. Dogs yelped when kicked because yelping was built into their mechanism ('programmed into them', we would say today). Mind was what distinguished humans from all other earthly beings, proposed the savant in a naturalization of the Christian doctrine of the uniqueness of the human soul.

While thus preaching the bleakest of dualisms, Descartes acknowledged that in going about his daily life, man does not constantly perceive himself as a self divided, composed of two completely disconnected halves (*res cogitans* and *res extensa*). Through pain, hunger, thirst and other such sensations, a person would find that he (that is, his *cogito*) was not only housed in his body but was so intimately united with it that the two seemingly composed a unity. This familiar experience could be explained only through the symbiotic interaction of soul and body: it was that for which Descartes had to account next.

His early *Règles pour la direction de l'esprit* (Rules for the Direction of the Mind: 1628) proposed that the five senses received external stimuli just as wax took an impression. This imprint was then instantly conveyed to the 'common sense', which functioned as a seal, and made its mark on the fancy or imagination. The retention of such images explained memory. The process also worked in reverse: the fancy could activate the nerves, which stemmed from the brain where the imagination was seated.

This account, however, explained nothing more than the mechanism for receiving sense impressions; acts of cognition and ratiocination were something different, 'purely spiritual, and not less distinct from every part of the body than blood from bone, or hand from eye'. The mind was thus duly honoured by the *Règles*, but in a way which restated rather than resolved the dualism at the core of Descartes's thought-world.

It was in the much later *Les Passions de l'âme* (The Passions of the Soul: 1649) that Descartes finally confronted the psycho-physiological ramifications of the rigid dualism premised by his mechanical philosophy. The soul – that is, the rational soul: the old Aristotelian vegetative and sensitive souls had disappeared in the body-machine – is indivisible and by nature independent of matter (extension). But there is one pocket of the brain, the pineal gland, a unitary structure seated in the mid-brain just behind the main ventricle, where the soul directly operates on the body. The slightest movements taking place in it 'may alter very greatly the course of these spirits; and reciprocally . . . the smallest changes which occur in the course of the spirits may do much to change the movements of this gland'. ('Spirits' here meant the animal spirits, understood, rather traditionally, as superfine fluids acting as intercessors between the senses and the brain.) The soul, via this pineal gland anchorage, operates throughout the rest of the body by means of the animal spirits in the nerves and blood. Thus, Descartes accounted both for the actions and perceptions arising from the soul, and also for those deriving from the body and the external world.

It was critical to Descartes to chalk out an absolute distinction between the autonomous actions of the soul and what was activated by the body, for fundamentals of responsibility and moral dignity were at stake. Clearly, acts which emanated from the soul were within its power (to perform or forgo). When passions generated in the body prevailed, it meant that proud *homo rationalis* had succumbed to low appetites or to illnesses, physical or psychiatric, as in the case of fever or delirium. Physical urges (hunger, lust and so on) were provocations to action, prompting conflicts between what they spurred the soul to do and its proper dictates (temperance, continence). What was novel to Descartes (by contrast with Plato) was the view that the soul was quite unitary; the body was a machine pure and simple and had no subaltern (Galenic) souls of its own; the animal spirits and other faculties by which the body channelled sense impressions were themselves attributes of the flesh. Hence, moral conflicts experienced by man within himself were strictly clashes between body and soul, and not between different parts of the soul. 'For there is within us but one soul,' he insisted.

The error which has been committed in making it play the part of various personages, usually in opposition to one another, only proceeds from the fact that we have not properly distinguished its functions from those of the body, to which alone we must attribute every thing which can be observed in us that is opposed to our reason.

Ultimately, it was the soul's job to determine action – freedom of the will was cardinal to Descartes, the supreme affirmation of human dignity.

The importance of Descartes lay in his boldly designating the soul as a philosophical rather than a religious principle, an immaterial thinking subject. In the process the *machina carnis*, the body machine, was laid bare for study in the naturalistic terms of the new science. While upholding the Christian soul, he transformed its status into the *cogito*, rendering it independent of divines and the ministrations of the Church. His was a soul for the thinking gentleman.

Through moves which proved epochal, the soul was thus naturalized and the self set on a rational basis. The 'I' stood matchless in all its glory. Small wonder that later generations spun a 'creation myth' around Descartes – he had single-handedly created modern man, rather as God's *fiat* had created Adam. The Cartesian explanation of the hinge of soul and body was, however, a blatant botch which never carried much credence even among sympathizers, leaving behind the embarrassing problem of the 'ghost in the machine'.

Descartes's English impact was potent, notably upon the Cambridge Platonists (discussed in the next chapter) and Sir Kenelm Digby, a gentleman-philosopher whose sponge-like mind soaked up the thinking of the age. Ardent in his admiration of Descartes while also highly devout (he was a convert from Anglicanism to Catholicism), Digby presented in his *Of Bodies* and *Of the Immortality of Man's Soul* (published as one in 1644) both a scientific account of man and also Christian pieties concerning the soul. Natural scientific in its approach, *Of Bodies* furnished boldly mechanical explanations. Unlike his contemporary Hobbes, however, Digby did not thereby deny the existence of anything beyond matter, or limit knowledge to sense experience. One of his aims, indeed, in representing the body as completely mechanical and fully explicable in terms of matter and motion was to point up the indispensability of an entity not thus explicable – that is, the soul.

His treatise on the soul was quite different in orientation and method, being based not on sense experience but on deductive reason. It cast the body, in a Platonic manner, as a clog to the soul. Human actions, argued Digby, proceeded from two principles, the understanding and the senses, identified respectively with soul and body and, by inference, with the archetypes of angels and animals. Thus, as for Descartes, moral conflict was waged between body and soul, not among various warring factions within the soul. Digby upheld the hierarchical principle of due subordination: reason was master of the senses and passions. Just as for Descartes, reason could effect no action, however, without assistance from those lieutenants, the animal spirits, pulsing from the brain; and Digby made much of the peril that the soul might be swayed by the imagination.

Such fears applied to the rational soul only in its imperfect, earthly sojourn. Its stay here was merely probationary, however: once emancipated from the body it would be purified. Digby's discourses on body and soul thus climaxed on a lyrical, almost mystical, note: the soul would ultimately be incorruptible in the highest degree: 'There can be no change made in her, after the first instant of her parting from her body; but, what happiness or misery betideth her in that instant, continueth with her for all eternity.'

Digby's hymn to the soul finds echo in the writings of the physician Sir Thomas Browne who, in *Religio Medici* (1642) and elsewhere, took fideistic pleasure in its mysteries. But all such homage to the autonomous and pre-eminent soul was brought down to earth by a fly in the philosophical ointment, Thomas Hobbes.

The short way, adopted in Hobbes's most important work, *Leviathan* (1651), and elsewhere, with all such high-flying metaphysical dualism was to cut the Gordian knot and deny that ontology. Man – indeed, nature at large – was wholly physical, entirely without an incorporeal element. No 'spirit' existed, as posited either by the Churches or by Descartes, and there were no 'clear and distinct' Cartesian ideas independent of sense experience. In his 'Objections' to Descartes's *Méditations philosophiques* (1641), Hobbes rebutted the Frenchman's tenet that knowledge of consciousness preceded sense-data.

It is not surprising that Hobbes was so bent on drastic philosophical cleansing. He had been driven to despair, indeed into exile, by the bitter carnage of the Civil War, which he blamed on the machinations of the clergy and their mystifying ideological formulas. To counter the diseases of devious dogmatism and the loose or crafty thinking upholding it, what was needed was the brisk purge provided by stringent doses of nominalism and materialism. Only then would all that specious talk of the 'immaterial' be recognized for what it was: vacuous, mendacious and deceitful: 'The *universe*', proclaimed Hobbes, 'is corporeall, that is to say, body; . . . and that which is not Body, is no part of the Universe.' The religio-political pay-off was dynamite: no immaterial spirit, no lords spiritual, no Church or supernatural realm as traditionally conceived. Long before Nietzsche, Hobbes philosophized with a hammer.

It was through materialist spectacles that Hobbes viewed human nature. Man was simply a machine, mere matter in motion; thoughts and feelings were jolts and reactions in the sense organs induced by external pressures and producing in turn those brain-waves called ideas. The imagination was the consciousness of ideas which lingered in the mind after the original stimuli had died away; and memory was their recollection ('decaying sense', in one of Hobbes's many memorable phrases). Such motions went on independently of speech, and hence, *pace* Descartes, were common to the animal kingdom, too. This mordant materialism which reduced emotions to motions was aimed at 'vain philosophy, and fabulous traditions' – like angels, demons and other 'abstract essences' bred by fevered imaginations.

Hobbes nowhere rejected the Christian revelation *per se*, but his attitudes and logic appeared to impugn it, and he was widely taken as a two-faced unbeliever, hypocritically quoting Scripture – as in the very title of his *magnum opus* – but subverting its truths. Though he affirmed God's existence, he denied that either the Deity or the soul was immaterial: incorporeal spirit – or incorporeal anything else for that matter – was 'unimaginable' and hence illusory. Glossing I Corinthians 15: 44 ('it is raised a spiritual body'), the great debunker stated that what St Paul there meant was 'bodily spirits. . . . For air and many other things are bodies, though not flesh and bone, or any other gross body to be discerned by the eye.' Asserting his allegiance to Scripture, Hobbes blamed the fiction of a separate or disembodied soul on the 'demonology of the Greeks'. It was his own reading, he proclaimed (presumably tongue in cheek), which was truly biblical: soul there was but breath, the life of the body. In the same vein, Hobbes nowhere denied the Christian doctrine of personal immortality. But once again, he insisted, the gospel had been perverted by the conniving clergy. The dead would indeed rise on the Last Day, and the faithful would receive eternal life. Man, however, was not immortal by virtue of his nature (the fallacy of Plato and all subsequent metaphysical theology), but by grace of a God whose essence was power.

Contemporaries mistrusted Hobbes's lip-service to Christianity: to deny the essential incorporeality and immortality of the soul – was this not to sap the faith? His short answer to the enigmas of Cartesian mind–body dualism – that there was no such autonomous thing as mind – was repugnant to his contemporaries; it was too belittling to human dignity and destructive of all morality. Nor did they endorse his view that 'immaterial substance' was 'unimaginable' and that only the 'imaginable' – that is, what was capable of being represented pictorially – was the stuff for discourse. After Hobbes, no one could ignore the spectre of libertine atheism conjured up by his denial of the soul's immateriality; indeed, Restoration rakes found in him a kindred spirit, exonerating their immoralism.

Hobbes threw down a further sly challenge to man's self-esteem. It concerned the status of a person. '*Persona* in latine', he commented,

signifies the *disguise*, or *outward appearance* of a man, counterfeited on the Stage; and sometimes more particularly that part of it, which disguiseth the face, as a Mask or Visard . . . So that a *Person* is the same that an *Actor* is, both on the Stage and in common Conversation; and to *Personate*, is to Act, or Represent himself, or an other.

How offensive to reduce a legal personage to an actor, impersonator or pretender! It was an issue taken up by Locke.

John Locke (1632–1704) was by far the most influential philosopher of the late seventeenth century. In his early years a conservative Oxford don, Locke was subsequently radicalized by the reactionary politics of post-Restoration years, and played a decisive role in the politics of the years following the Glorious Revolution of 1688, when he published key writings championing constitutional government, religious toleration, rational Christianity, liberal economics and currency reform. The coping-stone of his *œuvre* lay, however, in his vision of man.

His master-work, the *Essay concerning Human Understanding* (1690), set out a persuasive model of the new man for the new age, through a radical analysis of how the mind achieves sound knowledge. There were no *a priori* absolute verities, no eternal fitnesses or 'innate truths'. Far from affirming with Descartes that the mind possessed an intuitive knowledge of the indivisibility of the soul, Locke even doubted that we could know anything of its nature – hence, personal identity was a problem he had to address. Claims made from Plato onwards for objectively existing Ideas, self-evident to reason, did not square with experience; and the same held for Descartes's clear and distinct ideas. The inescapable fact of the kaleidoscopic diversity of human beliefs and opinions, at different times and in different places, made nonsense of all such claims. Take a new-born infant: was not its mind like an 'empty cabinet', a *'tabula rasa'*, or a piece of 'white Paper'? Knowledge was partial, and acquired only by experience, that is to say, through the five senses:

methinks, the *Understanding* is not much unlike a Closet wholly shut from light, with only some little openings left, to let in external visible Resemblances, or *Ideas* of things without; would the Pictures coming into such a dark Room but stay there, and lie so orderly as to be found upon occasion, it would very much resemble the Understanding of a Man.

Lack of certitude did not drive Locke, however, to scepticism, despair or a reactive rationalism. The experience of the senses led to the accumulation and consolidation of probable truths sufficient for God's purposes for man. Similarly, although no moral absolutes were graven upon the heart or head, the psychological mechanisms of pleasure and pain, desire and aversion, did in fact bring about a sound-enough practical grasp of good and bad, vice and virtue. Hence, touting the methods of empirical science as championed by Bacon and the Royal Society, Locke aimed to rescue epistemology and ethics from the follies of dogmatic error and rehouse them in solid structures, and his legacy to the eighteenth century was a cautious confidence in the educability of man as a progressive creature. Man was malleable, and he could change for the better.*

But what *was* man? What did Locke's empiricist critique of the Cartesian *cogito* – reason enthroned, like Louis XIV, as an absolute monarch – leave of the very concept of personal integrity and moral agency, all so proudly vaunted in the Cartesian 'I'? If the mind started

---

* Such views were possible because Locke played down the Fall; he resolutely insisted on the capabilities of human understanding. The Christian God could be known, as could nature and nature's laws. Locke was no sceptic; he sought not to deny truth, its pursuit or its attainability but to set it on a sound footing.

out blank, was a person irremediably a void – mere putty, or a puppet? Could there be any stable, constant, individual self at all? If there could, what was its nature and how did it grow? Not least, was there, as the Churches taught, a heaven-bound soul? Critics spied in Locke's thinking a dangerous and cynical relativism: might he be a Trojan horse for Hobbism?

Initial readers of the *Essay* noted Locke's relative silence – evasiveness? – on such issues. In response to his friend William Molyneux's urging that he should more fully address the question of the individual, he added to the second edition (1694) a new chapter entitled 'Of Identity and Diversity'. This amplified themes already introduced at the beginning of Book II, where Descartes's view that the mind never stopped thinking (advanced as confirmation of *res cogitans*, the lofty 'I') had been criticized. It was fallacious, countered Locke, to believe that the mind was always thinking. For when it did not think, it was aware of so doing, and there were obviously times when we had no inkling whatsoever of thinking taking place. Perceptions, he insisted, were self-reflexive: 'When we see, hear, smell, taste, feel, meditate, or will any thing, we know that we do so.' Hence it was 'impossible for anyone to perceive, without perceiving, that he does perceive'.

Experience was the *sine qua non* of knowledge, and self-consciousness accompanied every experience. So this feeling of perceiving-yourself-perceiving was such that 'in every Act of Sensation, Reasoning, or Thinking, we are conscious to our selves of our own Being'. The self-awareness which defined and sustained the ego was 'the condition of being awake'.

This conviction led Locke to radical conclusions as to the unity of wakefulness, perceiving and selfhood. In an aphorism which contemporaries found particularly teasing – it was also the nearest Locke came to a philosophical joke – he proposed that Socrates asleep might not be the same person as Socrates when philosophizing:

if the same *Socrates* waking and sleeping do not partake of the same *consciousness*, *Socrates* waking and sleeping is not the same Person. And to punish

Socrates waking, for what sleeping *Socrates* thought, and waking *Socrates* was never conscious of, would be no more of Right, than to punish one Twin for what his Brother-Twin did, whereof he knew nothing.

(Typically, for Locke, questions of identity ran into matters of public and legal accountability.)

Conversely, he suggested in a no less provocative thought-experiment about oneness or identity, that if two apparently different people shared the same consciousness, they should be considered the same person:

suppose the Soul of *Castor* separated, during his Sleep, from his Body, to think apart. Let us suppose too, that it chuses for its Scene of Thinking, the Body of another Man, *v.g. Pollux*, who is sleeping without a Soul: For if *Castor*'s Soul can think whilst *Castor* is asleep, what *Castor* is never conscious of, 'tis no matter what Place it chuses to think in. We have here then the Bodies of two Men with only one Soul between them, which we will suppose to sleep and wake by turns; and the Soul still thinking in the waking Man, whereof the sleeping Man is never conscious, has never the least Perception. I ask then, Whether *Castor* and *Pollux*, thus, with only one Soul between them, which thinks and perceives in one, what the other is never conscious of, nor is concerned for, are not two as distinct Persons, as *Castor* and *Hercules*; or as *Socrates* and *Plato* were?

The implications were mind-boggling.

Though Locke could not so easily be accused as Hobbes of atheistical mischief-making, this speculation certainly pulled the rug away from under all orthodoxy. Questions of fractured and multiple personality, with all their anarchic implications, were thus being raised, as early as the close of the seventeenth century, as the inevitable consequences of Locke's dethroning of the Cartesian *cogito*. Who then did wear the crown? Who was master of the house? Who was a pretender?

What lay at the heart of the matter, Locke avowed, was *continuity of consciousness*: it was therein — not in some property of the body — that sameness or unity lay. 'Had I the same consciousness, that I saw the Ark and *Noah*'s Flood, as that I saw an overflowing of the *Thames* last Winter, or as I write now,' he proposed in another outlandish but pointed thought-experiment,

I could no more doubt that I, that write this now, that saw the *Thames* overflow'd last Winter, and that view'd the Flood at the general Deluge, was the same *self*, place that *self* in what Substance you please, than that I that write this am the same *my self* now whilst I write (whether I consist of all the same Substance, material or immaterial, or no) that I was Yesterday. For as to this point of being the same *self*, it matters not whether this present *self* be made up of the same or other Substances . . .

Identity – the 'I' – was thus continuity of experienced consciousness or memory.

In his new chapter on identity and diversity, Locke drove further these meditations on being awake and asleep, on consciousness and non-consciousness, identity and fragmentation. His conclusion was that self-identity was the attribute of a being who 'has reason and reflection, and can consider it self as it self'.

Locke's account of what constituted a self was a remarkable break with that 'identity of substance' – the identity of the body based on physical continuity – which scholasticism had taken as the criterion of what made an individual. The implications were momentous. Since, for instance, the body was no longer the yardstick for the integrity of the self, the same body might be inhabited or haunted by multiple selves – as in the case of Socrates sleeping and awake. It sounds like a secular analogue of diabolical possession, close to certain modes of madness, and potentially no less disorienting.

Locke's equation of personhood with consciousness – in effect, he rewrote Descartes to read 'I am conscious, therefore I am, whoever it is I be' – comes across in his declaration that '*self* is not determined by Identity or Diversity of Substance, which it cannot be sure of, but only by Identity of consciousness'. And this is where his post-Hobbesian way of speaking of the 'person' came in: '*Person*, as I take it, is the name for this *self*. Where-ever a Man finds, what he calls *himself*, there I think another may say is the same *Person*.' Stretching back into the past and forward beyond the present, personhood was not fundamentally fixed in the ensemble of the flesh, in the face, torso and limbs, but was borne in the understanding or self-awareness, regarded as the 'totality of the Impressions, Thoughts, and Feelings, which make up a person's conscious Being'.

In thus making the self hinge on such potentially impermanent, ephemeral phenomena as 'impressions, thoughts, and feelings', Locke seemed to his critics to come perilously close to undermining it completely: did he not imply that the self was all in the mind? Locke, however, felt no cause for unease: far from opening the floodgates to scepticism, madness or unbelief, his was a nobler vision, rescuing and liberating the essential ego, the first person (or conscious selfhood), from the contingent and drossy encumbrance of mere corporeality. His doctrine was also, critically in Locke's eyes, a ringing refutation of Hobbesian materialism: man was not defined by the material body that Hobbes deemed was all there was. And Locke certainly showed no hesitation in affirming the actuality of the self as he portrayed it. 'For if I know *I feel Pain*,' he insisted, 'it is evident, I have as certain a Perception of my own Existence, as of the Existence of the Pain I feel. . . . Experience then convinces us, that *we have an intuitive Knowledge of our own Existence.*' Far from believing that he was dissolving reality away, Locke considered that he was offering a more valid and acceptable sense of the self: I am my consciousness, the sum total of my life experiences, or my memory; I am not circumscribed by my mortal coil.

Locke had his philosophical defenders. In the urbane style which Joseph Addison and Richard Steele made their trademark, his ingenious opinions were given an approving airing in the *Spectator* (see Chapter 7) – part of its publicizing of Locke's thinking at large. Critics, however, censured 'conscious selfhood' as a piece of philosophical impudence or as a covert *apologia* for moral relativism, religious heresy or intellectual irresponsibility at large. Tory satirists, in particular, as will be shown in Chapter 9, attacked it as a specious philosophical excuse for trendy self-indulgent permissive poppycock. With its hint that man is, or can reinvent himself as, whatever he likes, Locke's philosophy of the self was characterized by hardliners as all too typical of those wicked, Whiggish times and their pernicious descent into self-admiring narcissism.

To be sure, Locke's conviction that selfhood inhered in a consciousness which was, by his own admission, discontinuous (witness sleep) opened up all manner of tantalizing possibilities. Many such kites were flown by his gadfly friend and somewhat embarrassing supporter, Anthony Collins. The controversies which ensued between that gentleman lawyer-cum-freethinker and the rationalist Anglican divine Samuel Clarke brought those disturbing implications to the fore. In an exchange on the immortality of the soul, for which the matter in contention was personal identity, Clarke insisted (in rather Cartesian vein) that consciousness was a property *inherent* in the immaterial and indivisible soul. As such, it was a quality existing prior to and independently of *experience*. For the sceptical Collins by contrast, Lockean experience was all in all, no matter if it were discontinuous and fragmentary in nature. For Clarke the Christian rationalist, the omnipresence of the conscious mind confirmed the immortal soul, which was in its turn a proof of the Supreme Intellect. Deny this, and the whole edifice of objective truth would totter. Challenging these pieties, the impish Collins revelled in Locke's suggestion that consciousness, while assuredly coterminous with the self, was nevertheless intermittent: remember Socrates asleep. Thinking, stressed the Deist, following Locke, did not go on all the time: slumber, trances, coma, absent-mindedness and derangement all proved that perception, like matter itself, was interrupted and divisible. Golden opportunities opened up for the sceptical lawyer. 'Let us consider to what Ideas we apply the Term *Self*,' he proposed, giving such unsettling speculations a challenging spin:

If a Man charges me with a Murder done by some body last Night, of which I am not conscious; I deny that I did the Action, and cannot possibly attribute it to my *Self*, because I am not conscious that I did it. Again, suppose me to be seized with a short Frenzy of an Hour, and during that time to kill a Man, and then to return to my *Self* without the least

Consciousness of what I have done; I can no more attribute that Action to my *Self*, than I could the former, which I supposed done by another. The mad Man and the sober Man are really two as distinct Persons as any two Other Men in the World.

Here were unfolded some of the shocking implications of Locke's account of the self – implications that were never spelt out, of course, by that ultra-cautious philosopher. His freethinking friend's plausible forensic speculations not only problematized personal responsibility in the ethical and legal spheres, but also implicitly challenged Christian doctrines of divine accountability and punishment in the world to come.

The Clarke–Collins controversy fanned out. Joseph Butler, a Dissenter who had converted to the Church of England and was to climb to a bishopric, appended a dissertation 'Of Personal Identity' to his popular *The Analogy of Religion* (1736), dedicated to Clarke. Butler endorsed the latter's criticism of Collins. His views on the conscious self had baleful consequences, precisely because, according to the Locke–Collins line, 'personality is not a permanent, but a transient thing . . . no one can any more remain one and the same Person two Moments together, than two successive Moments can be one and the same Moment'. Believe that, and all would collapse in chaos!

Particularly worrying, Locke's notion that identity lay in 'conscious selfhood' seemed to threaten orthodoxy on the crucial matter of life after death. If your body was not your self, what did this mean for the Universal Resurrection? To this we shall return in Chapter 6.

5

SCIENCE RESCUES
THE SPIRIT

And new Philosophy calls all in doubt!

JOHN DONNE

Despite the fears of the metaphysical poet and Dean of
St Paul's, John Donne, other influential thinkers, as we have seen –
from his contemporary Francis Bacon through to Thomas Willis and
John Locke – believed that it was not the 'new philosophy' which was
truly disturbing and destructive: rather, science would come to the
rescue of truth, setting it at last upon rock-solid foundations after all
the centuries of scholastic castles in the air. Far from puncturing the
soul, science would breathe new life into ailing theories of the self.

The emergent Church, as indicated in Chapter 2, had consolidated
a corpus of philosophical theology which showed that Creation was
permeated by Holy Spirit and proved that the divine and immaterial
was superior to mutable and perishable matter. To explain man, the
offshoots of Platonism, Aristotelianism and Galenism which domi-
nated medieval and Renaissance university curricula taught of a nest
of life-bearing distinctive souls – rational, animal and vegetative –
which were the active principles of will, life, form, growth and
generation, operative through the medium of 'spirits', those superfine
fluids inherent in living bodies.

Above all, Christianity embraced the immaterial, eternal individual human soul, which gave man his unique place on the divine
Chain of Being. The twin doctrines of base flesh and the salvation of
the soul afforded solace and hope to the wretched feudal masses
overwhelmed by the insecurity of life and the certainty of death.

But, equally, they reinforced the authority of Church and State, by dictating inescapable accountability, the meting out of rewards and (especially) punishments for all eternity. Crime, sin and apostasy would mean not just the lash, the gibbet or the faggot in the here-and-now, but the doom of burning in hell everlastingly. Indeed, early modern heretics and Enlightenment freethinkers held that all those beyond-the-grave terrors had been cooked up in the first place by scheming churchmen to intimidate and fleece the laity: Christian eschatology and soteriology (the theory of salvation) thus served the powers that be very nicely.

This helps to explain why orthodox teachings about the spiritual realm came under such fire in England during the upheavals of the Civil War and Commonwealth (1642–60): after all, if there were no soul as taught in the catechism, there would be no hell – so what the hell? Ranters, Fifth Monarchists and other tub-thumpers bent on exploding the magic and majesty of power exposed the doctrines of eternal rewards and punishments as fictions fabricated by cunning clergy. Advocating agrarian communism, the Digger spokesman Gerrard Winstanley explained that heaven and hell were not in truth the shape of things to come but figurative – inner, subjective states: 'Why may we not have our Heaven here (that is, a comfortable livelihood in the Earth)?' Why indeed?

Symptomatic of this mutiny was the popularity of 'mortalism', the heresy that, upon death, the soul sleeps until the Last Judgement. 'Some believe', thundered a pillar of Puritanism, Edmund Calamy, in 1646, 'that the *Soul dyeth with the Body*', rising again only on the Day of Judgement. One notorious advocate of this 'soul-sleeping heresy' was Thomas Hobbes. Crucial to his dynamiting of priestcraft was rejection of the soul's intrinsic immortality. That fallacy – the doctrine that souls were incorporeal principles, living on after death by virtue of their inherent nature – had been smuggled in by the Church from the trash of Greek metaphysics. The Bible – Hobbes, of course, loved playing the Devil citing Scripture – gave not a word of warrant for any such natural immortality: in the sacred writings, 'soul' simply meant life or breath. As earlier discussed, the Hobbist denial of spirit was generally read as a veiled denial of God, and thus as a green light for 'anything goes' libertinism.

Mortalism not only squared with Hobbes's anticlerical immoralism. It also appealed to populists like the Levellers. Twisting Aristotle for his own ends, Richard Overton, for one, argued for the inseparability of body and soul, and of form and matter. The soul in reality was 'the internall and externall Faculties of Man joyntly considered': soul and body 'must as well end together as *begin* together; and *begin* together as *end* together. . . . they neither can *Be*, nor consist without other'. The soul could not naturally outlive the body; grace would come only on the Last Day. Such formulas of faith, which downplayed the separate soul, released the laity from the vice-grip of the Church.

What made mortalism so plausible, yet disturbing, was that it flowed inexorably from Luther's rejection of the popish doctrine of purgatory and the whole probationary palaver of indulgences, invocation of saints, passing bells, requiem masses and other abuses which it bred. For Protestants, there was no such place. In that case, demanded radicals, in what celestial way-station could the soul actually be lingering between death and the Last Trump? Mortalism's watertight logic on this point commended it to intellectuals like Milton, eager to cleanse Christianity of the dregs of popish hocus-pocus and 'vulgar errors', and it was also attractive to plebeian radicals because of its exposé of the outrageous prolongation of the power of throne and altar beyond the grave.

Nor was mortalism the only teaching which, in Christopher Hill's apt phrase, was turning the world upside down in the wake of the Civil War. The old order was also being defied, for instance, by all those antinomian preachers and self-styled 'saints' who claimed to be personally inspired with the Holy Spirit (again bypassing the clergy). Did not the Bible teach that to the pure all things were pure? Why then must free spirits obey the powers that be? The doctrinal, social and political anarchy thus brewing up gave the coming 'new philosophy' a particular appeal to those who saw in science a buttress of order, intellectual, social and cosmic alike.

*

In its account of the order of nature, the 'mechanical philosophy' sought to replace superannuated scholasticism with a fruitful utilitarian philosophy of works not words. But it was not merely a superior research tool; for its advocates, it had a nobler mission. Ultimately derived from Aristotle, the teachings of the 'schoolmen' – principally, of course, Roman Catholic priests – perpetuated the essential defects of that pagan: idolizing Nature as they did, their drift was materialistic and atheistic. Basic to such 'peripatetic' thinking was the commitment to a teleological, self-moving organic Nature: did that not mean, alleged critics, that spirit was subordinated to substance or matter, and God the Creator and Sustainer dethroned?

It was in part because of this anti-scholastic groundswell that the doctrines of Descartes, outlined earlier, initially won a warm welcome in England, notably among a clutch of Cambridge academics who were alarmed by common-man 'atheism' but equally disaffected with the hard-line Calvinism dominant in the 1640s. The Calvinists' doctrinaire, predestinatory denial of human free will, their conviction of radical sinfulness, was countered by these Cambridge 'Latitude men' or 'Latitudinarians' (the slur-words of their enemies) through appeal to the Christian humanist ideal of the dignity of man, and in particular to the image, derived from Proverbs 20: 27, of reason in man as the 'candle of the Lord', a natural light to complement the divine.

The divine Henry More, a fellow of Christ's College (Milton's Alma Mater), was one who in his youth had been tormented by the Calvinist threat of being predestined to hell. In 1653 he hailed Descartes, with whom he had been corresponding, as a 'sublime Mechanick' (that is, champion of the mechanical philosophy), 'a man more truly inspired in the knowledge of Nature, than any that have professed themselves so this sixteen hundred years'; and he declared himself 'ravished with admiration of his transcendent *Mechanical* inventions, for the salving the *Phaenomena* in the world'.

Cartesianism thus initially seemed just the ticket for More and his colleagues: its dualism sanctioned daring new explorations of nature while gloriously upholding reason and free will. It was rapidly to prove a false friend, however. It did not take long for More and other such 'men of latitude' to conclude that, despite its welcome anti-Calvinist endorsement of free will, the drift of Cartesianism, with its *a priori* tenet that nature was nothing but matter in motion, was to banish God from His Creation and thus serve as the slippery slope to unbelief. Reason was desirable, no doubt, but was not the Cartesianism brand which dictated mechanistic materialism blinkered, shallow and debasing? 'I oppose not rational to spiritual,' insisted another of the Cambridge Platonists, Benjamin Whichcote, 'for spiritual is most rational.'

Small wonder that by 1665 More himself was declaring to the Hon. Robert Boyle, doyen of the experimentalists and founder-fellow of the Royal Society, 'that the phaenomena of the world cannot be solved merely mechanically, but that there is the necessity of the assistance of a substance distinct from matter, that is, of a spirit, or being incorporeal'. Creation could not function by mechanical causes alone. In his *Enchiridion Metaphysicum* of 1671, More, by then also a fellow of the Royal Society, distanced himself huffily from the 'upstart Method of *Des Cartes*', explaining that his 'Mechanical Philosophy' was not at all 'the Experimental Philosophy' espoused by that august body. 'This Profession', he scoffed, Cartesianism in his sights, 'cannot rightly be called the *Mechanical Philosophy*, but the *Mechanical Belief or Credulity*.' Divorcing himself in this way from his former allegiance, More strategically rescued 'true' mechanical philosophy from the false (Cartesian) version of it, now exposed as being derived from those 'infidel' philosophers of Antiquity, Democritus, Epicurus and Lucretius.

This thumbs-down for Cartesianism owed much, of course, to the growing notoriety of the home-grown mechanist (and supposed atheist) Hobbes. Their teachings were poles apart. Hobbes was a 'naturalist', the Cambridge divines idealists; he posited an exclusively material world, they celebrated a universe vibrant with spirits; he postulated determinism in a mechanical order governed by iron laws, they portrayed man as a free agent within a vital, dynamic, 'plastic' nature. He accepted nothing transcendental, they savoured the delights of the divine.

In their mature writings, the Cambridge Platonists thus expounded doctrines which, while discrediting scholasticism, distanced themselves equally from Cartesian mechanism and its no less atheistical drift. In those times of exceptional freedom, proclaimed More, 'the Tempter would take advantage where hee may, to carry men captive out of one darke prison to another, out of *Superstition* into *Atheisme* it self'. True empirical study of nature was called for, since it was that which would reveal not only that there was a God but that Creation was spiritual through and through and that man had a soul and free will.

Nature's workings, More was convinced, could not be explained by the billiard-ball model of matter advanced by Descartes or Hobbes. It was of the essence of body that its 'parts cannot *penetrate* one another, is not *Self-moveable*, nor can *contract* nor *dilate* it self, is *divisible* and *separable* one part from another'. Given that matter was thus perfectly inert, something else must co-exist in nature besides, to account for its operations; and that was its opposite and complement, that is, spirit: 'I conceive the intire Idea of a *Spirit* in generall . . . to consist of these severall powers or properties, viz. *Self-penetration*, *Self-Motion*, *Self-contraction* and *Dilation*, and *Indivisibility*.' Generating activity as it did, it was 'plain that a *Spirit* is a notion of more perfection than a *Body*', insisted More, adopting the old Platonizing tendency to view the world in hierarchical, evaluative terms.

It was, moreover, fundamental to Platonism that the higher could never be engendered by, derived from, or explained in terms of, the inferior. Hence, spirit could not possibly be a product of matter, or order the outcome of chance. Such hierarchical anti-reductionism had crucial implications for More in his account of the human soul, in particular respecting the Hobbist doctrine that the mind was wholly determined and conditioned from without. '*The soul of Man is not* Abrasa Tabula,' insisted More (Locke, of course, was to take issue with this). Nor could the soul be an emanation or secretion of the body. 'I demand therefore', he silenced a potential reductionist objector,

> to what in the body will you attribute *Spontaneous Motion*? I understand thereby a power in our selves of wagging or holding still most of the parts of our Body, as our hand suppose or little finger. If you will say that it is nothing but the *immission* of the *Spirits* into such and such Muscles, I would gladly know what does *immit* these *Spirits* and direct them so curiously. Is it *themselves*, or the *Braine*, or that particular piece of the Braine they call the *Conarion* or *Pine-kernell* [pineal gland]? . . .
>
> If you say the *Brain* immits and directs these Spirits, how can that so freely and spontaneously move it self or another that has no Muscles?

Dissection yielded no evidence of the seat or operation of imagination, memory or any other mental or spiritual faculties: soul could nowise be reduced to brain. QED.

Intended as a refutation of 'atheism', a celebration of cosmic order and a defence of human dignity, *The True Intellectual System of the Universe* (1678) by More's colleague Ralph Cudworth offered a systematic refutation of rigid mechanism and endorsement of the spiritual as part of a vision of the Great Chain of Being or Scale of Nature, presided over by the Universal Mind. Claiming, in the subtitle to this vast mausoleum of erudition, that his was a work *Wherein, All the Reason and Philosophy of Atheism is Confuted; And its Impossibility Demonstrated*, Cudworth, Master of Christ's College, set out to prove the existence of a God defined as 'a perfect conscious understanding Being (or Mind) existing of it self from eternity, and the cause of all other things'. An incorporeal Deity, he stressed,

> moves Matter not *Mechanically* but *Vitally*, and by *Cogitation* only. And that a *Cogitative Being* as such hath a *Natural Imperium* over *Matter* and *Power* of Moving it without any *Engines* or *Machines*, is unquestionably certain, even from our own *Souls*: which move our Bodies and Command them every way, meerly by *will* and *Thought*.

God's relation to the universe was mirrored in the soul's relation to the body.

Taking his cue from Plato's *Timaeus*, Cudworth – reflecting, one surmises, upon his own experience as the Master of a Cambridge college – held that God presided over Creation not immediately but indirectly, through an intermediary 'plastic nature', a subordinate deputy executing His design. The voluntarist or Calvinist tenet that 'God himself doth all *immediately*, and as it were with his own hands, form the body of every gnat and fly, insect and mite' was demeaning to the Deity. The role of 'plastic nature', this subservient or executive instrument, moreover allowed the anti-Calvinist to resolve the old theodicy problem of why evil existed – surely God could not be its author? Nature's apparent imperfections, Cudworth insisted, were not of his willing, but arose from the inadequacies of that 'plastic nature' in the teeth of the 'indisposition' of matter (were the college porter and butler entirely trustworthy?).

While metaphysics was Cudworth's forte, he was not indifferent to facts. 'If there be once any Invisible ghosts or Spirits acknowledged as Things Permanent,' he asserted, 'it will not be easie for any to give a reason why there might not be one *Supreme Ghost* also, presiding over them all.' Those ghosts became crucial to the case against Descartes, against Hobbes, and against all other atheist onslaughts: they were scientific proofs of the spiritual.

Among the Cambridge divines, however, it was Henry More, as befitted a fellow of the Royal Society, who turned to what Robert Boyle would call 'matters of fact', so as to prove the spirit through science. In both the third book of his *An Antidote against Atheism* (1653) and throughout *The Immortality of the Soul* (1659), More presented accounts of witchcraft and possession, miraculous cures, '*Apparitions*', and such 'extraordinary effects' as 'speakings, knockings, opening of doores when they were fast shut, sudden lights in the midst of a room floating in the aire, and then passing and vanishing'.

On the trail of spiritual manifestations, divine and diabolical, More collaborated with a fellow enthusiast, Joseph Glanvill, an Oxford graduate and Somerset clergyman who devoted himself to promoting Baconian philosophy. His first book, *The Vanity of Dogmatizing* (1661), was an attack on the errors of the peripatetic philosophy; his *Plus*

Ultra (1668) extolled the new science; while his *Philosophia Pia* (1671) taught the harmony of science with Christianity.

Initially entitled *A Philosophical Endeavour towards the Defence of the Being of Witches and Apparitions*, Glanvill's demonology was greatly expanded to form his *Saducismus Triumphatus*, published posthumously by More in 1681.* The first part canvassed the theoretical possibility of witchcraft, the second mustered evidence for the reality of witches. Pitching into Hobbes's *a priori* denial of witchcraft, Glanvill denounced materialism as crude, bigoted and against the facts. There were many things beyond human reason – what vanity in dogmatizing! – while it was reasonable to believe in spirits on many grounds: well-attested experience, the weight of received opinion, and the gradated nature of the Chain of Being, rising from gross matter up to God. Glanvill also attacked Descartes – whom he too, like More, had initially admired – as a two-faced sophist who affirmed the existence of spirit while perversely excluding spirits from the world. If, as Christians held, the soul had an existence separate from the body, what was the problem about its being transported through the air, or even possessing another body? Descartes was thus a lurking Hobbist, and Hobbes a closet atheist.

To prove his point, Glanvill piled up reports to confirm that the soul acted upon its physical location. His aim was to show that spirit possession and fascination, albeit brought into disrepute by shady faith-healers and wild enthusiasts, should rightly become the territory, indeed the prize, of experimental philosophy. Himself a fellow of the Royal Society, Glanvill's sightings of the supernatural were received by that august body. Assuring the Society in 1682 that the soul had 'a much bigger sphere of influencing power, and thereby may extend it . . . even out of the Body', no less a scientist than Robert Hooke cited Glanvill's accounts of fortune-telling, mind-reading, and of what would later be called hypnotism.

Witchcraft was a phenomenon which Glanvill urged the Society

---

* The Sadducees, it will be remembered, were the influential Jewish group who denied the reality of spirits.

to study, in an impassioned plea prefixed to *A Blow at Modern Sadducism* (1668), where he pointed to the compatibility of its investigation with the Society's ethos of free inquiry. Between them, More and Glanvill came up with many sightings. In 1670 the former involved himself in 'psychic' phenomena at Cookhill Priory near Ragley Hall, the home of his cherished friend Anne, Lady Conwell. Through a stone slab in the floor of a cottage constructed in the abbey ruins strange sightings and callings were observed, and ghosts were said to glide through it. More had the slab lifted and boldly descended with a candle. Dripping water and whistling draughts might, More speculated, explain the sounds that distressed the cottagers, but his eagerness to lend credence to such phenomena was typical of his mind-set.

The principal supernatural phenomenon which came to his notice was that of the 'drummer of Tedworth'. In 1661 the Mompesson family of that Wiltshire village were persecuted by a drummer – they had, rumour had it, been stingy with alms – through loud bangings and other poltergeist-like noises. This business seemed to many, notably Glanvill who published it with great fervour, concrete evidence for the activity of spirits, and it was welcomed accordingly – by More as well – as a weapon against scepticism and mortalism.

The conviction that the new philosophy could confirm the spirit realm led to an outpouring of books, including Richard Bovet's *Pandaemonium, or the Devils's Cloyster, Being a Further Blow to Modern Sadducism* (1684), a work alluding to Glanvill and dedicated to More. The hope of proving the supernatural through science was no eccentric foible – it was common to the age and central to the endeavours of none other than Robert Boyle, the so-called father of modern chemistry.

As envisaged by that noble investigator, experimental natural philosophy required precise demarcation. It was to be sharply distinguished from neo-Aristotelian scholasticism and from every other '-ism' which falsely attributed to Nature what was properly to be credited to the will of God – ever the pious Protestant, Boyle was unswervingly hostile to concepts of Nature, not least Cudworth's

Neoplatonic 'plastic nature', which detracted from a proper appreciation of Divine majesty.

What then was the constitution of Nature? Boyle always returned to the primacy of matter and motion: perceptible ('secondary') qualities depended on the size, shape, motion and arrangement of the ('primary') component parts. There were no other hidden agents or occult forces: the workings of Nature were truly the will of God.

All his life Boyle was moved by religious impulses. His earliest writings were works of pious moral exhortation, before a second 'conversion experience' in the late 1640s – he had already experienced the conventional *religious* rebirth – turned him into the apostle of experimental science. Thereafter his fervent piety found expression mainly through the medium of natural philosophy, in such works as *The Christian Virtuoso* (1690–1). In his will he set up what became known as the Boyle Lectures, to be delivered annually from a London pulpit to teach how natural science led to Nature's God.

Boyle fretted about the threats which dogmatic rationalism posed for faith – like the Cambridge Platonists, he regarded humble reason as perfectly compatible with mysteries. Imperious rationalism was linked in his mind with the dismissiveness about the Resurrection and the immortality of the soul which he identified with such murky Renaissance figures as Pomponazzi, who in their turn had drawn their inspiration from Aristotle and the Greek atheists. Boyle thus shared the Cambridge Platonists' fear of the 'atheist' threat, singling out 'Socinians' (Arians) for over-reliance on reason. Strictly defined, Socinianism was the anti-trinitarian credo; more broadly, however, it was a smear word implying stiff-necked rationalism. Urging systematic investigation to quell such threats, Boyle held that observation and experiment proved the activities of 'spirit' in Nature, thus avoiding the dual pitfalls of materialist atheism on the one hand and the excesses of the enthusiasts on the other.

To counter such tendencies, Boyle touted the role of scientific research to support the plausibility of the Resurrection. 'We have really yet but a very small Insight into the true Nature of Bodys,' he insisted, addressing the case for the soul's immortality, '& a much lesser into that of Spirits.' His air-pump experiments, for instance, which proved, against scholastic precepts, the reality of the vacuum and the springiness of the air (hence 'Boyle's Law'), were assumed to confirm the presence of spirit in the atmosphere. Experimental 'pneumatics' (air studies) also showed that efficient causes might be not just material but vital and spiritual, analogous to the action of the human soul. Trials with phosphorus and other igniting and exploding chemicals similarly pointed to the presence of spirits. With a similar aim, in the mid-1670s Boyle published essays on celestial magnetism and alchemy.

Ever wary about his own reputation and fearful that adversaries would distort his meanings, Isaac Newton – himself a closet alchemist – predictably found Boyle's decision to publish such opinions rash: they were 'not to be communicated without immense damage', and he called his co-worker to 'high silence'. Yet the pious Boyle was not deterred from his mission to lay bare the spiritual world through science. In a letter 'Of celestial Influences or Effluviums in the Air', for example, he later offered an 'apology for astrology' which stressed the spiritual dimension: 'Our spirits are more near and more analogous to the nature of light than the air, so they must be more prone to and easy to be impressed than it.'

Boyle adopted a two-pronged strategy to validate and vindicate the spiritual. There were aspects of spiritual activity, particularly what fell within traditional 'natural magic', which could be harnessed by the new science. Once thus 'demonstrated' in the laboratory, spirit could be effectively integrated into Nature and hence natural philosophy. Experimental pneumatics or chemistry revealed at the bench the innate principles active in what had once been judged merely occult: instruments and apparatus showed spirits at work, the genie in the lamp.

Then there was a residue of 'supernatural phenomena', such as ghosts. While these eluded laboratory scrutiny, apparitions could be sufficiently affirmed and attested, in due Baconian manner, by authorized witnesses, and thus established as 'matters of fact'. Boyle shared Glanvill's and More's confidence as to the reality of witchcraft and similar phenomena that manifested God's (or Satan's) first-hand intervention in the world, making explicit his support for Glanvill's demonological project and plying him with verified accounts of witchcraft. Yet just as Newton chid Boyle, the latter in turn wagged his finger at Glanvill: he must be 'very carefull to deliver none but well attested narratives'.

Boyle continued to file such data for the rest of his life. Remarkable stories of supernatural powers appear in the notes made by Bishop Gilbert Burnet after a meeting with the aged experimentalist. Similar material was earmarked for a work entitled 'Strange Reports' which Boyle partly published. Lists of 'Supernaturall phaenomena' included 'A person that saw spirits in the day tyme', 'Apparitions in a magicall looking glasse', 'An absent witch tormented', and so forth.

Anxious to vindicate the new philosophy and to demonstrate God through it, yet temperamentally given to soul-searching, Boyle walked a tightrope. He deplored reductionist rationalism, with its atheistic undertow, and even entered into correspondence in the 1670s and 1680s with Quakers and other marginal figures – letters dismissed in an eighteenth-century inventory as 'Enthusiastic' and 'unintelligible'. Yet he was afraid – witness his caution to Glanvill – of appearing credulous and thereby risking discrediting his science.

Such fears were not Boyle's alone. Fellows of the infant Royal Society, while being prepared to use the methods and credit of science to authenticate the spirit world, were troubled lest the attempt would seem gullible, draw the ridicule of the wits around Charles II's court, and thus disgrace the enterprise. Just as Newton did not publish his alchemical experiments, the Royal Society did not follow up Glanvill's pleas to research witchcraft. Where, then, was the line to be drawn? Where did the spiritual forces of (lawful) natural magic and (satanic) black magic begin?

It was a question which perturbed Boyle. He was always fascinated by diabolical and magical phenomena, in 1658 sponsoring the English translation of a book by François Perreaud as *The Devill of Mascon*, and planning to publish a sequel to the collection of 'Strange Reports' dealing with 'Supernatural' phenomena. But he pulled back. One should beware of magic, he reasoned, not because it was false, but because, being real, it was too hot to handle.

Natural philosophers were thus in a cleft stick. Convinced that true science would disclose God's agency in Nature (and thereby prove the soul), they sought to naturalize the spirit by bringing it under laboratory control. Via the air-pump and the test-tube, spirits could be made visible and so be rendered safe and effective: good spirits would toe the line. Reactionary and bigoted divines who charged science with atheism could thus be rebutted: were not experiments the best way to give proof of the supernatural and so win over unbelievers?

But in speaking of spirits and the soul, immense risks lurked in mechanizing and rationalizing their action. The strategy had to be to undertake investigations to demonstrate the reality of spiritual activities without reducing these to the everyday and commonplace – for that way atheism, or at least Deism, lay.

It was the booby-trapped nature of that enterprise which gave Jonathan Swift such sport at the expense of the new philosophy. His *Discourse Concerning the Mechanical Operation of the Spirit* (1710) in particular felled both religious enthusiasts and natural philosophers with one stone: once the guileless mechanical philosopher naïvely reduced the soul to a cog in a machine, the Christian cause was lost – and natural philosophers were exposed as enthusiasts themselves, no saner than the sectaries. Did this not seem to bear out Sir Thomas Browne's fear that 'They who wou'd prove Religion by Reason, do but weaken the cause which they endeavour to support'?

And the dilemma worsened. For it soon ceased to be intellectually kosher or politically correct for progressives to look to the sighting of witches or ghosts: that path seemed to make too many concessions to credulity and to the enthusiasts. This inevitably left the human soul more vulnerable – or still more singular.

6

JOHN LOCKE REWRITES THE SOUL

> There is no need of debating the point about a man's
> being the same person with himself at the *present time,*
> because a man's own present consciousness will secure to
> him his own personal identity, though perhaps it will not
> confine it to himself alone. But the chief difficulty relates
> to his being the same with himself at *distant times.*
>
> ISAAC WATTS

Seeking a satisfactory sense of the self, Locke, as we have
seen, held that 'this personality extends it *self* beyond present Existence to what is past, only by consciousness'. The integrity of the self
from past to present thus lay not in the permanence of the flesh but
upon the fine thread of consciousness or memory. What, then, of the
future? What, to be precise, about that prophesied point when, at
the Last Judgement, we might reach the gates of the Kingdom of
Heaven?

Since the self was marked out 'only by Identity of consciousness',
Locke took the view that on the Last Day a person would be made
happy or miserable irrespective of 'in what Bodies soever they appear
or what Substances soever that consciousness adheres to'. Why
was he thus indifferent to, or impatient with, bodies ('scholastic
substances') beyond the grave? As a Christian he clearly held that in
the equation of identity with self-consciousness lay the best rebuttal
of materialism: whether Hobbes's corporeal God in a corporeal
heaven was in bad faith or a joke in bad taste, it needed to be seen
off. And as a Christian intellectual, Locke held the understanding to
be the supreme, the most divine part of a human.

Yet Locke's formulation did not spare him the bafflement or wrath of orthodox churchmen, for whom Holy Writ, divine justice and common sense clearly required the presence of the actual physical bodies of the departed present, in resurrected form, at the Last Judgement. How else, pray, was divine accountability to work? Edward Stillingfleet, Bishop of Worcester, was quick to contend that Locke's psychologizing of personal identity called into question the resurrection of the dead. Personhood could not be all in the mind: there needed to be material continuity, insisted the prelate, 'a *Vital Union* between the Soul and Body and the Life which is consequent upon it': bodily survival and revival were essential to divine sovereignty, in the last resort because it was upon the flesh of the damned that the Lord's retributive justice would ultimately be delivered.

In *The Bishop of Worcester's Answer to his Second Letter* (1697), Stillingfleet further criticized Locke's disembodied selfhood by appealing to St Paul, who unequivocally states that the dead will receive physical rewards and punishment proportionate to what they have done in the flesh ('every one may receive the things done in the body, according to that he hath done, whether it be good or bad': 2 Corinthians 5: 10). By implicitly questioning whether the dead would be resurrected in the same flesh as they had lived, Locke (accused Stillingfleet) contradicted the teachings of the Scriptures as well as eroding divine justice.

By the time *Mr Locke's Reply to the Right Reverend the Lord Bishop of Worcester's Answer to his Second Letter* appeared in 1699 – the controversy rumbled on and on – Thomas Beconsall, fellow of Brasenose College Oxford, had further argued, in a sermon on *The Doctrine of a General Resurrection: wherein The Identity of the Rising Body is asserted, against Socinians and Scepticks*, that Locke's account of personal identity allowed for 'no distinction between the Righteous and the Wicked':

For if the Wicked at the point of Death do not immediately vanish into Air, or if Mankind do not usually judge before-hand, and thereupon deny 'em the Office of Burial, or if the Allotments of Life and Damnation are not indiscriminately ascertain'd (to affirm any of which would be a gross a palpable Ab[s]urdity) then the Wicked must come forth of their Graves; and make their Resurrection, tho' a most Fatal one, even the Resurrection of Damnation.

Locke seemed to threaten due punishment of the wicked.

Three years later, Philip Stubbs, a former fellow of Wadham College, Oxford, similarly insisted that that final reunion of body and soul on which Locke hedged his bets was essential for the accomplishment of 'a compleat state of Happiness and Misery'. These were but some of the charges, predictably mainly from reactionary High Church Oxford, that were levelled against Locke (himself an Oxford graduate, but by then in bad odour at his Alma Mater for his political as well as religious liberalism) in defence of reincarnation.

The posthumous appearance in 1707 of Locke's *Resurrectio et quae sequuntur* added fuel to the flames. In this work he sketched the eschatological framework underpinning the views on identity and resurrection he had developed in the *Essay concerning Human Understanding*. While the righteous would be raised to immortality in a spiritual mould, sinners, Locke held, would be cast into hellfire, but not *everlastingly*: they would be spared that fate by being eventually annihilated.

The cat seemed out of the bag: critics took Locke's double-standard eschatology as evidence of his long-suspected heretical leanings: was he not too soft on sinners, letting them off the hook? Denial of the eternity of hellfire was common among Socinians (those who disbelieve the divinity of Christ). In 1719 the Oxford scholar Winch Holdsworth, in a defence of reincarnation, specifically dubbed Locke 'that Celebrated Writer of the Socinian Kind', and his heterodoxy on bodily identity was repeatedly censured as a threat to the Christian order: once question eternal punishment, and how would law and order be upheld? What then was to stop your servant ravishing your wife and filching your silver? To question bodily resurrection was as stupid as axing the gallows.

Locke, however, was not alone in his disquiet about traditional pulpit teachings on the afterlife. Indeed, the decades of amazing intellectual effervescence, or turmoil, around 1700 threw up a galaxy of new formulations about the Beyond. One contemporary who declared himself to be a true Christian yet whose views scandalized his age was John Asgill, a lawyer, commonwealthman and freemason who had the dubious distinction of being the first MP ever to be expelled from the House of Commons of Great Britain – that is, Parliament as convened after the 1707 Act of Union. The reason lay in the 'many profane and blasphemous Expressions' contained in his *An Argument Proving that According to the Covenant of Eternal Life Revealed in the Scriptures, Man may be Translated from Hence into that Eternal Life without Passing through Death*, published in 1700.

While it was certainly idiosyncratic, tongue-in-cheek even, Asgill's reading of the Bible had a certain Christian logic to it. His case for the escape from death proclaimed in his title hinged upon the doctrine of the Cross. Through Adam's sin, mortality had come into the world, but Christ had then been crucified to annul the law of death. So, subsequent to the Son's sacrifice, why should anyone ever perish? Believers in Christ's covenant need not die but should soar straight to heaven, like Elijah in his chariot of fire. Why then did people apparently go on dying? The reason was all in the mind: they died only because of their fear of death. 'I shall not go hence *by returning unto the Dust*,' proclaimed Asgill, 'but that I shall *make* my Exit by way of *Translation*, which I claim as a dignity belonging to that Degree in the Science of Eternal Life' that was broadcast in the Scriptures. The idea of a posthumous probationary period for the soul was unscriptural, smacking of the Romish abomination of purgatory, insisted the Pope-hating Asgill; the Kingdom of Heaven would be instantaneous for those with faith in simultaneous translation.

Asgill drove to its logical conclusion the mortalist exposure of Greek metaphysics and Catholic theology propping up an independent, immaterial soul untouched by the dissolution of the flesh. His was another blow struck against the clutches of power-mad Churches on the individual even beyond the grave. Eternal life must mean survival of body and soul conjoined: 'The Spirit is so perfectly mixed with, and diffused through the whole Body,' he insisted, touting a materialism that seemingly anticipated Priestley, 'that we can't now say which is *Spirit,* nor which is Earth, but the whole is *one intire living Creature.'*

Asgill's effusion was patronizingly dismissed by Daniel Defoe as the 'Enthusiasm of pious Lunacy', but there was method in his madness and, as is shown by his expulsion from the House of Commons, many judged such views not mad but bad. Not only were they heterodox but, like mortalism in general, they subverted the economy of posthumous judicial rewards and punishments which underwrote earthly law and order.

As ever in theological controversies, Asgill's attempted elucidations of the faith made confusion worse. If Christ, as Asgill held, had truly cancelled the Law of Death, then what possible necessity could there be – asked the quarrelsome Defoe – even for translation? 'We may as well *save God Almighty the Trouble,*' he exploded, 'abide where we are, and go all to Heaven at once.' Parliament chose not to wrangle; in April 1707 it ordered the burning of his book, on grounds of heresy. Around the same time he was, moreover, detained in the Fleet Prison for debt and, still confined, he died, it seems untranslated, thirty years later.

Asgill may have been a gadfly and trouble-stirrer but, even so, such matters as heaven and hell were a minefield. Take, from the other end of the ideological spectrum, Henry Dodwell. He refused to swear allegiance to William and Mary and was a renowned High Churchman, but was even so no pillar of orthodoxy. *An Epistolary Discourse, Proving from the Scriptures and the First Fathers, that the Soul is a Principle Naturally Mortal, but Immortalized Actually by the Pleasure of God to Punishment or to Reward, by its Union with the Divine Baptismal Spirit* (1706), was a statement of pious mortalism. God had created Adam out of the dust, afterwards adding his breath of life (*pneuma*), so that man became a 'living soul'. Hereafter, continued Dodwell, the Lord then superadded his divine breath (*pnoe,* imparted at baptism) which bestowed upon man the capacity for immortality. At the Fall, the *pneuma* had been lost and so post-lapsarian man became mortal; yet he retained the divine breath, conferred at baptism into the Church, so long as it pleased God to sustain it. Thus, as a result of Original Sin, man lost his *natural* immortality, yet was not thereby reduced to a Hobbesian state of non-existence at death, for souls *post mortem* were *supernaturally* sustained (by the sacrament of baptism). The divine breath, he explained in a later *Defence*, 'seems to be the *Principle* that enables *Humane Souls* to subsist in *Hades* in their *separate* State'.

Thus, in a curious convergence with the radical mortalists, Dodwell posited a naturally mortal soul. Unlike them, however, he championed a divine soul-life proceeding continuously after death, thanks to baptism. But, he had to ask, confronting one of the perennial stumbling-blocks to consensus over salvation, after death where exactly did this soul go? Tackling this 'temporary accommodation' predicament – one rendered controversial by the Protestant elimin-ation of purgatory – Dodwell held that the location after death of separate souls lay in transit stations in the firmament, equidistant between heaven and hell. The righteous and the wicked would occupy different quarters, the former being confined below the moon, the latter just above. In the lowermost zones of heaven, the less perfect would undergo expiation to prepare them for their promotion to the higher regions. Finally, on Resurrection Day, bodies would be levitated out of their earthly graves into the skies, to be reunited with the waiting souls. At that point, Dodwell maintained, 'our *Bodies* also will by him be made *Pneumatical*, when they are *fashioned like his glorious* Body'.

In asserting a *natural* mortality of the soul, Dodwell acceded to the commonsense logic of the mortalists. But his commitment to the vitality of the soul between death and the Last Judgement, buoyed up through God's spirit, was quite out of step with the politics of the mortalist tradition and reveals (as does his stress upon baptism) his High Church attachment to a visible hierarchy and God's ubiquitous and unceasing moral government of Creation.

Locke's fudge of the question of man's corporeal state in heaven – his preference for some nobler disembodied existence – obviously grieved many honest churchmen, fearful that this would erode proper accountability. But it did promise to solve, reduce or circumvent other nagging problems posed by the ambiguities of physicality in the afterlife.

The material minutiae of heaven and hell had always been contentious in the very gradual evolution of teachings as to these two locations over the centuries. Calvinist orthodoxy included the expectation – presumably attended with widespread *schadenfreude* – that the hosts of damned would far exceed the saved: 'many be called, but few chosen' (Matthew 20: 16) was a favourite text. In *An Enquiry into the Nature and Place of Hell* (1714), Tobias Swinden, a grand master of celestial arithmetic, expressed his outrage at the suggestion of the Continental theologian Drexelius that there would be a mere hundred thousand million lost souls in a hell just one German mile square. 'It is a poor, mean and narrow Conception,' he scoffed, 'both of the Numbers of the Damned, and of the Dimensions of Hell.' Hell had generally been assumed to be sited at the centre of the earth but, thinking big, Swinden transferred it to the sun, reasoning that terrestrial subterranean regions could not possibly house all the hordes of the reprobate.

Hard-liners had always relished the gory physicality of hell. 'We have heard . . . of some who have endured breaking on the Wheel, ripping up of their Bowels, fleaing alive, racking of Joynts, burning of Flesh, pounding in a Mortar, tearing in pieces with Flesh-hooks, boyling in Oyl, roasting on hot fiery Grid-irons, etc.' – thus John Shower fired up readers' fantasies in his *Heaven and Hell; or the Unchangeable State of Happiness or Misery for all Mankind in Another World* (1700):

And yet all these, tho' you should superad thereto all Diseases, such as the Plague, Stone, Gout, Strangury, or whatever else you can name most torturing to the Body . . . they would all come short . . . of that Wrath, that Horror, that inconceivable Anguish which the Damned must inevitably suffer every Moment, without any intermission of their pains, in Hellish Flames.

Hell's terrors could thus be represented as the bodily sufferings experienced this side of the divide writ large. 'If it be an intolerable thing to suffer the heat of the fire for a year, or a day, or an hour, what will it be to suffer ten thousand times more for ever?' demanded the Presbyterian Richard Baxter in *The Saints' Everlasting Rest* (1650). 'What if thou wert to suffer Lawrence's death, to be roasted upon a gridiron . . . If thou couldst not endure such things as these, how wilt thou endure the eternal flames?' Among traditionalists, anticipations continued of the future punishments in store for sinners – Englishmen who had stuffed their statute book with hundreds of capital crimes and who religiously turned up to hangings would hardly flinch at an unashamedly punitive ('vindictive' was their word) hell. Samuel Johnson's notion of damnation ('Sent to Hell, Sir, and punished everlastingly') is notorious.

What had always excited the most salutary horror was precisely that infinite quality of hell's torments: 'the great aggravation of this misery', gloated Baxter, 'will be its eternity'. But in the sunnier climate of all-is-for-the-best enlightened optimism, liberal Christians increasingly held that the eternal punishments which had been Christian orthodoxy at least since the Athanasian Creed (late fourth century) were inconsistent with a benevolent Father. Locke, as we have seen, came round to believing in a merciful obliteration for the damned. Archbishop Tillotson himself had been accused of doubting eternal torments. William Whiston, an Arian (disbeliever in the Trinity), Newton's successor as Lucasian Professor at Cambridge, declared, in *The Eternity of Hell Torments Considered* (1740), that such 'common but barbarous and savage opinions' were incompatible with divine love. In *Christianity as Old as the Creation* (1730), Matthew Tindal, a Deist (disbeliever in divine intervention), condemned those who 'impute such Actions' to God, for they 'make him resemble the worst of Beings, and so run into downright Demonism'. Milder expectations were evidently gaining ground among 'enlightened' Christians mindful of God's compassion as well as His power. Boschian evocations of devils roasting the wicked on a spit receded from Anglican pulpit oratory, while the clockwork universe of the new science eroded belief in the mundane powers of Satan and the reality of witchcraft – the Statutes relating to it were repealed in 1736.

Lenient divines thus mitigated hell's punishments for others; but for the individual, what truly counted were the expectations held out for the saved in the great habitation in the sky. At this point, Locke's questions about selfhood were terribly pertinent: in what guise would a person appear at the pearly gates?

Church orthodoxy had penal reasons – utter accountability – for stipulating the resurrected body's identity with the temporal. But what did that actually mean? Debate over the details of bodily survival had marked the Christian views on reincarnation since earliest times. Such matters as the preservation of hair and nails and many other distinctive physical features had kindled perennial disputes. Shall we have the same height, weight and age as we did at our death? Would diseases, deformities and decay disappear? Writing in 1650, the divine John Seager had stated that resurrected bodies would certainly consist of flesh and bones; yet, he conceded, heavenly eyes and ears, hands and feet would not need to be made of the same substance as our terrestrial torso.

Christian Platonists, for their part, were disposed to envisage the afterlife primarily as a spiritual abode. Holding that 'there is no *stable Personality* of a man but what is in his Soul', Henry More downplayed resurrection of the fleshly body, warts and all, in line with his notion of God's justice: 'for so shall the Body of an old man be punished for the sins of that Body he had when he was young'. More painted a delightful picture of this immaterial existence amid the heavenly hosts:

they cannot but enravish one anothers Souls, while they are mutual Spectators of the perfect pulchritude of one anothers persons and comely carriage, of their graceful dancing, their melodious singing and playing, with accents so sweet and soft, as if we should imagine the Air here of itself to compose Lessons, and to send for the Musicall sounds without the help of any terrestrial Instrument.

Ralph Cudworth similarly envisaged an essentially ethereal existence, in which heavenly selves would assume an angelic shape, with 'such a countenance, and so cloathed, as they'. Bathed in God's glory, the heavenly host, surmised Thomas Burnet, another of that group, would consist of a celestial gossamer 'as pure and thin, as the finest Air or Aether'.

In the new eighteenth-century climate which brought the flourishing of material and domestic culture and the cultivation of 'affective individualism', it is not surprising that man-centred rather than theocentric ideas of a future state made headway among believers at large. In the *Athenian Gazette*, set up in 1691 by John Dunton as the first ever question-and-answer magazine, in response to a reader's query: 'Are there sexes in heaven?', the columnist – perhaps Dunton himself – held in orthodox manner that all that was imperfect and accidental would be erased; hence sexuality would vanish – saucily adding: 'we won't add for another Reason what, as we remember, one of the Fathers has said – That *were there any Women in Heaven, the Angels cou'd not stand long*, but wou'd certainly be seduced from their Innocency, and Fall as *Adam* did.' This question of heavenly genders was to assume great personal poignancy for Dunton soon afterwards, however, upon the death of his beloved wife. In response, in 1698 he produced *An Essay Proving We shall Know our Friends in Heaven*, which held out the prospect of reunion. 'Her Death', he wrote, 'has made me so very melancholy, that I had pin'd away in a few days, had not the hopes of finding her again in Heaven, given me *some Relief.*'

As envisaged by Dunton, heaven was bound to involve the resumption of worldly familial relations. Epitomizing the new companionate marriage ideal, he maintained that since life in the here-and-now was not agreeable without familiar acquaintance, must that not be true of heaven too? 'Be assured,' he wrote, old friends 'will not be wanting in the Height and Perfection of all Glory, Bliss and Joy.' Moreover, to ensure personal identity, even *memories* of our own and our nearest and dearest's former lives would remain intact. Unlike the high-minded Cambridge Platonists on the one hand and such Calvinist killjoys as Baxter on the other, Dunton adjudged that we would know each other in a 'familiar' way. Though conjugal relations *per se* between husbands and wives would not be resumed – Jesus had said there would be no marriage in heaven – the distinction of the sexes would remain as before: 'the Soul . . . of the one is Resolute

and Constant, that of the other Light, Wavering and Changeable. . . .
The Soul of one takes a pride in being Grave and speaking little; the
other talks much, and cannot forbear *twatling upon every thing.*'

This homely heaven was not just a foible of Dunton's. The fantasy
of the New Jerusalem as an improved extension of everyday life
became widespread, with all its prospects, pleasures – and puzzles.
'My Grandmothers were old Women when *I* knew them,' pondered
Samuel Johnson's friend, Hester Thrale:

to *me* therefore they must at the Day of Judgement *appear* Old; how else
shall I know em? . . . to their Parents & Nurses however they must appear
Babies . . . while to the new-rais'd Eye of Husbands, Lovers, Friends &c.
who could recognize no possible Acquaintance either with the Crone or
Baby – Lucy Salusbury and Philadelphia Cotton must certainly be seen as
they were in Youth, Health, & Maturity.

All this might seem baffling, she mused, but it was in truth 'most easy
when we reflect on the Omnipotence of God's holy *Word* & *Spirit*'.

Many Georgian visions of heaven were conspicuously modelled
on the familiar life of this world. In 1703 William Assheton, the
Rector of Beckenham in Kent, wrote a short tract refuting those
schoolmen who believed that heavenly life consisted 'in bare speculation, gazing upon each other, and admiring each other's perfec-
tions'. With typical middle-class enthusiasm, Assheton asserted that
there would certainly be action as well as contemplation in heaven.
'Now we are not in the least to suspect, when such multitudes of
active beings are met together,' he surmised, 'that they will be idle;
but will incessantly be employed.' Since heaven was God's kingdom
it would moreover have, just like England, 'laws and statutes and
governors and subjects, and those of different ranks, orders, and
degrees'.

Influential in this conspicuous move away from the contemplative
vision of heaven (that of the Cambridge Platonists) to a more active
view, reflecting Protestant notions of virtuous work and energy, was
the Dissenter Isaac Watts. He filled the afterlife with saintly and

endless action and improving possibilities. In a best-selling funeral sermon delivered in 1722, entitled 'Death and Heaven; or the Last Enemy Conquered, and Separate Spirits Made Perfect', Watts described a heaven standing between the theocentric heaven of Calvin and the unashamedly anthropocentric heaven proclaimed by nineteenth-century books like *Heaven our Home* (a favourite of Queen Victoria). The orthodox considered that heaven was a place of contemplation and rest. Watts rejected this view. Christians accustomed to an active life would be disappointed with a passive beatific vision. 'When angels are so variously and delightfully employed in service for God, in his several known and unknown worlds,' reflected Watts, 'we cannot suppose the spirits of just men shall be eternally confined to a sedentary state of inactive contemplation.' Although contemplation 'is a noble pleasure', the very sight of the divine 'will awaken and animate all the active and sprightly powers of the soul'. A perfect instance of the Protestant work-ethic, Watts concluded that, rather than being confined to eternal meditation, the soul will 'set all the springs of love and zeal at work in the most illustrious instances of unknown and glorious duty'. Since fatigue was unthinkable in heaven, the saints would endlessly join in the work of God. 'Those spirits who have tasted unknown delight and satisfaction in many long seasons of devotion, and in a thousand painful services for their blessed Lord on earth,' Watts noted, 'can hardly bear the thoughts of paying no active duties, doing no work at all for him in heaven, where business is all over delight, and labour is all enjoyment.' Active Christians, who might have got bored with eternal meditation, would serve God 'perhaps as priests in his temple, and as kings, or viceroys, in his wide dominions'.

Also influential in England was the vision of Emanuel Swedenborg, who made London his second home and published many of his works there. Few Englishmen became true Swedenborgians, but his ideas point to changing outlooks, from the erstwhile primarily theocentric doctrine of heaven to a more domesticated model. In his *The Economy of the Animal Kingdom, Considered Anatomically, Physically, and Philosophically,*

Swedenborg suggested that only a thin curtain would divide heaven from earth, with heavenly life commencing straight after death, less as the antithesis of terrestrial existence than its continuation and completion. Although heaven remained the traditional garden of repose, the saints were now depicted as engaged in spiritual improvement. And finally, the traditional primacy of the beatific vision was replaced by an accent on human love, expressed through family, friends and neighbours.

Popular writers like Dunton were no longer prepared to let the clergy exercise a monopoly over matters transcendental, and began revamping heaven after their own image. Highly influential was Elizabeth Singer Rowe's *Friendship in Death*, a mailbag of letters from the dead to the living, which went through an impressive fifteen editions between 1728 and 1816, becoming a key source for popular views on the fate of the soul and fulfilling a role rather as spiritualism did later for the Victorians. Love, Rowe assured her readers, was the very essence of futurity. Altamont had died grieving for his dead wife Almeria. As he floats up to heaven, Rowe has the husband tenderly gushing,

The first gentle Spirit that welcom'd me to these new Regions was the lovely *Almeria*; but how Dazling! how divinely Fair! Extasy was in her Eyes, and inexpressible Pleasure in every Smile! . . . With an inimitable Grace she received me into her aetherial Chariot, which was sparkling Saphire studded with Gold: It roll'd with a spontaneous Motion along the Heavenly Plains, and stop'd at the Morning Star, our destin'd habitation. But how shall I describe this fair, this fragrant, this enchanting Land of Love!

Popular though such effusions proved, describing heaven nevertheless required tact, and authors had to steer a tricky course between extremes, so as to avoid creating more problems than they solved. It was easy for Pope to sneer at the proverbial North American Indian who thought that he would be reunited in heaven with his creature comforts –

> Go, like the Indian, in another life
> Expect thy dog, thy bottle, and thy wife . . .

– but how was Christian thinking superior? Quizzed whether negroes would arise on the last day, the *Athenian Gazette* responded: 'Taking then this blackness of the Negro to be an accidental Imperfection . . . we conclude thence, that he shall not arise with that Complexion, but leave it behind him in the darkness of the Grave, exchanging it for a brighter and a better at his return again into the World.' And what of all those other hoary objections to resurrection? What would be the fate at the Last Trump of corpses mutilated on the battlefield, dissected or cannibalized? And what about anomalies like Siamese twins, then much in the news? Lazarus Coloreda and his brother John Baptista, who grew from his navel, had been exhibited in freak shows around 1640. A query as to their fate was later posed to the *Athenian Gazette*. 'We find no lineaments of a Rational soul in *Baptista*, nor so much of the Animal as Brutes have,' the answer cautiously suggested:

his brother shall rise without him at the Day of Judgment, for there will be no Monsters at the Resurrection . . . but if he has a Rational Soul . . . then he will be ranked among Children, Fools and Ideots at the last Day; but will rise separate with a perfect Body, not with another Body, but the same specifick Body, adapted and fitly organised for a future State.

As will be discussed in Chapter 9, *The Memoirs of Martin Scriblerus*, authored by a bunch of Tory wits, gleefully burlesqued all such vain attempts to fathom the mystery.

It was James Boswell, however, who perhaps predictably got to the heart of the matter. If Christianity taught a rematerialization of our embodied selves in the afterlife, what would follow? That pious drunk and godfearing lecher got into a discussion on 'the subject of a future state' with the altogether more sceptical Lord Kames:

I said it was hard that we were not allowed to have any notion of what kind of existence we shall have. He said there was an impenetrable veil between us and our future state and being sensible of this, he never attempted to think on the subject, knowing it to be in vain. . . .

Boswell was never one to be fobbed off:

I told him how Maclaurin had pushed Sir John Pringle at Lord Monboddo's upon the subject, and had asked him what we were to have that could make us wish for a future state: 'Shall we have claret, Sir John?' 'I don't know but you may, Mr. Maclaurin.' 'Well,' said my Lord, 'it is true this body is put into the grave. But may we not have another film, another body, more refined? The ancients,' said he, 'all describe a future state as having enjoyments similar to what we have here. Let us lay aside the prejudices which we have been taught. Suppose we have other bodies. Why may we not have all the pleasures of which we are capable here? For instance, the pleasure of eating. Why not that, in a more delicate manner?' I mentioned, before he spoke of eating, our being told we are to have music. 'And,' said he . . . 'and there is another pleasure'; (I thought, though I divined what he meant clearly enough, that he should speak it out plainly, so waited in silence till he proceeded) 'why not have the pleasure of women?' 'Why not,' cried I, with animation. 'There is nothing in reason or revelation against our having all enjoyments sensual and intellectual.'

The irony, here revealed, of the orthodox Christian position on reincarnation was that it paradoxically seemed to sanction the flesh in all its unregenerate concupiscence.

This chapter has addressed a dilemma that had often been raised by the odd heretic but which was in the eighteenth century growing more insistent. In associating identity with consciousness – man is essentially his memory – Locke advanced a doctrine rather congenial to progressive aspirations and sensibilities. It accorded that self a heightened dignity (it resided in the mind), and elevated it above the base, vulgar and physical. For Locke at least it was Christian: that self was evidently the soul.

Such a view ran into trouble with the Churches, however, because its dematerialization of personal identity hazarded the key doctrine of the resurrection of the flesh, the heart of Christian soteriology and eschatology, to say nothing of popular hopes of an afterlife. *Prima facie*, it might seem paradoxical indeed that the teachings of the Churches should so insistently have clung to the indispensability of the flesh. The new thinking adopted by Locke and the intellectual élites established distance from a clerical creed which could now be spurned as pandering to the vulgar even as it served the interests of the powers that be.

PART II

MEN OF LETTERS

7

THE SPECTATOR: *THE POLITE SELF IN THE POLITE BODY*

There is nothing which I contemplate with greater pleasure than the dignity of human nature.

RICHARD STEELE

Hopes vied with fears in the breasts of late-seventeenth-
century Englishmen. Great expectations had been raised by the
Glorious Revolution of a final escape from the crises of the Stuart
century, with its bloody civil strife and wars of faith embroiling
Anglicans, Catholics, Puritans and militant sectaries. Charles Stuart,
Oliver Cromwell, God-intoxicated zealots and the 'infallible artillery'
of the church militant – all had to be consigned to the nightmare
past.

Concerns remained for the present, however. Tainted by the
louche glitter of the Merrie Monarch and the Catholic interlude of
James II, the court was distrusted as corrupt and disreputable. And
many an upright gentleman detested the 'great wen' – London,
resurgent, phoenix-like, after the Fire – as a sinkhole of vice, where
parvenu wealth strutted its stuff and such quackish financial innovations as the Bank of England and the Stock Exchange were rising,
like mushrooms on a dunghill, to threaten honest wealth.

And there was another equivocal novelty: Grub Street. Newspapers, pamphlets and magazines proliferated, especially once the
lapse of the Licensing Act in 1695 put an end to censorship; but
would all that ephemeral paper spread sense and civilization, or yet
more divisive folly? Claiming to harness the power of print to a
civilizing mission were Richard Steele, who founded the *Tatler*, and

Joseph Addison, his collaborator from 1711 on the *Spectator*. The mission of these magazines was to refashion man – and woman – for the bewildering post-1688 age of opportunity. It proved a turning-point: the press was in effect becoming the new pulpit, sermonizing lifestyle.

The first of a new breed of media-men, Addison and Steele set out to woo not just the capital's smart urbanites and the propertied classes of the shires but also those on the make who aimed to emulate their betters. They wrote to instruct old stagers and *nouveaux riches* alike how to conduct themselves in the new public sphere – how to want to be perceived and received. The *Spectator* thus held a mirror up to society, albeit one which broadcast new images rather than simply reflecting old ones. It was to be the inner censor of the new generation and its instructor.

The paper's literary trademark was 'Mr Spectator' himself, 'a Spectator of Mankind', silent, omnipresent but unseen in all the capital's coffee houses and clubs, theatres and taverns, nooks and crannies. His goal, Addison famously announced, was to rescue philosophy (rational thinking, that is) from obscure academic cloisters and libraries to dwell among this up-and-coming coffee-house and tea-table society, and he cloaked himself at such venues in his fictive presence. An all-observant censor, 'Mr Spectator' would seek out follies and foibles and then offer correctives.

Mr Spectator doubled as Mr Dissector, anatomist of the modern breast. In an image pioneered a century earlier by the metaphysical poets, various *Spectator* papers picture the wielding of a social scalpel, penetrating the veneer of fashionable social bodies to lay bare the diseased innards. In one vignette Addison imagined attending the dissection 'of a *Beau's Head*'. At first sight this looked just 'like the Head of another Man', but

upon applying our Glasses to it, we made a very odd Discovery, namely, that what we looked upon as Brains, were not such in Reality, but an Heap of strange Materials wound up in that Shape and Texture, and packed together with wonderful Art in the several Cavities of the Skull.

Two birds could be killed with one stone: that beau, and the by-then discounted philosophizings of Descartes:

The *Pineal Gland*, which many of our Modern Philosophers suppose to be the Seat of the Soul, smelt very strong of Essence and Orange-Flower Water, and was encompas'd with a Kind of horny Substance, cut into a thousand little Faces or Mirrours, which were imperceptible to the naked Eye; insomuch that the Soul, if there had been any here, must have been always taken up in contemplating her own Beauties.

Other hollows were 'filled with Ribbons, Lace and Embroidery' or with 'invisible Billet-doux, Love-Letters, pricked Dances, and other Trumpery of the same Nature'. And further:

There was a large Cavity on each Side of the Head, which I must not omit. That on the right Side was filled with Fictions, Flatteries and Falsehoods, Vows, Promises and Protestations; that on the left with Oaths and Imprecations. . . . the large Canal entered into a great Cavity of the Skull, from whence there went another Canal into the Tongue. This great Cavity was filled with a Kind of spongy Substance, which the *French* Anatomists call *Galimatias*, and the *English* Nonsense.

The anatomist then applied his knife to the heart of a jilt. This was found to have suffered 'Millions of little Scars, which seem'd to have been occasioned by the Points of innumerable Darts and Arrows'. The organ contained a liquor which had in it 'all the Qualities of that Spirit which is made Use of in the Thermometer, to shew the Change of Weather':

He affirmed also, that it rose at the Approach of a Plume of Feathers, an embroidered Coat, or a Pair of fringed Gloves; and that it fell as soon as an ill-shaped Perriwig, a clumsy pair of Shooes, or an unfashionable Coat came into his House. . . . Having cleared away the *Pericardium*, or the Case and Liquor above-mentioned, we came to the Heart itself. . . . Upon weighing the Heart in my Hand, I found it to be extreamly light, and consequently very hollow.

Autobiography was inscribed upon the flesh and, in pursuit of his vocation as censor and reformer, Mr Spectator thus played the part not just of all-seeing observer but of assistant surgeon.

Mention of Mr Spectator and Mr Dissector serves as a reminder that the running trope in the *Spectator* was 'all the world's a stage'. '*Totus mundus agit histrionem*', quoted Addison: everyone is a player, conjuring up a theatre of the world upon whose boards all must perform. Allusion to part-playing had ever been the weapon of stern moralists exposing insincerity and duplicity. As employed in the *Spectator*, however, the device was positive and edifying: modern man would do well to copy the actor who had mastered his lines and gestures, who possessed consummate stage presence and played his part word-perfect in life's comedy – good humour being as essential for Addison and Steele as for their contemporary, Lord Shaftesbury.

This social comedy, in other words, called for a transformed presentation of the self. Yesterday's men, readers learnt, had the wrong acting style: their looks were too grave, saintly, sombre, fastidious ('nice' in the old and strict sense – 'picky') and hotheaded, always standing upon their honour or quick to take offence; and there was more than a grain of truth in Hobbes's characterization of the solitary, poor, nasty and brutish quality of the human condition. An end to all such spleen! Spectatorial man would be an upbeat sociable performer, one of the troupe rather than a solitary, melancholy star. The newly eligible persona would display a refined yet relaxed public presence and man's potential would be polished up to perfection: 'I consider an Human Soul without Education like Marble in the Quarry, which shews none of its inherent Beauties, till the Skill of the Polisher fetches out the Colours, makes the Surface shine, and discovers every ornamental Cloud, Spot and Vein that runs thro' the Body of it.' That, in a nutshell, was the *Spectator*'s ambition, to fashion man anew. If Shaftesbury's good nature provided the raw materials, the polishing would be achieved through Lockean education.

Smoothing rough edges, Addison and Steele aspired to turn belligerent and vituperative antagonists into politically correct coffee-house conversationalists, and (respecting the fair sex) giddy fashion-mad flirts into sensible, well-informed creatures, who would grace their husbands and instruct their children. The strife and sorrow of old were not the inescapable legacies of Original Sin; they were self-inflicted and corrigible: 'Half the Misery of Human Life might be extinguished, would Men alleviate the general Curse they lie under, by mutual Offices of Compassion, Benevolence and Humanity.' The physician in Mr Spectator aimed to heal the disastrous ruptures of the 'divided society', those estranging Whigs and Tories, High and Low Church, town and country, gentry and commerce, men and women, by means of the creation of agreeable, conformist social actors. And complementing that call to social discipline, Mr Spectator also addressed another aspect of the human condition in need of remedy, the body itself, its nature and culture. The *Spectator* club was to be a coming together of gentlemen from all walks of life in happy harmony.

The human physique was glorious, declared Mr Spectator, and its Maker to be venerated. Even the pagan Galen 'could not but own a Supreme Being upon a Survey of this his Handywork', while 'since the Circulation of the Blood has been found out, and many other great Discoveries have been made by our Modern Anatomists, we see new Wonders in the Human Frame'. Attention was drawn to features of the body – the symmetry of eyes and ears, hands and feet, for instance – which optimized its functioning and served as sublime proofs of the Supreme Designer: 'Is it possible for Chance to be thus delicate and uniform in her Operations?' For further proof, readers were directed to that contemporary work of scientific popularization, Sir Richard Blackmore's didactic epic poem *Creation* (1712), 'where the Anatomy of the human Body is described with Great Perspicuity and Elegance'. 'Know yourself' included knowing your body. Handsome, harmonious, durable, adaptable to all needs and capable of self-repair, man's flesh and blood was in itself a hymn of praise to the Great Original.

How absurd, then, that through gluttony, drunkenness, luxury, ignorance, neglect and myriad other acts of commission and omission, God-given bodies were so abused. Commending moderation and temperance, a handful of *Spectator* papers were given over to correcting this deplorable situation. An inspiration to all should be the renowned Renaissance longevist, Luigi Cornaro, whose tale was told.

By the age of 35, this sixteenth-century Paduan nobleman found his physical constitution on the brink of ruin through sensual over-indulgence. Such desperate circumstances drove him to embrace a temperate life, and he rapidly recovered in what proved to be a quasi-religious conversion. Eventually, at the ripe old age of 83, he composed his *Discourse on the Temperate Life* (1550), which propounded his regimen of health; a second discourse was added at the age of 86, a third at 91 and a fourth at 95.

Despite his advanced years, insisted Cornaro, his senses remained tiptop; his teeth were well preserved, he could easily climb stairs and even mount his horse unaided. He waxed lyrical over the joys of life, his love of reading and writing, his discussions with scholars and artists, and, dearest to his heart, the company of his grandchildren.

The secret lay in dietary temperance. As one grew older, food intake had to be reduced, because 'natural heat' decreased in the elderly. In time, his diet came to consist of morsels of meat, bread and egg broth. 'I always eat with relish', he claimed, and 'I feel, when I leave the table, that I must sing.' The nobleman confidently predicted the extension of man's lifespan beyond the biblical 'three score and ten'. All could live to 100, while those blessed with a robust constitution could aspire to 120. The fact that this paragon of health passed away prematurely in 1565, at the disappointing age of 98, did not prevent the *Spectator* from holding him up as a shining example of man's power to take charge of his body and make it subserve the end of the good life – indeed it erroneously claimed he had lived to beyond 100. Cornaro's treatise, purred Addison, 'is written with such a Spirit of Cheerfulness, Religion, and good Sense, as are the natural Concomitants of Temperance and Sobriety. The mixture of the old Man in it is rather a Recommendation than a Discredit to it.' Go, and do thou likewise.

Excess was one of the *Spectator*'s great complaints – eat only one dish at a meal, avoid lavish sauces, do not gormandize. It also praised bodily hygiene, offering 'hints upon *Cleanliness*, which I shall consider as one of the *Half-Virtues*, as *Aristotle* calls them'. And, endorsing that drive towards stricter bodily control then so conspicuous, it commended propriety and sensitivity in physical comportment. A reader's letter – real or fabricated, who can say? – raised such sensitive issues: 'It is my Misfortune', opened the correspondent,

to be in Love with a young Creature who is daily committing Faults . . . [she] either wholly neglects, or has no Notion of that which Polite People have agreed to distinguish by the Name of *Delicacy*. After our Return from a Walk, the other Day, she threw her self into an Elbow Chair, and professed before a large Company, that *she was all over in a Sweat*. She told me this Afternoon that her *Stomach aked*; and was complaining yesterday at Dinner of something that *stuck in her Teeth*.

What was to be done? The joke was clearly equally on this insufferable hoyden and on the letter-writer for being such a wimp as to put up with her.

In pursuit of the well-tempered body, the *Spectator* made much of the need for physical exercise, grounding its advice on the lessons of the new mechanical philosophy – humoralist medicine was evidently pretty passé. 'I consider the Body as a System of Tubes and Glands,' declared Addison,

or to use a mere Rustick Phrase, a Bundle of Pipes and Strainers, fitted to one another after so wonderful a manner as to make a proper Engine for the Soul to work with. This Description does not only comprehend the Bowels, Bones, Tendons, Veins, Nerves and Arteries, but every Muscle and every Ligature, which is a Composition of Fibres, that are so many imperceptible Tubes or Pipes interwoven on all sides with invisible Glands or Strainers.

Once accept that the body was a machine, and was it not plain as a pikestaff that it should not be allowed to rust or seize up through disuse? 'There must be frequent Motions and Agitations, to mix, digest, and separate the Juices contained in it, as well as to clear and

cleanse that Infinitude of Pipes and Strainers of which it is composed.'
Exactly as it commended social energy, the *Spectator* likewise held that
physical activity was a prophylactic against weakness and lethargy.

And just as it sought to harmonize male and female, land and
trade, town and country, so as to restore social health, so too the co-
operation of body and mind was vital to create and sustain personal
well-being. Man being 'a Compound of Soul and Body', *mens sana in
corpore sano* was the watchword, and this required that animation without which, taught Addison, 'the Body cannot subsist in its Vigour, nor
the Soul act with Chearfulness'. Activity in the somatic economy
pepped up 'all the Faculties of the Mind, by keeping the Understanding clear, the Imagination untroubled, and refining those Spirits that
are necessary for the proper Exertion of our intellectual Faculties'.
Neglect this, and what was the result? 'The Spleen' – a disorder
'frequent in Men of studious and sedentary Tempers, as well as the
Vapours to which those of the other Sex are so often subject'.

A life of leisure (*otium*) might seem enviable, but the idle rich –
'those who are not obliged to Labour, by the Condition in which
they are born' – often suffered for lack of exercise and would become
'more miserable than the rest of Mankind, unless they indulge themselves in the voluntary Labour which goes by the Name of Exercise'.
Addison and Steele were no slavish advocates of the Protestant
Work-ethic, fetishizing labour in and for itself, but they did endorse
spirited exertion.

Hunting formed particularly valuable exercise; and one of the
members of the *Spectator* club, Sir Roger de Coverley, was applauded
for his pursuit of the chase. 'My Friend Sir ROGER', declared Mr
Spectator,

has been an indefatigable Man in Business of this kind, and has hung several
Parts of his House with the Trophies of his former Labours. The Walls of
his great Hall are covered with the Horns of several kinds of Deer that he
has killed in the Chace, which he thinks the most valuable Furniture of his
House, as they afford him frequent Topicks of Discourse, and shew that he
has not been Idle –

though a sentimental aside noted that the humane Sir Roger – anticipating Sterne's Uncle Toby? – could not bear to kill the prey he loved to hunt but kept them in a kind of retirement park. This form of 'labour', Addison noted, had the approval of the 'English Hippocrates', Dr Thomas Sydenham; and, he further insisted, 'that those Parts of the World are the most healthy, where they subsist by the Chace'. Drawing what became a familiar primitivist moral, he ruefully noted that 'Men lived longest when their Lives were employed in hunting', whereas town life and the civilizing process brought hazards for health.

So what was the man-about-town to do? Mr Spectator let readers into his personal secret: 'I exercise my self an Hour every Morning upon a dumb Bell that is placed in a Corner of my Room.' In his salad days he had even gone in for 'fighting with a Man's own Shadow'. This shadow-boxing consisted 'in the brandishing of two short Sticks grasped in each Hand, and Loaden with Plugs of Lead at either end. This opens the Chest, exercises the Limbs, and gives a Man all the Pleasure of Boxing, without the Blows.' Shadow-boxing, he sardonically added, might serve social purposes which went well beyond personal fitness: 'I could wish that several Learned Men would lay out that Time which they employ in Controversies and Disputes about nothing, in *this method* of fighting with their own Shadows. It might conduce very much to evaporate the Spleen.' The penchant for pugilism we associate with the buccaneering Byron can thus be traced back to the suave Mr Spectator.

Man being this 'compound of body and soul', it was necessary to work out, every day, with a 'double Scheme of Duties' to achieve fitness: 'thus employ the one in Labour and Exercise, as well as the other in Study and Contemplation.' Omit this, abandon yourself to idleness, excess and suchlike follies, and sickness would soon follow. And there lay the slippery slope to dependence upon doctors and medicine. 'Physick, for the most part,' pronounced Addison at his most preachy, 'is nothing else but the Substitute of Exercise or Temperance' – 'the Apothecary is perpetually employed in countermining the Cook and the Vintner'. These could be avoided by smart preventive action: had not Diogenes restrained a young man from going to a feast, saying that he was 'running into imminent Danger, had not he prevented him'? Today things were far worse: 'when I behold a Fashionable Table set out in all its Magnificence, I fancy that I see Gouts and Dropsies, Feavers and Lethargies, with other innumerable Distempers lying in Ambuscade among the Dishes.' Anti-doctor satire was fashionable – Samuel Garth's cynical *Dispensary* (1699) had just proved a best-seller – and the *Spectator* contributed to disabusing the public: 'we may lay it down as a Maxim, that when a Nation abounds in Physicians it grows thin of People.' Physicians, Addison went on, 'may be described like the *British* Army in *Caesar's* time: Some of them slay in Chariots, and some on Foot'. The threat of such practitioners was the best health warning of all.

No small contribution to preventive medicine was made by a healthy mind: morbid thinking imperilled the frail corporeal barque; weak minds bred ailing bodies. 'One of that sickly Tribe who are commonly known by the name of *Valetudinarians*' confessed to readers how he had ruined his health by bingeing on medical books:

I no sooner began to peruse Books of this Nature, but I found my Pulse, was irregular, and scarce ever read the Account of any Disease that I did not fancy my self afflicted with. *Doctor Sydenham*'s learned Treatise of Fevers threw me into a lingring Hectick, which hung upon me all the while I was reading that excellent Piece.

He then successively read himself into consumption (tuberculosis), gout, gravel and the stone. And a new complication followed, for he had been seduced by 'that Ingenious Discourse written by *Sanctorius*'.

An associate of Galileo, Santorio Santorio (Latinized as Sanctorius) was an early seventeenth-century pioneer of the new scientific medicine which set special emphasis upon measurement. He developed a thermometer to gauge bodily temperature, and his most influential book, *De Statica Medicina* (On Medical Statics: 1614) recommended other instruments besides – a pendulum for measuring pulse-rate, a hygrometer, a syringe to extract bladder stones and the 'pulsilogium', a pulse-watch.

His most ingenious device was the weighing machine or what came to be known as the Sanctorian Balance. Eating, writing and even sleeping in this complicated cage-like wooden contraption, Sanctorius monitored his body functions for some thirty years, documenting alterations in body-weight after dining, evacuating and exercising, and correlating these variables against his state of health. Discovering that the weight of his excreta was less than that of the food and drink he consumed, with no increase in his own weight to account for the difference, he explained the discrepancy in terms of 'invisible perspiration', traditionally judged a salutary way of sweating off internal toxins.

The *Spectator*'s valetudinarian imprudently took up this 'Mathematical Chair', so as 'to direct my self by a Scheme of Rules':

I used to Study, Eat, Drink, and Sleep in it; insomuch that I may be said, for these three last Years, to have lived in a Pair of Scales. I compute my self, when I am in full Health, to be precisely Two hundred Weight, falling short of it about a Pound after a Day's Fast, and exceeding it as much after a very full Meal; so that it is my continual Employment to trim the Ballance between these two Volatile Pounds in my Constitution. In my ordinary Meals I fetch my self up to Two hundred Weight and a half Pound; and if after having dined I find my self fall short of it, I drink just so much Small Beer, or eat such a quantity of Bread, as is sufficient to make my weight.

Eventually he reached the absurd point at which 'I do not dine and sup by the Clock, but by my Chair'. And the result? – 'notwithstanding this my great Care to ballast my self equally every Day, and to keep my Body in its proper Poise, so it is that I find my self in a sick and languishing Condition'. Hence he begged Mr Spectator 'to consider me as your Patient, and to give me more certain Rules to walk by than those I have already observed'. Recourse to the balance had evidently made him even more unbalanced than before.

If the perils of poring over medical books was an old humanist conceit, the weight-watching hypochondriac who reduced life to the quantification of inputs and outputs was new and suggestive – Swift would have relished it – of the evil genius of mindless mechanical materialism. How ominous that the Sanctorian slave wanted yet more rules! And how prophetic of future physical and dietary cultures in which all manner of artless attempts to monitor and manage in the name of health (or happiness, or beauty) ended up nightmarishly counter-productive and self-destructive.

People succumbed in myriad ways to the crotchets of the ill-managed mind. Visiting a friend, Mr Spectator noted, 'I had the Misfortune to find his whole Family very much dejected'. Why so? His wife had 'dreamt a very strange Dream the Night before, which they were afraid portended some Misfortune to themselves or to their Children'. And what further caused the 'settled Melancholy' disfiguring her face? 'We were no sooner sate down, but, after having looked upon me a little while, *My Dear*, says she, turning to her Husband, *you may now see the Stranger that was in the Candle last Night*.' Worse was to follow:

Soon after this, as they began to talk of Family Affairs, a little Boy at the lower end of the Table told her, that he was to go into Join-hand on *Thursday*. Thursday! says she, *No, Child, if it please God, you shall not begin upon* Childermas-day; *tell your Writing-Master that* Friday *will be soon enough.*

Ensnare yourself in such superstitions, Addison reflected, and you would end up making it a 'Rule to lose a Day in every Week'.

Worse still were those religious enthusiasts, who saw not just silly strangers in the candle but demons and visions everywhere. Spirits as such were no problem at all to Addison – quite the reverse: 'all the Regions of Nature swarm with Spirits,' he assured, echoing More or Glanvill. Indeed, with a nice touch, Mr Spectator imagined such higher beings overseeing humanity as an etherealized version of himself: 'we have Multitudes of Spectators on all our Actions, when we think our selves most alone.' Such spiritual beings, however, should not be the occasion for gloom: 'I am wonderfully pleased to think that I am always engaged with such an innumerable Society.' The spiritual should thus exalt man's sense of self-esteem.

Drawing on Locke's account of the (mis-)association of ideas, Addison explained how false beliefs about demons and devils arose out of the silly talk of vulgar nurses and servants. Errors took root which perverted true faith into superstition (indelibly associated with the papists), or that enthusiasm which was the mark of the Puritan. Committed as they were to the Anglican *via media*, Addison and Steele passionately condemned all that perverted faith.

Against such 'little horrors of imagination', the *Spectator* offered correctives. Lifting a tale from the newly translated *Arabian Nights*, it told of a hypochondriacal ruler cured by a wise physician not through medications as such, but by the imaginative counter-suggestion which formed the medicine of the soul:

He took an Hollow Ball of Wood, and filled it with several Drugs, after which he clos'd it up so artificially that nothing appeared. He likewise took a Mall, and after having hollowed the Handle, and that Part which strikes the Ball, he enclosed in them several Drugs after the same manner as in the Ball it self. He then ordered the Sultan, who was his Patient, to exercise himself early in the Morning with these *rightly prepared* Instruments, 'till such time as he should Sweat. When, as the Story goes, the Virtue of the Medicaments perspiring through the Wood, had so good an Influence on the Sultan's Constitution, that they cured him of an Indisposition which all the Compositions he had taken inwardly had not been able to remove.

Small surprise that one of the morals of the tale was 'how beneficial Bodily Labour is to Health, and that Exercise is the most effectual Physick'.

The radical prophylactic against the waywardness of the mind lay in an energetic reform of education, presently marred by false theory and lack of balance: 'The general Mistake among us in the Educating our Children, is, That in our Daughters we take Care of their Persons and neglect their Minds: in our Sons, we are so intent upon adorning their Minds, that we wholly neglect their Bodies.' As always, such divisions were damaging. Taking their cue, yet again, from Locke, it was explained that since boys and girls began with similar mental equipment, the *tabula rasa*, education for both must be rational and geared to the symbiotic cultivation of mind and body.

Passionate popularizers of Locke's philosophical and educational ideas, Addison and Steele took the gamble of putting across his controversial views on personal identity. As we saw in the previous chapter, these were a red rag to conservative bulls who feared they undermined the permanence of the self in an objective moral order. These speculations seem to have caused no worry to Addison and Steele, who cheerfully dramatized Locke's account of conscious self-hood by conscripting an episode from *The Persian Tales* (recently translated by Ambrose Philips), a tale of transmigrating spirits, re-animated bodies and mistaken identities.

Having learned from a dervish the trick of implanting his soul into a dead body, King Fadlallah enters the corpse of a deer. The cunning holy man then seizes the opportunity to occupy the king's newly vacant body, preventing him from repossessing it. Only after migrating through a succession of corpses and mistaken identities is Fadlallah able to regain his own flesh. Was not Locke then right? Bodies were contingent and even interchangeable appendages, rather like suits of clothes or disguises.

Prompted by this fable to address head-on the question of 'what it was that might be said to compose *personal Identity*', the *Spectator* knew where to look for the answer:

Mr. *Lock*, after having premised that the Word *Person* properly signifies a thinking intelligent Being that has Reason and Reflection, and can consider itself as itself; concludes, That it is Consciousness alone, and not an Identity of Substance, which makes this personal Identity of Sameness.

It went on to cite the discussion (quoted in Chapter 4) in the *Essay concerning Human Understanding* of the man who remembered both Noah's Ark and the recent flooding of the Thames, meant by Locke to show how, through the possession of memory, the self might transcend different embodiments and times.

Addison and Steele were thus the first champions of Locke's beguiling idea that consciousness, not substance, was the location of the person. They must have judged that this would strike a chord with their readers. Not, it must be emphasized, because of any pessimistic, cynical or subversive connotations it carried. Mr Spectator was not selling decadent rakery or Hobbesian libertinism, tempting readers to savour the bottomless depths of illicit fantasy; neither was he a Humean sceptic *avant la lettre*, casting aside the stable Christian absolutes with an 'anything goes' amoralism. Rather, exactly like Locke, Addison and Steele offered conscious selfhood as a more appealing and plausible rendering of identity. For them it was of a piece with Christian doctrine and Plato's avowal of the soul's supremacy over the passions.

Pondering 'the Immortality of the Soul' – that 'Subject upon which I always meditate with great Delight' – Addison insisted, sounding more conventional than Locke, that such eternal existence 'is the Basis of Morality, and the Source of all pleasing Hopes and secret Joys'. Were such hopes mere wish-fulfilment, or were there rational grounds for believing in that separate soul? One confirmation, he suggested, lay in dreaming. Some theories of dreams – the notion that they were 'Revelations of what has already happened in distant Parts of the World, or . . . Presages of what is to happen in future Periods of Time' – were extravagantly fanciful. But 'dreams may give us some Idea of the great Excellency of an Human Soul, and some Intimation of its Independency on Matter', for they attested an 'Activity which is natural to the Humane Soul', which 'the Power of Sleep' could not 'deaden or abate'; though a person might be 'tired and worn out with the Labours of this Day', this 'active Part in his Composition' was 'busie and unwearied'. Dreams might thus be deemed the 'Relaxations and Amusements of the Soul, when she is disencumbered of her Machine' or 'disengaged from the Body'. By implication, such an exercise of imagination could persist once the body was not slumbering but dead. Claims such as these, as we have seen, were hotly contested between Collins and Clarke.

Addison adduced further plausible grounds for the separate soul, derived from the enigma of mundane existence. Life was so short, he reflected, that 'a Man, considered in his present State, seems only sent into the World to propagate his Kind'. In other words, 'he does not seem born to enjoy Life, but to deliver it down to others' – almost a foretaste of the 'selfish gene'. Such a fate was not surprising 'in

Animals, which are formed for our use, and can finish their Business in a short Life'. But the brevity of man's earthly sojourn seemed, *prima facie*, a blemish in the divine scheme, for 'a Man can never have taken in his full measure of Knowledge, has not time to subdue his Passions, establish his Soul in virtue, and come up to the Perfection of his Nature, before he is hurried off the Stage'. Would the Divine Dramatist thus bring the human drama to such a botched and premature finale? Was it not far more likely that terrestrial life was just a prologue? Nearly a century later, Godwin came up with similar musings, but reached very different conclusions.

As will be evident from Addison's slighting reference to the animal kingdom, on the soul the *Spectator* endorsed age-old 'human excep-tionalism'. This conviction was justified through an anthropological and historical tenet popular in the century to come: belief in the unique and separate human soul was embraced by modern, pro-gressive, civilized minds. 'THE *Americans*' – that is, native American Indians –

believe that all Creatures have Souls, not only Men and Women, but Brutes, Vegetables, nay even the most inanimate things, as Stocks and Stones. They believe the same of all the Works of Art, as of Knives, Boats, Looking-glasses: And that as any of these Things perish, their Souls go into another World, which is inhabited by the Ghosts of Men and Women.

Such animistic opinions were, of course, 'absurd', insisted Addison, oozing a condescending cultural chauvinism. Yet, in a typical enlight-ened gesture, he also confessed that 'our *European* Philosophers' of former times had embraced 'several Notions altogether as improb-able'. Platonists – the master himself seemed exempt – 'entertain us with Substances and Beings no less extravagant and chymerical', while 'many *Aristotelians* have likewise spoken as unintelligibly of their substantial Forms' – that stock gibe against scholasticism. Wherever it was to be found, such animism was symptomatic of a primitive mentality. Modern reason knew better – that human beings, and they alone, possessed an immortal soul.

*

The *Spectator* created and publicized an eligible persona for the new, post-1688 public: man as a sociable being. This modern self rested upon a healthy and disciplined body. And that, in turn, would sustain a healthy mind, one which avoided ensnarement in phantasms and which, in the Lockean dispensation, would prove capable of continuous adaptation to the exigencies of a challenging but opportunity-rich environment. Man thus became not just a sociable animal but a progressive one, too. Spectatorial man, conditioned to play his part in the public sphere, became one of the preferred fashionings of the self. What made its stress on appearances, on the presentation of the self, so acceptable was Addison and Steele's skill in convincing their readers that what lay beneath, to be presented, was a noble and estimable self.

8

SHAFTESBURY AND MANDEVILLE

The turmoil of the seventeenth century prompted the disturbing question: had Aristotle been mistaken to call man a social and political animal? If so, what then did human nature truly comprise?

One response, prompted by the Civil Wars, was that of Hobbes: man was inherently an aggressive loner, *homo lupo lupus*. Fear and the belligerence it bred made political society no better than a ceasefire, a defensive compact of atomized antagonists trying to make their lives somewhat less solitary, poor, nasty, brutish and short than in that dire 'war of all against all' which was the state of nature.

Hobbes painted life black – he was a secular Calvinist, peddling his own version of Original Sin – and the legacy he left to later philosophers was dismal indeed. But was man truly such a wretch? If so, could anything be done about it, except endorsing that reign of prophylactic terror set out by the author of *Leviathan*? Two who grasped the nettle were the 3rd Earl of Shaftesbury and Bernard de Mandeville.

It must be rare for one philosopher to be present at another's birth, but that is just what happened in 1671 in the case of Anthony Ashley Cooper, 3rd Earl of Shaftesbury, whose nativity was attended by John Locke, secretary and personal physician to the baby's grandfather, the leading Whig statesman of the day. Locke's advice was soon to guide the 1st Earl during the Exclusion Crisis and their subsequent exile in the Dutch Republic. As well as being the key philosopher of Whiggery and liberal individualism, Locke became the grandson's tutor.

Following his return to England after the Glorious Revolution of 1688, the noble teenager devoted himself to prolonged study of the Greek and Latin authors, with particular attention to Plato,

Xenophon and the great Stoics – Cicero, Seneca, Epictetus and Marcus Aurelius. The Whig principles he inherited were strengthened by readings in the English republicans, especially James Harrington; and he also evidently read widely in divinity, being attracted to latitudinarian divines like John Tillotson, then Archbishop of Canterbury, whose rational theology, faith in human reason and distaste for dogmatism appealed to the young Earl's cool and classical temper. Most congenial of all were the Cambridge Platonists, notably Benjamin Whichcote and Ralph Cudworth who deemed the standards of good and evil absolute and immutable, not relative or (as for the Calvinists and Hobbes) dependent simply on God's will. His preferred authorities espoused a benevolist concept of the Deity, a respect for human reason in its quest for truth, and an optimistic affirmation of man's natural sociability and predisposition to good.

Shaftesbury was affronted by Hobbes's view of man as fundamentally selfish, by his nominalist denial of inherent and disinterested goodness, and by his *apologia* for absolutism as the only recourse in a wicked world. He owned first editions of his tutor's *Essay concerning Human Understanding* and the *Two Treatises of Government* (both 1690), evidently read soon after publication, and Locke may have tried out on his pupil some of the educational ideas expounded in his *Some Thoughts Concerning Education* (1693). Deeming the new-born mind a sheet of blank paper, wholly indeterminate and plastic, it followed for Locke that education was all, nurture counted for far more than nature: 'of all the men we meet with, nine parts of ten are what they are, good or evil, useful or not, by their education.' His aristocratic tutee may not have found these egalitarian views wholly palatable, and a sometimes tense relationship developed between tutor and pupil and, more broadly, between certain of Locke's teachings and the identity to which the young Earl aspired.

In most ways, Shaftesbury turned out the wished-for product of his model education. His politics were to remain impeccably Whig, his hatred of Catholicism and the Stuarts lifelong and passionate; he detested absolutism's trammelling of the mind; and he proved the staunchest advocate of English liberty – 'We are now in an Age', he proclaimed, 'when *Liberty* is once again in its Ascendant. And we are our-selves the happy Nation, who not only enjoy it at home, but by our Greatness and Power give Life and Vigour to it abroad.' Yet through temperament – he was languid and aloof – and the accidents of health – he grew up weak and asthmatic – he avoided the life of politics as pursued by his grandfather, becoming instead reclusive, given over to bookish and aesthetic pursuits.

While impeccably Whiggish, Shaftesbury nevertheless in some ways revolted against Lockean indoctrination – indeed, he occasionally attacked his 'foster-father' in a manner plainly Oedipal; ' 'twas Mr. Lock', he griped in 1709, 'that struck at all Fundamentals, threw all *Order* and *Virtue* out of the World, and made the Very Ideas of these . . . *unnatural* and without foundation in our Minds.' What were his grounds for believing this? It was Shaftesbury's accusation that 'Virtue according to Mr. Lock, has no other Measure Law or Rule, than Fashion & Custome'. Locke had no doubt questioned the dogma that moral absolutes were graven on the mind – all came from experience – but the Hobbist gibe would have made the tutor turn in his grave.

Shaftesbury patently had no sympathy for those egalitarian elements in Locke (and before him, Hobbes) which levelled all innate attributes. Ever the aristocrat and connoisseur, his thinking exuded self-possession in the inherent superiority of the polite cultured gentleman. 'To *philosophize*, in a just Signification, is but to carry *Good-Breeding* a step higher,' he proclaimed: 'For the Accomplishment of Breeding is, To learn whatever is *decent* in Company or *beautiful* in Arts: and the Sum of Philosophy is, To learn what is *just* in Society, and *beautiful* in Nature, and the Order of the World.' No breeding, no philosophy – no justice or beauty, nothing fine.

Hobbes had made it virtually incumbent upon his successors to adopt, in their rebuttals, the analytic and anatomical method which he had wielded to such effect. It was essential to dissect the social animal, reduce it to its elements, and determine what made the human machine tick. Shaftesbury took up the challenge. Although not personally devoted to natural science – unlike Locke, he had no medical training – he was fascinated by self-anatomy. In the century after Vesalius, 'anatomizing' had become a popular literary and philosophical genre, both in the sense of grasping a subject through formal partition and division, as in Robert Burton's *The Anatomy of Melancholy* (1621), and also in the sense of prying beneath the surface to unveil hidden truths and lance festering sores – for instance, Philip Stubbs' *The Anatomy of Abuses* (1583). Self-anatomy, introspection into one's own body (*autopsy* in the literal sense), was the vogue: 'I have cut up mine owne *Anatomy*,' declared John Donne in his *Devotions*; 'dissected myselfe, and they are got to read upon me.'

Performing such a philosophical 'autopsy', to bare the nature of the self, was also crucial to Shaftesbury's philosophical enterprise, in fulfilment of the oracle's decree: 'That celebrated *Delphick* Inscription, RECOGNIZE YOUR-SELF, was as much as to say *Divide your-self*, or BE TWO. For if the Division were rightly made, all *within* would of course, they thought be rightly understood, and prudently managed.'

At the age of 23, Shaftesbury disclosed to Locke, with a fine rhetorical flourish, his commitment to this holy grail of *nosce teipsum*. 'What I count True Learning, and all wee can profitt, is to know our selves,' he declared:

Whilst I can gett any thing that teaches this; Whilst I search any Age or Language that can assist mee here; Whilst such are Philosophers and Such Philosophy, whence I can Learn ought from, of this kind; there is no Labour, no Studdy, no Learning that I would not undertake.

But the Cartesian version of this journey into the interior – Descartes's much-trumpeted 'discovery' of the ultimate Archimedean point in Reason – was, laughed Shaftesbury, quite fatuous:

'TWILL not, in this respect, be sufficient for us to use the seeming *Logick* of a famous Modern, and say, '*We think*: therefore *We are*.' Which is a notably invented Saying, after the Model of that like Philosophical Proposition; That '*What is, is*.' – Miraculously argu'd! 'If *I am; I am*.'

Descartes claimed to be on a truth trip, but he was just going round in solipsistic circles. One had to revert one stage further – the real problem was: 'What constitutes the *we* or *I*?' And this once more raised Locke's question of the integrity, constancy or oneness of the first person pronoun: whether, as Shaftesbury powerfully put it, 'the I of this instant, be the same with that of any instant preceding, or to come'. With this still unsolved, the ego in the *cogito* counted for nothing.

Introspection bred doubts and led Shaftesbury to recurrent ruminations on the theme of 'Who am *I*?', even driving him to the conclusion that 'I [may] indeed be said to be lost, or have lost My Self.' A continuing motif of the speculations recorded in the privacy of his notebooks was the unending quest for self-understanding: 'What am I? who? whence? And to what or whom belonging? with what or whom belonging to me, about me, under me?' The speculations of a discerning individual given over to introspection, Shaftesbury's self-probings could be radical in their implications. In his publications, and all the more so in his confidential manuscripts, there flowed streams of consciousness, reflection and commentary, expressive of his grasp of the mercurial and broken nature of consciousness: ever-changing, impulsive, revelatory, quixotic and even self-contradictory in both mood and content. Shaftesbury found the creative quality of his own sensibility engrossing – he grew self-absorbed. Brooding upon it and recording it, it was living proof to him of the presence, power and uniqueness of the human soul that his mind was a spring, forever bubbling up with passions and *aperçus*.

Shaftesbury had no dread that, at least for noble souls, the flighty and fragmentary quality of consciousness would spell danger. Unlike Collins and other subversive freethinkers, he had not the slightest polemical itch to show that the fleeting character of the mind was evidence of somatic dependence or sickness – that the soul was simply a secretion of the brain which fluctuated, and might perish, with the body. Neither did he entertain fears that the self would crash in consequence of imperfections of memory – indeed, he took issue with Locke's grounding of 'conscious selfhood' on continuity of memory: what counted was the spirited blaze of the moment. 'Notable reasoners about the nice matters of identity', he noted, with a hint of a sneer towards his tutor,

affirm that if memory be taken away, the self is lost. And what matter for memory? What have I to do with that part? If, *whilst I am*, I am but as I should be, what do I care more? and thus let me lose *self* every hour, and be twenty successive selfs, or new selfs, 'tis all one to me.

Aristocratic cool indeed! Was it not the privilege of a lord to lose himself once in a while, and reinvent himself as he pleased? The status, indeed stateliness, of a nobleman shielded the Earl from the risk of personality disintegration: did he not have a title, a pedigree, a stately pile? Whatever his state of mind, the gentleman in him commanded respect. It was almost as though only the insecure bourgeoisie had the need for something so prosaically reassuring as that insurance policy, continuity of personhood.

Shaftesbury was lastingly charmed by the flair and creativity of his genius. Although he was no Christian, his idealistic, Neoplatonic theosophy dwelt upon the glories of the Deity, the beauties of Creation, and the unbridled participation of the noble soul therein, those 'Things of a *natural* kind: where neither *Art*, nor the *Conceit* or *Caprice* of Man has spoil'd their genuine order'.

The converse of this elevation of the lofty brilliance of the mind lies in the pungent distaste Shaftesbury so often expressed for the flesh. 'SHOU'D One, who had the Countenance of a Gentleman, ask me', he recorded with disdain, 'Why I wou'd avoid being *nasty*, when nobody was present' – what he is talking about is blowing his nose in private – 'In the first place I shou'd be fully satisfy'd that he himself was a very nasty Gentleman who cou'd ask this Question; and that it wou'd be a hard matter for me to make him ever conceive what *true Cleanliness* was.' However, he continued, showing contempt for both his body and his imagined interlocutor,

I might, notwithstanding this, be contented to give him a slight Answer, and say, ' 'Twas because I had a Nose.' Shou'd he trouble me further, and ask again, 'What if I had a Cold? Or what if naturally I had no such nice

Smell?' I might answer perhaps, 'That I car'd as little to see myself *nasty*, as that others shou'd see me in that condition.' But what if it were *in the Dark*? Why even then, tho I had neither Nose, nor Eyes, my *Sense* of the Matter wou'd be still the same; my Nature wou'd rise at the Thought of what was sordid: or if it did not; I shou'd have a wretched Nature indeed, and *hate my-self* for a Beast.

As this highly revealing instance shows, the Platonist and the fastidious nobleman thus joined in their aversion to the squalor of snot – that too too solid flesh: sparks of the intellect might happily intrude upon Shaftesbury, but not emunctory emissions.

In similar vein is the emphatically heretical memo he penned under the entry for *Somation* (a word seemingly of his own invention, presumably referring to bodily business):

A wretchedly foolish and selfish human creature thinks he has to do with his body and that it is still some part of himself and belonging to him even when he is out of it. A wiser mortal thinks his body no part of himself and belonging to him even when he is out of it. But a truly wise man thinks his body no part of himself nor belonging to him even whilst in it.

Such extravagant sentiments have a touch of the Pythagorean, and evoke classical asceticism of various strands. Shaftesbury, it is clear, far more trenchantly than Locke, derided the old doctrine of substantial form, that is, the body as the *sine qua non* of personal identity. 'Why this hankering after the flesh? this clinging, this cleaving to a body?', he demanded, a neo-pagan sounding bizarrely like some Puritan tub-thumper:

What art you afraid should be taken from thee? what art thou afraid of losing? *Thyself*? What is then lost? A tooth? Wilt you go out for a tooth? Go then? A hand, a leg, a whole body, and what more? Is not this the furthest? and is not this in reality less still than the tooth?

Such clinging to the flesh made no sense, because 'self lies not in the body'. For 'I (the real I) am not a certain figure, nor mass, nor hair, nor flesh, nor limbs, nor body; but mind, thought, intellect, reason'.

Here was the Lockean doctrine of 'conscious selfhood' taken to rather extreme (and evidently élitist) lengths: the nobleman clearly regarded his flesh as a bridgehead of vulgarity distressingly lodged within himself.

What was of prime importance for Shaftesbury was the disciplined self-control imparted by reason. ''Tis the known Province of Philosophy to teach us *our-selves*,' he explained in his significantly titled *Soliloquy* (1710), 'keep us the *self-same* Persons, and so regulate our governing Fancys, Passions, and Humours.' Not the flesh but philosophy was the sure guarantee of sameness and oneness. And the goal of such self-command was the attainment of perfect autonomy: 'a MIND, by knowing *it-self*, and its own proper Powers and Virtues, becomes *free* and independent. . . . The more it conquers in this respect the more it is its own *Master*.' Along parallel lines, he remarked in some drafts that 'He who has once form'd himself . . . He, and He alone, is truly Free.'

Shaftesbury aimed to vindicate human nature against misanthropic detractors – both secular Hobbesians and Calvinists who, by treating man as fallen and predestined, outrageously rendered God vindictive and vengeful – they proceeded, he remonstrated, '*as if Good-Nature, and Religion, were Enemies*'. So negative was their idea of God that it made them in effect 'Daemonists' – worshippers of a malevolent deity.

Owing much to the Cambridge Platonists, Shaftesbury's vindication of God and human nature expressed itself in a double thrust. He invested deeply in loveliness of form; human nature would be perfected when it truly appreciated the beauties of Creation. 'O glorious *Nature*! supremely Fair, and sovereignly Good!', he apostrophized,

All-loving and All-lovely, All-divine! Whose Looks are so becoming, and of such infinite Grace; whose Study brings such Wisdom, and whose Contemplation such Delight; whose every single Work affords an ampler Scene, and is a nobler Spectacle than all which every Art presented!

He was hardly less of an enthusiast for man-made splendours – noble houses, classical sculpture, painting in the grand manner, epic poetry.

The vocation and perfection of the great-souled man lay in aesthetic projects and cultural accomplishments. Virtue, knowledge and beauty formed a club of the good – the only trinity Shaftesbury ever acknowledged: 'For all Beauty is Truth. True Features make the Beauty of a Face; and true Proportions the Beauty of Architecture; as true Measures that of Harmony and Musick.'

With comparable intentions, he was, furthermore, ardently committed to the vindication of man as a social animal, in the Aristotelian tradition. Refuting the Hobbesian *homo lupo lupus* while also distancing himself from Locke's *tabula rasa*, Shaftesbury aimed to show that man was born gregarious. And through the polish produced by sociability, he could be perfected: 'If *Eating* and *Drinking* be natural, *Herding* is so too. If any *Appetite* or *Sense* be natural, the *Sense of Fellowship* is the same.'

A keyword in this philosophy was sympathy, indeed something close to Marcus Aurelius' Stoic ideal of a universal sympathy. '*To sympathize*, what is it?', he inquired; 'To feel together, or be united in one Sence or Feeling – the Fibers of the Plant sympathize. The Members of the Animal sympathize. And do not the heavenly Bodyes sympathize? why not?' In brief, both aesthetically and socially, Shaftesbury aimed to be the vindicator of human nature.

In practical terms what this meant was a stalwart advocacy of 'good humour', especially to keep at bay that melancholy which was the malady of the élite and the fanaticism infecting the vulgar. Whereas religious zeal all too readily triggered morbid preoccupations and deeds, religion ought to be a matter of the reasonable and the rapturous: 'Good Humour is not only the best Security against Enthusiasm, but the best Foundation of Piety and true Religion.'

In holding that human nature was to be championed not just against Hobbists and Calvinists but also against the vulgar, Shaftesbury (like Mr Spectator) donned the guise of a doctor of society, diagnosing social pathologies and probing their root causes. 'The Human Mind and Body are both of 'em naturally subject to Commotions,' he thus observed, 'and as there are strange Ferments in the Blood, which in many Bodys occasion an extraordinary Discharge;

so in Reason too, there are heterogeneous Particles which must be thrown off by Fermentation.' The great-souled man was, axiomatically and self-evidently, worlds apart from the herd: magnanimity was inherently noble. Shaftesbury nevertheless devoted much energy to anatomizing and vilifying the masses. Blind creatures of habit, they were incurably subject to dire psycho-pathological disorders which made them project their narrow-mindedness upon the universe: themselves racked by fear, they responded by fantasizing a terrifyingly malign universe.

It was notably in *Characteristicks of Men, Manners, Opinions, Times*, his study of enthusiasm, published in 1711 in reaction to the eruption of godly hysteria among the Camisards, the so-called 'French Prophets', that Shaftesbury exposed deranged fervour in the religious sphere. Drawing on Lucretius, Epicurus and other classical philosophers, he exposed false faiths as the emission of dark and distorted imaginings. Twisted fancy conjured up visions of mean and vindictive deities who sported with defenceless man and demanded blood and sacrifice to satisfy their petty whims. What produced these sick men's dreams? The body was to blame. Unhealthy flesh bred vapours and other internal disturbances; these occluded the brain, which then distorted sense inputs, the result being a distorted perversion of reality. Here also lay the explanation, according to Shaftesbury, in a typically erudite digression, of 'panic':

We read in history that Pan, when he accompanied Bacchus in an expedition to the Indies, found means to strike a terror through a host of enemies by the help of a small company, whose clamours he managed to good advantage among the echoing rocks and caverns of a woody vale. The hoarse bellowing of the caves, joined to the hideous aspect of such dark and desert places, raised such a horror in the enemy, that in this state their imagination helped them to hear voices, and doubtless to see forms too, which were more than human: whilst the uncertainty of what they feared made their fear yet greater, and spread it faster by implicit looks than any narration could convey it. And this was what in after-times men called a *panic*.

Shaftesbury detested vulgar anthropomorphism in religion, in whatever manifestation. He warned against crude portrayals of God in man's image, as warped by cramped and peevish minds, but he also deplored the gross anthropomorphic tendencies of orthodox piety: 'Dost thou, like one of those Visionaryes, expect to see a Throne, a shining Light, a Court & Attendance? is this thy Notion of *a Presence*? and dost thou wayt till then, to be struck and astonish'd as the Vulgar are, with such appearances & Shew? – Wretched Folly!' In a similar context, Cudworth had quoted Xenophanes. 'If Oxen, Lions, Horses and Asses, had all of them a Sense of Deity, and were able to Limn and Paint, there is no question to be made, but that each of these several Animals would paint God according to their respective Form & Likeness, and contend that he was of that shape & no other.' Petty-minded men thus made monsters out of their own minds. By contrast, much as for the Cambridge Platonists, Shaftesbury's Deity was an Ideal Presence everywhere immanent and all-perceiving.

The defence of religion mounted in Shaftesbury's *Characteristicks* in the dialogue between Philocles and Theocles had a view to demonstrating such a 'universal Mind'. That Mind sustained the cosmic order, which supported the social order, which in turn guaranteed noble minds their autonomy. Shaftesbury endorsed Locke's refinement of the self into consciousness, but took it further: man could devote his energies to knowing himself, and to being himself, provided that he was truly patrician.

One who crossed swords with Shaftesbury was the controversialist, Bernard de Mandeville. The Whig aristocrat and the Rotterdam-born physician-satirist shared certain commitments; both espoused post-1688 Whig values, both championed Great Britain and the United Provinces against the Sun King and rejoiced in political freedom; both hated 'gravity' and pretentiousness, and deflated them with ridicule. But there the similarities ceased. Sprung from the bourgeoisie, Mandeville's sympathies were populist through and through: unlike the remote Earl, he prided himself upon being street-wise and plain-speaking.

Shaftesbury-mouthpieces were introduced into various of Mandeville's writings, and made to spout high-flown and disinterested sentiments which eulogized human nature. 'His Notions I confess are generous and refined,' Mandeville conceded, and he did not condemn such altruistic views:

This Noble Writer (for it is the Lord *Shaftesbury* I mean in his Characteristicks) Fancies, that as Man is made for Society, so he ought to be born with a kind Affection to the whole, of which he is a part, and a Propensity to seek the Welfare of it. The attentive Reader, who perused the foregoing part of this Book [Mandeville's *Fable*], will soon perceive that two Systems cannot be more opposite than his Lordship's and mine.

His Lordship's system, however, was pie in the sky; it failed the reality test.

In stark contrast to the head-in-the-clouds idealist, Mandeville stubbornly portrayed himself as the voice of feet-on-the-ground realism. '*ONE of the greatest Reasons why so few People understand themselves*', he expostulated, '*is, that most Writers are always teaching Men what they should be, and hardly ever trouble their Heads with telling them what they really are.*' And what they really were, at bottom, were Hobbesian egoists.

It is, of course, hardly an accident that this man who loved playing the no-nonsense realist was a practising physician and medical author, professionally inured to the blunt truths of the flesh. He gloried in strutting around in the persona of a hardbitten dissector of human nature, one of 'the curious, that are skill'd in anatomizing the invisible Part of Man'. 'Could we undress Nature', he explained – Mandeville habitually conflated the medical and the sexual – 'and pry into her deepest Recesses, we should discover the Seeds of this Passion before it exerts it self, as plainly as we see the Teeth in an Embryo, before the Gums are form'd' – an unusually chilling image.

Though initially (like so many others) a champion of Descartes, Mandeville learnt from experience that strict mind–body dualism was an obstacle to understanding. It was impossible to make progress in fathoming man without paying close attention to the flesh and its ceaseless symbiosis with thought. The body was forever influencing the mind, and vice versa. 'When a Man is overwhelm'd with Shame,' for instance, 'he observes a sinking of the Spirits; the Heart feels cold and condensed, and the Blood flies from it to the Circumference of the Body; the Face glows, the Neck and Part of the Breast partake of the Fire.'

To ignore or disdain the flesh in the manner of Shaftesbury was myopic folly or hypocrisy. As a doctor of society, it was his job to be concerned, Mandeville insisted, with the actual operations of bodies individual and politic, with social functioning and breakdown, with how dysfunctions could be cured or palliated by the expert. 'Laws and Government are to the Political Bodies of Civil Society', he programmatically announced at the opening of his *magnum opus*, 'what the Vital Spirits and Life it self are to the Natural Bodies of Animated Creatures.' In the body politic and natural alike the master anatomist discovered that huge consequences stemmed from the petty and seemingly trivial – 'small trifling Films and little Pipes that are either over-look'd, or else seem inconsiderable to Vulgar Eyes'.

The doctor's solution to the enigma of human nature was spelt out clearly in his *The Fable of the Bees: Or the Knaves Turn'd Honest* of 1714, an extended reworking of 'The Grumbling Hive', some doggerel rhyming couplets published nine years earlier. The *Fable* presented a cautionary tale of how a prosperous, acquisitive commercial society (London, Amsterdam) could be brought to its knees by a sudden conversion to 'honesty' – that is, as understood in Christian or classical terms, the pursuit of self-denial and austere virtue.

The ultimate motive force behind society, revealed the *Fable*, was pure Hobbesian self-interest. The outcome did not have to be Hobbes's state of terror, however, for the trick of society lay in converting basic survival instincts (eat or be eaten) into less socially destructive – indeed socially beneficial – vices, for instance, envy and avarice, and the love of honour, glory and reputation. Practices were devised whereby, without abandoning one whit of their essential egoism – quite impossible! – people made themselves socially useful, by masking it. Indeed, it was greed, vanity and *amour propre* which actually kept the social merry-go-round turning – they provided work and created wealth through the intricate mechanisms whereby social ostentation, display and eminence supplanted naked physical aggression. Rank, ostentation, ornament, equipage, fame, titles and suchlike show and splendour provided the psychological satisfactions necessary to displace gross violence while gratifying the 'odious part of pride'. Among these artificial virtues which society affected, honour was crucial: 'In great Families,' he bantered, 'it is like the Gout, generally counted Hereditary.'

Transvalued into enlightened self-interest and clad in conventional mores and pious clichés, self-seeking did not, in short, have to be malignant: in fact, the astute would prize it as the very yeast of society. The war of all against all was socialized into emulative competition – flaunting more liveried servants or a finer taffeta gown than your neighbours. Once harnessed, selfishness worked to the general good, vice became a virtue, and private vices, public benefits. High-minded moralistic platitudes filled the air – it was all hypocrisy, but *that* hypocrisy was salutary because it was an open secret. The art of conflict management was down to the craftiness of the astute politician, resourceful in channelling gut urges into artificial wants.

> Thus every Part was full of Vice,
> Yet the whole Mass a Paradise;
> Flatter'd in Peace, and fear'd in Wars,
> They were th'Esteem of Foreigners,
> And lavish of their Wealth and Lives,
> The Ballance of all other Hives.
> Such were the Blessings of that State;
> Their Crimes conspired to make 'em Great.

What was the secret, the grand arcanum, of the thriving hive? Vice made the world go round – or, translated from Christian censure into plain English, self-interest:

> Thus Vice nursed Ingenuity,
> Which join'd with Time and Industry,
> Had carry'd Life's Conveniences,
> It's real Pleasures, Comforts, Ease,
> To such a Height, the very Poor
> Lived better than the Rich before,
> And nothing could be added more.

What happened, by contrast, at that fateful moment when the 'knaves turn'd honest', revealed Mandeville, was that the new honesty precipitated social collapse. The ban on egoism and the craving for honour and glory meant that emulativeness vanished, and with it socio-economic ambition and the social integration that brought. All returned to acorns and frugality.

A choice was thus presented: either accept human nature (egoism) as Nature dictated and civilize it to general advantage, or embrace the superhuman rectitude of the rigorist morality-mongers, and accept the ruinous social consequences. (As part of his campaign to expose the sanctimonious and their double-think, Mandeville dropped innuendoes that the 'honesty' plank was itself a yet more pernicious mode of hypocrisy.) His own preference was clear: people should get real:

> Then leave complaints; Fools only strive
> To make a great an honest hive . . .
> Fraud, luxury and pride must live
> While we the benefits receive.

Mandeville, in other words, would deny his contemporaries any easy moral self-congratulation:

> T'enjoy the world's conveniences,
> Be famed in war, yet live in ease,
> Without great vices, is a vain
> Eutopia seated in the brain.

Mandeville's anatomical realism extended beyond showing how greed was good. His *The Virgin Unmask'd: Or, Female Dialogues Betwixt an Elderly Maiden Lady, and her Niece, On several Diverting Discourses on Love, Marriage, Memoirs, and Morals, &c. of the Times* (1709) and *A Modest Defence of the Public Stews* (1724) addressed hypocrisies about sex – the denial of desire – in particular the social charade of female 'virtue'. Despite pretences about their modesty, women were as lascivious as men, revealed Dr Mandeville, echoing the frankness, or misogyny, of the Restoration. Animal urges ruled – it was all a matter of reproductive biology or 'the Constitution of Females'. 'A View of the Fortifications, which Nature has made to preserve their Chastity' was provided by the cynical physician, so as to explain 'the Reason why it so often surrender'd':

Every Woman who is capable of Conception, must have those Parts which officiate, so fram'd, that they may be able to perform whatever is necessary at that Juncture. Now, to have those Parts so rightly adapted for the Use which Nature design'd them, it is requisite that they should have a very quick Sensation, and, upon the Application of the *Male Organ*, afford the Woman an exquisite Pleasure; for, without this extravagant Pleasure in Fruition, the recipient Organs could never exert themselves to promote Conception.

Biologically, in other words, women had thus to be libidinous for reproduction to work. Socially speaking, good order – the marriage market, the transfer of property, the need for legitimacy – required checks on that libidinousness:

To counterballance this violent natural Desire, all young Women have strong Notions of Honour carefully inculcated into them from their Infancy. Young Girls are taught to hate a *Whore*, before they know what the Word means; and when they grow up, they find their worldly Interest entirely depending upon the Reputation of their Chastity.

Since women were always on heat and no more 'naturally' chaste than men, 'artificial chastity' had to be inculcated, to produce and preserve 'actual chastity'.

Lubricity, male and female alike, must (like the economy) be socially managed, for the naked and unrestrained expression of lust (as of power or greed) brought social catastrophe, not least rape and other casual sexual violence. For such reasons, matrimony had been introduced, and, so as to avoid women being cheapened, their virtue – in other words, their chastity – became prized as a precious commodity, to be traded on the marriage market at the best price. Women must be taught the (cash) value of virginity – or its semblance.

In his *Modest Defence of the Public Stews*, Mandeville similarly proposed public provision of prostitutes as the optimal way of protecting all the aforesaid 'virtuous' women, while assuaging the lusts of throngs of men like sailors, newly arrived in port, for whom some 'drain' or 'sluice' was imperative.

Mandeville's thinking and language were wilfully gross – how that *enfant terrible* must have loved shocking Shaftesbury! Love was reduced to the purgation of lust, viewed in terms of the hydraulic systems imagined by iatromechanistic medicine. Marriage was a nice problem in commodity demand and supply. Practical solutions must be found to matters which would not go away: the body would have its way. Like Freud, Mandeville taught that no good would come of repressing human nature.

The quarrel between Mandeville and Shaftesbury might be glossed as follows: for the former *all* humans unfailingly behaved as the *vulgar* did for the latter. Mandeville regarded the idealized version of disinterested human nature advanced by Shaftesbury (at least for his peers) as yet another form of hypocrisy or false consciousness, maybe even a product of self-delusory zeal. Overall, pessimistic realism was the best policy; what counted was self-awareness and social management. 'The Rules I speak of', he declared, 'consist in a dextrous Management of our selves, a stifling of our Appetites, and hiding the real Sentiments of our Hearts before others', for '*private Vices by the dextrous Management of a skilful Politician, may be turn'd into publick Benefits*'.

This chapter's juxtaposition of Shaftesbury and Mandeville highlights certain tensions prominent in the rethinking of identity at the dawn of the eighteenth century. The Hobbesian spectre loomed – man reduced to beast or machine, to anti-social egoism. And, in the light of Locke's model of the mind as a blank sheet of paper, how plausible was Shaftesbury's counter-attempt to give the mind a Neoplatonic hue, possessed of an innate beauty of thinking, a generous self, a sociable affinity? Would that prove tenable? Or was it just aristocratic confidence – indeed, a confidence-trick – tempting the likes of honest Mandeville to put in the boot?

What is perhaps most significant is one final thing these writers shared: Christianity as such had become irrelevant to both. With Shaftesbury and Mandeville, we are dealing in the realms of philosophy, medicine and science. The Christian immortal soul, set its grand eschatological narrative of sin and redemption, has been left behind.

9

SWIFT AND THE SCRIBLERANS: NIGHTMARE SELVES

* THERE is in Mankind a certain   *   *   *

*   *   *   *   *   *   *   *   *

Hic multa   *   *   *   *   *   *   *

desiderantur.   *   *   *   *   *   *   *

*   *   *   *   *   *   *   *   *

*   *   *   And this I take to be a clear Solution of the Matter.

JONATHAN SWIFT

Satire deflates and debases. It is an art which topples greatness, undermines pretension and punishes pride by revealing the low in the pretendedly high, the filth in the pure, the folly in reason. This belittling trick deploys telescopic lenses which picture the human as lesser and lower, or as a machine or beast, driven by depraved desires. Satire reduces what purports to be subtly superior to a repertoire of stigmatizing symbols and cardboard cut-outs, turning character into caricature, signalled by exaggerated physiognomical distortions – the huge nose, gaping mouth and bloated belly, or comparable animalistic traits. In this humbling of the complex into the simplistic, satire finally reduces the mind, soul or spirit to that flesh which always bespeaks inferiority on the Chain of Being.

The effect may be all the more biting when the satirist is himself a fervid Christian, because the preacher's business, no less than the satirist's, may be to lash vanity and hypocrisy, to expose the Pharisee masquerading as the godly, to prick pride, and bring man down to his true fallen self, a stinking sink of sin.

Jonathan Swift was both a satirist and a clergyman of the Church of England. His savage indignation was of the savagest: who else could have suggested, in *A Modest Proposal*, that the solution to Ireland's demographic problems was to tuck into its babies? – 'a young healthy Child, well nursed, is, at a Year old, a most delicious, nourishing and wholesome Food; whether *Stewed, Roasted, Baked*, or *Boiled*; and I make no doubt that it will equally serve in a *Fricasie*, or *Ragoust*'.

Such ferocity owes something (much, surely) to accidents of biography, right from his strange start in life. Born in Dublin in November 1667, some months after the death of his father, baby Jonathan was immediately carried off to Whitehaven in Cumbria by his nurse, where she kept him for three years, quite out of contact with his family; meanwhile, the infant's mother betook herself to Leicester, where she remained for the rest of her life – her son did not see her again until he was 22.

Swift was sent to school in Kilkenny – he loathed it – graduating to Trinity College, Dublin, where he proved an unruly student. During King William's wars, he feared trouble as a Protestant when the deposed Catholic James II invaded Ireland, and he fled to England, first to his mother in Leicester, and then to Moor Park in Surrey, home of the diplomat Sir William Temple, who took the young man on as his secretary. It was there that he met Esther Johnson (Stella), the 8-year-old daughter of one of the servants.

In the early 1700s Swift spent much of his time in London, where he wormed his way into the company of coffee-house wits and politicians, and, beginning to publish political tracts, won a reputation as a controversialist. His glory days were between 1710 and 1714, when he threw in his lot with the Tories. They fell, however, and with the Hanoverian succession the Whigs assumed permanent power. That put paid to Swift's glittering career. He gloomily returned to Ireland to take up a position as Dean of St Patrick's Cathedral in Dublin, and a permanent bitterness set in: 'I reckon no man is thoroughly miserable unless he be condemned to live in Ireland.'

Thither his two great admirers followed him: first Stella, and later the more insistent Vanessa. On the face of it, he treated both women abominably, but both loved him unstintingly. He spent most of his adulthood in communication with them, and much psycho-biographical ink has been spilt debating what he was up to: did he have sexual relations with them? Did he embark upon clandestine matrimony – with one, or even both? Swift was secretive about his passions, and he handled his women with deep ambivalence, reserve and a style of jokey infantilization suggestive of profound fear both of the feminine and of his own emotional and sexual wants – in short, of intimacy. Misogyny marks the searing disgust driving such poems as 'The Lady's Dressing Room' (1730), 'A Beautiful Young Nymph going to Bed' and 'Strephon and Chloe' (1731), all of which dissect women's defects with unconcealed gusto. The 'heroine' of the second of these is an ageing strumpet who uses every cosmetic aid to conceal the ravages of time and the pox, and Swift puts on a display of clinical relish in baring the underlying horrors:

> Then, seated on a three-legg'd Chair,
> Takes off her artificial Hair:
> Now, picking out a Crystal Eye,
> She wipes it clean, and lays it by.
> Her Eye-Brows from a Mouse's Hyde,
> Stuck on with Art on either Side,
> Pulls off with Care, and first displays 'em,
> Then in a Play-Book smoothly lays 'em.
> Now dextrously her Plumpers draws,
> That serve to fill her hollow Jaws.
> Untwists a Wire; and from her Gums
> A Set of Teeth completely comes.
> Pulls out the Rags contriv'd to prop
> Her flappy Dugs and down they drop.

'Never be taken in by false appearances' was Swift's habitual satirical message. 'In most Corporeal Beings, which have fallen under my Cognizance, the Outside hath been infinitely preferable to the In,' he elsewhere proclaimed; 'Last Week I saw a Woman flay'd, and

you will hardly believe how much it altered her Person for the worse.'
The sordid reality beneath the mask haunted him: was all civilization
just dirt and derangement at heart?

Hacking deep into human nature, Swift exposed and explored the
tensions between body and soul, flesh and spirit, that are thematic to
this book, overtly highlighting those questions of identity – who does
man think he is? – so fiercely debated in the Augustan decades.
Evidently man was not the *homo rationalis* he pretended to be but
rather, at best, *homo rationis capax* – a creature capable of rationality,
though by implication falling short.

His 'anthropological' satire appears as its most diagrammatic in
Gulliver's Travels, published in 1726. Once you had the idea of the big
men and little men, commented Dr Johnson, everything else followed. True, but Johnson abhorred Swift, and *Gulliver* is, in reality,
more subtle and rewarding than that.

The voyage to Lilliput is primarily a kick at that arch butt of the
Tories, Robert Walpole – who could take the rap for Swift's enduring
Hibernian exile. Walpole, the great manager and his supporting
'Robinocracy', are reduced to Lilliputian littleness, and the ecclesiastical disputes of the day are sent up in the rancorous but asinine
conflicts between the Big-Endians and the Little-Endians. In the first
book, Gulliver, a ship's surgeon, himself serves as a paragon of honest
humanity and decency, exposing the Machiavellian diplomacy and
politicking of the Lilliputians, whose rapacity and cunning are panto-
mimed by their stature: dwarfishness is a sure sign of a mean mind
and base motives.

The satire takes a new twist when, on his second voyage, Gulliver
visits Brobdingnag, whose inhabitants tower above him. The boot is
now on the other foot, and it is Gulliver who is exposed as diminutive
of stature and understanding alike. The Brobdingnagians furthermore excite Swift's disgust at the flesh. Their very grossness exagger-
ates all the minute flaws and hideousness normally concealed from
the eye by the limitations of human vision – as it were, they expose
themselves – as Gulliver is reduced in the hands of his captors to a
baby, pet or mannikin.

Not least, Gulliver/Swift is repelled at being turned into an impotent object of sexual desire by the lusts of the gigantic bosomy Brobdingnagian matrons: 'Their Skins appeared so coarse and uneven, so variously coloured when I saw them near, with a Mole here and there as broad as a Trencher, and Hairs hanging from it thicker than Pack-threads; to say nothing further concerning the rest of their Persons.' In one episode, he barely escapes being eaten alive by a large infant who is pacified only by 'the last Remedy', a 'monstrous Breast'. Later, an even more 'horrible Spectacle' threatens to engulf him, a cancerous breast 'swelled to a monstrous Size, full of Holes, in two or three of which I could have easily crept, and covered my whole Body'.

Though Swift is manifestly revolted by the flesh, any possibility of escaping it (seemingly Shaftesbury's solution?) is scotched by the third book, the visit to Laputa. The islanders themselves aspire to transcend the flesh by losing themselves in lofty reasoning and recasting the sensory world all around into the abstractions of natural philosophy, quantity and geometry, rather as the advocates of the 'new philosophy' blotted out 'secondary' for 'primary' qualities. In the process, however, they hubristically blind themselves to reality and are useless at elementary practicalities – a trait Swift always mocked, despising as he did the myopic vanity of high-flown speculators. Small surprise that their wives slip off to have sex with males from a neighbouring island: their own husbands have lost touch with what makes them human.

In having Gulliver ridicule the futile attempts of the Laputans to divest, or rise above, the flesh, was Swift obliquely reflecting upon his own flawed and frustrating strategies for containing the old Adam? Fairly accepting of the most noxious Lilliputian and the grossest Brobdingnagian, Gulliver (and perhaps Swift) maintains that he has never seen 'a more clumsy, awkward, and unhandy People' than the Laputans – they were, in fact, the most 'disagreeable Companions' he had ever met.

Equally it may be no accident that the third book of the travels also features the wretched Struldbrugs, the people who have discovered the secret of how to avoid the fruits of the flesh, death. The price, however, for their fabulous longevity is that they inescapably grow thoroughly melancholy and wretched:

When they came to Fourscore Years, which is reckoned the Extremity of living in this Country, they had not only all the Follies and Infirmities of other old Men, but many more which arose from the dreadful Prospect of never dying. They were not only opinionative, peevish, covetous, morose, vain, talkative; but uncapable of Friendship, and dead to all natural Affection, which ever descended below their Grand-children. Envy and impotent Desires, are their prevailing Passions. . . . The least miserable among them, appear to be those who turn to Dotage, and entirely lose their Memories; these meet with more Pity and Assistance, because they want many bad Qualities, which abound in others.*

Idealized in the 'golden age' myth of the Greeks and the astonishing spans of Methuselah and other Old Testament patriarchs, longevity had ever had its allure, and a tradition of prolongevist writings had grown up, including those (as we have seen) of Luigi Cornaro. Swift countered by displaying the consequences of a thoughtless and short-sighted quest for longevity, for the Struldbrugs had achieved long life without permanent youth, fitness, vitality or, above all, good nature. Their extra years merely brought them the pains of crotchetiness and senility. Their decayed flesh and crabby minds were portrayed with a mixture of pity – in anticipation, doubtless, of his own coming old age – vehement disgust, and the perhaps orthodox Christian conviction that embodiment was a life sentence. If the Laputans, intent on obliterating their carcasses, were the most 'disagreeable' of Gulliver's discoveries, the Struldbrugs were the most 'mortifying' – and, predictably, 'the Women more horrible than the Men'. The Laputans' futile dreams of transcendence were exacerbated by the Struldbrugian nightmare of everlasting mortality.

The culmination of the satire against human pretensions is, of course, the fourth voyage to the land of the Houyhnhnms and Yahoos

---

* Swift had a terror of ageing – and rightly so as he did indeed grow senile.

– it is the philosophical key to *Gulliver's Travels*, because it poses the key dilemma of *homo rationis capax*. Gulliver finds, to his consternation, that the creatures who are rational and graced by many of the qualities honoured in mankind – generosity, dignity, peaceableness, sociability – are not human at all but equine. Indeed, the Houyhnhnms, being horses, cannot even read, but they do speak, and they talk reason unlike anybody else Gulliver meets on his voyages into the unknown – that is, Swift's travels in his moral imagination.

Mistrusting as he did the prating din of rival creeds, Swift gives these rational horses no books: they gain all the wisdom they need from nature. They cannot understand why Gulliver is so ashamed of some parts of his body as to fear nakedness. They have no words for disbelieving, because lying is to them unknown – language is for communicating one's thoughts, why should it be used for concealment? 'To clear up which' – as so often, Gulliver is here apologetically doing his gullible best to make them grasp why human society was so vice-ridden – 'I endeavoured to give him some Ideas of the Desire of Power and Riches; of the terrible Effects of Lust, Intemperance, Malice, and Envy. . . . After which, like one whose Imagination was struck with something never seen or heard of before, he would lift up his Eyes with Amazement and Indignation.'

Life among the Houyhnhnms is idyllic. Gulliver soon accustoms himself to a simple diet of grain, herbs and milk, 'and I cannot but observe, that I never had one Hour's Sickness' – Swift, like Addison, held most illness resulted from over-eating and drinking, and bad medicine. Although like a Yahoo in physique, Gulliver is not treated as such, because he is endowed with reason, and he enters into discussion of affairs back in Europe with a wise Houyhnhnm. The latter is appalled to learn that in the recent war against France, 'about a Million of Yahoos might have been killed'. Gulliver relates the causes of wars – ambitions, jealousies and such vain quarrels as 'whether Flesh be Bread, or Bread be Flesh: Whether the juice of a certain Berry be Blood or Wine' – not forgetting to boast of the vast ingenuity that goes into the making of 'Cannons, Culverins, Muskets,

Carabines, Pistols, Bullets, Powder, Swords, Bayonets', and so on. Although he detests Yahoos, the Houyhnhnm no more blames them than a bird of prey, because they are devoid of reason and so lack choice. When a creature blessed with reason misuses it, however, he makes things 'worse than Brutality itself'.

In starkest contrast to the wise and gentle Houyhnhnms are the loathsome Yahoos. These bestial beings with human traits – they are vicious, violent, aggressive and filthy in their habits – attack Gulliver and shit on him from the trees. It dawns on him that Yahoos are in essence humans minus (the capability for) reason. If to be human is to be a compound of mind and body, all is currently bemusing, because it is the horse, the Houyhnhnm, who is rational and the Yahoo, the humanoid, who is animalistic.

Bemused is how Gulliver himself ends up, because he returns to London from the land of the Houyhnhnms seething with loathing for his own race. On meeting his wife and children once more, he is disgusted by their touch, stench and habits: 'As soon as I entered the house, my wife took me in her arms, and kissed me; at which, having not been used to the touch of that odious animal for so many years, I fell in a swoon for almost an hour.' 'During the first year' he is back in England,

I could not endure my Wife or Children in my Presence, the very Smell of them was intolerable, much less could I suffer them to eat in the same Room. To this Hour they dare not presume to touch my Bread, or drink out of the same Cup; neither was I ever able to let one of them take me by the Hand. The first Money I laid out was to buy two young Stone-Horses, which I keep in a good Stable, and next to them the Groom is my greatest Favourite; for I feel my Spirits revived by the Smell he contracts in the Stable. My Horses understand me tolerably well; I converse with them at least four Hours every Day. They are Strangers to Bridle or Saddle; they live in great Amity with me, and Friendship to each other.

Gulliver is clearly out of his mind: who but a lunatic would talk to horses? Yet he is a madman who has seen to the bottom of things. Misanthropy seems the rational course.

If in *Gulliver's Travels* the satirical tropes are big-and-little and animal-and-human, in *A Tale of a Tub* Swift essays a different repertoire to dissociate, defamiliarize and deflate. There, it is clothes which conceal, reveal and symbolize the inner man, and the human paradox.

A Tale of a Tub shows how Christians are no Christians. Above all, it exposes the splits between Catholicism, Lutheranism and Calvinism, signified respectively by three heroes, Peter (standing for St Peter and Catholicism), Martin (Luther or Lutheranism) and Jack (Jean Calvin or Puritanism). Each is identified by his coat, and their respective claims to truth are flagged by the paltry insignia of external fashion – holy faith is worn on the sleeve and has been reduced to squabbles over buttons and lapels: '*That Fellow . . . has no Soul; where is his Shoulder-knot?*' As often, Swift recruits an unreliable narrator (the 'Hack') to convince the reader of the rationality of such a reduction:

what is Man himself but a *Micro-Coat*, or rather a compleat Suit of Cloaths with all its Trimmings? As to his Body, there can be dispute; but examine even the Acquirements of his Mind, you will find them all contribute in their Order, towards furnishing out an exact Dress: To instance no more; Is not Religion a *Cloak*, Honesty a *Pair of Shoes*, worn out in the Dirt, Self-Love a *Surtout*, Vanity a *Shirt*, and Conscience a *Pair of Breeches*, which, tho' a Cover for Lewdness as well as Nastiness, is easily slipt down for the Service of both.

The *Tale* expressed Swift's particular detestation for bigots and zealots who were convinced that they, and they alone, possessed a corner on truth – by dint of divine authority in the case of the Catholic Church, or the Bible, as with Protestants. Fearful of the legacy of antinomian mechanic preachers and the presence of the 'French prophets' (who provoked Shaftesbury to his *Letter concerning Enthusiasm*), Swift, like so many contemporaries, lampooned perverted religion as a disgusting physical pathology: all that spiritual 'inspiration' was nothing but disorders of the guts. The promptings of (holy) spirit were nothing other than the animal spirits, all jarring and at cuffs.

The same was done with political greatness. Louis XIV was elsewhere shown by Swift to be not a true Sun King but a gilded meteor which had already passed its zenith:

> Giddy he grows, and down is hurled
> And as a mortal to his vile disease,
> Falls sick in the posteriors of the world.

And this 'vile disease'? A sly footnote informs us that it was a *fistula in ano*, that royal ailment suffered by Louis XIV, which for Swift said it all: all his glorious schemes emitted from his lowest and vilest orifice, the Sun King was a pain in the arse. Power lust was but a madness arising from a somatic pathology, as vapours arose from the bowels and nether regions to cloud the mind. Flesh was the great leveller:

The very same Principle that influenced a *Bully* to break the Windows of a Whore, who has jilted him, naturally stirs up a Great Prince to raise mighty Armies, and dream of nothing but Sieges, Battles and Victories. . . . The same Spirits which in their superior Progress would conquer a Kingdom, descending upon the *Anus*, conclude in a *Fistula*.

Such was the gross origin of the imperial itch: the root cause was anger, and that was basically choleric humour. And, addressing religious enthusiasm, Swift declared, ambivalently, that the corruption of the senses was the generation of the spirit: all that pretended to nobility was merely a symptom of some internal disorder. In a 'Digression on Madness', Swift has his unreliable narrator insist that such craziness is itself of great benefit to mankind – for were not imperial conquerors, the founders of new religions, and the framers of new discoveries in philosophy all out of their minds?

In Section VIII of the *Tale*, the Hack proudly introduces the learned Aeolists who maintain 'the original cause of all things to be wind' – their interpretation of the '*anima mundi*; that is to say, the spirit, or breath, or wind of the world'.* Soul is thus by implication dissolved by that philosophical sect into a load of hot air. And this

---

* Swift is here playing philologically on the etymology of inspiration: *spiro*: I breathe.

disturbing possibility is returned to in *The Mechanical Operation of the Spirit*, a satire against canting Quakers claiming to be inwardly possessed by the voice of God and to speak with divine tongues. Once again, Swift dwells on the somatic pathology which makes the human machine emit such senseless noises in perfect assurance that they are the revelations of truth – that is, 'enthusiasm', which 'may be defined, *A lifting up of the Soul or its Faculties above Matter*'. There are, assures the Hack, developing the conceit,

three general Ways of ejaculating the Soul, or transporting it beyond the Sphere of Matter. The first, is the immediate Act of God, and is called, *Prophecy* or *Inspiration*. The second, is the immediate Act of the Devil, and is termed *Possession*. The third, is the Product of natural Causes, the effect of strong Imagination, Spleen, violent Anger, Fear, Grief, Pain, and the like. These three have been abundantly treated on by Authors, and therefore shall not employ my Enquiry. But, the fourth Method of *Religious Enthusiasm*, or launching out the Soul, as it is purely an Effect of Artifice and *Mechanick Operation*, has been sparingly handled.

He would, however, change all that.

This device enables Swift to fell two foes with one stone: he targets those bogey men, the antinomian free spirits who claimed to 'ejaculate' transcendental truth, while, at the same time, he mocks those equally vain physiologists who believed their mechanical science encompassed the whole truth of the human animal.

Swift enjoys toying with hazardous speculations as to the corporeal springs of consciousness. It was 'the opinion of choice *Virtuosi*, that the Brain is only a Crowd of little Animals', he teases,

but with Teeth and Claws extremely sharp, and therefore, cling together in the Contexture we behold, like the picture of *Hobbes's Leviathan*. . . . That all Invention is formed by the Morsure of two or more of these Animals . . . That if the Morsure be Hexagonal, it produces Poetry; the Circular gives Eloquence; If the Bite hath been Conical, the Person, whose Nerve is so affected, shall be disposed to write upon the Politicks; and so of the rest.

Zealous scientists were the brethren of canting zealots: both set themselves up (or were set up by Swift) as infallible oracles. He had not a grain of sympathy for religious enthusiasts, but he found equally foolish the medico-scientific materialism encouraged by Descartes and Hobbes – man reduced to machine. Anybody who thus collapsed the truly complex into the simple was a fool. He who reduced the fake complex to its core was a satirist devoted 'to the universal improvement of mankind'. Mankind, for Swift, was certainly in need of it.

Another project with which Swift was involved – how extensively is debatable – was *The Memoirs of Martinus Scriblerus*, a further satire on learned folly cobbled together by a club of Tory wits, headed by the Scottish physician, John Arbuthnot. 'The design', recalled Alexander Pope, 'was to have ridiculed all the false tastes in learning, under the character of a man of capacity enough that had dipped in every art and science, but injudiciously in each.'

The theme inspiring the mock-serious *Memoirs* is that rather Lockean question, the making of a man, the fabrication of an individual: what is it to assume an identity, to be Martinus Scriblerus himself and no one else? A virtuoso in rhetoric, anatomy, classical learning and natural philosophy, Martinus is displayed as a wonder – yet an enigma: is he nothing other than the sum of the inputs stuffed into him from infancy (his 'programming', as we would say)? Does he have a real identity, or is he but an artificial construct, some android, automaton or a monster? Is he purely and simply the product of his education, that Lockean dream? And, if so, does that leave him lacking in some *je ne sais quoi*, some essential interiority? Or, as postmodernists might hold, is the self something which, in any case, exists only when discursively constructed: is Martinus Scriblerus nothing other than what is being memorialized? And if so, where does that leave the memorializing persona? As ever, Augustan satirists make merry with the spectre of infinite regress, and the threat to the bedrock of truth posed by unreliable memorialists as well as unreliable autobiographers like Gulliver.

Martinus Scriblerus – Martinus presumably because of Martin

Luther and the Protestant ego, Scriblerus as one afflicted by the itch of writing, that disease pitilessly mocked by Swift and others – is the darling son of Cornelius, a doting father whose fond ambition it is to rear a prodigy of greatness. Having established Martinus's noble genealogy, the *Memoirs* proceed to document the pedagogical labours of his pedantic parent, who has trustingly combed the educational treatises of the ancients to learn how to fashion the perfect specimen: 'The good Cornelius also hoped he would come to stammer like Demosthenes, in order to be as eloquent; and in time arrive at many other Defects of famous men.'

Martinus was thus the ultimate hothouse creation, formed after the dreams and schemes of a father engulfed in erudition and deaf to common sense – Cornelius was clearly the inspiration for Walter Shandy. His project of building a model man is burlesqued as a quintessentially *modern* imbecility, through Cornelius himself is, ironically, an idolater of the ancients.

Through a series of droll chapters, the *Memoirs* dwell on the physical and medical nostrums which dominate Cornelius's heroic man-building (to devote so much attention to mere matters of the body is itself a mark of the misguided). The father is obsessed, for example, by food: the right diet will be the making of the model man – long before Feuerbach, he knew that man is what he eats. Cornelius has also got it into his head to perform prophylactic surgery, a most idiosyncratic alternative to circumcision. His pride and joy, he is persuaded, will be the better for the removal of his 'spleen' – both the bodily organ and the temperament. The literal-minded Cornelius is so short-sighted as to imagine that a constitutional trait can be rectified by a physical cut – in any case, what presumption, to think that mankind is wise enough to redesign the God-given!

Receiving medical instruction as part of his higher education, Martinus himself gets involved in a comic dissecting 'accident' – one grosser than those described in the *Spectator*. Intending to perform an autopsy, he buys the corpse of a criminal, and instructs his servant to deliver it:

As he was softly stalking up stairs in the dark, with the dead man in his arms, his burthen had like to have slipp'd from him, which he (to save from falling) grasp'd so hard about the belly that it forced the wind through the *Anus*, with a noise exactly like the *Crepitus* of a living man.

Is there, this cameo prompts, truly any distinction between a living and a dead man's fart, and so by implication between farting and speaking, between sound and speech, between the animate and the deceased?

While a medical student, Martinus toys with various modish systems of medical reductionism which Arbuthnot and his friends clearly scorned. Ambitious to explain the dispositions of the mind in somatic terms, he considers (in a way reckoned by the wits to be shallowly reductionist) '*Virtues* and Vices as certain Habits which proceed from the natural Formation and Structure of particular parts of the body', much as 'a Bird flies because it has Wings, and a Duck swims because it is web-footed'. Various conclusions are drawn by our hero.

1st, He observ'd that the Soul and Body mutually operate upon each other, and therefore, if you deprive the Mind of the outward Instruments whereby she usually expresseth that Passion, you will in time abate the Passion itself; in like manner as Castration abates Lust.

2dly, That the Soul in mankind expresseth every Passion by the Motion of some particular *Muscles*.

3dly, That all Muscles grow stronger and thicker by being *much us'd*; therefore the habitual Passions may be discerned in particular persons by the *strength* and *bigness* of the Muscles us'd in the expression of that Passion.

Rather as with phrenology later, the exercise of the body was here, albeit satirically, being touted as the royal road to the perfection of the soul.

Such speculations as to body–mind interaction naturally plunge Martinus into what we have seen was one of the great debates of the time, the soul's location. Was Descartes right to quarter it in the pineal gland? At first Martinus 'labour'd under great uncertainties'

– 'sometimes he was of the opinion that it lodg'd in the Brain, sometimes in the Stomach, and sometimes in the Heart' – but then he changes his mind: 'Afterwards he thought it absurd to confine that sovereign Lady to one apartment, which made him infer that she shifted it according to the several functions of life: The Brain was her Study, the Heart her State-room, and the Stomach her Kitchen.' Then he comes round to Willis's view:

He now conjectured it was more for the dignity of the Soul to perform several operations by her little Ministers, the *Animal Spirits*, from whence it was natural to conclude, that she resides in different parts according to different Inclinations, Sexes, Ages, and Professions. Thus in Epicures he seated her in the mouth of the Stomach, Philosophers have her in the Brain, Soldiers in their Hearts, Women in their Tongues, Fidlers in their Fingers, and Rope-dancers in their Toes.

And finally it is back to Descartes, 'dissecting many Subjects to find out the different Figure of this Gland':

He suppos'd that in factious and restless-spirited people he should find it sharp and pointed, allowing no room for the Soul to repose herself; that in quiet Tempers it was flat, smooth, and soft, affording to the Soul as it were an easy cushion. He was confirm'd in this by observing, that Calves and Philosophers, Tygers and Statesmen, Foxes and Sharpers, Peacocks and Fops, Cock-Sparrows and Coquets, Monkeys and Players, Courtiers and Spaniels, Moles and Misers, exactly resemble one another in the conformation of the *Pineal Gland*.

Yet more animal satire reminiscent of Swift.

Speculations as to the soul's embodiment inevitably led to all the issues raised in the Locke controversy: if Locke were right that the personality lay in 'conscious selfhood' – one seemingly rather contingent and precarious – where did that leave the soul?

Setting the cat among the pigeons, the Scriblerans concocted spoof letters from a 'Society of Freethinkers', which reproduced and mock-seriously endorsed Collins's arguments against Clarke, designed to sabotage the Christian/Cartesian doctrine of an immortal, immaterial ever-thinking soul. The fictitious society's Secretary opened by bluntly admonishing Martinus for wasting his genius 'in looking after that Theological Non-entity commonly call'd the *Soul*' – what was it but a 'Chimera', upheld only by 'some dreaming Philosophers' and other 'crack-brain'd' fellows'?

Playing devil's advocate, the Scriblerans gave seeming endorsement to the Secretary's Collinsian disproof of the Clarkean soul. And as he successively dismissed the Christian rationalist's main points, the ever-conscious soul was reduced to a figment of the imagination.

The first of Clarke's 'Sophisms' refuted was the contention 'that *Self-consciousness* cannot inhere in any system of Matter, because all matter is made up of several distinct beings, which never can make up one individual thinking being'. Here lay what Clarke considered his trump card – 'self-consciousness' is undivided, and hence matter, being divisible, could never unite diverse acts into those of 'one individual thinking being'. The Secretary took Collins's counter – thought is divisible and consciousness can emerge from the combined operation of all the particles of a thing, that is, thinking matter – and drove it to its logical extreme, through the use of a 'familiar instance':

In every *Jack* there is a *meat-roasting* Quality, which neither resides in the Fly, nor in the Weight, nor in any particular wheel of the Jack, but is the result of the whole composition: So in an Animal, the Self-consciousness is not a real quality inherent in one Being (any more than meat-roasting in a Jack) but the result of several modes or qualities in the same subject.

The 'familiar instance' was, of course, meant to be ludicrous, but it was prophetic of the monistic materialism of the future.

What was so wrong, asked the Secretary, with a soul marked by changeability not permanence? It was just like the stocking of the notorious old miser Sir John Cutler, which, though endlessly darned, still remained the item of hosiery he wore:

Sir John Cutler had a pair of black worsted stockings, which his maid darn'd so often with silk, that they became at last a pair of silk stockings. Now supposing those stockings of Sir John's endued with some degree of

Consciousness at every particular darning, they would have been sensible, that they were the same individual pair of stockings both before and after the darning; and this sensation would have continued in them through all the succession of darnings; and yet after the last of all, there was not perhaps one thread left of the first pair of stockings, but they were grown into silk stockings, as was said before.

What would Locke have made of the self-consciousness of a sock?

Consciousness *à la* Locke was, held the freethinkers, the *sine qua non* of personality, even though that self-presence might well be intermittent, and its organic substrate (like the worsted-cum-silk) something whose very physicality changed all the time. Mutability was impishly being represented as inherent to the soul's very being. The subversive implications of such views, derived from Locke via Collins, are plain: what it is to be a human has become remarkably nebulous. Like Swift in his *Mechanical Operation of the Spirit*, the Scriblerans were targeting the pretensions of those modern philosophers who nonchalantly sacrificed time-honoured and lofty ideals of humanity for modish speculations potentially destructive of all moral order.

The shocking dissolving of personality prompted by freethinking was further teased out in the facetious account of Martinus's marriage. Martinus falls in love with Lindamira, one of a pair of Siamese twins exhibited at a freakshow. As was discussed in Chapter 6, conjoined twins were in the news and attracting debate, the model in this case being a set of twins, Helena and Judith, displayed in London in 1708. Born in Hungary, they were united at the buttocks and they shared a common vagina and rectum. Following popular folklore, it was held that their malformation was the result of their mother's having seen, during gestation, a pair of monstrous dogs joined with their heads in opposite directions. The twins attracted the attention not only of scientists and sightseers but also of the wits. 'Here is the sight of two girls joined together at the back,' remarked Swift, 'which, in the newsmonger's phrase, causes a great many speculations; and raises abundance of questions in divinity, law, and physic.'

In the rodomontade offered in the *Memoirs*, Martinus, to the freakshow owner's chagrin, elopes with Lindamira, her sister Indamora perforce accompanying. To obtain redress, the proprietor takes Martinus to court, on the grounds that, given the manner in which the two are joined, every time Martinus exercises his conjugal rights over the former he commits bigamy (and incest) with the latter. To complicate matters, the owner marries Indamora off ('while her sister was asleep') to the black prince Ebn-Hai-Paw-Waw, another member of the travelling show, provoking Martinus to cross-petition for relief from this unforeseen extension to his already tense ménage.

The court case was particularly complicated in Cartesian and Christian terms, because Lindamira and Indamora constituted, if two selves, something more than one and less than two bodies. How many souls were they? Was it a case of two souls housed in a single body, like Locke's example of Socrates awake and Socrates asleep? Did both of the souls, or individuals, equally exercise legal proprietorship over the whole of the conjoint body, or only over certain demarcated parts of it? Since the law treated the wife as her husband's property, the court had to decide whether, as Martinus maintained, the twins together 'constitute but one wife', or whether, as the black prince's counsel maintained, they were 'two distinct persons' and could thus be owned and enjoyed by two husbands at once. Crucial to the forensic reasoning was the familiar question of where in the body lay the soul, specifically the female soul.

The sticking-point proved the pudenda. Martinus's lawyer, Dr Pennyfeather, maintained that as Lindamira–Indamora 'hath but *one* Organ of Generation, she is but *one individual Person*, in the truest and most proper sense of Individuality'. One organ of generation equalled one person, because it equalled one soul; and the genitals, he maintained, were the seat of the soul in women – was not that manifest from the tyranny sex exercised over them? 'Where there is but one Member of Generation,' the learned doctor contended, 'there is but one body, so there can be but one Soul; because the said organ of Generation is the Seat of the Soul.' He went on to reassert the theological doctrine of traducianism: 'it has been the opinion of many most learned Divines and Philosophers, that the Soul, as well as Body, is produced *ex traduce*' (that is, through the act and organs of generation). This was specially true of women!

To resolve these ticklish questions, recourse was finally had to the traditional jury of matrons, who examined the twins and determined that 'the Parts of Generation in Lindamira and Indamora were distinct'. On that basis the judge decided that they could be the property of two husbands, while warning the brothers-in-law to take care lest they slid into adultery or incest. Thankfully, all was resolved when a higher court decided to dissolve both marriages 'as proceeding upon a natural, as well as legal Absurdity'.

The tale of Martinus and the Siamese twins betrays flagrant chauvinist bias and that prurient fascination with the minutiae of female sexuality typical of the misogynistic Swift and his cronies. Profound questions were nevertheless being raised as to the integrity of the self, the relations of mind and body, and the boundaries between one person and another, indicative of the climate of problems created by the new personality philosophy floated by Locke – the *Memoirs* in fact specifically added gender to the melting-pot. The arguments raised there, and in Swift's satires, in a facetious tone, so as to sabotage trendy views, were rapidly destined to become the radical staples of the next generation.

IO

JOHNSON AND
INCORPORATED MINDS

The great business of his life was to escape from himself;
this disposition he considered as the disease of his mind.

SIR JOSHUA REYNOLDS

At first glance the life of Samuel Johnson reads as a classic moral tale of Smilesian self-help, exertion triumphant over adversity. Born in 1709 in provincial Lichfield, he grew up sickly, being taken at the age of 3 by his mother to London to be cured by Queen Anne's 'royal touch' of the 'king's evil' (scrofula): physical illness thereafter dogged his long but painful life.

Poverty forced him to leave Pembroke College Oxford without a degree, and the next two decades brought unremitting struggle. Moving in 1737 to London, he obtained employment on the *Gentleman's Magazine* as a hack writer and parliamentary reporter, before his career as a man of letters was given a decisive boost when he was commissioned to prepare a *Dictionary of the English Language*, which was eventually published in 1755. Meanwhile he began to appear in print in his own right. *London*, a savage satirical poem on the 'great wen', appeared anonymously in 1738; and eleven years later he published the equally sombre *The Vanity of Human Wishes*, an imitation of the tenth satire of Juvenal, expressive of his own dark vision of human folly. A year later, he began to bring out the *Rambler*, a magazine in the *Spectator* mould (though entirely without its insistent cheeriness) which ran didactic essays on morals, manners and religion. This was followed in 1758 by the *Idler*, equally moralistic in its commentaries on human failings, and one year later by his only extended work of fiction, the moral fable *Rasselas*.

Johnson's later years were crowned by his *Lives of the English Poets* and his edition of Shakespeare, monumental feats of scholarly criticism. By then he had gathered into the informal group known as the Club the leading literary figures of the day, and not only received a government pension (1762) but (posthumously) was the subject of the first immortal biography of a British man of letters, James Boswell's *The Life of Samuel Johnson* (1791). Overall, a success story, indeed, it seems. But that was only the public face of the 'great cham of English letters': there was an inner Johnson racked by anxiety that he could never be what he knew he should be, a rational Christian properly in control of himself.

Throughout his periodical writings and in the opinions recorded by Boswell, Johnson repeatedly and unambiguously gave expression to a Christian ideal of a divine order in which God had given man free will so that his immortal half could triumphantly master the flesh. It is a world view fleshed out and authenticated by the learned citations which permeate the *Dictionary* – no disinterested compendium of definitions but a covert primer in Johnsonian tenets, a citadel of traditional learning buttressing his own views on human nature and conduct.

As the *Dictionary* abundantly shows, Johnson was a dualist through and through: body and soul were ontologically distinct, and the human amalgam was an 'incorporated mind' – the phrase confirms how he prioritized the spirit. Just like Descartes or Samuel Clarke, he held that the soul never slept: 'That the soul always exerts her peculiar powers, with greater or less force, is very probable.'

The *Dictionary* treated the rational soul as categorically different from the 'sensible soul' found throughout the animal kingdom, and also from the senses among humans. Isaac Watts was here quoted, separating *soma* from soul: 'As we learn what belongs to the body by the evidence of sense, so we learn what belongs to the soul by an inward consciousness.' For Johnson, the soul was neither the agent nor the object of mere sense, and it emphatically had no base-camp in the body. 'That the soul and angels have nothing to do with grosser locality is generally opinioned' – it is Joseph Glanvill who is being quoted.

The main bodily whereabouts touted for the soul were the pineal gland, the blood and the brain. Johnson referred to belief in the first under 'pineal', but the brain was the proposed locale which got most attention in the *Dictionary*, and that view was treated with some ridicule. Glanvill was quoted again, characterizing the brain as a 'quagmire', with a '*clammy*' consistency unsuitable for 'supporting the motion of thought'; the High Church divine Jeremy Collier was hauled in to endorse this in an even more contemptuous strain: 'The brain . . . looks like an odd sort of bog for fancy to *paddle* in.' The brain was doubly ripe for the *Dictionary*'s raillery: not only was it a false address for the immaterial soul, it also betokened intellectual arrogance.

The soul–body distinction was absolute, and the temporal union of the two was, in Johnson's view, a mystery beyond human understanding. Man 'is compounded of two very different ingredients, spirit and matter' – it is Jeremy Collier who is again being ventriloquized – 'but how such unallied and disproportioned substances should act upon each other, no man's learning yet could tell him'. Johnson himself further endorsed this unequivocal divide between body and soul in his definition of 'life' as 'union and co-operation of soul with body', and in his denotation of 'trance' as 'a temporary absence of the soul from the body'. The soul–body link was prominent in the inventory of human ignorance – and one which also served to confirm the wisdom, power and glory of God. In some quotations the soul was even depicted as being in immediate communication with the celestial world, almost closer to God than to man: 'Our souls, piercing through the impurity of flesh' – here Johnson is quoting Sir Walter Raleigh – 'behold the highest heavens, and thence bring knowledge to contemplate the everduring glory and termless joy.' It is noteworthy that, although Johnson quoted extensively and approvingly from Locke in the *Dictionary* – he was his favourite philosopher – he did not include any of his more subversive and heretical views, such as 'thinking matter' or conscious selfhood.

Johnson thus advanced a noble vision of man. It was one quite removed from the Enlightenment belief in a natural science of man and also from enlightened expectations of human happiness, a point bluntly made by his moral tale *Rasselas*.

Son of the Prince of Abyssinia, Rasselas is confined in a valley where he lives free of all vexations. Despite these utopian delights, however, he is not happy, and this prompts him to ponder the grand questions of life: 'Every beast that strays beside me has the same corporeal necessities with myself. . . . I am hungry and thirsty like him, but when thirst and hunger cease I am not at rest.' To resolve his questions and discover what life is truly like, Rasselas concludes that he must escape from this 'happy valley'. But how? Turning to the 'new science', he consults an expert full of wonderous plans for flying chariots. He will build an escape machine – on condition that none shall be allowed to copy it. But when constructed, the machine merely flaps its wings uselessly and dives, Icarus-like, into the lake. In this ominous false start there lay a moral; had the prince been alert, it would have spared him his trip.

Rasselas next meets the poet Imlac, who describes life in the world beyond. And eventually he shows the prince the way to escape. Taking with them his sister and her lady-in-waiting, they go first to Cairo, where they see men living in carefree gaiety, but Imlac warns that this is illusory: 'There is not one who did not dread the moment when solitude should deliver him to the tyranny of reflection.' In disgust he turns away from so thoughtless a life.

Next he meets a rationalist philosopher, who explains how happiness consists in following the dictates of reason. Imlac, however, soon disabuses him: these theorists 'discourse like angels, but they live like men'. Watching the reactions of one to the death of his daughter, Rasselas sees how worthless is his philosophy.

What, then, of the pastoral idyll, with smiling shepherds tending their frisking flocks? This bucolic bliss proves as illusory as the palace of Reason once Rasselas finds 'that their hearts were cankered with discontent', for 'they considered themselves as condemned to labour for the luxury of the rich'. Nor is the hermit's cave any better, since a recluse confesses he has been able to shun the world's vices only by avoiding it altogether: 'My fancy riots in scenes of folly, and I lament that I have lost so much, and have gained so little.'

Continuing his quest for the grand arcanum of happiness, Rasselas concludes that it must lie in power: how splendid to rule a kingdom and make all one's subjects happy! But he is soon cured when he sees a once-powerful provincial governor being led in chains.

Contemplate the pyramids, Imlac tells him, 'the most pompous monuments of Egyptian greatness'. Men are little concerned with the present: they spend their time either regretting the past or laying plans for the future, and that is even true of the Pharaohs:

A king, whose power is unlimited and whose treasures surmount all real and imaginary wants, is compelled to solace, by the erection of a pyramid, the satiety of dominion and tastelessness of pleasures, and to amuse the tediousness of declining life, by seeing thousands labouring without end, and one stone, for no purpose laid upon another.

And thus the pyramids stand as timeless monuments to the futility of absolute power.

Finally the prince is taken to meet one who has spent all his life in the study of astronomy: here, surely, must true happiness lie! Moreover he claims astonishing powers: he can direct the weather and control the course of the sun – at his command the Nile will flood. But in exercising such measureless powers, he has made the melancholy discovery, that if he makes the rain fall here, deserts appear somewhere else. Man, it seems, can never see the consequences of his actions, and good intentions are not enough. The astronomer is obviously crazy. 'Of the uncertainties of our present state,' observes Imlac, 'the most dreadful and alarming is the uncertain continuance of reason.' And if reason is so undependable, how much more so is imagination, which leads men to dream up airy schemes for improvement which are little better than madness.

The final chapter is a 'Conclusion, in which Nothing is Concluded'; but all have learnt one thing, that whatever goals man sets himself, none will ever be fully attained. Like *Candide*, *Rasselas* teaches the vanity of human ambitions and traces the bounds of reason. Johnson distanced himself from fatuous Enlightenment notions of progress: a sombre acceptance of human limitations followed from his vision of the dignity of the soul and the burdens of free will. Yet even these proved elusive.

In June 1766 Henry and Hester Thrale unexpectedly called on their new friend Johnson, then in his mid-fifties, and were horrified to find him grovelling before a clergyman, 'beseeching God to continue to him the use of his understanding'. The embarrassed minister fled, whereupon Johnson cried out 'so wildly' in self-condemnation that Henry Thrale 'involuntarily lifted up one hand to shut his mouth'.

He was in the throes of mental collapse. Indeed, for all his renowned John Bull qualities, the great bear was no stranger to depression, that 'general disease of my life'. 'My health has been, from my twentieth year, such as has seldom afforded me a single day of ease,' he reflected in old age, and though he certainly did not escape *physical* ailments – chronic bronchitis, gout, dropsy, a stroke – it was clearly his melancholy which he had in mind.

His spirits first failed him in 1729. Kicking his heels at his parental home (that 'house of discord'), Johnson sank into suicidal lethargy, 'overwhelmed', Boswell put it, 'with an horrible hypochondria, with perpetual irritation, fretfulness and impatience; and with a dejection, gloom and despair, which made existence misery. From this dismal malady he never afterwards was perfectly relieved.' What intensified melancholy's terrors was the clumsy interference of his godfather, Dr Swynfen: the young Johnson was aghast to hear that doctor's prognosis of probable future madness. Profound melancholy crushed him again after the death of his wife Elizabeth (Tetty) in 1753 and then once more during the 1760s. On one occasion in 1764, for example, Dr Adams found him 'in a deplorable state, sighing, groaning, talking to himself, and restlessly walking from room to room'.

Welcomed into the Thrales' household and brightened by Boswell, Johnson enjoyed something of an Indian summer, but even then the spectre of breakdown continued to haunt him. In 1768 he entrusted a padlock to Hester Thrale's care, and three years later jotted in his diary: '*De pedicis et manicis insana cogitatio*' ('an insane thought about fetters and manacles'). Mind-forg'd manacles were paralysing him with fears of ruin and future confinement, culminating in 1773 in a terrible letter written in French to Hester Thrale, begging her to exercise discipline and governance over his 'fancied insanity'.

Johnson saw himself as the victim of a 'vile melancholy, inherited from my father'. 'When I survey my past life,' he confided to his diary on Easter Day 1777, 'I discover nothing but a barren waste of time with some disorders of body and disturbance of the mind, very near to madness.' Such reflections were not incidental flourishes but a regular minor key. Following his exposure of *The Vanity of Human Wishes*, *Rasselas* had been, as we have seen, a sustained anatomy of self-delusion, lacking even *Candide*'s guarded optimism about cultivating gardens; and the lay sermons of the *Rambler* and the *Idler* exposed both the 'vacuity of existence' and the pathology of escapism.

For certain of Johnson's contemporaries, the blues were a treasured identity badge. The new men of feeling prized self-absorbed melancholy as the poet's genius or the spring of sensitivity. Boswell (as we shall see) freely indulged his sensibilities in this direction. Johnson, however, would have no truck with this 'foolish notion that melancholy is a proof of acuteness'; as can be seen in his attack on Soame Jenyns, he detested whatever trivialized real suffering. Boswell might think he could safely cultivate his 'turn for melancholy', because (he had it on medical advice) melancholy was a distemper quite distinct from derangement proper. But Johnson had no such confidence, dreading melancholy as the slippery slope down into the very abyss of lunacy. The distinction was paper-thin – in fact, all in the mind. And, as Hester Thrale pointed out, such fears further fuelled his anxieties: 'Mr Johnson's health had always been bad since I first knew him, and his over-anxious care to retain without blemish the perfect sanity of his mind, contributed much to disturb it.'

Thus Johnson's melancholy was no mere literary caprice, it suffused the man. Everyone found him bizarre: peculiar in bulk, demeanour, gait, reactions. In dubbing him 'a respectable Hottentot', Lord Chesterfield aptly if snootily evoked the wild man within, a caged animal charged with pent-up energy: Ursa Major. Overbearing, dictatorial, truculent, a boor who talked for victory, tossing and goring his adversaries, Johnson united pride with abjection, lethargy (lying abed till the afternoon) with bouts of physical frenzy (an habitual midnight rambler, he was still climbing trees in his fifties). Always 'in extremes', he wolfed down his food ('madmen are all sensual') or was mortifyingly abstinent: what always escaped him was steady moderation.

The strain of living 'in extremes' etched itself onto his very appearance, for all to see. Running into Johnson for the first time, Hogarth 'perceived a person standing at a window in the room shaking his head and rolling himself about in a strange ridiculous manner, and concluded that he was an ideot'. Fanny Burney was no less staggered. 'He is, indeed, very ill-favoured, tall and stout but stoops terribly', she wrote: 'He is almost bent double. His mouth is almost constantly opening and shutting as if he were chewing. He has a strange method of frequently twirling his fingers and twisting his hands. His body is in constant agitation, see-sawing up and down.' By middle age, Johnson had developed a repertoire of fantastic tics, spasms and mannerisms – 'a convulsionary' was Thomas Tyers' verdict, evidently with religious fanatics in mind. 'He often had convulsive starts and odd gesticulations,' observed his stepdaughter, Lucy Porter, 'which tended to excite at once surprise and ridicule' – muttering under his breath, kneading bits of orange peel together, making clucking noises, obsessively fingering posts as he lurched along the street. 'He had another particularity,' added Boswell,

some superstitious habit, which he had contracted early, and from which he had never called upon his reason to disentangle him. This was his anxious care to go out or in at a door or passage, by a certain number of steps from a certain point, or at least so as that either his right or left foot (I am not certain which), should constantly make the first actual movement when he came close to the door or passage.

Johnson was thus riddled with phobias and grotesque compulsions. He even developed superstitions like fretting over adding milk to his tea on Good Friday, and Mrs Thrale sometimes discovered him buried in fantastical arithmetic:

When Mr Johnson felt his fancy, or fancied he felt it, disordered, his constant recurrence was to the study of arithmetic; and one day that he was totally confined to his chamber, and I enquired what he had been doing to divert himself, he showed me a calculation which I could scarce be made to understand, so vast was the plan of it, and so very intricate were the figures: no other indeed than that the national debt, computing it at one hundred and eighty million sterling, would, if converted into silver, serve to make a meridian of that material, I forget how broad, for the globe of the whole earth, the real globe.

Here is a man *sui generis*, deaf to polite mores, oppressed by bugbears: 'The great business of his life', judged Reynolds, 'was to escape from himself; this disposition he considered as the disease of his mind.' For Johnson thought himself prone to derangement: 'I have been mad all my life, at least not sober.' How are we to explain this melancholy?

Common sense suggests a simple solution: no wonder Johnson was odd and melancholy, he had good reason. He was a man apart, scarred from birth by physical stigmata, big-boned and clumsy, blighted by scrofula, half-blind in his left eye and half-deaf in his left ear. Yet he also – overcompensation? – towered above his fellow schoolboys in acuteness, memory, argumentation and powers of speech. Always different, he could not shake off the dread of isolation or the torment of talent thwarted, and his fighting instinct never relaxed. Starting out in life as 'nothing and nobody', hating his Oxonian poverty (where he was 'rude and violent', his companions mistaking his 'bitterness' for 'frolick') but then humiliated by being forced to quit, he spent the bloom of youth adrift and then failed as a schoolmaster. And when he finally found his feet it was by undertaking soul-destroying Grub Street hack-work. In a poignant aside in *The Lives of the English Poets*, he wrote of Pope that he 'was one of those few whose labour is their pleasure'. For Johnson, by contrast, hounded by publishers and creditors, labour was a trial, even a curse; and unlike his erstwhile pupil David Garrick, who had trudged with him to London to seek his fortune, recognition came late to Johnson: 'Slow rises worth, by poverty depress'd,' runs the *leitmotif* of *London.* Until he was in his fifties, he was struggling for life in the water, being arrested at least once for debt, and want dogged him till the granting of his pension. Moreover, after the death of Tetty grief and loneliness became his companions. Proud and combative, Johnson sometimes exulted in a triumph, as in his rasping put-down to Lord Chesterfield; but life always threatened to become stale, flat and wearisome.

Johnson believed his wretchedness, far from being exceptional, was the true human epitome: 'Every man will readily confess that his own condition discontents him.' It was a theme of which he never tired: 'the general lot of mankind is misery,' explained his *Life of Mr Richard Savage*, it is 'the condition of our present state, that pain should be more fixed and permanent than pleasure'; 'life', he instructed Boswell, 'is progress from want to want, not from enjoyment to enjoyment.' So many disappointments rained down as to be bearable only when gilded by pretence: 'The world, in its best state, is nothing more than a large assembly of beings, combining to counterfeit happiness which they do not feel, employing every art and contrivance to embellish life, and to hide their real condition from the eyes of one another.' Did he here betray fear that someone, somewhere, was genuinely happy? But if he was suspiciously swift to prick others' illusions, his scorn for the glib optimism of such coxcombs as Soame Jenyns was surely merited. In *A Free Inquiry into the Nature and Origin of Evil* (1757), Jenyns had argued in favour of the Leibnizian doctrine of cosmic optimism as versified in Pope's *Essay on Man*: all was for the best, and such supposed evils as illness and disability were only apparent, being integral to the grand scheme of benevolence instituted by a omnipotent Deity. Johnson damned Jenyns's views as specious rationalizations which made a mockery of suffering, and exposed such 'philosophy' as trivializing, an insult to real affliction.

Why was Creation so 'full of calamity'? Stupidity, ignorance, greed and tyranny must all shoulder some blame – affording in turn some prospect of remedy (hence his incendiary toast: 'Here's to the next insurrection of the negroes in the West Indies'). But most evil was woven into the very fabric of the post-lapsarian world. For Johnson subscribed to Original Sin – 'the natural depravity of mankind' – and grudgingly respected Mandeville's cynical realism. Asked by Lady Macleod whether man was naturally good (as held by Shaftesbury, Addison and other enlightened thinkers), he snapped, 'No, Madam, no more than a wolf,' an echo of the Hobbesian *homo lupo lupus*, which she found 'worse than Swift' – a response that must have been a sore point with Johnson, since he reviled the Dean's misanthropy ('a life wasted in discontent'), surely seeing too much of himself in that fellow Christian pessimist.

'When an offer was made to Themistocles', *Idler* readers were told, 'of teaching him the art of memory, he answered, that he would rather wish for the art of forgetfulness.' Johnson sympathized: consciousness – of how reality was more to be endured than enjoyed – was indeed a millstone. Johnson was melancholy because the world gave him every reason to be.

True. Yet that was not the whole truth, and not all who trod life's treadmill sank into his intermittent paralysis of the will. Johnson himself recognized that his despondency was not normal; he saw himself as sick, alluding frequently to his 'diseased mind'. So what disease did he have? Various commentators have asserted that his disturbances had an organic seat – and in his *Dictionary* Johnson himself favoured physical aetiologies, defining melancholy as 'a disease, supposed to proceed from a redundance of black bile'. Modern physicians have diagnosed Johnson as suffering from cerebral palsy, epilepsy, De La Tourette's syndrome, or, echoing contemporaries, St Vitus's Dance. It is important, however, not to lose sight of the fact that Johnson himself denied that his tics and mannerisms were somatic. Asked why he made such gestures, he answered: 'from bad habit' – a view borne out by Sir Joshua Reynolds, a member of the Club who wrote a 'Memoir' of Johnson after his death. He judged that 'Dr Johnson's extraordinary gestures were only habits in which he indulged himself at certain times. When in company, where he was not free, or when engaged earnestly in conversation, he never gave way to such habits, which proves that they were not involuntary.'

In truth, Johnson's trouble was basically psychological. He knew the causes well enough. 'Johnson's own sense of the working of the human imagination', Walter Jackson Bate has written, 'probably provides us with the closest anticipation of Freud to be found in psychology or moral writing before the twentieth century'; as an anatomist of the psyche, Johnson was profoundly perceptive. Few paid greater tribute to desire, or saw more clearly that deprivation and frustration reduced people to endless yearning, and that longings themselves festered. How alarmingly did imagination build crazy castles out of its own fictions! How the rationalizing mind masked its true intentions ('we are seldom sure that we sincerely meant what we omitted to do')! No wonder he dreaded the tyranny of dreams, warning Mrs Thrale that she should make her son tell her his dreams: 'the first corruption that entered into my heart was communicated in a dream.' When she tried to draw out of him what it was, he rejoined: 'Do not ask me,' and walked away in agitation.

Attuned thus to the psyche's undercurrents, it is not surprising that Johnson had some inkling of how he was his parents' child: 'I have often heard him lament', wrote Frances Reynolds, 'that he inherited from his Father, a morbid disposition both of Body and Mind. A terrifying melancholy, which he was sometimes apprehensive bordered on insanity.' Problems lurk here: how far was Johnson blaming his father, identifying with him, or excusing himself? Moreover, it is not certain that, however bumbling, henpecked and distant, Michael Johnson was particularly melancholy. But Johnson resented his lack of the right start in life, his physical handicaps being compounded with social inferiority: 'when I was beginning in the world,' he insisted to Fanny Burney, 'I was nothing and nobody.'

It cannot have been a sunny childhood. His parents, recalled Johnson, had little pleasure of each other. They were old when he was born – his father 54, his mother 40 – and remote, and three years later a younger brother, Nathaniel, came along: Johnson's silence about Natty speaks volumes.

Johnson resented his father's slide from affluence and, like Gibbon, loathed being paraded by him like a performing seal for his precocious talents. Later in life, he was overtaken by guilt towards his father, in his seventies performing an extraordinary act of atonement. 'I was disobedient,' he explained to Boswell, refusing to help at his father's bookstall:

Pride was the source of that refusal, and the remembrance of it was painful. A few years ago, I desired to atone for this fault; I went to Uttoxeter in very bad weather, and stood for a considerable time bareheaded in the rain, on the spot where my father's stall used to stand. In contrition I stood, and I hope the penance was expiatory.

And he found his mother petty, impossible to satisfy and punitive. She it was who warned him about hell before his third birthday, and, as he told Boswell, 'Sunday was a heavy day to him when he was young. His mother made him read "The Whole Duty of Man" on that day.' Longer-lived and more demanding, his mother was less easily exorcized. Once installed in London, Johnson did not once make the journey back to Lichfield in the nineteen years which remained of her life. On hearing she was dying, he did not speed to her bedside but plunged into writing *Rasselas*, exculpating himself by earmarking the proceeds for her funeral. If he felt love for her, it was clearly a devotion overlaid and warped by other emotions; not once in his diaries and prayers did he call her 'dearest', though commonly using the term for his female friends. His unresolved relations with her may have influenced his choice of a wife twenty-one years his senior, and led to his habit of filling his house with such dependants as the blind and grumpy Anna Williams, surrogate parents to care for by way of penance.

Johnson was preoccupied by idleness. It had of course been yoked with melancholy in medicine and culture ever since Antiquity, and the Church held sloth (*acedia*) to be one of the deadly sins. Johnson's experiences were doubtless coloured by such traditional associations, but they also deviated from the mainstream in important ways. If the *Rambler* and *Idler* followed Addison and Steele in painting a sick parade of the idle rich, it was in a completely different register that Johnson's mental health was threatened. Idleness was not having nothing to do, but being unable to face having to do too much, under the unforgiving rebuke of the text Johnson had engraved on his watch and doubtless also on his mind: 'that night cometh, when no man can work.' Johnson was no Chesterfieldian man of leisure, with time on his side, enjoying a balanced diet of recreation. Quite the reverse; in the prime of life, pride and poverty had driven him into gargantuan projects, writing the parliamentary reports and reams of other journalism for the *Gentleman's Magazine*, compiling his *Dictionary*, producing whole magazines single-handedly, churning out the lives of the poets and editing Shakespeare. His daily bread was monstrous toil, menial, grinding, against the clock; the lexicographer was indeed a drudge. Mutinying against the humdrum, tedious and burdensome, and with few personal comforts, Johnson's psyche was sorely tempted by idleness.

And he fought such seductive sirens. 'To have the management of the mind', he told Boswell, 'is a great art, and it may be attained in a considerable degree by experience and habitual exercise.' But could he attain it himself? It was a dilemma he dramatized through the character of 'Sober' in the *Idler*. A man of 'strong desires and quick imagination', 'Sober' seeks solace in 'love of ease', particularly in 'conversation; there is no end of his talk or his attention; . . . for he . . . is free for the time from his own reproaches'. The cameo pictured no Horatian happy mean in sight for the subject of this obvious self-portrayal. 'Sober's' desires and imagination 'will not suffer him to lie quite at rest', but rather leave him 'weary of himself'. Above all, he cannot bear to be alone with his thoughts. For 'there is one time at night when he must go home, that his friends may sleep; and another time in the morning, when all the world agrees to shut out interruption. These are the moments which poor Sober trembles at the thought.' Johnson precisely.

Fleeing from toil, left to his own devices, his conscience would begin corrosive self-accusations, arraigning himself for shilly-shallying, wasting his life, and sinking into vacuity. Thus the temptations of escape from daily despair ended in further paralysis. 'My indolence, since my last reception of the Sacrament,' he confessed to his diary on 21 April 1765, 'has sunk into grosser sluggishness, and my dissipation spread into wilder negligence. . . . A kind of strange oblivion has overspread me, so that I know not what has become of the last year.' Self-reproach became the signature of his life. His diary for 7 April 1776 reads: 'My reigning sin, to which perhaps many others are appendant, is waste of time.' And resolutions of reform littered his pilgrim's way like accusing signposts ever since, as early as his twentieth year, he had chivvied himself: 'I bid farewell to Sloth.'

Johnson dreaded idleness so powerfully because it handed a blank cheque to the demons of imagination. The 'vacancies of life' thereby activated the old peripatetic principle that 'Nature abhors a vacuum', crowding the unoccupied brain with 'vain imaginations'.

Johnson was obviously perturbed by the content of the phantasms streaming into his head. Soon after Tetty's death he referred to being 'depraved with vain imaginations' (sexual fantasies). Beseeching God to 'purify my thoughts from pollutions', he was relieved to find at Easter 1753 that at church he was not 'once distracted by the thoughts of any other woman'. Over the years he was to brood guiltily on the past, and wishfully about the future: 'no mind is much employed upon the present,' reflects Imlac in *Rasselas*, 'recollection and anticipation fill up almost all our moments.'

But Johnson's terror did not lie simply in *what* he imagined, but in the very act of surrender to intrusive fictions and fantasies. Driven by the 'hunger of imagination', he dreaded succumbing to a never-never land of wishes. Open the sluice-gates to the fancy and he would drown in make-believe. At times he feared such a fate was actually overtaking him, as his self-control began to buckle: 'I had formerly great command of my attention,' he wrote in 1772, 'and what I did not like could forbear to think. But of this power which is of the highest importance to the tranquillity of life, I have for some time past been so much exhausted.'

The mad astronomer episode in *Rasselas* is Johnson's imaginative exploration of this doom. The sage's solitary fantasizings about the heavens have turned monstrous, his yearnings for knowledge have swollen into *idées fixes*: 'All other intellectual gratifications are rejected,' explains Imlac,

the mind, in weariness of leisure, recurs constantly to the favourite conception, and feasts on the luscious falsehood whenever she is offended with the
bitterness of truth. By degrees the reign of fancy is confirmed; she grows
first imperious, and in time despotic. Then fictions begin to operate as
realities, false opinions fasten upon the mind, and life passes in dreams of
rapture or of anguish.

Johnson was thus haunted by dread that his 'mind corrupted with an inveterate disease of wishing' would cease to be under his control, in defiance of God's command.

The dread of fantasy supplanting reality, the rule of reason over-thrown by the dictatorship of delusion, was not, of course, uniquely Johnsonian – far from it. He was, among other things, introspecting within a paradigm of insanity brought into focus and prominence by Locke's *Essay concerning Human Understanding* (discussed in Chapter 4). Madness, as Chapter 18 will explore, had traditionally been regarded as stemming either from constitutional imbalance of the humours, particularly black bile, from ruling passions or from diabolical pos-session. Locke, by contrast, contended that it was essentially a ques-tion of intellectual *delusion*, the capture of the mind by false ideas concatenated into a logical system of unreality. Because knowledge sprang from sensations, ideas accurately reflecting reality had to be gradually pieced together out of fragmentary sensations, and were hence at best probable and provisional. The scope was huge for mistaken sensations or false associations, warped by fear, hope or other passions, to occlude the mind with error. While not using precisely his terminology, Johnson endorsed Locke's view that mad-ness was essentially 'in the mind', being consequential upon 'volun-tary delusion'. The sleep of reason allowed the fancy to spawn monsters. It was a prospect which tallied with his traditional Christian sense of human frailty, and his distrust of egoism, pride and presumption: 'There is no man whose imagination does not sometimes predominate over his reason, who can regulate this attention wholly by his will, and whose ideas will come and go at his command. . . . All power of fancy over reason is a degree of insanity.'

It was precisely this despotism of imagination which haunted Johnson. Indulging idleness to escape the gloomy round would prove but a leap out of the frying pan. Impressed early in life by *The Anatomy of Melancholy*, he knew the wisdom of Burton's adage, 'Be not solitary, be not idle', advising *Rambler* readers that 'that mind will never be vacant, which is frequently recalled by stated duties to meditations on eternal interests'. Otherwise a descent was in the offing: 'Idleness produces necessity, necessity incites to wickedness, and wickedness again supplies the means of living in idleness.'

Johnson was thus ensnared. Incapable through poverty, situation and temperament of assimilating himself into genteel leisure, unable to meld learning and sociability in Addisonian moderation, he lurched from melancholy toil to melancholy indolence, fearing all the time that that way madness lay.

Why could Johnson not drag himself out of this slough of despond? The answer lies in that religion which might, for another man, have been his lifeline. Johnson's melancholy was ultimately religious melancholy. Religion, after all, was in his blood. His mother had dinned *The Whole Duty of Man* into him in early childhood, that work of piety spreading its vision of sinful man humbled by a God of Justice, omnipotent and vengeful, dictating duties for man to obey, without respite, to stay his sin. This message – which young Sam resented, leading to scoffing in his teens – finally seized his heart when he was 'overmatched' at the age of 20 by William Law's *A Serious Call to a Devout and Holy Life*. Under this rule of Law, Johnson was to remain to the end of his days overawed by the terrors of sin, death and damnation.

He could not get death off his mind. 'Is not the fear of death natural to man?' Boswell asked him, equally death-obsessed. 'So much so, Sir,' replied his mentor, 'that the whole of life is but to keep away the thoughts of it.' Johnson strove mightily enough to fend it off. Sometimes, when Boswell raised the issue, he bellowed him down. Little things triggered great fears. When Bennet Langton drew up his will, Johnson made hysterical sport of him all day. Being 'of dreadful things the most dreadful', as he put it in the *Rambler*, the fear of death was naturally 'the great disturber of human quiet'. Johnson's dread of extinction became obsessive, and, as he well knew, it ate the soul: 'Fear, whether natural or acquired, when once it has full possession of the fancy, never fails to employ it upon visions of calamity, such as, if they are not dissipated by useful employment, will soon overcast it with horrors, and embitter life.'

Christianity gave Johnson the prospect of managing mortality, a revelation of triumph over the Grim Reaper, an earnest of life eternal. But only at a terrible price, that of obeying William Law's injunction to keep the mind so 'possessed with such a sense of [death's] nearness that you may have it always in your thoughts'. Perpetually thinking about death was harrowing. For Johnson's was a God of wrath: 'The quiver of Omnipotence is stored with arrows, against which the shield of human virtue, however adamantine it has been boasted, is held up in vain.' God racked mankind with superhuman duties, and punished the sinful by damning them. And when, in the midst of a conversation in Oxford, recorded by Boswell, the 'amiable' Dr Adams reminded him that God was infinitely good – it was all to no avail:

JOHNSON. 'That he is infinitely good, as far as the perfection of his nature will allow, I certainly believe; but it is necessary for good upon the whole, that individuals should be punished. As to an *individual*, therefore, he is not infinitely good; and as I cannot be *sure* that I have fulfilled the conditions on which salvation is granted, I am afraid I may be one of those who shall be damned.' (looking dismally.) DR. ADAMS. 'What do you mean by damned?' JOHNSON. (passionately and loudly) 'Sent to Hell, Sir, and punished everlastingly:' DR. ADAMS. 'I don't believe that doctrine.' JOHNSON. 'Hold, Sir, do you believe that some will be punished at all?' DR. ADAMS. 'Being excluded from Heaven will be a punishment: yet there may be no great positive suffering.'

We have already encountered the rising debate over the eternity of hell. No less alarmed than Johnson, Boswell could not resist following the question up, searching for consolation: 'But may not a man attain to such a degree of hope as not to be uneasy from the fear of death?'

JOHNSON. 'A man may have such a degree of hope as to keep him quiet. You see I am not quiet, from the vehemence with which I talk; but I do not despair.' MRS. ADAMS. 'You seem, Sir, to forget the merits of our Redeemer.' JOHNSON. 'Madam, I do not forget the merits of my Redeemer; but my Redeemer has said that he will set some on his right hand and some on his left.' – He was in gloomy agitation, and said, 'I'll have no more on't.'

It is a rather shocking exchange. *Timor mortis conturbat me* obviously applied just as strongly to Johnson as it did to any medieval poet or preacher; and much as he might have wished to embrace a less awful option, he clearly feared that his companions' more liberal doctrines revealed not just a denial of Scripture but man's sorry capacity for self-deception. Indeed, he was eternally suspicious of all convictions of a better future, which he was apt to dismiss as 'visionary'.

For Johnson the possibility of hell was at least preferable to the probability of oblivion. The wavering Boswell was less certain, and on one occasion he 'endeavoured to maintain that the fear of it might be got over' by rather tactlessly bringing up the opinions of Johnson's *bête noire*, the sceptic and unbeliever David Hume:

I told him that David Hume said to me, he was no more uneasy to think he should *not be* after his life, than that he *had not been* before he began to exist. JOHNSON. 'Sir, if he really thinks so, his perceptions are disturbed; he is mad; if he does not think so, he lies. . . .' BOSWELL. 'Foote, Sir, told me, that when he was very ill he was not afraid to die.' JOHNSON. 'It is not true, Sir. Hold a pistol to Foote's breast, or to Hume's breast, and threaten to kill them, and you'll see how they behave.' BOSWELL. 'But may we not fortify our minds for the approach of death' . . .

How dare Boswell of all people lecture Johnson about the need to strengthen his mind!

To deny the fear of dying was, for Johnson, hypocrisy, bluster or madness. When a certain Mrs Knowles tried to hearten him, saying that death was but 'the gate of life', Johnson insisted 'No rational man can die without uneasy apprehension'. She did her best:

Mrs. Knowles. 'The Scriptures tell us, "The Righteous shall have *hope* in his death".' Johnson. 'Yes, Madam; that is, he shall not have despair. But, consider, his hope of salvation must be founded on the terms on which it is promised that the mediation of our Saviour shall be applied to us, – namely, obedience, and where obedience has failed, then, as suppletory to it, repentance. But what man can say that his obedience has been such, as he would approve of in another, or even in himself upon close examination, or that his repentance has not been such as to require being repented of? No man can be sure that his obedience and repentance will obtain salvation.' ... Boswell. 'Then, Sir, we must be contented to acknowledge that death is a terrible thing.' Johnson. 'Yes, Sir, I have made no approaches to a state which can look on it as not terrible.' Mrs. Knowles (seeming to enjoy a pleasing serenity in the persuasion of benignant divine light): 'Does not St. Paul say, "I have fought the good fight of faith, I have finished my course; henceforth is laid up for me a crown of life"?' Johnson. 'Yes, Madam; but here was a man inspired, a man who had been converted by supernatural interposition.' Boswell. 'In prospect death is dreadful; but in fact we find that people die easy.' Johnson. 'Why, Sir, most people have not *thought* much of the matter, so cannot *say* much, and it is supposed they die easy. Few believe it certain they are then to die; and those who do, set themselves to behave with resolution, as a man does who is going to be hanged: – he is not the less unwilling to be hanged.' Miss Seward. 'There is one mode of the fear of death, which is certainly absurd: and that is the dread of annihilation, which is only a pleasing sleep without a dream.' Johnson. 'It is neither pleasing, nor sleep; it is nothing. Now mere existence is so much better than nothing, that one would rather exist even in pain, than not exist.'

The views of the pious Mrs Knowles – that God had set out in the Bible the prospects of a future existence secured through Christ's sacrifice – Johnson's brain no doubt subscribed to. But his gut reaction was to resist the reassurance, presumably because of his profound suspicion of being taken in by what, in others, he would have dismissed as false hopes, sentimentality or muddle-headedness.

Yet did not Johnson himself often clutch at straws? That is evident, for example, in his ardent but old-fashioned belief in spirits, ghosts and other signs of the supernatural – precisely as upheld a century earlier by the likes of Henry More, Joseph Glanvill and Robert Boyle. By Johnson's lifetime such views were considered archaic, plebeian, fanciful or Methodistical. Johnson, by contrast, battled against those who, in that enlightened age, argued the diabolical and spiritual away. As recorded by Boswell in his *Journal of a Tour of the Hebrides* (1785), he was having supper with some of the leading Scottish *literati*:

Mr. Crosbie said, he thought it the greatest blasphemy to suppose evil spirits counteracting the Deity, and raising storms, for instance, to destroy his creatures. – JOHNSON. 'Why, sir, if moral evil be consistent with the government of the Deity, why may not physical evil be also consistent with it? It is not more strange that there should be evil spirits, than evil men: evil unembodied spirits, than evil embodied spirits. And as to storms, we know there are such things; and it is no worse that evil spirits raise them, than that they rise.' – CROSBIE. 'But it is not credible, that witches should have effected what they are said in stories to have done.' – JOHNSON. 'Sir, I am not defending their credibility. . . . You must take evidence: you must consider, that wise and great men have condemned witches to die.' – CROSBIE. 'But an act of parliament put an end to witchcraft.' – JOHNSON. 'No, sir; witchcraft had ceased; and therefore an act of parliament was passed to prevent persecution for what was not witchcraft.'

Johnson was thus desperate to believe. But the belief which became imprinted on him was that of the onerousness of God's 'call', a *via crucis* of religious duties – prayers, fasting, church attendance, Bible reading, soul-searching – from which he equally continually shied away, because they all brought him inescapably face-to-face with his own worthlessness, not least his 'idleness'. Objectively, Johnson's morbid anxiety about wasting time was completely irrational and makes sense only under the ultimata of religious terrorism, under the lash of a divine taskmaster. With prayer upon prayer he abased himself: 'O Lord, enable me by thy Grace to use all diligence in redeeming the time which I have spent in Sloth, Vanity, and wickedness.' But successive promises of reformation only exposed his inability to amend. The demands were superhuman: how could he rise at six, as he continually pledged, when the dread insomnia kept him awake till deep into the early hours? How could he be dutiful in soul-searching when it brought to light nothing but fresh proofs of wickedness? In turn this produced more guilt, further confessions of 'manifold sins and negligences', spawning yet more 'oppressive terrors'.

Religion thus proved a torment, and Johnson never found peace. Mrs Thrale knew it only too well. As she perceived, it was precisely Johnson's religion which triggered his fears of madness: 'daily terror lest he had not done enough originated in piety, but ended in little less than disease. . . . He . . . filled his imagination with fears that he should ever obtain forgiveness of remission of duty and criminal waste of time.' And Johnson himself was helplessly aware how he made rods for his own back, notably by his 'scruples'. To assuage guilt, strengthen his resolve and placate the Deity, Johnson habitually bound himself by vows, which he called 'scruples'. As with his nervous tics and mannerisms, these resolutions temporarily relieved tension and acted as charms against further backslidings. But they too had their revenges. For the very act of making them created guilt, aware as he was of their superstitious, quasi-magical nature ('a vow is a horrible thing . . . a snare for sin'); and he was still guiltier about not keeping them: 'I have resolved till I am afraid to resolve again,' he confessed, in despair, in 1761.

Johnson was utterly tenacious of his reason; nothing meant more to him. People of other temperaments or convictions could ache for its eclipse, but Johnson's creed forbade such euthanasia of the spirit, since he believed it his cardinal responsibility to 'render up my soul to God unclouded'. He consistently esteemed the mind infinitely above the body. The physical was as nothing: 'I would consent to have a limb amputated,' he characteristically confided to Dr Adams, 'to recover my low spirits.' When he suffered a stroke, his real fear was for his mental powers, which he tested by composing a thematic Latin prayer:

> Summe Pater, quodcunque tuum de corpore Numen
>> Hoc statuat, precibus Christus adesse velit;
> Ingenio parcas, nec sit mihi culpa rogasse,
>> Qua solum potero parte, placere tibi.

('Almighty Father, whatever the divine Will ordains concerning this body of mine, may Christ be willing to aid me with his prayers. And let it not be blameworthy on my part to implore that thou spare my reason, by which faculty alone I shall be able to do thy pleasure'.)

Johnson gave up the medically prescribed opiates on his deathbed, to pass over with his mind clear.

Religion thus made the mind a jewel of infinite price, confirming Johnson's intuition that whatever he was, he was it through his mind. But he also knew only too well that 'of the uncertainties of our present state, the most dreadful is the uncertain continuance of reason'. And it was religious terrors precisely which raised those storms that risked his reason. With what enormous pathos of other possible lives unlived we find him writing: 'If I had no duties, and no reference to futurity, I would spend my life in driving briskly in a post-chaise with a pretty woman, but she should be one who could understand me, and would add something to the conversation.'

Johnson had a truly remarkable memory; no one read more widely and loved conversation and controversy. It was through the breadth and depth of his mind that he vindicated his existence to himself. Famously, when Oliver Goldsmith suggested that his Club should be broadened on the ground that 'there can be nothing new among us: we have travelled over one another's minds', Johnson was indignant, retorting: 'Sir, you have not travelled over *my* mind, I promise you.' Johnson thus represents the putative triumph of mind over body, but one which never freed itself from the paralysing fear of extinction.

*

The life of James Boswell offers an interesting pendant to that of his hero. The son of a pious Presbyterian mother and a domineering, authoritarian father, Boswell, like Johnson, had etched onto his infant imagination a Calvinist message of human sinfulness and divine punishment, from whose terrors he desperately tried to escape.

Seeking diversion, he came to London in his early twenties, aspiring to be a man of fashion, a man of the world, a man of letters. The tensions between his early indoctrination and his emancipatory aspirations explain his repeated bouts of frantic sexual release and the worsening drinking problem recorded in the journals he kept from the 1760s. He suffered nineteen bouts of the clap up to his death – indeed, he probably died of complications from those disorders.

In a man sprung from an ancient Scottish family, enjoying some professional success and blessed with a fragrant wife, such recklessness surely suggests that Boswell was driven by compulsive psychological forces, and by an equal compulsion to record his experiences. Returning to London, for instance, in November 1762, he made a beeline for his previous partners, but they had all flown. So he had to look elsewhere, as he confided to his journal on 25 November – only this time he meant to take precautions, going into amatory battle 'in armour', that is, wearing a condom:

I was really unhappy for want of women . . . I picked up a girl in the Strand; went into a court with intention to enjoy her in armour. But she had none. I toyed with her. She wondered at my size, and said if I ever took a girl's maidenhead, I would make her squeak. I gave her a shilling and had enough command of myself to go without touching her. I afterwards trembled at the danger I had escaped.

This was only the beginning of a career, too extensive to chronicle here, devoted to whoring, accompanied by that passion for alcohol celebrated in his published essays. 'I do fairly acknowledge that I love Drinking,' he wrote in one of his journalistic efforts, 'that I have a constitutional inclination to indulge in fermented liquors, and that if it were not for the restraints of reason and religion I am afraid I should be as constant a votary of Bacchus as any man.' It was, in fact, alcoholism which hastened his death.

Like Johnson, Boswell was tortured by a fundamental fear of death. He sought reassurance of any kind from anyone. He harassed the dying David Hume. The sceptical *philosophe*'s calm at his impending demise from liver cancer drove Boswell ever more distraught: he wanted to see in the unbeliever the fear which gripped himself. In vain he tried to make Hume reveal some spark of faith. At the sceptic's imperviousness, Boswell became increasingly desperate:

I . . . felt a degree of horror, mixed with a sort of wild, strange, hurrying recollection of my excellent mother's pious instructions, of Dr. Johnson's noble lessons, and of my religious sentiments and affections during the course of my life. I was like a man in sudden danger eagerly seeking his defensive arms.

The thought of somebody dying without dread was unbearable.

Boswell was irresistibly drawn to public executions. Such solemn occasions called to mind the reality of death – they were meant to – yet they were also fascinating to him. With voyeuristic horror, he felt compelled to see what actually happened as living human flesh became a lifeless corpse. Afterwards, he would be driven to drinking and whoring in hopes of obliterating these sights and their phantoms from his mind.

Desperately seeking escape from the lessons of his upbringing and hoping to reinvent himself, Boswell wrote himself endless instructions, telling himself who to be. Basically, he wished always to be Boswell, the sum total of his moments of consciousness – there lay the proto-Romantic in him – but he was never certain of his own nature for long. Insecure in his hold on his identity, he sought figures from whom he could draw strength and other qualities which would define and enhance him. 'Be vigorous. Be Temple,' he adjured himself (Temple was a close friend). And he had many such models, who were remarkably various. Johnson was to the fore. But so were Addison, Steele, Shakespeare, Isaac Walton, Donne and Demosthenes (we remember

Cornelius Scriblerus's wishes for his son). Nor did he confine himself to actual persons – over and again, Boswell cast himself in fictional roles. Now he was the hero of a novel, now 'a morose don' or an amorous Spaniard, now a man of pleasure, a castaway, an officer on campaign, or even Prince Hal. Above all, Captain Macheath, the highwayman hero of *The Beggar's Opera*, exercised a perennial fascination over him. A prisoner whom Boswell visited on the eve of his execution was described as 'just a Macheath. He was dressed in a white coat and blue silk vest and silver, with his hair neatly queued and silver-laced hat, smartly cocked.' The hanging the next day of this dashing figure so depressed Boswell that he could not sleep alone, and he shared a bed with his friend Erskine. But Macheath, if not the felon, was to rise again in the person of Boswell, who, for an evening, styled himself 'Macdonald' and took two streetwalkers to a tavern. Partly facetiously, but seriously as well, Boswell thus tried on a wardrobe of togs and accessories, so as to make his mark as a player on the stage of life.

Another form of instruction was the 'Inviolable plan' Boswell wrote out to curb the terrible bout of melancholy he suffered on arrival in Utrecht: 'Learn *retenue*. Pray do. Don't forget in Plan . . . Read your Plan every morning regularly at breakfast, and when you travel, carry it in trunk. Get commonplace book . . . The more and oftener the restraint, the better. Be steady.' Under the instructions of Johnson, he told himself that control was paramount: 'what may be innocent to others is a fault to you till you attain more command of yourself. Temperance is very necessary for you, so never indulge your appetites without restraint.'

Boswell wanted to make a gentleman of himself, but also knew that this was a role, and he recognized the near impossibility of carrying it off. One consequence was that on beginning to write a newspaper column, he styled himself *The Hypochondriack*. Hypochondria spelt that supersensitivity of mind and feelings which gave Boswell his sense of superiority, and would thus make him part of an élite authorized to comment on the human condition.

Just as Johnson suffered from the 'black dog', Boswell, too, had long periods in which his mind was dominated by depression. Whereas Johnson, however, advocated fighting it, Boswell was more inclined, characteristically in the newer age of sensibility, to wallow and glory in it, as proof of membership of the fashionable culture of suffering and supersensitivity. Johnson was moralistic about melancholy, Boswell, by contrast, self-revelatory. In one extraordinary essay, he confessed that, though he was in the depths of depression, he would share it with his readers, so as to relieve himself, demonstrate his candour – or maybe even help them understand their own condition:

The Hypochondriack is himself at this moment in a state of very dismal depression, so that he cannot be supposed capable of instructing or entertaining his readers. But after keeping them company as a periodical essayist for three years, he considers them as his friends, and trusts that they will treat him with a kindly indulgence. . . .

Instead of giving this month an essay published formerly, of which I have a few, that after a proper revision I intend to adopt into this series, I have a mind to try what I can write in so wretched a frame of mind; as there may perhaps be some of my unhappy brethren just as ill as myself, to whom it may be soothing to know that I now write at all.

In Boswell may be seen the new intense, introspective, self-revelatory identity of the late Enlightenment. The imperfections of self are no longer, as in Johnson, being fought, but are being exposed and, perhaps, enjoyed.

I I

EDWARD GIBBON:
FAME AND MORTALITY

The life of the historian must be short and precarious.

EDWARD GIBBON

As well as being the author of the monumental *Decline and Fall of the Roman Empire*, which appeared in six volumes between 1776 and 1788, Edward Gibbon was the historian of a different, but no less taxing, subject: himself. His *magnum opus* complete, he soon turned autobiographer – indeed, several times over, for he produced six different drafts of his memoirs, and several further fragments besides, between 1788 and 1793. Had he not been cut off prematurely by death at the age of 56 in the following year, the autobiography might well have proliferated, becoming ever more unfinished, out-Shandying *Tristram Shandy*. The historian of Rome evidently found imagining himself trickier than appraising an empire.

Why? As a historian, Gibbon stated himself honour-bound to present his life, both to himself and to the supposed public, so as to meet the scholar's criterion of 'naked, unblushing truth, the first virtue of more serious history'. But he was evidently also intent upon crafting a psychologically gratifying version of the self, painting a canvas which presented a favourable, even flattering, face to the world which made sense to its author of his own existence. It was to be warts and all, but the warts had to be good ones. Not least, Gibbon felt obliged, at the outset, to justify so vain an undertaking as autobiographizing: what made man unique in Creation, he explained, were the powers of memory and the recognition of one's wider place in time and space, within the grand scheme of things:

Our imagination is always active to enlarge the narrow circle in which Nature has confined us. Fifty or an hundred years may be alotted to an individual; but we stretch forwards beyond death with such hopes as Religion and Philosophy will suggest, and we fill up the silent vacancy that precedes our birth by associating ourselves to the authors of our existence.

Gibbon the author needed to situate himself amid 'the authors of [his] existence': to know his place – 'beyond death' included – helped to transcend it. By contributing to commemoration, autobiography was an assertion of the dignity of man, or a proper expression of self-esteem. Such a sentiment could have come from Johnson and, like him, Gibbon believed that one of the duties and privileges of the classically educated man lay in enlarging the mind, soaring above the vulgar immediacy of the here and now and triumphing over mortality.

Unlike Johnson, however, Gibbon was a man of the Enlightenment, specifically an unbeliever. Whereas the former's sense of self was gloomy – and rightly so, he would have insisted, given man's fallen state – the latter was disposed, temperamentally and philosophically, to optimism, albeit an optimism cloaked in the defensive and distancing self-mockery which was second nature to the 'lord of irony'. Adopting an upbeat stance justified the course of a far from conventional existence. The brave or strained cheerfulness of the *Memoirs* attempted to digest a rather wayward life into a coherent teleology, a well-constructed drama with a beginning and a middle (if the end was judiciously left open). In justifying the ways of Gibbon to the world, the author of his being wished to convey the sense that, against the odds, the pieces had all fallen into place. Apparent false starts and dead ends all had their reward, nothing had been wasted. The 'all is for the best'-ism of Pope's *Essay on Man* –

> All Nature is but art unknown to thee
> All chance direction which thou can'st not see –

was here applied to the historian's life, with the autobiographer arrogating to himself God's position of narrative omniscience. Young

Gibbon blundered his way through his early years, but some higher destiny (if scripted only by a picaresque sense of artistic form) was guiding him through the vicissitudes of things. Deceptive in informality and irony, this was autobiography in the mock-heroic, Olympian mode, with the author standing back from himself, in the autumn of life, objectively to vindicate his existence.

The autobiographer's task was in this case made simpler yet more taxing by the fact that Gibbon could not be of public interest except as the author of the *Decline and Fall* – he was hardly a man known for military or amatory conquests or for memorable opinions *à la* Johnson – he was a poor conversationalist – and a parliamentary career which involved not a single speech would have had little more than curiosity value. What any reader would want to know was what fitted him to write such a sublime work. He had the sense to recognize that therein lay the mystery and fascination of his life.

Hence Gibbon informs us, without further ado, that he is writing 'the history of my own mind', a phrase pregnant with Lockean (or Sternean) associations. 'The public is always curious', he opens confidently, or seeking to reassure himself, 'to *know* the men who have left behind them any image of their minds.' How did that mind become so stocked and skilled that it could produce a masterpiece? This is what he would relate, 'that one day his mind will be familiar to the grandchildren of those who are yet unborn'.

The making of Gibbon's mind was not as one might expect: there was no lengthy and meticulous apprenticeship, such as that enjoyed by Milton. Surprisingly, the *Memoirs* tell of a Shandean chapter of accidents: a tale of a curious infancy which grew odder as childhood slipped into adolescence. Neglected by his inattentive parents (Gibbon conveys his sense of grievance that they were inordinately wrapped up in each other) and brought up through a string of haphazard expedients, he became a freakish child, shown off by his father for his precocity in abstruse scholarship ('my sleep has been disturbed by the difficulty of reconciling the Septuagint with the Hebrew computation'). Packed off at the age of 14 to university by a proud but perplexed father, 'I arrived at Oxford with a stock of erudition that might have puzzled a Doctor, and a degree of ignorance of which a school boy would have been ashamed'. His comically absurd Oxford adventures – they are worthy of Evelyn Waugh – and above all his sense of even more grievous neglect then 'bewildered' him into the 'errors of the Church of Rome'. That blundering religious conversion brought his expulsion from an Alma Mater which was no more a mother to him than his real mother, followed by the Swiss exile dictated by his apoplectic father. The ministrations of Monsieur Pavilliard, his tutor in Lausanne, finally gave him his long overdue formal education (how odd to get one's drilling in Locke in Switzerland!). And much more besides which was strange followed in a chequered tale that led up to the historian's fateful decision: 'It was at Rome on the fifteenth of October 1764, as I sat musing amidst the ruins of the Capitol while the barefooted fryars were singing Vespers in the temple of Jupiter, that the idea of writing the decline and fall of the City first started to my mind.' Accident upon accident, yet something predestined too: 'my own religious folly, my father's blind resolution produced the effects of the most deliberate wisdom.' It was that blend of forces which propelled the Roman Empire, too.

A motif thus emerges which artistically shapes the *Memoirs*: apparent mishaps, mistakes or setbacks all work out for the best: waywardness and inadvertence produce order, every cloud has a silver lining, every mischance is a blessing in disguise. Indeed, by way of a pre-emptive strike, so as not to tempt fate, or critics, Gibbon presented himself as a lucky man. 'I have drawn a high prize in the lottery of life,' he declared:

The far greater part of the globe is overspread with barbarism or slavery: in the civilized world the most numerous class is condemned to ignorance and poverty; and the double fortune of my birth in a free and enlightened country in an honourable and wealthy family is the lucky chance of an unit against millions.

Lacking official providential guidance, the unbeliever's life is salvaged by good fortune.

The *Memoirs* laid bare the logic of events: the most unlikely or (at first sight) unpropitious events contributed to create the optimal circumstances, environment and stimulus for ripening his mind and forwarding his initially unrecognized grand project. He even benefited, he tells us, from the most improbable escapade in the life of that diminutive (four feet eight inches) fat man known unkindly as 'Mr Chubby-Chub', his spell in the militia: 'The discipline and evolutions of a modern battalion gave me a clearer notion of the Phalanx and the Legion, and the Captain of the Hampshire grenadiers (the reader may smile) has not been useless to the historian of the Roman Empire.' Gibbon frequently needed to induce a smile, so as to disarm resistance to his none too likable characteristics, notably his barely veiled and rather ruthless egoism.

Having slipped the clutches of Oxford and Catholicism, Gibbon explained his escape from the entanglements of matrimony when his father in effect vetoed his proposed union with Suzanne Curchod ('I sighed as a lover, I obeyed as a son'); and some years later a timely parental demise once again rescued him from the prospect of 'penury' and gave him sufficient income to buy the time and books needed for composition. Great works of literature, the historian realistically if self-justifyingly insists, require the right support-systems – those he inherits or carves out for himself:

Yet I may believe and even assert that in circumstances more indigent or more wealthy, I should never have accomplished the task, or acquired the fame, of an historian; that my spirit would have been broken by poverty and contempt; and that my industry might have been relaxed in the labour and luxury of a superfluous fortune. Few works of merit and importance have been executed either in a garret or a palace.

In a word, his life-story turned out to be a tale of growing autonomy, flowering into the independent self. If the attention given in the *Memoirs* to childhood shows that Gibbon bought Locke's notion that early years were crucial in personality formation, he certainly did not subscribe to the fashionable sentimentalization of childhood as an age of innocence – 'where ignorance is bliss, 'tis folly to be wise', sang Thomas Gray: 'I am tempted', countered Gibbon, 'to enter a protest against the trite and lavish praise of the happiness of our boyish years, which is echoed with so much affectation in the World. That happiness I have never known; that time I have never regretted.' Gibbon painted his life as a deliverance from childhood dependence into the freedom which came with mental maturity. The death of his father, the consequent acquisition of an independent income (fortune was his fortune), and the establishment of a position in the world together provided the platform for his adult achievements: 'Freedom is the first wish of our heart; freedom is the first blessing of our nature: and, unless we bind ourselves with the voluntary chains of interest or passion, we advance in freedom as we advance in years.'

Gibbon thus represents himself primarily as a man of intellect, and his autobiographical artistry shows how that mind had achieved autonomy, and how, by accident and design, luck and judgement, it had been destined for authorship. And what of the body in this fashioning of the self? Matters physical are strictly subordinate to the true business of his life: as a child 'the dynasties of Assyria and Egypt were my top and cricket ball', and thus it remained: he had no bodily attractiveness, sporting prowess or martial honours to boast.

'The pains and pleasures of the body how important soever to ourselves are an indelicate topic of conversation,' he confides and, respecting matters corporeal, he wanted discreetly to draw the curtain. Gibbon evidently felt less than comfortable about his body, and the *Memoirs* resort to distancing, ironizing, self-exculpatory evasion when matters of the flesh crop up. He will not, unlike certain autobiographers, he promises the reader, document in nauseating detail all his youthful ailments, nor will he emulate Montaigne's preoccupation with his every bowel motion. The obligation to 'naked, unblushing truth' did not extend to the whole truth. And yet, the very act of mentioning such unmentionables drew attention to them; and in truth his *Memoirs* proudly dwelt on the plethora of childhood illnesses from which he suffered. His beloved aunt, Miss Catherine Porten – 'the true mother of my mind' –

has often told me with tears in her eyes, how I was nearly starved by a nurse that had lost her milk: how long she herself was apprehensive lest my crazy frame, which is now of common shape should remain for ever crooked and deformed. From one dangerous malady, the small-pox, I was indeed rescued by the practice of inoculation. . . . I was successively afflicted by lethargies and feavers; by opposite tendencies to a consumptive and a dropsical habit; by a contraction of my nerves, a fistula in my eye, and the bite of a dog most vehemently suspected of madness.

In short, the boy 'swallowed more Physic than food', and the preservation of our young hero (how like the Shandean homunculus!) from turning into an 'illiterate cripple' was almost miraculous. While protesting that he did not 'wish to expatiate on so disgusting a topic', he nonetheless insisted that the 'school of learning' was less familiar to him than 'the bed of sickness'.

As ever, however, such calamities proved fortunate. It was this bed of sickness which gave him the leisure to indulge in that 'free desultory reading' which 'I would not exchange for the treasures of India'. The result? Before he proceeded to Westminster School (which he loathed as much as Locke had done)

I was well acquainted with Pope's Homer, and the Arabian Nights-entertainments, two books which will always please by the moving picture of human manners and specious miracles. The verses of Pope accustomed my ear to the sound of poetic harmony: in the death of Hector and the shipwreck of Ulysses I tasted the new emotions of terror and pity, and seriously disputed with my aunt on the vices and virtues of the Heroes of the Trojan War.

Filling his imagination, the images garnered from that early reading gave him his enduring vision of history as pageantry and performance, his sense of the human drama. Thus, the defects of his body were the making of his mind. And then – lucky Gibbon again – the 'mysterious energies' of Nature turned him into a healthy adult.

Even his adult illnesses were seen, if not quite as lucky breaks, at least as conducive to his choice in life. The principal malady he acquired later in life was gout. Gout, of course, is a story in itself, being the keynote malady of eighteenth-century gentlemen and men of letters, the lord of diseases and the disease of lords, one of those rare afflictions it was a positive 'honour' to acquire, it being a mark of good family and fine living. Gibbon cannot have been displeased to have his gentlemanly credentials confirmed by the onset of the gout.

First stricken in 1772, at the age of 35, he described it as a 'dignified disorder'. In succeeding years the bouts grew more frequent. 'The *Gout has* attacked my left foot,' he informed his friend Lord Sheffield in December 1774, as he was completing the first volumes of the *Decline and Fall*. The sceptical historian coped with 'that imperious Mistress' in part by shrugging it off with *risqué* humour. 'I suffer like one of the first Martyrs,' he told Sheffield in the following year, 'and possibly have provoked my punishment as much.' The ex-Captain of the grenadiers also had a line in military metaphors: 'the Gout has behaved in a very honourable manner,' he told his friend on another occasion, 'after a compleat conquest, and after making me feel his power for some days, the generous Enemy has disdained to abuse his victory or to torment any longer an unresisting victim.'

In Gibbon's metaphoric arsenal, gout might be an honourable enemy, but it could be an inexorable foe. 'So uncertain are all human affairs,' he explained to his stepmother a couple of months later, 'that I found myself arrested by a mighty unrelenting Tyrant called the Gout.' Occasionally he might call an attack 'almost agreeable', presumably having in mind the theory construing gout as a relief agency, a healthy discharge, not unlike a nosebleed. Ever optimistic, he stated of one fit that it had set him on the road to health: 'the body Gibbon is in a perfect state of health and spirits as it is most truly at the present moment, and since the entire retreat of my Gout.'

If not a blessing, gout could at least be facetiously passed off as one of the many bearable evils of mortal life:

When I was called upon last February for my annual tax to the Gout, I only paid for my left foot which in general is the most heavily assessed: the officer came round last week to collect the small remainder that was due for the right foot. I have now satisfied his demand, he is retired in good humour, and I feel myself easy both in mind and body.

One of the ostensible reasons for migrating in 1783 to Lausanne was to recruit his health – that famed Swiss mountain air! – and, once there, high above the lake, he presented himself as reaping the rewards. He gave his stepmother a flattering prospect of his improved health, attributing it to his compliance with the regime advocated by the orthodox physician William Cadogan: the air, he proclaimed, 'is excellently suited to a gouty constitution, and during the whole twelfthmonth I have never once been attacked by my old Enemy. Of Dr Cadogan's three rules, I can observe two a temperate diet and a easy mind.' The third of the rules, so striking by its absence, was exercise: in matters physical Gibbon was notoriously lazy.

His health was good, he liked to boast to his stepmother – presumably whistling in the dark – and 'though verging towards fifty I still feel myself a young Man'. The attacks, however, worsened. As ever, he put on a brave face: affliction was the mother of fortitude – 'My patience has been universally admired.'

From 1790 – the midst of his autobiographizing era – his health was deteriorating fast. The ambiguity of his mode of life, the discrepancy between reality and self-image, is captured by passages in letters written towards the end. 'My MADEIRA is almost exhausted,' he informed Lord Sheffield, 'and I must receive before the end of the autumn, a stout cargo of wholesome exquisite wine.' Meanwhile this man, his gout worsening and so desperate for drink, was reassuring his stepmother: 'My health is remarkably good.'

Bespeaking the self-image of an eighteenth-century gentleman, Gibbon's gout suited his lifestyle perfectly, making destiny his choice. And it was a malady he could flaunt: since it spared his 'more noble parts' – studied ambiguity again – it was not demeaning; and it called up hidden reserves of character. So long as he could banter about gout, the historian could ignore more serious complaints in the claim, or pretence, that his body was doing its job: 'The madness of superfluous health, I have never known; but my tender constitution has been fortified by time: the play of the animal machine still continues to be easy and regular.'

For the enlightened philosopher no less than for the Christian saint or sinner, in other words, the body should be essentially subordinate and secondary, a means to an end: out of sight, out of mind. Gibbon neglected the Addisonian advice of following the chase – except briefly to oblige his father (Hampshire's hunting sorts were bores); and, contrary to Doctors Cheyne and Cadogan's warnings, he spurned exercise. Furthermore, sex too ('the grosser appetite') appears to have left him cold: 'I was not very strongly pressed by my family or my passions to propagate the name and race of the Gibbons.' So striking is the lack of evidence of sexual activity that historians disagree whether his bent was straight or gay.

But to say that Gibbon saw himself above matters of the flesh is in no way to imply that he was an ascetic. He never dallied with the image, beloved of the Renaissance, of the lean and shrunk-shanked scholar, possessed of infinite *Sitzfleisch* and inured to pain. In *The Anatomy of Melancholy* (1621) Robert Burton had painted the classic cameo of the scholars' melancholy. 'They live a sedentary, solitary life, *sibi & musis*, free from bodily exercise, and those ordinary disports which other men use,' a lifestyle which '*dries the brain and extinguisheth natural heat; for whilst the spirits are intent to meditation above in the head, the stomack and liver are left destitute, and thence come black blood and crudities by defect of concoction.*' Melancholy and spleen, those stigmata of true scholarly dedication, inevitably followed.

That was not for Gibbon. He valued the new enlightened image of the man of letters who was also a man of the world. Thinking was too important to be left to crabbed and crackbrained dons – it must be rescued from those 'monkish' Oxbridge cells which (his experience showed only too well) bred morose idleness. What was needed, according – as we have seen – to such enlightened figures as Lord Shaftesbury and Joseph Addison, was politeness not pedantry. 'The separation of the learned from the conversable world', lamented the Scottish philosopher David Hume, putting in a plea for this modernization of the intellectual, had been 'the great defect of the last age'; learning had 'been as great a loser by being shut up in colleges', while philosophy had gone to ruin 'by this moping recluse method of study'. Things, however, were on the mend. 'Men of letters in this age have lost in a great measure that shyness and bashfulness of temper which kept them at a distance from mankind.' As a fellow man of the Enlightenment – one unreserved in his admiration for Hume the historian – Gibbon clearly agreed: how odd to imagine that great works of the mind came from peevish spirits in sickly bodies in musty surroundings? Once installed in the West End of London after his father's death, he could 'divide the day between Study and Society', advantageously to both.

Gibbon cultivated ease, and made much of such 'solid comforts of life' as 'a convenient, well-furnished house, a domestic table, half a dozen [!] chosen servants, my own carriage, and all those decent luxuries whose value is the more sensibly felt the longer they are enjoyed'. Deprived of the 'indispensable comfort' of a servant when banished to Switzerland, so much did it irk him that he actually recorded the fact in his *Memoirs*. Ever 'helpless and awkward', Gibbon liked his 'earthly blessings' and enjoyed flaunting himself as the quintessential Georgian man of sense, taste and refinement. All that notwithstanding, the prime function of bodily comforts, in his complacent vision, was to nurture the mind. His first 'joy' on inheriting his father's wealth was to lay out 'a bank-note of twenty pounds for the twenty volumes of the Memoirs of the Academy of Inscriptions'.

While Gibbon thus represented his body as subordinate and disci-plined, a means to an end, a 'machine' best neither seen nor heard, it may be psychologically revealing about his authentic relationship with his body – one tenser and less under control than he liked to admit – that he visualized his mind and matters intellectual in rather lurid corporeal idioms. His library was his 'seraglio' and the books he authored were his 'children'. Respecting his first publication, he alluded, with awkward affectation, to 'the loss of my litterary maidenhead'. Reading was the consumption of literary 'food', gratification of his 'insatiable appetite' for study. Greed – *bodily* greed, that is – was clearly not something to boast of – Gibbon, as caricatures make clear, grew inordinately fat. Intellectual voracity, by contrast, might be admitted, if with the usual self-exonerating irony. 'From the ancient, I leaped to the modern World,' he thus describes his childhood reading diet, 'many crude lumps of Speed, Rapin, Mezeray, Davila, Machiavel, Father Paul, Bower &c. [chroniclers and historians] passed through me like so many novels, and I swallowed with the same voracious appetite the descriptions of India and China, of Mexico and Peru.' Greed was good so long as it was for matters mental.

Gibbon tells readers he is giving them the 'naked truth', but his relationship to his body was evidently unresolved, and the naked flesh does not come across in his *Memoirs*. For while he refers to his gout (a good disease), he does not mention the complaint which indirectly killed him, his hydrocele – an enlargement of the scrotum (another swelling): evidently a 'bad', humiliating and frightening condition.

Gibbon was obviously ashamed about that particular protuberance. It grew bigger and bigger and, as contemporaries noted, he pretended to be unaware of it – though it drew attention to itself not only on account of its magnitude, but because it interfered with urination: he reeked and his presence became disagreeable. He would 'undraw the veil before my state of health', he stated in a letter to Lord Sheffield, 'though the naked truth may alarm you more than a fit of the Gout. Have you never observed through my inexpressibles a large prominency circa genitalia?' He had, he added, 'strangely neglected' it 'for many years' – the 'strangely' speaks volumes, and the resort to euphemism and Latin is telling. And how could Sheffield not have noticed it? Presumably its being connected with his genitals (one of those 'more noble parts'?) made it such a source of mortification, and it evidently forced him, finally, to think once again about the disorders and disintegration of the flesh – and to contemplate dissolution.

Gibbon was no Christian – he may have embraced some Deistic

belief in a presiding Intelligence but there is no sign that he imagined any mode of life after death. Indeed, his sneering and scathing attitude to Christianity made the doctrine of personal immortality a vain and laughable superstition, as shown by his treatment of his pious maiden aunt Hester. That 'holy Virgin' was a follower of William Law, the man whose *A Serious Call to a Devout and Holy Life* had 'overmatched' Samuel Johnson:

Her only study was the Bible with some legends and books of piety which she read with implicit faith: she prayed five times each day; and, as singing, according to the Serious Call, is an indispensable part of devotion, she rehearsed the psalms and hymns of thanksgiving, which she now, perhaps, may chant in a full chorus of Saints and Angels.

The prospect of extinction obviously exercised Gibbon, as it did Johnson, and the *Memoirs* were, among other things, his attempt to come to terms with mortality. Death – the death of others – was a natural fact to be coolly accepted: he would 'not pretend to lament' the five brothers who died in infancy, and he also brushed aside the death of his father ('The tears of a son are seldom lasting').

Facing his own future, Gibbon notes that although the 'evening' years might be the best time of life, he had doubts about the rosy picture of old age presented by Fontenelle, the French man of science who lived into his hundredth year. 'I must reluctantly observe, that two causes, the abbreviation of time and the failure of hope, will always tinge with a browner shade the evening of life.'

The 'play of the animal machine' remained fine, Gibbon assured his readers – somewhat disingenuously to say the least – and 'probability' was on his side: 'this day may *possibly* be my last: but the laws of probability, so true in general, so fallacious in particular, still allow me about fifteen years'. Yet, as he admitted, 'probability', though strong in the general case, was meaningless in the specific. That abbreviation of time was worrying. 'The present is a fleeting moment: the past is no more.' The older one grew, the less each passing year signified:

The proportion of a part to the whole is the only standard by which we can measure the length of our existence. At the age of twenty, one year is a tenth perhaps of the time which has elapsed within our consciousness and memory: at the age of fifty it is no more than a fortieth, and this relative value continues to decrease till the last sands are shaken by the hand of death.

In any case, there was less to look forward to, as 'time and experience' had 'dampened' anticipations 'by disappointment or possession'. 'After the middle season,' as he put it in one of his hierarchical metaphors, 'the crowd must be content to remain at the foot of the mountain; while the few who have climbed the summit, aspire to descend or expect to fall' – another decline and fall. Attempting to put his prospects in order, Gibbon explained his intimations of immortality: 'In old age, the consolation of hope is reserved for the tenderness of parents who commence as new life in their children; the faith of enthusiasts who sing Hallelujahs above the clouds; and the vanity of authors who presume the immortality of their name and writings.' The sentiments could have been Johnson's, but the register would have been quite different: how Gibbonian to compare himself to his aunt!

This chapter has examined a different sort of text: an autobiography. It has explored how a supremely literary individual, late in life, portrayed himself – conceived the relation between his mind and body – largely with a view to constructing an enduring public image. Gibbon was a man publicly happy to ignore his mortal coil. There is no immortal soul – and no tears are lost over that. There remains nevertheless a hope of immortality through 'litterary . . . fame'. He would not go to heaven; indeed his last years on earth, spent above the lake at Lausanne, would at best be a state of being 'alone in paradise'. But his books might last, including the *Memoirs* written 'that one day his mind will be familiar to the grandchildren of those who are yet unborn'. His mind will thus live on.

PART III
THE FRAILTY OF THE FLESH

12

THIS MORTAL COIL

After Death, nothing is

ROCHESTER

The Churches, as we have seen, taught that death closed a mundane life that was brief and wretched and opened the portal to life eternal. It was not extinction but metamorphosis. Death was thus not to be feared but welcomed, and ample testimony has come down of Christians eagerly embracing the Churches' notion of a 'good death', as encoded by the *ars moriendi*.

But there was more to it than the art of dying well as an audition for life eternal. Be it one's own death or that of others, dying involved an intricate and solemn fabric of social beliefs, procedures and expectations aimed at the safe passage of the decedent, some of which will be touched upon below. Elaborate preparedness was a necessary defence, with mortality always threatening and its management so crucial. Funerals were celebrated with far more pomp than marriages or baptisms, while the new secular cultural media accorded mortality new openings, not least magazine obituary columns and tear-jerking novels.

Everyman was forced to walk in the valley of the shadow of death. In the churchyard on Sunday, parishioners saw death all around: tombstones commemorating grandparents, parents, brothers and sisters who had perished in infancy, and not least their own offspring. As amply confirmed by sermons and pious works of religious comfort, and by the testimony of letters, diaries and funerary art, death loomed large in public culture and often governed individual minds. The Black Death of the mid-fourteenth century and subsequent outbreaks of plague lasting down to 1665 had, of course, cast a long, dark shadow, and their aftermath was the culture of the Dance of Death, the worm-corrupted cadaver, the skull and crossbones and the charnel house. This was reinforced by a theology which held death to be the wages of sin and, especially for those embracing Calvinist predestinarianism, stressed that for perhaps the great majority it would literally inaugurate the endless torments of hellfire.

Boldly challenging the comforting Roman Catholic doctrines of efficacious deathbed repentance, Protestant voluntarism stressed how the divine arrow could pierce at any moment, out of the blue. Hence, the pious Christian must needs be composed for that event – Bishop Ken warned: 'Live ev'ry day as if 'twere thy last.' Indeed, such *ars moriendi* handbooks as Jeremy Taylor's *Holy Dying* taught that ripeness was all; it 'must be the business of our whole Lives to prepare for Death', proclaimed William Sherlock's influential *A Practical Discourse Concerning Death* (1690).

The deathbed confrontation was bound (and was meant) to be awesome and overwhelming: 'death is a fearful thing', blabbed Claudio in *Measure for Measure* ('to die, and go we know not where'), calling to mind similar chilling passages from *Hamlet*. It had to be faced head-on and vanquished. This public face inured believers to trauma: panic was obviated because religious practices and cultural resources girded the faithful against the Arch-foe. Family prayers, fasting, devotions, Bible-reading and so forth, both before and at the deathbed, were designed to fortify believers as they came to die the good death.

The business of dying in early modern England predominantly involved a religious rite, the liberation of the soul from its carnal prison, and its escape, it was hoped, into the heavenly hosts. The seventeenth-century deathbed of the Puritan Philip Henry offers an exemplar of this well-staged drama. Sensing death coming over him, Henry took elaborate farewells of his family, bestowing upon them religious blessings and warnings, and repeatedly uttering pious ejaculations, mixed with prayers and Scripture texts. 'His Understanding and Speech continued almost to the last Breath,' concluded his biographer. 'One of the last words he said, when he found himself just ready to depart, was *O Death, where is thy* —— with that his speech falter'd and he quickly expired.' His death was exemplary and was written up as such.

Sudden deaths, which threatened this choreographed good death, were dreaded. But they were common. Letters and diaries tell sad stories of tragic drownings, falls, fires, firearms explosions, mishaps with tools, knives, poisons, and ubiquitous traffic spills. From its opening issue in 1731, the *Gentleman's Magazine* carried a column headed 'Casualties', meaning strokes of fate. Readers of the February number encountered someone drowned in Islington ponds, one man dropping dead of an apoplectic fit, two murdered in their beds, a pair suffocated while digging a pit, a coal-dealer falling out of a lighter, an attorney tumbling into a fire, a man drowned in the Thames, another in Queenhythe dock, a city butler, just fired, who slit his throat, a servant's arm broken after a granary collapsed, a house-fire by the River Medway, another in a Stratford corn-mill, a silk-weaver who cut his throat, a drunken clock-maker likewise, a labourer slaying his children, a man gored by an ox in Cheapside, and, completing the carnage, an Oxford student who lurched off Bottley Bridge and met a watery end. In the March number we find an Eton scholar stabbing his chum to death with a penknife (on the playing fields?), and the burning of the Duke of Beaufort's seat, with much loss of life. None of these people had a good death.

Appalled by the waste of life, enlightened thinkers abandoned fatalism for self-help, taking in the process steps which some saw as a blasphemous challenge to the inscrutable ways of God. Smallpox inoculation was introduced – though it met resistance from the Calvinist Scottish kirk, since it seemed to gainsay Providence. First-aid techniques were pioneered. First-aid manuals go back as far as Stephen Bradwell's *Helps for Suddain Accidents* (1633), but it was enlightened practicality and consumerism which got first-aid organized, not least through the sale of ready-made medicine chests and of instruction manuals for the public. In his best-selling *Domestic Medicine* (1769), William Buchan condemned the 'horrid custom immediately to consign over to death every person who has the misfortune by a fall, or the like, to be deprived of the appearance of life'. Many lives, he believed, could be saved and all, if properly trained, could save lives: 'every man is in some measure a surgeon whether he will or not.' Through such developments, death was beginning to be taken out of the hands of God.

Another resource lay in the hospital movement. Between 1720 and 1745 five great new London hospitals were founded through bequests and private philanthropy: the Westminster, Guy's, St George's, the London and the Middlesex; provincial and Scottish infirmaries followed. Every hospital made provision for emergency and casualty admissions. Exclusively targeted at accidents was the Institution for Affording Immediate Relief to Persons Apparently Dead from Drowning, founded in 1774 – in 1776 it changed its name to the Humane Society and from 1785 it became Royal. The Society's aim was to teach rescue techniques, especially in case of accidents with water. It also supplied equipment, awarded prizes and published pamphlets which advocated mouth-to-mouth resuscitation, tobacco clysters, electric stimulation and the importance of keeping warm. In winning publicity for itself, the Humane Society found an eager organ in the *Gentleman's Magazine*. Inspired by the Society, newspapers began to carry advice for dealing with accident victims. 'A correspondent has communicated the following directions for the recovery of persons seemingly drowned,' *Jopson's Coventry Mercury* told its readers on 31 May 1784:

In the first place, strip them of all their wet cloaths; rub them and lay them in hot blankets before the fire: blow with your breath strongly, or with a pair of bellows into the mouth of the person, holding the nostrils at the same time: afterwards introduce the small end of a lighted tobacco-pipe into the fundament, putting a paper pricked full of holes near the bowl of it, through which you must blow into the bowels.

Exactly paralleling the new concern with ascertaining the true signs of death and snatching back the 'apparently dead' was growing anxiety about premature burial. The fear of being buried alive became a public issue after Jacques-Bénigne Winslow, Professor of Anatomy in Paris, published in 1740 a paper on the uncertainty of the signs of death: absence of pulse or breathing were not to be taken as definite marks – the onset of putrefaction alone was a reliable indicator of irreversible dissolution. 'Lifeless' patients who could not safely be declared dead should be subjected to resuscitation procedures: tickling the nose with a quill, shrieking into the ears, cutting the soles of the feet with razors, inserting needles under the nails or thrusting a hot poker up the anus. Burial should be delayed.

Increasingly, the dying left explicit requests to ensure that they were not buried alive. Some asked for their hearts to be cut out, others to be embalmed. Miss Beswick, an elderly lady who died in Manchester, left 20,000 guineas to her doctor, Charles White, on condition that she was never buried.

Fired by experience with the apparently drowned and the prematurely buried, bold spirits mooted the taboo prospects of actually bringing people back from the dead, for instance through electric shocks. In this connexion, Galvani's celebrated experiments proved particularly 'galvanizing'. In 1792 this Italian naturalist described experiments in which the legs of dead frogs were suspended by copper wire from an iron balcony; as the feet touched the iron uprights, the legs twitched. These sensational experiments – life seemingly being restored to the incontrovertibly dead – were followed up by his younger contemporary Alessandro Volta. The connexions between electricity and the stuff of life implied by such researches proved highly charged, to say nothing of the apparent blasphemy involved in the possibility of 'resurrection' by human means.

Such Promethean hopes came to experimental fruition on humans in London on 17 January 1803, when Giovanni Aldini applied galvanic electricity to the corpse of the murderer Thomas Forster, whose newly hanged body had been rushed from Newgate to an anatomy theatre. When wires attached to a galvanic pile were hooked up to the criminal's mouth and ear, 'the jaw began to quiver,' so it was reported, 'the adjoining muscles were horribly contorted, and the left eye actually opened.' Applied to the ear and rectum, the wires 'excited in the muscles contractions much stronger . . . as almost to give an appearance of re-animation'. Such experiments encouraged literary and artistic fantasies in the Gothic mode, most celebratedly in Mary Shelley's *Frankenstein* (1818), which pursued the idea not of reanimation but of creating life out of inert matter *de novo*.

All such endeavours – from reviving the drowned to reanimating the dead – heightened speculation as to precisely what death was. What it *signified* had always been crystal clear to Christians: the portal to life eternal, and theologians had taught that death occurred thanks to the soul leaving the body. But medicine and science had traditionally been relatively reticent about specifying the nature of death, or what exactly happened at the moment of extinction. In the context of apparent death by drowning, especially, questions now arose about the timing and mechanism of the separation of body from soul, and about what we would call near-death experiences.

The eminent doctor John Fothergill offered his 'Observations' on a case reported by a surgeon who had inflated the lungs of a man suffocated by fumes in a coal mine, thus restoring him to life. The Quaker physician stressed the usefulness of what would later be called artificial respiration in cases of suffocation from noxious vapours, drowning, lightning, and so forth. To know whether an individual were truly a victim, death's signs had to be known, and its mechanisms understood. 'It does not seem absurd', he taught,

to compare the animal machine to a clock; let the wheels whereof be in never so good order, the mechanism complete in every part, and wound up to the full pitch, yet without some impulse communicated to the pendulum, the whole continues motionless . . . Inflating the lungs, and by this means communicating motion to the heart, like giving the first vibration to a pendulum, may possibly, in many cases, enable this something to resume the government of the fabric, and actuate its organs afresh . . . this case suggests, viz. the possibility of saving a great many lives, without risking any thing.

Through such speculations, death was beginning to be stripped of its mystery.

Might the 'dead' themselves have something to report? Narratives had occasionally been published of coma and prolonged sleep. Every year on his birthday, a certain Nicholas Hart – so an early eighteenth-century pamphlet related – was wont to fall so deeply asleep that he could not be awakened. His long sleeps captured the attention of 'Divines, Scholars, Gentlemen, and Physicians' who congregated to attend his awakening and sat 'about his Bed, to hear and take down what he would say when he came out of his trance'. Hart told them that his long sleep coincided with a journey of his soul into the afterlife: brought to the gates of heaven, he had attended the judgement of the souls of the newly dead. For five days a year Hart was thus turned into a prophet – or some said, a charlatan.

When physicians associated with the Royal Humane Society came to ponder and write up 'near-death' experiences, however, their framework was different from Hart's pious narrative, for they dwelt upon matters physiological and pathological. The more materialist doctors involved with the Society claimed that the air (oxygen) or electricity effective in recovering the quasi-dead indicated that the principle of life lay in those substances. The implication that such rescues could be used as 'natural experiments' into the nature of life and death was, in turn, deprecated by conservative churchmen, fearful of a medical take-over of one of the Christian mysteries. Certain radicals linked the rescue of the apparently dead to the resurrection of Christ; the orthodox deplored such thinking as blasphemy.

Amid such medico-scientific speculations, the cultural aspects of death were also coming under scrutiny. Despite the expunging of purgatory from Protestant theology, popular lore continued to hold that the soul remained in contact with the body for a while after death and that the behaviour of family and friends could affect the fate of the dead person's soul. In this belief lay one reason why the corpse remained at home until the funeral, during which time respectful visitors partook of specially prepared food and drink, often placed directly on the coffin. 'Watching' a corpse, or keeping vigil prior to burial, remained an important mark of respect, and 'waking' was popular in Irish, Welsh and Scottish communities, a noisy ceremony staged on the eve of the funeral, supposed to protect the corpse from evil spirits – as well as providing emotional release.

Deathbed folklore treated of the departure of the soul from the dying person. A wraith, disguised as a small animal, might first appear as a herald of death. The soul was widely thought to fly off in the shape of a bird. A corpse which failed to manifest rigor mortis was particularly feared as a mark of an unquiet spirit, and such 'undead' beings might stir, leading to disrupted graves (explaining why suicides were buried at crossroads, outside consecrated ground, with a stake through their heart: to prevent their souls from 'walking'). To prevent such commotions, 'sin-eaters' might be employed to remove the sins of the departed. 'In the county of Hereford,' reported the seventeenth-century antiquary John Aubrey,

it was an old custom at funerals to hire poor people, who were to take upon them the sins of the party deceased . . . The manner was that when the corpse was brought out of the house and laid on the bier, a loaf of bread was brought out and delivered to the sin-eater, over the corpse, as also a mazard bowl of maple, full of beer (which he was to drink up), and sixpence in money, in consideration whereof he took upon him, *ipso facto*, all the sins of the defunct and freed him or her from walking after they were dead.

Not least, ghosts remained a powerful force in popular culture – indeed, as we have seen, such élite figures as Joseph Glanvill, Henry More and other fellows of the Royal Society went ghost-hunting in expectation that authenticated sightings would give scientific backing to the existence of the spiritual realm, confuting Hobbesian 'atheism'.

Enlightenment thinking brought detached analysis, however, of all such associations, cultural accretions and 'superstitions' connected with the dying process. Comparative accounts were complied of divergent practices at different times and places, so as to lay bare the underlying rationales and psychological constraints. In his *Lectures on the Sacred Poetry of the Hebrews* (1787), the Anglican divine and Hebrew scholar Robert Lowth advanced radical speculations on the origins of beliefs about dying and the afterlife. Affirming naturalistically that 'the incorporeal world' had its source in 'things corporeal and terrestrial', he held that the ancient Hebrews' understanding of death emerged from mundane reflections on the condition and resting place of corpses. The Jews derived their ideas of the afterlife, he stressed, from 'what was plain and commonly understood concerning the dead, that is, what happened to the body'. Since it was plain that 'after death the body returned to the earth, and that it was deposited in a sepulchre . . . a sort of popular notion prevailed among the Hebrews, as well as among other nations, that the life which succeeded the present was to be passed beneath the earth'. The Jewish idea of an afterlife was but a ghostly, or fantasized, version of the condition of the body after death, while the dark world of Sheol, the descriptions of the souls inhabiting it, and the journeys of the dead to the pit, were poetic elaborations on the disposition of the body in the grave. In other words, the key to religious myths about death and immortality lay in recognition that the source of all spiritual imagery was the corpse, as mediated through speech and funerary ceremonies. Rather radically for a divine, Lowth thus implied that Judaeo-Christian teachings about death and the afterlife were rationalizations of interment practices, not *vice versa*.

In a comparable way the gentleman-philosopher Abraham Tucker showed in his *The Light of Nature Pursued* (1768) how beliefs about death emerged from rather elementary associations of ideas. Frightening indeed was 'the melancholy appearance of a lifeless body, the mansion provided for it to inhabit, dark, cold, close and solitary, are shocking to the imagination; but it is to the imagination only, not the understanding, for whoever consults this faculty will see at first glance, that there is nothing dismal in all these circumstances.' Tucker's thinking was evidently underpinned by Locke, who had argued in his *Essay concerning Human Understanding* that the fear of darkness was not a natural condition, but arose from bedtime stories told by 'foolish' maids to innocent children:

The *Ideas* of *Goblines* and *Sprights* have really no more to do with Darkness than Light; yet but a foolish Maid inculcate these often on the Mind of a Child, and raise them there together, possibly he shall never be able to separate them again so long as he lives, but Darkness shall ever afterwards bring with it those frightful *Ideas*, and they shall be so joined that he can no more bear the one than the other.

It was that irrational fear of darkness which sparked fears of one's fate *post mortem*.

To learn how to die with composure, it was necessary, reasoned Tucker, to overcome the nightmarish phantasms associated with funerary rituals, and the attendant palaver of hell, damnation and demons. Indeed, non-Christian burials became not uncommon, as in the funeral of John Underwood of Cambridgeshire, reported in the *Gentleman's Magazine* in 1733, in which the requiem involved the singing of the thirty-first Ode of Horace, after which the mourners were invited to take a glass of wine and then instructed to forget the departed.

'A desire of preserving the body seems to have prevailed in most countries of the world,' noted Mary Wollstonecraft, reflecting on some embalmed corpses she came across in Norway, while travelling on a business mission for her American lover, Gilbert Imlay, and the experience provoked a flood of musings typical of the late Enlightenment mind.

When I was shewn these human petrifactions, I shrunk back with disgust and horror. 'Ashes to ashes!' thought I – 'Dust to dust!' – If this be not dissolution, it is something worse than natural decay. It is treason against humanity, thus to lift up the awful veil which would fain hide its weakness. The grandeur of the active principles is never more strongly felt than at such a sight; for nothing is so ugly as the human form when deprived of life, and thus dried into stone, merely to preserve the most disgusting image of death.

This led her into meditations on the 'melancholy' thereby produced, though it was one which 'exalts the mind':

Our very soul expands, and we forget our littleness; how painfully brought to our recollection by such vain attempts to snatch from decay what is destined so soon to perish. Life, what art thou? Where goes this breath? this *I*, so much alive? In what element will it mix, giving or receiving fresh energy? – What will break the enchantment of animation? – For worlds, I would not see a form I loved – embalmed in my heart – thus sacrilegiously handled!

She also mused on the reaction these corpses provoked in her sensibilities in respect of her expectations of the general resurrection of the dead:

I could not learn how long the bodies had been in this state, in which they bid fair to remain till the day of judgment, if there is to be such a day; and before that time, it will require some trouble to make them fit to appear in company with angels, without disgracing humanity.

Wollstonecraft was a pious Anglican, but evidently for her Church dogma could no longer be taken on trust, to the letter: it had to be mediated through the expectations of the sensitive mind; significantly, what she wrote was 'without disgracing humanity' rather than 'without offence to God': even the afterlife had now become anthropocentric. With her fragile and faltering relationship with Imlay in mind, she finally asked:

without hope, what is to sustain life, but the fear of annihilation – the only thing of which I have ever felt a dread – I cannot bear to think of being no more – of losing myself – though existence is often but a painful consciousness of misery; nay, it appears to me impossible that I should cease to exist, or that this active, restless spirit, equally alive to joy and sorrow, should only be organized dust – ready to fly abroad the moment the spring snaps, or the spark goes out, which kept it together. Surely something resides in this heart that is not perishable – and life is more than a dream.

Among the élite, overtly pagan attitudes towards death and dying grew more conspicuous. Enlightened philosophers set out to teach how to die by providing an alternative, rationalist idea – that the dead were beyond death: *la mort n'est rien*. The Providence-challenging concept of 'natural death' became more widely accepted. Approaching dissolution, Hume notoriously bantered with Adam Smith as to how he lacked any good excuse for delaying embarkation upon Charon's boat across the Styx:

I thought I might say to him, 'Good Charon, I have been correcting my works for a new edition. Allow me a little time that I may see how the public receives the alterations.' But Charon would answer, 'When you have seen the effect of these, you will be for making other alterations. There will be no end of such . . .'

Among such pagan-minded gentlemen, death ceased thus to be the ultimate enemy, demanding heroic acts of resolution, faith and penitence. Instead, dying came to be widely treated as an easy passing, a final sleep. Laurel wreaths replaced the traditional death's head on tombs, funeral tablets trumpeted earthly virtues rather than divine justice, and the Gothick paraphernalia of yew trees and screech owls – the props of Thomas Gray's *Elegy Written in a Country Church-Yard* – transformed death from transcendental trauma into an essentially human morality drama which taught that the paths of glory lead but to the grave.

At the same time, death's scenario grew more secular in another way: it was becoming medicalized. Doctors changed the face of death, not by reducing its ravages or by actually (despite aspirations) increasing longevity, but by playing their part in forging new coping strategies.

Traditional medical etiquette had required that the mortally ill person be informed of his likely fate by his physician. Then, his part in the proceedings complete, the physician would withdraw, leaving the dying person to compose his mind and his will, and to make peace with God and his family. The Stuart practitioner Thomas Willis quit his patients after 'giving them over': 'He groaned horribly like a dying man . . . then judging the issue to be settled I bade farewell to him and his friends. At evening he died,' conclude his notes on one of his patients. The doctor's departure was not due to callous indifference, but rather to a sense of place, proper resignation and dignity. Physic was for the living. Dr Robert James's *Medicinal Dictionary* (1743), a huge medical compilation, has no entry for death.

The eighteenth century brought the development of the medical management of death at the bedside. 'When all hopes of revival are lost,' declared Dr John Ferriar, 'it is still the duty of the physician to sooth the last moments of existence.' The doctor should decide: 'it belongs to his province, to determine when officiousness becomes torture.' For Ferriar, the physician's continued presence in the position of authority was vital, not least to curb the excesses of nurses and servants who were paid to keep watch, with their violent and often cruel folk routines with the dying. Not least, such old women allegedly pronounced people dead prematurely.

According to the new medical protocols, the doctor must manage the actual process of ceasing to be. Early in the nineteenth century, Henry Halford stressed that the physician's true task must be to 'smooth the bed of death', or in other words, to undertake the management of pain, thereby overcoming fear and restoring tranquillity, orchestrating an end which would be serene and blissful. The suave Halford became the most sought-after physician of his age precisely because his patients had confidence that through generous medication he would not let them die in agony. Rumour had it that a 'lady of the highest rank ... declared she would rather die under Sir Henry Halford's care than recover under any other physician'.

The eighteenth century brought a growing medical interest in death. In 1761 Giovanni Morgagni, Professor of Anatomy at Padua, published *De Sedibus et Causis Morborum* (On the Sites and Causes of Disease) in which he correlated the *post mortem* pathological findings of almost 700 patients with the clinical course of their illnesses. For many lay people, however, such medical scrutiny was rather sinister. Autopsies could represent an assault upon the dead which was both disrespectful and (in the common imagination) also spiritually dangerous, since it condemned them to wander, mutilated and with identity lost, through eternity. In any case, autopsy was tainted because it was the official fate of criminals: after 1752 Parliament allowed judges to order anatomical dissection for the corpses of executed murderers.

From its beginnings in Renaissance Italy, public dissection of felons was staged as an official exhibition, held annually during carnival: ritualization within the upside-down world of that festival sanctioned the evident sacrilege of violating dead bodies. In England, dissection was publicly authorized in 1564, when the Royal College of Physicians obtained a grant of four corpses yearly. The opening up of the body in the anatomy theatre provided a showcase for medicine, conspicuously laying bare the errors of hidebound Galenism. Cutting up malefactors, however, indelibly tarred a medical procedure with the brush of violence and the violation of taboos, kindling intense and enduring grassroots distrust of dissection.

The 'Tyburn riots' staged against the surgeons in Georgian England show the fierce resistance of common people to having their deceased comrades carted off to Surgeons' Hall and subjected to the profanations of the dissectors – a revulsion caught by Hogarth in the final engraving of his 'Four Stages of Cruelty' series, where the murderer Tom Nero is being anatomized by the surgeons: was not medical dissection nothing but brutality writ large and given an official blessing? Public disquiet mounted further against the practice in the light of the sordid and illegal involvement of anatomists with grave-robbers or 'resurrection men' (a fascinating colloquialism!).

Quality cadavers were much less likely to meet such a fate – they seldom dug up the rich, 'resurrectionists' explained to a parliamentary committee, 'because they were buried so deep'. Yet this did not stop scare stories about the illegal procurement of bodies and grave-robbing. Such allegations provoked Thomas Hood's ironic 'Mary's Ghost: A Pathetic Ballad'. Her grave rifled and her remains dealt out among the anatomists, poor Mary's ghost addresses her fiancé:

> I vow'd that you should have my hand,
>   But fate gives us denial;
> You'll find it there, at Dr Bell's
>   In spirits and a phial.
>
> I can't tell where my head is gone,
>   But Doctor Carpue can:
> As for my trunk, it's all pack'd up
>   To go by Pickford's van.

> The cock it crows – I must begone!
> My William we must part!
> But I'll be yours in death, altho'
> Sir Astley has my heart.

With the dead, medicine seemed to be pre-empting the hand of God.

Changing attitudes towards suicide offer a final instance of a withdrawal from traditional Christian teachings. Throughout Christian history 'self-murder' had been both sin and crime, an offence against God and King, the business of courts ecclesiastical and civil. Since Tudor times juries had routinely returned verdicts of *felo de se* (wilful self-murder), imposing severe posthumous punishments: the suicide was denied Christian burial, the corpse being interred at a crossroads, a stake through the heart; and the felon's property was forfeit to the Crown. This cruel treatment expressed Protestant theological rigorism – suicide as a wilful mutiny against God – while also marking the tenacious assertion of royal rights under the new monarchy. Puritanism redoubled the punitiveness.

As in so many other walks of life, the new temper of the Restoration brought a transformation. It soon become standard for coroners' courts to reach a *non compos mentis* verdict, regardless of any real history or independent sign of mental instability in the victim: was not suicide itself sufficient proof of derangement? This 'medicalization' or 'psychologization' of self-destruction sanctioned a churchyard burial and put a stop to the escheat of the victim's possessions – a notable assertion of community will against the Crown at the very moment when Locke was affirming the natural right to property.

Shifting philosophies of the self, in any case, led the élite to commend 'Antique Roman' attitudes that approved suicide as noble-minded. On 4 May 1737, having loaded his pockets with rocks, Eustace Budgell, a former contributor to the *Spectator*, drowned himself in the Thames. Found on his desk was a suicide note: 'What Cato did, and Addison approved, cannot be wrong.' David Hume and others offered enlightened defences of suicide, and fashionable society meanwhile condoned the deed, holding that death was preferable to dishonour and, ever eager to outflank bigotry, enlightened opinion abandoned punitiveness for pity. The poet Thomas Chatterton, who poisoned himself at the age of 17, provided the perfect role model for the Romantic suicide cult. And even Pope had asked:

> Is it in heav'n a crime to love too well?
> To bear too tender, or too firm a heart,
> To act a Lover's or a *Roman's* part?
> Is there no bright reversion in the sky,
> For those who greatly think, or bravely die?

Crucial to this reconceptualization of suicide was the rise of print culture and its final triumph over the pulpit. The role heretofore played by the Church in fixing its meaning – overwhelmingly punitive – was usurped by the media, whose line was humanitarian through and through. Newspapers and magazines turned suicides into 'human interest' stories, indeed sensations, and encouraged vicarious, often morbid, public involvement, with the printing of suicide notes, last letters and tales of blighted love. Here, as elsewhere, the media gave voice to secular meanings, expressive of enlightened 'humanitarian narratives'. Like living itself, suicide was secularized. This shift in status from pariah, malefactor or sinner to object of pity, evident in the cases of suicides (and also the insane), was mirrored in many other walks of life, where behaviour which had heretofore attracted blame now found ambivalent exculpation in victim status.

Considerable transformation thus occurred in beliefs about death and the rituals which expressed them. The melodrama of the Christian 'good death' receded, to be replaced in many cases by the ideal of a calm departure (like falling asleep); to some degree the presence of the clergy yielded to the physician in attendance. For some brave spirits and freethinkers, to face death without the Christian calling on God was a bold and unflinching declaration and test of a new code of life and sense of self. As is suggested by Mary Wollstonecraft's reflections, death became newly experienced less as the portal to life eternal than as a framing device on life.

13

FLESH AND FORM

Typically of the theosophies and philosophies emerging from the Eastern Mediterranean in the Roman era, Christianity problematized the flesh, and down the centuries graphic rhetorics of denunciation harped on the associations between flesh, sex and sin. 'I come from parents who made me a condemned man before even I was born. Sinners begot a sinner in sin, and nourished him in sin,' declared Hugh of St-Victor in the early twelfth century:

I received nought from them but misfortunes, sin, and the corrupt body I wear. I hurry to those who have already departed through the death of their bodies. When I look at their graves, I see nothing but ashes and worms, stench and horror. That which I am now, they once were. What am I? A man born of a slimy humour, for at the moment of conception I was conceived out of a human seed. This form then coagulated and, in growing, became flesh. After which I was thrown out into the exile of this world, wailing and crying.

A hundred years later, posing the same 'what am I?' question, Pope Innocent III, too, vilified salacious flesh with no more mercy:

Man is formed of dust, mud, ashes, and, what is even viler, of foul sperm . . . Who can ignore the fact that conjugal union never occurs without the itching of the flesh, the fermentation of desire and the stench of lust? Hence any progeny is spoiled, tainted and vitiated by the very act of its conception, the seed communicating to the soul that inhabits it the stain of sin, the stigma of fault, the filth of iniquity.

To contain the flesh, the early Church commended asceticism, desert fathers mortified the flesh, medieval holy men and women, saints and mystics suffered heroic denial and legendary feats of fasting, while ordinary Christians were required to follow suit according to their lights – for instance through the discipline of Lenten abstinence.

The shifts of temper associated with Protestantism, rationalism and capitalism did not so much supersede traditional suspicions about the flesh as bring new suspicions about the suspicions. Was not spectacular fasting itself a manifestation of vainglory, or perhaps of sickness? Were not many traditional reports of triumphs over the flesh, as recorded in lives of the saints, incredible, superstitious and thus at risk of scandal? In any case, was it not all rather misguided? For Protestants, the preferred discipline of the body did not take the form of pious infirmity but of regular labour in one's calling, while the Catholic celebration of chastity and virginity yielded to praise of godly procreation and parenthood. Marital sex became a God-given solace: the genuine Christian should produce and reproduce.

Established Christian asceticism was thus not so much abandoned as rationalized and naturalized in emergent early modern practices of bodily control. By the long eighteenth century, medicine, cleanliness and hygiene (including sexual) became prime vehicles of the regulation of flesh which if corrupt and fallen could also be seen as a glorious gift of God. Building for instance upon William Harvey's demonstration in his *De Motu Cordis* of the functions of the heart as a pump, advances in physiology boosted confidence that the machinery of the body was becoming understood, thereby encouraging the cultivation of a genre of sacred anatomy which proclaimed that the organism, properly investigated by science, would further reveal God's design in the perfect proportions and divinely crafted contrivances of the *machina carnis*. If it was highly dishonourable, as Robert Boyle reflected, 'for a Reasonable Soul to live in so Divinely built a Mansion, as the Body she resides in, altogether unacquainted with the exquisite Structure of it', that great experimenter and others were striving to overcome such lamentable ignorance. Science was discovering the new-found lands of the great bodily systems, and (as we have seen with Addison and Steele) popularizers trumpeted news of what had, till recently, been *terra incognita*. Cited in the *Spectator*, the versified anatomical descriptions presented by Sir Richard Blackmore in *Creation* represent the most august, if hopelessly fustian, example of pious veneration of the divine handiwork:

> The salient point, so first is called the heart,
> Shap'd and suspended with amazing art,
> By turns dilated, and by turns comprest,
> Expels, and entertains the purple guest.
> It sends from out its left contracted side.

What admirable proofs of the wise and benevolent Contriver were the heart and the vascular system!

Daily life remained a grind for the great majority in the eighteenth century. Most power was still muscle power; long childbearing careers were the curse women bore (many could not take the strain and died prematurely); cold, damp, overwork and poor diet were ubiquitous. But whereas the thrust of medieval Christian teachings lay in resignation and the tropes of heaven, a new stress was emerging upon the right, and the responsibility, of the cultivation of vigorous health.

Christian piety had always poured scorn on undue concern for the welfare of the body as vanity: consider the lilies of the field, take no thought for the morrow, God will provide – the thread of life depended upon grace and the mysteries of Providence. Eighteenth-century Christians, however, cast aside certain vestiges of medieval mortification and unconcern for the welfare of the flesh. The Anglican clergy were prominent in founding hospitals and promoting smallpox inoculation – traditional Calvinists, we have seen, viewed this as defying Providence – while John Wesley, the founder of Methodism, wrote the century's most popular medical self-help text, *Primitive Physick* (1747). Dissenters, too, moved with the times. 'Lord teach me to prize health,' beseeched the Presbyterian, Richard Kay, in the 1730s, then just beginning a brief career as a physician in Lancashire (death from fever cut him off in his thirties). A century later, the Cambridge churchman Charles Kingsley averred that there was actually 'something impious' in that 'neglect of personal health' which the 'effeminate ascetics' of the Oxford Movement enjoined to prove their unworldiness: a complete reversal of values. For 'muscular

Christians' like Kingsley, a healthy body was the vessel, and the mark, of a healthy soul: *mens sana in corpore sano*. Physical feebleness was a perverse affectation which smacked of monkish popery; God's work needed strength and energy.

If the rational Christian thus had a duty to foster health, how precisely was it to be safeguarded and improved? Advice filled the air, and home-care books flooded the market. Works like John Burton's *Treatise on the Non-Naturals* (1738) and John Arbuthnot's *An Essay Concerning the Nature of Aliments* (1731) explained to the educated the ideas behind health care, while Wesley's *Primitive Physick* told the poor how to look after themselves with little more than a pot of honey, a string of onions, a pitcher of cold water and a besom.

The *sine qua non* for positive health, everybody understood, lay in establishing and maintaining a robust constitution that would serve as an investment and security against illness. Contrariwise, a corrupt constitution was as disastrous for the individual as for the body politic. Specific spasms and bouts of disease were alarming, but nothing boded worse than the erosion of one's very system. 'I wish I could speak more favourably of poor Clarke,' Edward Gibbon confided to his friend Lord Sheffield, 'but . . . his Constitution is broke up.' Such vitiation was irremediable. 'My constitution will no longer allow me to toil as formerly,' complained the asthmatic surgeon and author Tobias Smollett. What did he mean? 'I am now so thin you would hardly know me. My face is shrivelled up by the asthma like an ill-dried pippin, and my legs are as thick at the ancle as at the calf.' In his novel *Humphry Clinker* (1771) particularly, Smollett showed bodily disease and disorder fuelling weakness of character and bad behaviour.

The constitution was the reservoir of inner strength and resistance, that vigour which abounded when all one's organs co-operated effectively, directed by the mind through sprightly animal spirits. Life was a flame – a favourite metaphor – which should burn bright and hot, and one's constitution was the tallow, the oil and the wick. If one lacked a good constitution in the first place, or if it fell into decay with time or was wrecked by reckless living, medicines would not avail when infection or affliction struck. Doctors were thus seen as secondary, auxiliaries useful largely by dint of their capacity to give good health advice and to prescribe drugs which would reinforce spontaneous, internal powers of recuperation – the 'healing power of nature'.

Thus, the constitution was the very foundation of individual well-being (the political analogy with the British Constitution was clear). Suffering from 'scurvy', some non-specific form of skin complaint, Isabella Duke told her physician – none other than the philosopher John Locke – that she had no hope of recovery from her specific ailment, 'unless it be by mending the Habit of my Body in general, and sweetning my Blood'.

To enjoy this good constitution, sound foundations had to be laid in infancy and consolidated in youth. The plan spelt out by Locke himself in his *Some Thoughts Concerning Education* (1693) commended early hardening of the young, and hence still pliable, body. Nothing could be worse than spoiling the new-born with cosseting, for 'cockering and tenderness' would create and then confirm physical frailty in the infant, thereby spawning spindly, hothouse youths destined to turn into lifelong valetudinarians dependent on stimulants and medicines.

Babies, according to Locke and his army of followers, needed a cool environment, loose clothes, freedom of movement and simple nourishment (initially, the mother's breast). In time they should be systematically exposed to a more bracing regime, including unheated bedrooms, going barefoot, cold-water bathing and even – Locke's rather fiendish suggestion – wearing shoes that would 'leak water' when it rained. (His disciple James Nelson thought this a bit much.)

This 'hardening' regime had powerful emotional and ideological resonances, chiming among other things with the fashionable bucolic myth that peasants, forced to live hard, must be healthier and more resilient than the pampered urban rich, and belief in the healthiness of the 'noble savage'. The Newcastle engraver and nature-lover Thomas Bewick praised the 'hardy inhabitants of the fells' of Northumberland who, 'notwithstanding their apparent poverty', were able to 'enjoy health and happiness in a degree surpassing that of most other men'. Constitutional 'hardening' long enjoyed an English vogue as the best way of 'immunizing' the body. 'Delicacy', warned *On the Management of Children* by 'Seymour' (*nom de plume* of Sir John Hill), 'is the Portent of a thousand Mischiefs.'

By avoiding mollycoddling and trusting to nature, a stout constitution could be established as a treasure-chest of health. How could such 'stamina' be safeguarded throughout adult life? As attitudes and actions show, many believed the answer lay in faithfully following a health regime. It was vital that each department of life – diet and dress, the ensemble of activities making up the day – should be ordered in light of their health implications, so that each element should be beneficial, and the whole would provide a balanced economy of living. Nothing could be taken for granted, everything counted. Rich or poor alike, each individual had the power in myriad minor ways to promote healthy living – or hazard it. 'I'm a great friend to Air,' recorded Lady Mary Coke, delighted to get back into her own home 'where I might have as many windows op'ned as I pleased'. While visiting Lady Lucy Howard, 'I was of infinite use both to her & her House,' this bossyboots reported, 'by opening all the windows, which were as closely shut as if it had been the coldest day in Winter, but I suppose you know She has always a fire in her Bed Chamber the hottest day in summer; how can She have her health with such management?' Evidently Lady Mary was a good Lockean.

From the Greeks onwards, doctors had systematized all the items of vital importance to healthy living and dubbed them collectively the 'non-naturals'. There were said to be six in all, thus tabulated by the fashionable Bath physician George Cheyne: '1. The Air we breathe in. 2. Our Meat and Drink. 3. Our Sleep and Watching. 4. Our Exercise and Rest. 5. Our Evacuations and their Obstructions. 6. The Passions of our Minds.'

One of the prime reasons why people diarized so religiously was to keep track of physical routines, with a view, if necessary – as all too often! – to shaming themselves into mending their ways. It was possibly with an eye to health that a few diarists – Robert Hooke for example – also recorded their orgasms and other sexual activities, often indicated by a cryptic symbol. Best theory had it that too much and too little sex were equally debilitating, though ideas about what frequency was ideal differed. Increasing numbers – like the *Spectator*'s hypochondriac – weighed themselves regularly, even though this frequently makes sorry reading, for it was commonly, as with Sir Joseph Banks, his wife and his sister Sophia, a tale of gravitation to obesity – by 1794, Sophia was fourteen and a half stone, and her brother far heavier: no wonder his gout worsened. When John Baker depressed the scales in 1772, he admitted 'I was then extremely fat and weighed above 15 stone, I think, 10 pounds'. According to Thomas Short, physician and attentive social observer, writing in 1727, it was an age of eating: 'I believe', he asserted, 'no Age did ever afford more Instances of Corpulency than our own.' England was becoming a nation of fatties.

Health freaks and worriers made free in their advice to others as to how to protect it. 'My deare Ned,' Lady Brilliana Harley cautioned her son, 'be carefull of yourself, and forget not. Doo exersise; for health can no more be had without it, then without a good diet.' Among the non-naturals exercise went with moderation: 'Be temperate in all things in your diet,' William Penn admonished his children, 'for that is physic by prevention.' 'Exercise and application', Thomas Jefferson told his daughter, 'produce order in our affairs, health of body and cheerfulness of mind.' The pursuit of health thus required the same sort of eternal vigilance as did maintenance of the purity of the soul.

The classic give-away sign of a vitiated constitution lay in wasting. The flesh fell off the old – the chief image of the elderly was a withered state, all skin and bones. The flesh might also waste among the young, however. Teenaged girls suffering from what was known as the 'green sickness' or chlorosis wasted away, it was often said out of frustrated sexual longing (marriage was the remedy). The parallel to such a maid was the male adolescent who declined, allegedly as a consequence of 'self-abuse' – eighteenth-century physiology taught that the vital fluid which was the flame of life dwelt in the semen. Seminal loss consequent upon compulsive masturbation was regarded as peculiarly depletive. A youth who 'was observ'd to Manstrupate very often' shortly 'died of a deep Consumption, having lived till he became like a Ghost, or living Skeleton', reported *Onania*, the most popular of a multitude of sensationalist warnings. James Graham, the vocal sexual pioneer of the 1780s, dubbed such self-abusers 'poor creeping tremulous, pale, spindle-shanked wretched creatures who crawl upon the earth, spirting, dribling, and drawing off, alone'.

Thus associated with weakness, physical and moral, thinness was also derided because it was the mark of penury. Stoutness, by contrast, was esteemed as the mark of the wealthy: there was no honour in poverty, but amplitude was appreciated. Portraits of the Restoration and Augustan eras show Englishmen proud to display a good *embonpoint* or an ample corporation, while fleshiness in females was suggestive of allure and fertility.

Such ingrained preferences for the fat over the thin were also reinforced by patriotic prejudice. Cartoon caricatures took comic pride in the ever corpulent John Bull, in sharp contrast to the onion-nibbling, starveling French peasant, a bag of bones, or the effete, effeminized Versailles courtier, dolled up in the latest foppish fashions but, insect-like, without an ounce of flesh, signifying a lack of virility.

Traditional wisdom maintained that this healthy constitutional stoutness and strength were upheld by a hearty appetite, especially for red meat. The Englishman's proverbial love of roast beef was thus not mere patriotism, gluttony or fantasy, but positively therapeutic. Energetic trenchermanship was a prudent form of preventive medicine. 'He that does not mind his belly will mind nothing,' ran Samuel Johnson's dictum, perhaps hinting at the old proverb, 'The belly carries the legs and not the legs the belly.' Designated by Edward Jenner the 'grand Monarque of the Constitution', the stomach needed to be active and toned up so as to digest the copious amount of food required to concoct the blood, spirits and humours which animated the limbs. Hence the preferred victuals were strong and savoury, and the beef, beer and burgundy diet of the rich was evidently more invigorating than the insipid gruel and water of the poor. 'My Stomach brave today,' purred Parson Woodforde in 1795, 'relished my dinner.' Rarely a day went by without his logging what he ate. Indeed, his ultimate diary entry before his death culminates with a last supper: 'Very weak this Morning, scarce able to put on my Cloaths and with great difficulty, get down Stairs with help . . . Dinner to day, Rost Beef etc.' John Locke was equivocally informed by a correspondent that his wife, 'in order to her health [*sic*] . . . is enterd into a course of gluttony, for shee is never well but when shee is eating'.

This model of the healthy body as a vital economy, demanding energetic and regular replenishment of stimulus, was widely accepted by the medical profession itself, culminating in the controversial Edinburgh medical theorist John Brown, who stressed that life itself was a 'forced state', maintained only by external stimulus (see below, Chapter 21). Dr Thomas Trotter endorsed the advice of the Venetian longevist Luigi Cornaro who prescribed two cordial glasses of wine a day for those aged 40, four at 50, and six at 60 – proof that the much-prized moderation in no way implied abstinence – while Dr Peter Shaw wrote a book in 1724 to prove *Wine Preferable to Water*, indeed *A Grand Preserver of Health*. Alcohol was perhaps the prime item in the entire *materia medica*. For long Parson Woodforde swigged a medicinal glass of port as 'a strengthening Cordial twice a day'.

Hearty eating and drinking in turn required equally energetic waste disposal. Constipation with its putrefying excrements and indurated faeces would, all agreed, produce gastric ferments, flatulence and bile, leading, many feared, to intestinal poisoning. Hence the popular physiology of the non-naturals attended to evacuations no less than to appetites. Purging with laxatives was the panacea, but sweats, emetics and blood-letting were important auxiliaries.

An entrenched medical materialism thus pictured the pulsating body as a through-put economy; its well-tuned functioning depended upon generous input and unimpeded outflow. Circulation was the key, as with the economy at large; stagnation was an evil. This need for positive stimulus had to be squared, however, with other age-old doctrines – both medical and religio-moral – of temperance, moderation and the golden mean. Might not the drive to tank up the system sanction greed and so precipitate pathological excess? 'I verily beleeve [Dr Baines] will kill himself ere long by his intemperance,' lamented Anne Lady Conway, a close friend of the Cambridge Platonists and hence one disposed to beware the snares of carnal appetites. Similar fears were often expressed in reaction to what an early Georgian pamphlet denounced as 'the present luxurious and fantastical manner of Eating'. Notorious for such indigestible favourites as pudding, the English were, as the saying went, digging their graves with their teeth. 'Purging and vomiting almost the whole day,' lamented Parson Woodforde on 18 July 1786, 'I believe I made too free Yesterday with Currant Tarts and Cream &c.'

It was a common tale, even down to the ominous 'etcetera'. John Carrington learnt the hard way when his love of 'Butock of beef' destroyed first his stomach and then his health. At one dinner, his diary reveals, he pigged himself with 'Roasted hear & a hasht hear & boyled Sholdr of Motton & onions, puding etc. . . . Plenty of punch & good company', but justice proved summary: 'Theese fine made dishes did not agree with me, purged me very much all next day, I am for plane food.' Too late, however! Over the next few months, entry after entry reads 'canot eate nor drink', 'no stomake to eat', and so forth. His constitution was destroyed; decay set in, and he died.

If serious eating was parlous, gross drinking proved still more constitutionally destructive. Erasmus Darwin dubbed alcohol 'the greatest curse of the Christian world'; and no wonder, for oceans were swallowed, and not just during the gin craze. Sylas Neville recorded bottle days while a medical student in Edinburgh: 'Sun. Sep. 17. Dined at the Fox & Goose, Musselburgh. . . . Lucky I did not go yesterday, as a company of only 8 or 10, chiefly Shiel's friends, drank 27 bottles of claret & 12 of port, besides Punch, & were all beastly drunk.' Such drunkards 'died by their own hands', opined

Steele's *Tatler*. The irony of toasts was not lost on the Georgians: 'to drink health is to drink sickness.' For, stated George Cheyne, 'running into *Drams*' was ruinous; 'neither *Laudanum* nor *Arsenick* will kill more certainly, although more quickly'. And who knew better of the dangers of dissipation than that Scottish physician who wrestled all his life to restrain the appetites which he knew were medically so lethal?

Born in Aberdeen in 1673 and trained at the University of Edinburgh in Newtonian science and mechanistic medicine, Cheyne migrated to London to make his fortune as a physician. He rapidly established a name as a witty man-about-town with 'Bottle-Companions, the younger Gentry, and Free-Livers'. Gaining a reputation as 'a Scotchman with an immense broad back, taking snuff incessantly out of a ponderous gold box', he hobnobbed in coffee houses and taverns with a free-living crowd (as was the custom among young physicians), so as to get himself known and build up a trade, 'nothing being necessary for that Purpose, but to be able to *Eat* lustily, and swallow down much *Liquor*; and being naturally of a large *Size*, a cheerful Temper, and Tolerable lively *Imagination* . . . I soon became caressed by them, and grew daily in *Bulk* and in Friendship with these gay Gentlemen.' The consequence, however, was that he grew 'excessively fat, short-breath'd, lethargick and listless'. Fearing for his life, he quit London and put himself on an austere (greens, milk and seeds) diet, until he saw his podgy flesh melt away 'like a Snow-ball in Summer'. Over the years, Cheyne's weight was to go up and down with monotonous frequency.

His worst crisis came around 1720, when, experiencing 'a Craving and insufferable Longing for more Solid and Toothsome Food, and for higher and stronger Liquors', he became a three-bottle man and blew up to thirty-two stone (some 450 pounds), eventually needing a servant to walk behind him carrying a stool, on which to recover every few paces. His legs erupted in scorbutic ulcers; erysipelas and gout followed; and he took refuge in the 'slow poison' of opiates. At his grossest, he confessed, he 'went about like a Malefactor condemn'd', his gluttony producing 'Giddiness, Lowness, Anxiety,

Terror', 'perpetual Sickness, *Reaching, Lowness, Watchfulness, Eructation*', and a nervous hypochondria which 'made Life a Burden to myself, and a Pain to my friends'. In old age, he recalled his worst crisis:

I had been so exceedingly fat, and overgrown beyond any one I believe in Europe, that I weighed 34 Stone, this had so stretched my Skin and Belly, that when I was shrunk to a common Size by many repeated Vomits, want of Sleep, a perpetual Lowness, Loss of Appetite, and Inability to digest any Thing but Milk and Bread, my Gouts fell out through the Cawl where the Spermatic Vessels perforate it and made a kind of Wind Rupture which was some Years a Breeding unheeded.

Cheyne proved one of the most widely read prophets against physical excess in what was becoming a weight-watching age. Being a doctor, he largely expressed his warnings in medical terms, explaining in a series of books, including *The English Malady* (1733), based upon his own experience, how corpulence produced derangements of the digestive and nervous systems which impaired not only health but mental stability. Tension or laxity of the nervous system produced anxiety, the horrors, sleeplessness, nightmares and fear of death. Excesses of the flesh bred infirmities of the mind.

Cheyne's call to medical moderation was, however, also an expression of a mystical Christian Platonism trained at the emancipation of the spirit – he can thus be thought of as recasting traditional Christian bodily anxieties into physiological and medical idioms. For Cheyne, the flesh was indeed the spirit's prison house. Excessive flesh encumbered the spirit; burning it off emancipated it.

Following the teachings of the German mystic Jakob Boehme, he imagined prelapsarian bodies innocently feeding on 'Paradisiacal Fruits'. After the Fall, the flesh of the newly carnivorous humans had been subjected to the laws of corruption of matter. Addressing '*Expiation, Purification,* and *progressive Perfection*', his works aimed at recovering the purity of the prelapsarian body. So, through keeping the 'pipes' of the body clear of 'peccant Humours', vegetarian diet also relieved fallen humanity from 'the present *load of corruption*' and soothed the 'mortal Distemper' which had afflicted sons of Adam ever since the Fall. The ritual of weighing the soul was an iconographic topos familiar to Christianity from the ceremony of the weighing of sins at the Last Judgement.

Cheyne's views grew influential, and his correspondence with the printer and novelist Samuel Richardson shows his attempts to encourage moderation in his friends and patients by encouraging them to eat less, avoid fermented liquors and exercise more, for example through riding. A 'staunch Epicure' given to overwork, Richardson was urged by Cheyne to relax, diet and exercise – upon the 'chamber horse' if he would not go outdoors; he himself rode it 'an Hour every Morning', noted Cheyne, and found 'great Benefit'. The contraption involved a long board supported on each end, with a chair in the middle which bounced up and down.

Cheyne's books were extremely popular and many later medical thinkers echoed his calls to temperance, with added intensity. Moderation would overcome that classic Georgian disorder, the gout, proclaimed Dr William Cadogan. If the turn towards regulating the flesh was decidedly health-oriented, however, it also became part and parcel of a wider movement, expressive of preferred cultural ideals and personal identities. A sign of this lies in the rise of principled ethical vegetarianism in the second half of the eighteenth century (until then there were only vegetarians by necessity, only those who could not afford meat). Joseph Ritson, for example, held that because dead meat itself was corrupt, it would stir violent passions, whereas greens, milk, seeds and water would temper the appetite and produce a better disciplined individual. In *A Vindication of Natural Diet* (1813), Percy Bysshe Shelley argued that meat-eating turned people sanguinary. Vegetarianism also wore a humanitarian hue – it was cruel for humans to slaughter animals merely for food.

Fatness and thinness, as we have seen, had always raised questions of preferred or prescribed body image, personal and public. The truly obese had always been objects of literary and artistic satire – for grossness bespoke greed, lack of self-control and the vulgarity of temper associated with low life. But in traditional national, social and occupational stereotyping a certain stoutness was a positive property, betokening not just healthiness but the rock-solid strength of the gentleman, yeoman farmer, magistrate or citizen. The able lawyer should be rotund, because he must have a solid grounding in reality and not be easily swayed. 'Bottom' was a desirable character trait, signifying guts, backbone or courage, sound fundamentals.

Other occupations, of course, might require a decorous thinness. The honest clergyman – witness Sterne's Parson Yorick – was expected to be fleshless, because ascetically floating up heavenwards: the lard-tub friar or podgy parson had been, from time immemorial, a figure of fun and contempt. Academics, too, were expected to be somewhat emaciated, living as they did on pure thought, in their heads, aspiring to the purely intellectual. The great Sir Isaac Newton supposedly often went without his dinner, not descending to thinking about mere matters of the flesh. Yet the scholar's thinness, that mark of mind, was also reputedly a source of melancholy, illness and discomfort – thus a highly ambiguous serio-comic conventional sign, respectful yet dismissive at the same time.

The years after 1750 were to bring a trend of profound importance for the future: thinness steadily became fashionable in a public arena in which fashion itself was acknowledged to be exerting an ever greater sway. For both males and females, the cut of sartorial styles had long been ample. In post-Restoration female fashions, a cur-vaceous softness at large, and specifically in the breasts – whose snowy, swelling amplitude was endlessly celebrated in erotic art, bawdy tales and medico-scientific writing on motherhood – domi-nated sartorial shapes. Petticoats and gowns proliferated, mirrored by various other forms of swollen display, for example, the preference in the age of Queen Anne for enormous wigs. The swagger portraits of the era of Kneller and Lely were meant to make people look big.

In the latter decades of the century, however, litheness became chic and fashion directed itself to the slim look. Breeches began to give way to trousers and trousers grew tighter; military uniforms became particularly thigh-hugging in the Napoleonic wars. And, in the 1790s, in the wake of the French Revolution, the old layered petticoats, hoops and corsets yielded to lighter fabrics, such as muslin,

for female attire, worn directly over the skin, revealing and emphasizing bodily contours. The new fashions were kind to the young, cruel
to age.

The fashion for thinness, and all it implied about enslavement
to fashion, was criticized by many, including the Bristol physician
Thomas Beddoes, a sharp and radical social observer. It was, in his
view, destructive of health. How bizarre that bright young things,
seeking public attention, positively sought to look tubercular, as if
delicacy and a tenuous grasp on life made them all the more appealing
– indeed, sexy!

Through association with fine sensibility and the cult of youth, the
tubercular look – indeed tuberculosis – was becoming positively *de
rigueur*. 'Writers of romance', wrote Beddoes, '(whether from ignorance or because it suits the tone of their narrative) exhibit the slow
decline of the consumptive, as a state on which the fancy may
agreeably repose, and in which not much more misery is felt, than
is expressed by a blossom, nipped by untimely frosts.' The preposterous idea had taken root that 'consumption must be a flattering
complaint', associated as it was with superior imagination, talents
and discrimination.

Many doctors and critics accused trend-setting élites of pursuing
pernicious lifestyles which sacrificed health to fashion. Mad for the
mode, high society was decking itself out in the injurious 'light dress'
that was all the rage in the Revolutionary 1790s. And such sartorial
frivolity was just the tip of the iceberg. For the 'method of education'
that was *à la mode* in polite circles aimed to turn children into
weaklings. Seduced by the siren sensibility and neglecting the sound
advice of Locke, parents made their progeny serve time as 'poor
prisoners' in draughty boarding schools. Thereafter, adolescents, by
then 'weak, with excess of sensibility', were allowed to lounge around
at home on sofas, reading 'melting love stories, related in novels'. All
such diversions designed to 'exercise the sensibility' proved 'highly
enervating'. Not surprisingly, thanks to this 'fatal indolence', 'the
springs of their constitution have lost their force from disuse'. A
further insidious danger to the flesh derived from sedentariness: the

solitary vice. Beddoes judged onanism the predictable outcome of the irresponsible cocktail of mollycoddling, absurdity and neglect which passed for a polite upbringing.

In the process whereby a girl was 'manufactured into a lady', parents positively delighted in delicacy. Thin being fashionable, such darlings were allowed to get away with finicky eating. Hoodwinked by pseudo-medical faddery – were they all reading Cheyne? – parents were encouraging vegetarianism, 'believing that they thus render the constitution a signal service'. All such foibles had to be abandoned, insisted Beddoes, looking to medieval forebears as models. They hunted, fought, hawked, and did without 'effeminate' carriages. 'The general diet of former centuries was more invigorating', for the 'opulent of both sexes, appear to have participated rather more largely of animal food', often breakfasting 'upon a fine beef steak broiled'. By contrast with the preciosities of the fastidious – 'it is upon the lilies of the land, that neither toil nor spin, that the blight of consumption principally falls' – far healthier were labourers who pursued heavy physical exercise, drank with gusto and, above all, were lusty carnivores.

The vitiated taste for the slimline and slender which Beddoes deplored is indeed a lifestyle watershed. It marks the moment when fashion began that infatuation with youth, with its innocence, spontaneity and unspoilt beauty, which has grown (admittedly unevenly) ever more marked over the last two centuries. Increasingly, the fascinating personality was youthful rather than mature, spirited rather than wise, sensitive rather than sober, budding rather than formed: 'Bliss it was in that dawn to be alive, / But to be young was very heaven': the youth cult is evident, not just in Wordsworth but in many of the writings of the time, for example in William Blake's *Songs of Innocence*, in the broader Romantic idealization of the child, and (as we shall see in Chapter 25) in Byron's dread of ageing. Flesh was acceptable only so long as it did not yet bear the signs of decay.

This attests a great transformation. Traditional religion professed a profound and principled ascetic suspicion of and revulsion against the flesh. These precepts coexisted with arguments in favour of the healthiness and social eligibility of bulk: weight carried weight. That whole congeries of values was now in question. The Christian distrust of the flesh was undermined, but only to be transvalued and reborn in the guise of fashion's horror at excessive ponderousness, especially when associated with ageing and decline. In the process there arose a new cult of the lithe, limber, slim body indicative of delicacy and fineness of sensibility. Through the modern cult of youth, the body was becoming an object of worship through its initiation into a disappearing act. No longer despised, the body was becoming a tyrant in a new puritanism.

14

PUTTING ON A FACE

Ask a toad what beauty is, the supreme beauty, the *to kalon*. He will tell you it is his lady toad with her two big round eyes coming out of her little head, her large flat snout, yellow belly, brown back. Interrogate a Negro from Guinea; for him beauty is a black, oily skin, sunken eyes, and flat nose.

VOLTAIRE

Looks, so the previous chapter suggested, obviously count in the creation of identity. Appearances are insignia of reality, expressions speak louder than words, a person's mind or soul can be read from their expression – such views are perhaps coterminous with social experience itself, one of those sign-systems indispensable for communication and coherence.

A multiplicity of disciplines has attempted to codify such commonplaces. Stressing the parallels between microcosm and macrocosm, Greek thinkers held that the human form corresponded systematically to the ideal forms and hidden geometrical harmonies of the cosmos at large: man was in some sense the measure of all things, a kind of natural ruler. In a chapter of his *De Architectura* dealing with temple design, the Roman architect Vitruvius (first century BC) commended the use of certain archetypal shapes and natural proportions in building. Declaring it the measure of perfection, he inscribed the body of a male with limbs outstretched within the primary geometrical shapes of the square and circle. This perfectly circumscribed figure ('Vitruvian Man') in turn generated various further sets of proportions. It provided, for example, a guide for column design – columns being the closest architectural analogue to the body. There were, according to Vitruvius, nine head-heights in the total height of the well-proportioned figure; the height of a column should therefore be the equivalent of its 'capital' (Latin: *caput* = head) multiplied by nine. Different column types (Doric, Corinthian, and so on) were to be read as expressive of human diversity, male and female, young and old, plain and fancy. Such ideas were elaborated in the Renaissance: Filarete, for example, treated doors and windows as 'orifices'. As man was patterned on the heavens, so the city and its buildings should be reflections of the human. Traditions were thus inaugurated which were to exercise sway over artistic imaginations and practices long beyond the Renaissance. It was this body classical which bore the *imprimatur* of art, defining the golden and the ideal world as proposed by Michelangelo and enshrined in later centuries in the academic tradition of the canons of beauty.

The Greeks had also outlined a science of physiognomy, later often but wrongly given the authority of Aristotle. Particular facial features and their characteristic expressions – the chin, brow, smile, lips, eyes – vouchsafed evidence of inner states within the mind or soul. Likenesses between human and animal features provided further clues: did not some faces bear close resemblance to wolves, lions, tigers, asses, apes, cats and curs? Did not the animal kingdom in general imitate the human? The Aesopian inference was evident. Committed as it was to humoralism, as discussed in Chapter 3, classical medicine also saw 'complexion', the outward quality imprinted on the skin, as indicative of inner humoral balance and hence of temperament. Overall, one's fortune lay in one's face: physiognomy was destiny.

Christianity, for its part, upheld broadly similar doctrines as to natural signs and the inner and outer. Nature was the book of God, and appearances spoke truth – did not the Bible teach that man was made in God's image? The doctrine of signatures elaborated in Renaissance botany and natural history likewise provided keys to the reading of signs planted in creation – the meaning, use and purpose of a plant or mineral were visible in the signatures that it bore, a natural hieroglyphics stamped upon it by God: there were sermons in stones.

Popular folklore and learned medicine alike furthermore held that 'monsters' or 'freaks' – babies born with blemishes or supernumerary limbs – revealed the secret sin or crime which had marked their conception. If a baby was born with feral features, was it not because, in the throes of passion, the woman was fantasizing about copulating with an ape? The power of the unruly and lurid female imagination to imprint itself upon the foetus amounted to another way in which the inner inscribed itself upon the flesh.

Acting theory, likewise, held that specific gestures and postures adopted on the stage naturally conveyed precise dramatic emotions or meanings. By way of parallel to theatrical rhetoric, it was also held that signing formed a natural language of the deaf, universally intelligible, transcending the arbitrary particularities of national tongues. The deaf and dumb worldwide could thus speak effortlessly to each other, through natural expressiveness, in a way impossible at a meeting of English, French and Germans who could hear.

Classical teachings about painting, too, codified in the Renaissance and given a broad circulation in Georgian England through the Royal Academy, mirrored acting theory by holding that particular poses, demeanour and facial expressions faithfully conveyed specific emotional and mental states. Endorsing physiognomy, the aesthetics of painting schematized commonplace intuitions that beauty of figure and countenance were expressive of goodness of soul, whereas an ugly face, or a deformed body, bespoke the knave. In the language of art and life alike, purity, nobility, virtue and health were all distinguished by beauty; ugliness was the mark of Cain.

Within this universal sign-grammar of good and bad, particularities of body incarnated and encoded specific differences of personality, type or rank. Thus, males not only had bodies that were distinctive from females, but they also revealed discrete characters: a man was not merely male biologically, but *masculine*. Similarly, it was no accident that the upper ranks of society were literally taller –

superiority of height enshrined and blazoned forth superiority of spirit: the lower classes were meant to look up to their betters.

Aesthetic conventions routinely portrayed 'lowlife' characters as low of stature and marked by grotesquely inferior bodies that displayed vulgar and disgusting features, such as the buttocks. By contrast, upper-class physiques were classically marked by loftiness, straight noses, high brows and a sense of self-contained, self-assured prepossession, utterly unlike the porous permeability of the bodies of the low with their gaping mouths and anuses, ever gobbling up too much food and drink, and letting off excessively – farting, shitting, pissing, vomiting, sweating and swearing. Everything picturable told its story in moral and artistic world views in which soul endlessly inscribed itself through the *soma*. If 'high art' standardly affirmed such aesthetics of identity, all could of course be mined and subverted by caricaturists, who exploited the exaggerations of the grotesque for comic and satiric effect.

This entrenched notion that appearance revealed nature was mirrored and extended by wider studies of human types. 'Anthropology' had been a term initially applied to studies of mankind in general, but by the eighteenth century it was becoming more specifically associated with accounts of non-Europeans, especially the 'savages' encountered on exploration of the Americas, Africa and the Pacific. The breathtaking physical diversity of mankind had always made travellers' tales and folklore a source of 'wonder' – all those tribes like the Tartars with heads like dogs, or those who wore their heads beneath their shoulders – but attempts were increasingly made in the Enlightenment to classify them more philosophically, principally on the basis of schemata of different physical types and appearances, and to grade them on scales of the civilized and the savage within the Chain of Being.

One criterion in such differentiations was alleged proximity to other primates – a reprise of the old animal physiognomy. Humans bore evident similarities to the gibbons, orang-utans, chimpanzees ('pongos') and gorillas – themselves barely distinguished – which had recently come to the notice of Europeans. Did mankind descend imperceptibly into such primates? Whites were evidently superior, but negroid types were lower, their wiry hair, darker skins, prognathous jaws, lower brows and so forth clearly flagging them as more 'brutish'. Were they perhaps products of miscegenation with monkeys, and hence not to be sharply differentiated from them at all?

The gradation of human types must have a story to tell. Physical difference had customarily been explained by the Genesis narrative. In the dispersal of tribes consequent upon Noah's Flood and the Tower of Babel, corruption had set in, resulting in a confusion of degenerate tongues and cultures, while, thanks to the curse of Ham, those descending from his seed had sunk into blackness and barbarity.

The stadial sociologies of progress developed in the Enlightenment in turn shaped anthropology, replacing degeneration from Paradise with man's progress from primitivism. This enlightened 'rudeness to refinement' frame of reference (examined more fully in Chapter 19) manifestly challenged the biblical account, questioning as it did regression from an initial Edenic state.

Racial differentiation – 'why were some peoples black?' was how the question was loaded – grew more sharply problematized in an age of imperial expansion and the apogee of the slave trade. Various solutions were suggested. Some held that negritude was a product of living under the tropical sun, a perhaps *beneficial* adaptation to a fierce climate – an environmentalist solution chiming with monogenesis and Lockean malleability models. But if negroes had truly been blackened by exposure to the burning sun, why did their descendants not then lighten when they came to live in colder climes?

Such pigmental indelibility spelt polygenism for some: blacks formed a distinct species altogether, a separate creation. Addressing the 'Diversity of Men and Languages' (in his *Sketches of the History of Man*, 1774), the Scottish judge Lord Kames was one who, wrestling with human variety, concluded that there must have been multiple special creations, hinting that blacks might be related to orang-utans and similar great apes then being unearthed in tropical forests. Various implications might follow from polygenism: it might mean that blacks were permanently different, indeed inferior, yet uniquely adapted to tropical living – one way in which apologists could rationalize slavery. Opponents of racial prejudice and emancipators of slaves reasserted the classical doctrine of the uniformity to human nature. Skin pigmentation was accidental and superficial – only skin-deep, as we might say. Quizzed whether blacks would arise on the Last Day, that pioneering magazine, the *Athenian Gazette*, responded, as we saw in Chapter 6, that the blackness would be left behind when they died – a view echoed in Blake's 'The Little Black Boy':

> My mother bore me in the southern wild,
> And I am black, but O! my soul is white.

If compassionate, Blake clearly believed white was best.

In short, the belief was prevalent and powerful in all manner of discourses, both humoralism and its successors, that physique at large, and in particular the face and its expressions, were signatures of the self within: personality was stamped upon and radiated out from the body. But such convictions were also being intellectually questioned and threatened by events.

For one thing, Cartesian mind–body dualism in the broadest sense posed deep threats. Descartes's radical severance of mind and body, psyche and *soma*, imputed the fundamentals of physiognomy. If mind were disembodied – nothing more than a ghost in the machine – how could scrutiny of the casing of the machine tell one about the ghost?

Many material and cultural developments were lending weight to this subversive possibility. It had always been acknowledged, of course, that reading character might present difficulties, rather like peering though a glass darkly; but what if looks were actually designed to lie? How could physiognomy cope with systematic hypocrisy of countenance?

This was a predicament explored by Georgian novels. From Henry Fielding to the Gothic vogue, they abound with good-natured if guileless heroes and heroines who put their trust in faces, believing, with the Old Man of the Hill in *Tom Jones*, 'a good Countenance is a

Letter of Recommendation'. But the invariable moral was that such natural physiognomists were hopelessly, indeed culpably, credulous. In that novel, Squire Allworthy (names also conventionally told stories) is taken in by the odious Blifil:

Mr *Allworthy* certainly saw some Imperfections in the Captain; but, as this was a very artful Man, and eternally upon his Guard before him, these appeared to him no more than Blemishes in a good Character; which his Goodness made him overlook. . . . Very different would have been his Sentiments, had he discovered the whole.

No accident, surely, that *Blifil* is an anagram of *ill fib* – the name in its own way is as deceptive as the face.

For Fielding, only bitter experience in the lying ways of the world would teach the lesson. Watching *Hamlet* with Tom Jones, the old-stager Partridge scrutinizes the face of Claudius, and exclaims: '. . . how People may be deceived by Faces! *Nulla fides fronti* [Put no trust in the face] is, I find, a true Saying. Who would think, by looking in the King's Face, that he had ever committed a Murder?' The ostensible culprit in all this was knavery, or rather the latest fashions in knavery. Unlike traditional devil figures, the new villain haunting Georgian letters was an ingratiating, specious, two-faced Tartuffe, as Anglicized in Joseph Surface in Sheridan's *The School for Scandal* (1777) – his name, if not his face, gives him away.

Worse still, Georgian opinion was appalled to find itself at the mercy not merely of brazen monsters and bare-faced hypocrites, but of the man of the world; for the man of mode was the man behind the mask. Hobbes, it will be recalled, chillingly stated that 'a *Person* is the same that an *Actor* is, both on the Stage and in common Conversation; and to *Personate*, is to Act, or Represent himself, or an other'; and the religious radical Thomas Tryon chillingly noted that only one type of person lacked that ability to impersonate, possessing rather a character utterly transparent: and he was the madman:

For when men are so divested of their *Rational Faculties*, then they appear naked, having no *Covering*, Vail or *Figgleaves* before them, to hide themselves in, and therefore they no longer remain under a Mask or Disguise but appear even as they are, which is very rare [with] any that retain their *Senses* and *Reason*.

Was it not a strange paradox indeed that the defining character of rational (Hobbesian) man should be his ability to deceive?

Fashion became a dominant feature of eighteenth-century culture, and many critics deplored the consequence, the swirl of fluctuating façades threatening traditional values which had prized port and bearing as manifestations of worth, birth and virtue. Time was, the nostalgic held, when it was impossible to confuse the titled, the gentry and the masses – they looked so different. But could not mere moneybags now mount the grand show of conspicuous consumption traditionally assumed to be exclusive to pedigree, lineage and good breeding? The authenticity of pomp seemed endangered by inflation and devaluation – its signals reduced to a fashion parade. Appearances were sowing confusion. Lord Chesterfield observed that a true gentleman held that the show made by clothes was paltry indeed; nevertheless, one had to dress well, for it was the only way to attract the attention which true gentility deserved.

Meanwhile this critical devaluation of traditional grandeur triggered a frantic search for subtler status signatures which wealth alone could not command. Therein lay the putative allure of fashion for the *beau monde*: would not only the best-bred have the discrimination – denied to Mr Money – to appear not just opulent but tasteful? For, as Hazlitt later put it, 'fashion is gentility running away from vulgarity'. Of course, in the 'continual flux and reflux of fashion' it was all too easily a matter of man of mode today, *démodé* tomorrow. Staying smart – sporting the right look – had to become a fine art. It was no accident that the dandy was about to make his appearance.

Down the ages countless Jeremiahs had, of course, lamented the spread of luxury and its attendant social pretensions and confusions. What is particularly noteworthy of the Georgians, however, is how they were hoist with their own petard, both loving and hating the Vanity Fair of Bath or Vauxhall, their new dream-world of signs. It was they who, even as they indulged the snobbish ostentation of dressing up their servants in their cast-offs, complained that, through such 'levelling in dress', the maid could no longer be distinguished from her mistress. It was they who went in for slumming, Regency beaux dressing down and visiting Whitechapel. It was they who gambled on the Exchange, grabbing South Sea stock, yet bemoaned how paper wealth was a delusion, a mere bubble, lacking substance.

As with the faces of the fake coins flooding the market, so too with human faces; counterfeiting threatened all. Take female beauty. Georgian aesthetics and erotics glamorized fine ladies into sex objects, trained to adopt a femininity that was designed to gratify the male gaze – traditionally that had been the stigma, or prerogative, of actresses and whores. Ladies – respectable ladies, that is – were now making themselves up ever more extravagantly with powder, paint, patches and puffs – such phrases as 'make-up' and 'making a figure' convey the artifice of it all. Nature's face became invisible behind the painted one – for eighteenth-century cosmetics, just like stage make-up, were caked, elaborate and garish of hue. Nature's face disappeared, too (as we have seen Swift complaining), behind visors, wigs, jewels, masks, fans, lace, gauze and other paraphernalia meant to conceal age, wrinkles and pock-marks, and to tantalize all at once.

Public – that is, *male* – ambivalence about make-up shows in one specific physiognomic anxiety. The test of a lady's modesty proverbially lay in her capacity to blush: she who could not blush was the lady without shame. But the woman who wore rouge (or as we say today, 'blusher') wore an imitation blush, which all too readily camouflaged lost innocence, hiding the bare-faced cheek of the shameless woman. 'When a Woman is not seen to blush,' opined Fielding, 'she doth not blush at all.'

And so the Georgian belle figured as a creature of art, such as was parodied as Lady Stucco, an off-stage character in *The School for Scandal*, 'made up of paint and proverb'. Indeed, as cartoonists never tired of revealing, such a woman was forever displaying herself actually making herself up, or holding court *en déshabillé* at her toilette, where she would perform the rites of 'making her face' (more sexual innuendo, for 'making faces' was colloquial for having sex).

The quintessence of this man-made, made-up milieu was the vogue for the masquerade, damned by Addison as a front for 'assignations and intrigues'. The itch to go incognito, perhaps even cross-dressing, seemed to many the depth of decadence: no longer the proud escutcheon of self, one's appearance was merely a device for going hidden, trying out new identities, revelling in confusion, surprise and deceit – a delicious danger, naughty but nice. The masquerade might be taken as the materialization of Locke's destabilizing of identity: there, multiple personality was not merely possible, it was mandatory.

In this way, fashion threw down the gauntlet to conventional physiognomical wisdom. What was to be done, was there a remedy? One much touted antidote was the maxim to put one's trust not in faces but in actions. 'By their Fruits you shall know them'; thus Fielding quoted Scripture in his *Essay on the Characters of Men* (1743); or, in more homely terms, 'handsome is that handsome does'. In the end, it would be the deeds of a Blifil – or of those other objectionable characters in *Tom Jones*, Square or Thwackum – which would give the lie to the specious promises of their oily words and plausible faces.

If looks thus denied any earnest of personality, perhaps the best way of weighing up characters was indeed literally to weigh them up. This whimsical suggestion came from John Clubbe, a quirky antiquarian, who, despairing of conventional physiognomy and seeking an alternative 'Key to every Man's breast', decided, as a good Newtonian, that the way to tell the light- from the heavy-hearted was through the 'Mechanical Apparatus' of a magnetic weighing-machine, which would 'weigh men in the balance' to gauge their 'intellectual Gravity'. The suggestion itself was light-hearted, but it carried a graver purpose. For gravity of demeanour was an imponderable of great physiognomical ambivalence, precisely because, as Lord Shaftesbury had observed and Fielding had quoted, 'Gravity is of the Essence of Imposture'. It was the grave-faced gentleman, in the opinion of Sterne's Parson Yorick, who was the real hypocrite – and

Yorick, more than a little phthisical, hated naught so much as the grave.

As Clubbe's black humour suggests, the prospects for a true physiognomy looked slim. Tristram Shandy himself pondered the difficulty of 'taking a man's character'. Had 'Momus's glass' but been set up 'in the human breast', it would all be so easy, for in that case it would be possible to see into a man's soul without any difficulty. 'But this is an advantage not to be had by the biographer . . . our minds shine not through the body, but are wrapt up here in a dark covering of uncrystallized flesh and blood.' But that was impossible, and perhaps just as well, given the sinister resonances of 'taking a man's character'. (Momus, the ancient god of fault-finding, wanted a window in man's breast through which his thoughts could be seen.)

Not surprisingly, then, many Georgians opted, not for an alternative physiognomy, but for alternatives to physiognomy, techniques for managing social intercourse amid the faceless crowd. One solution was to embrace the idea of the world as a stage: 'The World hath been often compared to the Theatre,' opens the seventh book of *Tom Jones*. Men and women were simply players, acting their parts, mouthing their lines. In this *theatrum mundi*, transparency and intelligibility would no longer have to rely upon a penetrating physiognomical gaze. Rather, what was needed, precisely as the *Spectator* had advocated, was shared texts and agreed performing styles and stage directions. Each must act out his presentation, not of the self but of his role in the text of life. Not sincerity, but keeping up appearances, looking the part, following good form – these were what counted.

Early in the century, of course, Bernard de Mandeville had given the theatre of the world a more cynical twist. *The Fable of the Bees* had argued that the hypocrite was not a *personally* depraved parasite, for social morality itself was one gigantic collective sham, the name of the game, the *comme il faut*. Morality was a tacit compact to camouflage lust, pride and selfishness behind a veil of decency. Hence morality was 'Cant', a 'Deceit', 'Cheat' or 'counterfeit Gravity' for form's sake, in which all undertook 'a dextrous Management of ourselves', 'hiding the real Sentiments of our Hearts before others', thereby gaining our desires without losing face 'in the Eyes of the World'. The 'Mask Hypocrisie' was thus not society's solvent but its cement.

The socially acceptable epitome of Mandeville's philosophy lay in Lord Chesterfield's advice to his son. Chesterfield bade young Philip pay lip-service to the rules of the game. Yet his view of conduct befitting a gentleman also shows an interesting twist. For Chesterfield judged expressiveness of countenance to be hopelessly vulgar. Never be seen laughing, he admonished, for laughter betrayed rusticity – and carious teeth – and involved a 'shocking distortion of the face'. The most a gentleman should do is smile (he should never show his teeth). Chesterfield was, in fact, advocating something more shady than that: that his son for private gain should undermine the public style of acting. 'Make yourself absolute master ... of your temper and your countenance,' he advised, 'so far, at least, as that no visible change do appear in either, whatever you may feel inwardly.' The point was precisely to be inscrutable, illegible, and thus to defy the *voir*, *savoir* and *pouvoir* of others:

A man who does not possess himself enough to bear disagreeable things without visible marks of anger and change of countenance ... is at the mercy of every artful knave, or pert coxcomb; the former will provoke or please you by design, to catch unguarded words or looks by which he will easily decipher the secrets of your heart.

Self-possession was thus the ultimate challenge to physiognomy.

Chesterfield, however, was widely dismissed as a poseur. Fresh cultural currents were flowing from the mid-eighteenth century, aiming to put corrupt society back in touch with nature, with true feelings, spontaneity and the heart. The revised doctrines of physiognomy advanced by the Swiss pastor Johann Caspar Lavater attempted to overcome its problems by holding that true physiognomy must focus not upon the labile and factitious features of the face – smiles, scowls, pouts, grimaces, sneers – but rather on permanent anatomical features – jaw structure, nose and ear size, brow angle and so on – over which the individual had no manipulative control but which had been created by God and Nature as a legible public language.

Novelists and painters endorsed Lavaterian views by continuing, with great consistency, to portray the good, noble and heroic as beautiful and fair of countenance, and villains as dark and disfigured. Few eighteenth-century sitters wished to have themselves depicted by face-painters warts and all, in the Cromwellian manner, and that is true even of self-portraits, as is shown in Sir Joshua Reynolds's idealizations of himself. Such preferences could be rationalized by arguing that idealized presentations were uplifting and therefore carried moral force. But the underlying issues had become hotly debated. For example, in William Godwin's novel *Things As They Are* (1794, later retitled *Caleb Williams*), the gentlemanly and aristocratic Falkland is fair of countenance but, as Williams himself discovers, he has a hidden flaw – his appearance flatters to deceive. Caleb Williams has a noble soul, though one encased within an unprepossessing demeanour.

In short, the relationship of personality to physique remained fraught. Conventional wisdom taught that appearance was legible – experience warned otherwise. Meanwhile, a succession of would-be sciences of physical appearance, from physiognomy to physical anthropology, staked their claims to explicate the dark secrets.

15

SEXING THE SELF

You think she's false
I'm sure she's kind,
I take her body
You her mind.
Which has the better bargain?

WILLIAM CONGREVE

In his *Essay concerning Human Understanding*, Locke took up the challenge of the nature of the person, one thrown down by Hobbes in his comments on the 'persona' quoted in the last chapter. Addressing subjectivity, Locke equated 'person' with conscious self-hood, continuity of consciousness capable of representing itself to itself. Given that that '*self* is not determined by Identity or Diversity of Substance . . . but only by Identity of consciousness', he declared that '*Person* . . . is the name for this *self*'.

That seemed to account for the person of 'man', tacitly male. What, however, about that of a woman? All too easily might she experience herself as no person at all. Dated March 1768, the very first entry in Fanny Burney's journal is thus addressed 'To A Certain Miss Nobody'. 'A thing of this kind ought to be addressed to some-body,' she pondered:

I must imagine myself to be talking – talking to the most intimate of friends – to one in whom I should take delight in confiding, and remorse in concealment: – but who must this friend be? . . . To *whom*, then, *must* I dedicate my wonderful, surprising and interesting Adventures? . . . – Nobody!

To Nobody, then, will I write my Journal! since to Nobody can I be wholly unreserved – to Nobody can I reveal every thought, every wish of my heart, with the most unlimited confidence, the most unremitting sincerity to the end of my life!

Alongside this self-negating diary of a female nobody, other takes were possible on the status of female personhood – or the lack thereof. In the 1790s the pioneer feminist Mary Wollstonecraft deplored the fact that women were admired pre-eminently for their 'person' – what was most conspicuous about them. What she meant by that, of course, was far from Hobbes's or Locke's meaning: it was the *figure*. Her *A Vindication of the Rights of Woman* (1792) explained that the 'person' of a woman was 'idolized', that is, respected only for its 'sexual character'. It was an admiration which paradoxically cheapened and weakened those upon whom it was bestowed: for Protestants, nothing was more detestable than idolatry.

For Wollstonecraft, public – that is, male – fixation upon the female 'person' entailed and sustained the subjection of women. In a provocative but sinister conspiracy, men sought women for their physical charms, and women colluded with flirtatious looks and demeanour so as to secure the most eligible males in the marriage market. In this matrimony game, a mode of sexual selection, the stakes were high, but the rules were devised by males, and they held all the trump cards.

How had that situation come about? The eighteenth century brought many attempts to explain – and that usually meant endorse – the relations between the sexes historically, perhaps the most thorough coming from William Alexander. In his *History of Women*, published in three volumes in the 1770s, this obscure Scottish surgeon maintained that the difference between the sexes was not just a matter of timeless biology: the sexes were essentially socially constructed – indeed, quite specifically, womanhood was of men's making. Men were always grousing about women, he noted, 'without examining how far these complaints are well or ill founded, we shall only observe, that in cases where they are well founded, when we trace them to their source, we generally find that source to be ourselves'. Women were thus products of patriarchy – men got the women they deserved. It was therefore time that they were not reviled but understood. That is what Alexander set out to do.

The evolutionary account he unfolded was significantly grounded in the histories of wealth, property and law set out by the social theorists of the Scottish Enlightenment. John Millar's *Observations Concerning the Distinction of Ranks* (1771), the essay 'Of the Progress of the Female Sex' in Lord Kames's *Sketches of the History of Man* (1774) and William Robertson's *History of America* (1777) laid the foundations for Alexander's view that, considered as a commodity, women had become, thanks to successive stages of development, more highly valued. Deploring the plight of the sex in 'barbarous' societies, all such writers designated the 'savage' woman as slave or drudge. 'To despise and degrade the female sex', explained Robertson, 'is the characteristic of the savage state in every part of the globe.'

Millar theorized the historical evolution of women in society. Primitive males were marked not by the 'passions of sex' but by 'mere sensual appetites'. The hardships of savage life deprived them of the leisure for 'cultivating a correspondence with the other sex', while the lack of economic and social stratification allowed free and tyrannical access to women through rape and conquest. Speculating about the place of women, on the basis of his voyage to Tahiti with James Cook, Joseph Banks similarly reflected how, in Africa and the Americas, women were treated solely as beasts of burden. 'Can love exist in countries where women are beasts of burthene,' he asked: 'I think not.'

With the rest, Robertson interpreted the subsequent private ownership of women (within matrimony) as a milestone of progress, proof of a new male 'attachment' to the female sex – a dramatic advance upon the 'dispassionate coldness' of the primeval savage. The advent of private property in women was a stage along the road to improvement: 'In countries where refinement has made some progress, women when purchased are excluded from society, shut up in sequestered apartments and kept under vigilant guard of their masters.' Transformed into private property, women's value rose as objects of jealous care – a marked advance, he insisted, over their 'beast of burden' status in savage society.

The privatization of women as exclusive personal belongings thus accorded them a role, however passive, in social progress; for as wives they could inspire the ripening of male sentiments and passions, even if they hardly developed into higher beings themselves. The sex was thus instrumental in bringing about the ends of progress. Feminine affection and maternal love were typically treated by Kames, Millar and Robertson as biological constants: womankind had been quasi-civilized all along, naturally possessing as she did a soft and docile sensibility, esteem for which grew with the refinement of males. Thanks to the woman, it was thus the male who truly rose from savagery to civility.

In proceeding to trace the 'gradual progress of women from their low state in savage life to their elevated station in civilized nations', Kames too made it clear that he believed that women's 'progress' consisted not primarily in any (self-)improvement of their own faculties and prospects but rather in the increased regard for their qualities entertained by men. In the Scottish conjectural scheme of history, women were thus credited as essential, but passive, bearers of civilization.

Two factors were particularly singled out in such accounts of 'improvements' in the standing of women: the role of material enrichment, and the impact of chivalry. To Millar, it was only with the later (feudal) stages of material development, accompanied by advances in property law and inequalities of property and rank, that there emerged a true enhancement of women's status, and sufficient peace and leisure to permit warm imaginations to focus on those charming objects of desire. The triumph of chivalric ideals with their cult of love had further brought that 'great respect and veneration for the female sex' which had so transformed European manners.

Not until the emergence of commercial society, however, did 'women become, neither the slaves, nor the idols of the other sex', but 'friends and companions' in the blossoming of the modern, domesticated family, when the sexes, while differentiated by a division of labour, were united by 'esteem and affection'. Only in modern refined society, Kames emphasized, had women achieved – that is, been granted – the regard which assured them enhanced status. 'One will not be surprised', he commented, 'that women in Greece were treated with no great respect by their husbands. A woman cannot have much attraction who passes all her time in solitude: to be admired, she must receive the polish of society.' Modern times had carved out influential public spaces and roles for them. All such analyses may be read as the cynical Mandeville's fable history of the prizing of women seen through rose-coloured spectacles.

In his elaboration of such themes, Alexander essentially concurred. Among primitives, woman was a work slave: sexual slavery followed. Early women were also objects of sexual trading. Becoming the property of males, they had no rights of their own but acted as an improving ferment. With the general progress of society, he explained, women gradually acquired influence and status in developments facilitated by changing manners and morals, new cultural ideals and, through a complicated symbiosis, legal arrangements. In a series of chapters titled 'Of the Treatment, Condition, Advantages and Disadvantages of Women, in Savage and Civil Life', Alexander drew upon the materialism of the 'four stages' theory of social development common to Millar, Smith and others, to chart the progress of the sex 'from slavery to freedom'.

Like Millar, he made much of the impact of courtly love. By idealizing the maiden, making her inaccessible, and requiring honour and valour on the part of the male suitor, medieval minstrelsy produced a cult of pure love – as distinct from gross possession or gratification – which idealized the female. Chastity commanded greater respect, and the love object was less to be enjoyed than worshipped – a development paralleling the cult of the Virgin in medieval Catholicism.

In his own century, Alexander pointed out, important changes were afoot. The softening of manners inherent in the transition from a warrior to a polite urban society exalted the role of woman as hostess, home-maker, mother and educator. Heightened domesticity gave her, if not the whip-hand, at least greater sway. Women polished society, and society, in return, granted them higher status. Only in Europe (as opposed to primitive societies) were women neither 'abject slaves' nor 'perpetual prisoners', but rather 'intelligent beings'. Refinements in the treatment of women were thus benchmarks of progress.

Such developments, so complacently applauded by magnanimous male theorists, might be experienced by women not as progress, however, but at best as a mixed blessing and, at worst, highly deleterious: new refinement was just old slavery writ large. The implication grated that the sex's nature and destiny were subordinate to pleasing males and improving society. All too readily did such views sanction doctrines of the complementarity of the sexes which were barely disguised justifications for enduring male supremacy – 'You must lay it down for a Foundation in general', taught Viscount Halifax in his *Advice to a Daughter* (1688), 'that there is *Inequality* in the *Sexes*, and that for the better Oeconomy of the World, the *Men*, who were to be the Lawgivers, had the larger share of *Reason* bestow'd upon them.' Such naked expression of male superiority ceased to be politically correct in the eighteenth century, but the Scottish physician John Gregory, the English writer James Fordyce and other authors of influential advice books for women continued to insist that the finest contribution women could make to society was to grace it by their superior sensibilities: through their placidity and compliance, the fair sex should be a softening agent.

Jean-Jacques Rousseau's influential educational manual, *Émile*, was comparable in its drift. The boy Émile was to be brought up as active, rational and assertive; complementing him, his sister Sophie should be yielding, loving and nurturing – indeed, specifically child-like: it was for men to exercise their reason, women to feel. It was through such accommodation of opposites that the wisdom of sexual difference would best be fulfilled.

Resenting and resisting such blatant sexism or rationalizations of gender difference, many women turned to Locke's model of the mind as a *tabula rasa* – the mind had no sex – and the view expressed in his *Some Thoughts Concerning Education* of the essential mental identity of boys and girls – by consequence of which there should be 'no great difference' in the training of the sexes. Calling on parents to reject 'the absurd notion, that the education of females should be of an opposite kind to that of males', the Whig Catharine Macaulay out-Locked her hero by arguing unambiguously for unisex education. 'Let your children be brought up together,' she declared, 'let their sports and studies be the same; let them enjoy, in the constant presence of those who are set over them, all that freedom which innocence renders harmless, and in which Nature rejoices.' Girls should receive a no less intellectual education than boys was also the view of Richard and Maria Edgeworth's *Practical Education* (1802).

Few women went so far as Macaulay, however, in seemingly collapsing male and female identities. Many favoured some version of the division of sexual labour as envisaged by the Lockean *Spectator*, which conferred a civilizing mission upon the sex. Urging improved female education, Addison and Steele called upon the fair to comport themselves more rationally, so as to be true companions to their husbands and proper examples to their children. Girls should be brought up as rational creatures, not to qualify them for professional careers or the senate, but because reasonable women made the best wives and mothers. If Swift mocked Addison for 'fair sexing it', prominent ladies applauded his stand. 'The Women have infinite obligation to him,' the bluestocking Mrs Elizabeth Montagu complimented Addison:

before his time, they used *to nickname Gods creatures, & make their ignorance their pride*, as Hamlet says. Mr. Addison has shown them, ignorance, false delicacy, affectation & childish fears, are disgraces to a female character . . . He does all he can to cure our sex of their feminalities without making them masculine.

From the pious Mary Astell onwards, whose *Some Reflections upon Marriage* (1697) exposed women's continuing marital 'slavery', a succession of articulate women voiced an idea of female identity in which women should be esteemed primarily for their minds. Astell's prime call was for better education, to ensure women's maturity as moral and spiritual agents: cultivation of the mind was a God-given right and duty.

Elizabeth Carter and the other vocal bluestockings of the Georgian century presented women as polite, genteel and inherently no less intelligent than men. Preferring the life of the mind, piety and sociability, they had no ambitions for professional and political emancipation. And sexuality needed to be treated with extreme caution, since all too often sexual reputation had proved the sex's weak spot. When, for example, Catharine Macaulay married a man half her age, most of her circle cut her: yielding to such irrational infatuation was perceived as letting the side down.

It is in the light of such diverse options that Mary Wollstonecraft's profound dissatisfaction with the available female personas is best assessed. Born in 1759, the second of seven children, Wollstonecraft might have enjoyed the prospects of a comfortable existence, as her paternal grandfather was an affluent silk-master. But his will made provision only for her elder brother and her father, a tyrant who squandered his share of the inheritance. The rank injustice of this – and of so many of her other formative experiences – was not lost on her.

In her late teens she became a lady's companion in Bath – a humiliating experience – returning home in the latter part of 1781 to nurse her ailing but self-pitying mother. The following spring she lived with the Bloods, the impoverished family of her dearest friend, Fanny, leaving them in the winter of 1783 to assist her sister Eliza and her new-born daughter. Hatching a plan to establish a school, the two sisters moved to Newington Green, just north of London, where Mary met the Revd Richard Price, head of the thriving local Dissenting community.

In November 1785 Wollstonecraft set sail on what was to be a wretched trip to Lisbon, where Fanny was expecting her first child. On board she struck up a friendship with a consumptive man whom she nursed day and night for nearly two weeks. All such experiences gave the settings and much of the content for her first novel, *Mary, a Fiction* (1788) – loaded title!

Mary, a piece of self-analysis and fantasy, offers a portrait of a heroine possessed of impressive intelligence and social graces despite a defective upbringing. She feels that life owes her something better than the trials she has to endure: she is at odds with her parents, with her status as a newly-wed, and even with the friend (modelled on Fanny) to whom she devotes herself until her death (like Fanny) from consumption.

Attractive to men, the fictional Mary (barely veiled if somewhat wishful autobiography) enters into flirtatious relationships with several – despatched abroad immediately after the wedding, her husband's only role in the story is to permit (or stymie) other romantic possibilities. She relishes the unvarnished manners of literary men 'past the meridian of life, and of a philosophic turn'; and is moved by an unprepossessing but sensitive invalid, Henry, and his passionate embraces. 'Have I desires implanted in me only to make me miserable?' she asks: 'can I listen to the cold dictates of prudence, and bid my tumultuous passions cease to vex me?' Nowhere is adultery defended in so many words, but the implication is that feeling rather than convention is the honest guide to conduct. Sensibility, 'the most exquisite feeling of which the human soul is capable', is not to be tarnished by the slur of gross sensuality. Published three years after it was written, *Mary* was Wollstonecraft's first attempt to debate out loud the ambiguities of female identity, its perils and possibilities. Her later didactic writings suggest that she drew back from this endorsement of passion as a potential solution or course of action.

On her return from Lisbon, Mary found her school in complete disarray, and her financial difficulties parlous; and, partly to relieve her financial plight, she penned *Thoughts on the Education of Daughters: With Reflections on Female Conduct in the More Important Duties of Life* (1787). Covering such topics as 'Moral Discipline', 'Artificial Manners', 'Boarding-Schools' and 'On the Treatment of Servants', this short book reveals the profound influence of Locke's educational thinking on her conception of moral discipline and how to inculcate it. Parents had to ensure that 'reason should cultivate and govern those instincts which are implanted in us to render the path of duty pleasant – for if they are not governed they will run wild; and strengthen the passions which are ever endeavouring to obtain dominion – I mean *vanity and self-love*'. Girls must be made resilient in the face of life's inevitable vicissitudes: there would be no shortage of them. Her later anthology, *The Female Reader; Miscellaneous Pieces in Prose and Verse; Selected from the Best Writers and Disposed under Proper Heads; For the Improvement of Young Women* (1789), taught similar sternly improving lessons.

Until then, Wollstonecraft's writings had mostly been of a moral hue, but Burke's *Reflections on the Revolution in France* (1790) infuriated her, and her rapidly penned rejoinder, *A Vindication of the Rights of Men*, exposed it as a self-serving parade of rhetoric from a man blighted with a 'mortal antipathy to reason'. Wollstonecraft's Burke was infatuated with Marie-Antoinette (whom she considered devoid equally of virtue and sense), besotted with rank, contemptuous of the people and silent about the oppressive laws which compounded their misery.

Her masterpiece, *A Vindication of the Rights of Woman*, berated for the servitude of her sex politicians, parents, preachers, schoolmasters and -mistresses, tutors and governesses, and such sexist authors as Rousseau, Dr Gregory, Dr Fordyce and Lord Chesterfield. Its social and political proposals ranged from civil and political rights for women down to the details of the school curriculum.

Women must learn autonomy, mastering skills to support themselves and their children. Marriage, she argued, ought to be based on friendship rather than sexual attraction (or, as she now characteristically put it, 'mere animal desire'). What made women's position in the existing social order so radically disadvantaged and unsatisfactory was that they were encouraged (by men; that is to say, by the system) to play the coquette, which, by bringing to the fore qualities that were sex-specific and eroticized rather than human, won them short-term attention. Society would have them flaunt their charms as 'alluring mistresses', by inducing them to behave in childish, kittenish or flirtatious ways.

A vitiated model of female modesty was thus exploited in which chastity – or the reputation for possessing it – was all-important, and this in turn made conquest supremely enticing to predatory men. Women, in other words, had been reduced to coveted sexual challenges and catches, pawns in a game of seduction, resistance and conquest. The status progress trumpeted by Alexander, Kames and Millar was merely a sham: in actuality, modern marriage was no better than 'legal prostitution'. A woman might thus exercise a fleeting sexual power but overall the role was degrading, setting centre-stage as it did an animal passion which would be temporary and should be subordinate. Wollstonecraft wanted something better for her sex: 'I do not wish them to have power over men; but over themselves.'

Encouraging the giddy girl and the spoilt and pettish coquette, sexual power weakened and cheapened women. In her didactic works and later fiction, Wollstonecraft censured the married woman – her main model was Lady Kingsborough, to whose children she had served as governess between 1787 and 1788 – who divided her time between her mirror and the salon, succumbed to every fad, and was flirtatious and unfaithful in thought yet too timid to risk her reputation by taking a lover. Having farmed out her infants to wet-nurses, such a creature showed no true interest in them on their return, fearful lest her daughters should outshine her; she could not concentrate long enough to improve herself by reading; she affected physical frailty, feigned illness to gain attention, lacked all decorum before her husband, children and servants, and feared not God but the loss of her looks. Dependent upon men's favours, such women were no friends to their own sex. From her own mother onwards, she had seen far too much of such frailties all her life.

In her bid to reform her sisters, Wollstonecraft could not sufficiently stress the ephemeral and overrated nature of sex and romance: 'Love, considered as an animal appetite, cannot long feed on itself without expiring,' she explained:

when even two virtuous young people marry, it would, perhaps, be happy if some circumstances checked their passion . . . If sexual desire is part and parcel of a human's life it should ideally lead rather quickly to the state of considered reflective, rational friendship between the male and the female.

The romanticization of women, regarded by Alexander, Kames and Millar as a kind of empowerment (they would, wouldn't they?), in reality thrust two qualities – or rather vices – to the fore. First, ignorance: it was the uneducated and irrational woman who gratified male wants. What was to blame here was 'a false system of education' put about by

men who, considering females rather as women than human creatures, have been more anxious to make them alluring mistresses than affectionate wives and rational mothers; and the understanding of the sex has been so bubbled by this specious homage, that the civilized women of the present century, with a few exceptions, are only anxious to inspire love, when they ought to cherish a nobler ambition.

That defect was to be countered by the rational education of girls on a basis of history, biography, geography, science, domestic physiology and true morality, to which end Wollstonecraft did her didactic bit with her high-minded *Thoughts on the Education of Daughters*.

The other great vice – itself the product of irrationality and encouraged by men – was vanity, that is, preoccupation with 'person' or appearance. This gave women the reputation – alas, all too richly deserved – of being the 'frivolous sex'. 'They spend many of the first years of their lives in acquiring a smattering of accomplishments,' Wollstonecraft priggishly lamented,

meanwhile strength of body and mind are sacrificed to libertine notions of beauty . . . And this desire making mere animals of them, when they marry they act as such children may be expected to act: – they dress; they paint, and nickname God's creatures. – Surely these weak beings are only fit for a seraglio!

The pitiful marriage of ignorance and vanity produced an 'artificial weakness' in ladies which encouraged in them 'a propensity to tyrannize, and gives birth to cunning, the natural opponent of strength'.

Preoccupation with 'person', and the cultivation of alluring appearances dictated by fashion, could, furthermore, be detrimental to health. Like Thomas Beddoes (as discussed in Chapter 13), Wollstonecraft told of women who prided themselves upon their weakness and pallor, so as to gain celebrity. 'I once knew a weak woman of fashion,' she claimed,

who was more than commonly proud of her delicacy and sensibility. . . . I have seen this weak sophisticated being neglect all the duties of life, yet recline with self-complacency on a sofa, and boast of her want of appetite as a proof of delicacy that extended to, or perhaps, arose from, her exquisite sensibility.

The solution to this obsession with 'person' or the body was the cultivation of the mind. For 'in what does man's pre-eminence over the brute creation consist? The answer is as clear as that a half is less than the whole; in Reason.' Rationality in women was all too often scanted, even by the high-minded. Milton, she complained, 'tells us that women are formed for softness and sweet attractive grace' – 'I cannot comprehend his meaning,' she spat, 'unless, in the true Mahometan strain, he meant to deprive us of our souls, and insinuate that we were beings only designed by sweet attractive grace, and docile blind obedience, to gratify the senses of man when he can no longer soar on the wing of contemplation.' Perhaps that was what Milton meant when he wrote, of 'our first parents': 'He for God only, she for God in him'.

The avidity of her sex's absorption in the physical, their preference of body over mind, grieved Wollstonecraft. In truth, everything which drew attention to the flesh was potentially ensnaring for them. In a passage with an almost hysterical ring, she exposed the evils of schoolgirls sharing washing facilities or a common bedroom:

In nurseries, and boarding-schools, I fear, girls are first spoiled; particularly in the latter. A number of girls sleep in the same room, and wash together. And, though I should be sorry to contaminate an innocent creature's mind by instilling false delicacy . . . I should be very anxious to prevent their acquiring nasty, or immodest habits; and as many girls have learned very nasty tricks, from ignorant servants, the mixing them thus indiscriminately together, is very improper.

The result was that, from childhood onwards, women grew too preoccupied with matters of the flesh: 'women are, in general, too familiar with each other, which leads to that gross degree of familiarity that so frequently renders the marriage state unhappy.'

Foundations were thereby laid in youth, she continued in a highly charged and rather misogynistic passage, for that seductive but fatal absorption in the bodily which entrapped women as inferiors. 'Nasty customs' resulted 'which men never fall into':

Secrets are told – where silence ought to reign; and that regard to cleanliness, which some religious sects have, perhaps, carried too far, especially the Essenes, amongst the Jews, by making that an insult to God which is only an insult to humanity, is violated in a beastly manner. How can *delicate* women obtrude on notice that part of the animal oeconomy, which is so very disgusting? . . . After their maidenish bashfulness is once lost, I, in fact, have generally observed, that women fall into old habits; and treat their husbands as they did their sisters or female acquaintance.

Through such over-familiarity, women discovered they could insinuate themselves into men's affections with 'bodily wit' and similar 'intimacies'. In short, she concluded, 'they are too intimate. That decent personal reserve which is the foundation of dignity of character, must be kept up between woman and woman, or their minds will never gain strength or modesty.'

Not least, the pervasive physicality of a girl's upbringing readily led to the evil of masturbation and other 'nasty indecent tricks' learnt from each other, 'when a number of them pig together in the same bed-chamber'. Like many in her day, Wollstonecraft believed that self-abuse became compulsive, thereby rendering women reliant upon sexual gratification in a way sure to encourage an unhealthy dependency upon male attentions. The sex thus made chains for itself.

Wollstonecraft, it must be stressed, was no prude. Since the supreme duty of a woman was to be mother to her children – in a social capacity, mother to the nation – she wanted girls to be educated with a rational awareness of the biological essentials for rational motherhood, including a knowledge of the facts of life: 'Children very early see cats with their kittens, birds with their young ones, &c. Why then are they not to be told that their mothers carry and nourish them in the same way? . . . Truth may always be told to children, if it be told gravely.'

If there is an element of 'the lady doth protest too much' in all this it is because of the deep tensions between precept and practice in Wollstonecraft's life (Boswell offers a parallel). For the author who warned against the perils of sexual passion was also the woman who thrust her attentions upon the married Henry Fuseli and flung herself at the adventurer Gilbert Imlay (and twice attempted suicide after he rejected her).

The dilemmas of Mary Wollstonecraft also epitomize the paradoxes of female identity. Should a woman be just like a man? Were women in some crucial way different? Should such differences be cultivated or obliterated? Should the relations between the sexes be based essentially upon high-minded friendship? Should sex be discounted – in effect, as her husband William Godwin wished, disappear? Did they possess finer sensibilities? What, in short, did women want?

No conclusive answers emerged. What is abundantly clear, however, from the musings and meditations of such women as Mary Wollstonecraft is that women had never before set their own agenda. The perennial and unquestioned despotism of men – in scripting women's roles – must end. They must henceforth be the mistresses of their own destinies. Women could never control their bodies until they first took possession of their minds.

16

TELLING YOURSELF

How provoking it must have been when Thomas Hobbes noted, as we have seen, that our word 'person' was derived from the Latin for 'Mask or Visard . . . So that a *Person* is the same that an *Actor* is'. For actors had never been held in good odour – it was on account of the 'immorality' of the stage for such reasons that the Puritans had closed the theatres down. More broadly, the status of 'acting' or 'playing a part' had always been deeply dubious in Judaeo-Christian (and above all Protestant) cultures desperately fearful of idolatry and similar abominations. Edward Gibbon was amused to quote from his aunt's favourite writer, William Law, ranting about the evils of the theatre: 'The actors and spectators must all be damned: the play-house is the porch of Hell, the place of the Devil's abode, where he holds his filthy court of evil spirits: a play is the Devil's triumph; a sacrifice performed to his glory, as much as in the Heathen temples of Bacchus or Venus &c. &c.' Amateur theatricals would soon prove the downfall of the sexual morals of the younger Bertrams in Jane Austen's *Mansfield Park*.

On the stage, the subversive implications of 'playing a part' have always been explored and exploited through the devices of disguise and mistaken identity, transformation, the classic bed-trick, and such like. Theatrical make-believe revealed how temptingly easy it was to slip out of one part and into another (all it needed was a change of mask and costume); Boswell might actually become Macheath. It also brought to prominence the disturbing reality of illusion: now one saw Hamlet, now one saw Garrick. All these worries had, of course, long been harped on by preachers and moralists eager to expose not just theatres as such but the great 'theatre of the world'. And they were especially voiced in the emergent post-Restoration pleasure society in London and the provinces, in which drama flourished and the tricks of the stage seemed to be pervading the wider world, not least through that abomination of abominations, the masquerade, where everyone could act whatever part they liked, masked and in disguise, for an evening.

If fundamentalists, steeped in the Old Testament, were particularly disturbed by the lies and blasphemy of the stage, even the business of telling one's own story was not unproblematic within Christian values (in popular speech, 'telling stories' remains a common euphemism for lying). For were not pride and vanity – blowing one's own trumpet – among the most heinous vices?

Yet there was a solution of sorts, for Christianity itself had furnished a story of its own, the master-narrative of the salvation of the individual soul, the Bible story of the creation, fall and redemption of Adam and his seed, pictorialized throughout medieval and Renaissance art and versified from Dante to Milton. From medieval times, Catholicism 'humanized' the Christian truths, emphasizing the idea of the immanence of the divine in the human in the cults of the Virgin, the Christ child and *Corpus Christi*, God made flesh. Saints' lives proliferated, and transcendental experiences were recorded by mystics such as Dame Julian of Norwich or her admirer, Margery Kempe of King's Lynn. Kempe's narrative, the very first autobiography in the English language (not written down by herself but dictated to a priest), recounted the story of her trials, temptations and final redemption in the eyes of the Lord. Meanwhile, the office of confession was designed to elicit truthful accounts of the state of one's soul, with a view to contrition, penance and the forgiveness of sins.

In parallel movements, Renaissance humanism sanctioned the growth of self-portraiture and autobiography. The latter genre had many sources and models, notably Augustine's *Confessions*, in which the Bishop of Hippo charted his route from paganism, through heresy, finally to true faith. There were also exemplary humanist reflections upon the self, particularly the writings of Petrarch and Pico Della Mirandola, who set the soul within the divine Chain of

Being, required to fulfil its potential in the order of things as a spiritual being temporarily hitched to a physical body. In more sceptical vein, the essays of Michel de Montaigne in sixteenth-century France raised doubts about the status of the self. His *'que sçais-je?'* – what do I know? – carried the implication that man does not possess true self-knowledge intuitively: humble scepticism is perhaps the basis for Christian piety. Writing or painting oneself could thus be legitimate if it were undertaken in the name of truth, or by way of example, instruction or confession.

While scourging that ultimate scandal, egoism, Christianity thus paradoxically encouraged its highest and most overt manifestation – the notion that God's very design lay in the salvation of the individual soul: Christ died for *my* sins. But to achieve salvation it was crucial to possess the true faith or grace: to tell God and the world of one's sins and doubts, failings and faith, could thus become one of the highest Christian duties, a great act of witness.

The Stuart century brought the flourishing of the genre of spiritual autobiography, particularly among Puritans, providing a framework for highly charged individual experiences. Take for instance George Trosse. Born in Exeter in 1631 into a wealthy family of Anglican lawyers, Trosse later looked back at his youth as a Sodom of sin – a 'very Atheist', he had followed every 'cursed, carnal principle' which had fired his lusts.

Pricked by a 'roving Fancy, a Desire to get Riches, and to live luxuriously in the World', as he recorded in his autobiography, Trosse travelled abroad to enjoy the 'unregenerate World; the Lusts of the Flesh, the Lusts of the Eyes, and the Pride of Life', being led into 'great Sins and dangerous Snares', and indulging in 'the most abominable Uncleannesses' short of 'compleat Acts of Fornication'. Even grave illness did not lead him to think on death and damnation, or on the merciful Providence which had spared him.

Eventually he returned home, a notorious sinner against all the Commandments, enslaved to a licentiousness which had hardened his heart. A crisis ensued. After one particularly gross drinking bout, he awoke hearing 'some rushing kind of Noise' and seeing a 'shadow' at the foot of his bed. 'I was seiz'd with great Fear and Trembling,' Trosse recalled. A voice demanded: 'Who art thou?' Convinced it must be God, he contritely replied, 'I am a very great Sinner, Lord!', and fell to his knees and prayed. The voice proceeded. 'Yet more humble; yet more humble.' He removed his stockings, to pray upon his bare knees. The voice continued. He pulled off his hose and doublet. Warned he was still not low enough, he found a hole in the floor and crept into it, praying while covering himself in dirt.

The voice then commanded him to cut off his hair, and at this point he anticipated it would next tell him to slit his throat. Spiritual illumination now dawned: the voice was not God's but the Devil's! Knowing he had 'greatly offended', he finally heard a call: 'Thou Wretch! Thou hast committed the Sin against the Holy-Ghost.' Falling into despair – the sin against the Holy Ghost was reputed to be unpardonable – he wanted to curse God and die, and his head exploded with a babel of clamouring voices, making a 'Torment of my Conscience'.

Buffeted by further voices and visions, Trosse fell into a 'distracted Condition'. His friends, fortunately, knew of a physician of Glastonbury in Somerset who was 'esteem'd very skilful and successful in such Cases'. There they carried him by main force, strapped to a horse; he resisted with all his might, believing he was being dragged down into the 'Regions of Hell'. Voices taunted: 'What, must he go yet farther into hell? O fearful, O dreadful!' The Devil, Trosse later recalled, had taken complete possession.

He identified the Glastonbury madhouse with hell, seeing its fetters as satanic torments and his fellow patients as 'executioners'. Eventually, however, though long seeking 'revenge and rebellion' against God, he grew more tranquil, largely thanks to the doctor's wife, 'a very religious woman', who would pray with him until his 'blasphemies' began to subside. Finally, 'I bewail'd my Sins', and he was thought to have recovered enough to return to Exeter.

Alas! Like the proverbial dog to his vomit, he returned to his old ways. This time, however, the fight with the Tempter was in the open. He now applied to godly ministers for guidance in removing his 'great Load of Guilt'. Carried once again to Glastonbury, he 'rag'd against God', believing that he had sinned once more against the Holy Ghost, but the doctor 'reduc'd [me] again to a Composedness and Calmness of Mind'.

Even then, his regeneration was not complete, for his faith was but 'Pharisaical'. Backsliding, he was induced to return for a third time to Glastonbury. Finally, and this time permanently, 'God was pleas'd, after all my repeated Provocations, to restore me to Peace and Serenity, and the regular Use of my Reason'. A man reborn, Trosse went off to study at Oxford. With divine assistance, he was called to the ministry, and he became a pious Nonconformist preacher. He told the world his story in *The Life of the Reverend Mr George Trosse: Written by Himself* – it was published posthumously in 1714 – so that others could know God's mercy and be able to bring themselves back from the brink.

Among the many contemporary tellings of the self through the Christian narrative of sin and redemption, the most influential were the writings of the tinker John Bunyan, a Baptist. Persecuted in the repressive atmosphere after the Restoration he wrote his classic works in Bedford Gaol: as so often, the imprisonment of the flesh was the emancipation of the spirit. *Grace Abounding to the Chief of Sinners* (1666) told of a reformed sinner, and, in allegorical mode, *The Pilgrim's Progress* (1678) narrated the snares besetting the Christian. For Bunyan, the pilgrim's road to the Celestial City winds through Vanity Fair, where Christian and his companion Faithful are pelted by the mob, set in irons, and hurled into a cage as a public spectacle. Faithful is sentenced to be burnt at the stake, and though Christian escapes and 'came to a delicate plain, called Ease', this is more the beginning of his trials than the end: 'at the farthest side of that plain was a little hill called Lucre', and beyond lay Doubting Castle.

As autobiography, *Grace Abounding* is remarkable for what it does *not* tell us about Bunyan – we do not even find out the name of his wife. Everything is excluded from this spiritual autobiography but what touches on his inner life, the trials he underwent and their meaning, the spiritual battlefield on which he was assailed. Even at the tender age of 9 or 10, Bunyan was afflicted by dreams of devils – indeed, he wished himself a devil, so that he might be tormentor rather than victim. The first great crisis occurred after his marriage. One Sunday, he heard a sermon on Sabbath-breaking, and 'at that time I felt what guilt was, though never before, that I can remember'. By afternoon, he had shaken off his agony, but he could not escape it for long, for

the same day, as I was in the midst of a game at Cat, and having struck it one blow from the Hole, just as I was about to strike it the second time, a Voice did suddenly dart from Heaven into my Soul which said, *Wilt thou leave thy sins and go to Heaven, or have thy sins and go to Hell?* At this I was put to an exceeding Maze. Wherefore, leaving my Cat upon the ground, I looked up to Heaven, and was as if I had, with the Eyes of my understanding, seen the Lord Jesus looking down upon me, as being very hotly displeased with me, as if he did severely threaten me with some grievous Punishment for these and other my ungodly Practices.

Bunyan leapt to the conclusion that he was quite beyond redemption. 'Wherefore I found within me a great desire to take my fill of sin, still studying what sin was yet to be committed, that I might taste the sweetness of it.' For two years he was convinced of inescapable damnation. He tried to make sense of all that happened to him, including his dreams. He once found himself alone and cold at the foot of a walled mountain on whose sunny slopes sat the blessed people of Bedford he so envied. After some searching, he discovered 'a narrow gap, like a little doorway in the Wall', and at last managed to pass through it. Every new conviction of salvation brought with it new trials and new temptations to blaspheme, as it were to test God's love.

Spiritual autobiographies in this mould continued to be written through the eighteenth and nineteenth centuries, above all by those marginalized Protestant Dissenters who had been excluded (by fiat and choice) from Vanity Fair. Experiencing persecution by the powers of darkness and loathing for the vanities of the world, such pilgrims held that intense individual experience with God was paramount: the term 'experimental' was used to signify that such autobiographies were the product of true 'experience'.

The rich print-based cultural world of the Georgian era also produced, by way of parallel but also critique, many variants upon the genre. Swift and other satirists mercilessly guyed the unlettered self-importance of the peddlers of such soul-food, exposing their humility and self-laceration as an egregious and obnoxious form of self-advertisement (*s'excuser, c'est s'accuser*). Such Puritan hypocrites as Joseph Surface in Sheridan's *The School for Scandal* litter Georgian plays and novels – they were one of the stock butts for an age rejoicing in its escape from moral rigorism.

A secular, comic and satirical alternative to the Christian salvation story was Henry Fielding's *A Journey from This World to the Next* (1743), in which the just-deceased narrator takes us with him on a sardonic tour of the underworld. Inspired by the Greek satirist Lucian, in whose *Dialogues of the Dead* the greats of the ancient world gathered in the nether regions to discuss the vanities and follies of humankind, the satiric journey into the nether regions was a common literary device. In Fielding's variant of the 'News from Hell', a boat filled with the spirits of the recently deceased forms the forum for a discussion of the transitory nature of life.

Fielding's narrator from beyond the grave is deadpan: 'On the first of *December* 1741, I departed this Life, at my Lodgings in *Cheapside*.' The world he leaves behind, without sorrow or regret, contains little but a host of uncaring relatives squabbling over the will and a sozzled old woman watching the corpse – shades of Hogarth. The narrator is then conveyed by Mercury to a coach in which other spirits are awaiting transportation to Elysium, and from them he hears sordid tales of how they in turn left the wicked world behind. The cumulative effect of this – and of the ensuing encounters with the City of Diseases, the Palace of Death, the Wheel of Fortune, the Court of Minos, and with Elysium itself – is to confirm 'the Vanity, Folly, and Misery of the lower World, from which every Passenger in the Coach expressed the highest Satisfaction in being delivered'.

In a key episode, the travellers come to a crossroads, and have to choose between two paths. One is almost impassable, while the other affords the most pleasant of prospects. Yet great crowds are attempting to negotiate the bad highway, and only a few proceeding along the good one. We learn that the obstructed road is the path to greatness, and the clear road leads to goodness.

The much-debated rise of the novel at this time sustained the intensity of the scrutiny into character and motives typical of the Bunyanesque spiritual autobiography, while transvaluing it into secular and psychological terms. Comparable themes were to the fore: the innocent making his or her way in a wicked world, trials of goodness, transformations from ignorance and folly to wisdom, learning the hard way, the innocent abroad – all appear, in the comic register, for instance, in another work of Fielding's, *Joseph Andrews*.

There had always been romances and picaresque tales, but novels seemed something new (hence the name). Their 'realism' gave them a potent appeal, in particular, perhaps, among less sophisticated readers: 'I have heard a party of ladies discuss the conduct of the characters in a new novel,' divulged Robert Southey, 'just as if they were real personages of their acquaintance.' Enlightened psychological analysts pondered as to what precisely gave these products of the imagination such an air of reality. 'The frequent Recurrency of an interesting Event, supposed doubtful, or even fictitious,' reflected David Hartley, paying tribute to the power of the imagination, 'does, by degrees, make it appear like a real one, as in Reveries, reading Romances, seeing Plays, &c.' In daydreaming about a fiction, brooding upon an episode could make it seem true.

Within the novel a newish, and often purportedly autobiographical, mode developed: fiction masquerading as confession. Classic are the first-person narratives of Daniel Defoe – Moll Flanders telling her story in *The Fortunes and Misfortunes of the Famous Moll Flanders* (1722), for instance, is a woman of the world fighting for survival in wicked and mercenary times. Fictionalized from the real story of the castaway Alexander Selkirk, *Robinson Crusoe* presents a hero washed up on a desert island with virtually nothing except his wit and will, to spin a civilization out of himself. Crusoe is the ultimate self-made man, half Christian pilgrim and half entrepreneur, who becomes a king – the ultimate childish fantasy of omnipotence. Scores of novels fictionalized, often in the first person, the saga of the individual confronted by the evil and the powerful, having to learn the ways of the world in order to survive. Sentimental novelists in particular often drew on personal experience. Left by her husband with several young children, Charlotte Smith projected herself as a shabby-genteel heroine in a hateful world. In novel after novel, such as *Emmeline* (1788) and *The Young Philosopher* (1798), her heroines suffer at the hands of legal chicanery and male power, be it that of fathers, ghastly husbands, lawyers, conniving parsons and all manner of other blackguards and bullies.

Apt for exploring the personality under pressure was the epistolary novel, notably Samuel Richardson's *Pamela* (1740), the story of a servant girl made good, and *Clarissa, or The History of a Young Lady* (1747–8), the tragedy of a lady from a genteel family brought to ruin, rape and death at the hands of a rake. The secret of epistolary novels lies in the dissection of the mind not just of the heroine (or less frequently hero) but also of the other correspondents; the novel thereby becomes a vehicle for analysing the interacting psychologies of many protagonists.

Confession, autobiography and fiction merged above all in the writings of Jean-Jacques Rousseau. His *Émile* showed the development of the self through the process of education; *Julie; ou la Nouvelle Héloïse* probed the tangled twists of love and loyalty; above all his autobiographical *Confessions* – a work widely found deeply shocking – justified a self who was neither a model Christian pilgrim nor even a worldly success. *Confessions* was, self-confessedly, about a character neither good nor exemplary whose chief claim to fame was uniqueness. His ringing 'if I am not better, at least I am different' became the late-Enlightenment credo, before inspiring Romanticism. In Addison's eyes, as we have seen, one's duty had been to sparkle as a convivial conformist; in the gospel according to Jean-Jacques, it was in the unbiddable rough diamond that true value lay. The spirit of nonconformity became *de rigueur* and self-preoccupation was prized.

The new privileging of inner experience subverted hard-and-fast classical distinctions between the inner and the outer, fact and fantasy, and invited readers to remake themselves as originals, following inner promptings – with a little help from fictional stimulus material.

The self which loomed so large in autobiographical writings and pseudo-autobiography justified his (or occasionally her) existence primarily in terms of uniqueness rather than exemplary quality. The lives of the saints thus gave way to fictional protagonists as the role models upon whom people would fix and plot their experiences and responses. It is significant that Boswell would urge himself to be Macheath: he never aspired to be St Jerome. The non-commendable became exemplary, and in an age of print, fiction supplied the new role models.

Critics exposed the subversive power of fiction, offering as it did seductively dangerous models for life: the rakish hero, the bewitching lost soul, the woman or man of sensibility justifying all in terms of exquisitely uncontrollable feeling – or even something more brazen still, as in John Cleland's *Memoirs of a Woman of Pleasure*, the best-selling story of Fanny Hill. In the sensibility wave, many readers lost themselves in private fiction, an imaginative collusion with writers. By fantasizing about themselves or fictionalizing their own lives, novelists created texts of the imagination which fed their readers' fancies. Fiction thus emerged as a fertile medium for 'rethinking the self'.

The novelty of the culture the novel created should not be over-looked. For the first time ever, a mass public was identifying itself imaginatively with the fortunes of fictional folks like (or, at least, imaginably like) themselves. The old injunctions to obey the Commandments, to behave like the saints or the exemplary figures of Graeco-Roman antiquity (Horatius, Pericles, Xenophon – all the role models so crucial to Cornelius Scriblerus), were now challenged by the possibility of vicarious imaginative engagement with whatever was picked off the circulating library shelves. It became so easy to fantasize being someone else. That had always been condemned as envy or vain imagination: now it was the ordinary expectation and experience of every novel reader, for it was through such fictions that the secular voyage into the interior was pursued and popularized.

The upstart genre of the novel also marks a decisive embourgeoisement and feminization of culture. With the likes of Charlotte Smith, Maria Edgeworth, Amelia Opie and Mary Brunton penning the best-sellers around 1800, this was the first time that women had made a prime contribution, through the printed word, to the shaping of public manners and morals. As will be clear, it is primarily with the growing prominence of fiction, notably the novel, that the self-identity of women has become an issue in this book.

The novel attracted popular bewilderment and reactionary venom:

> 'Tis NOVEL most beguiles the Female Heart.
> Miss reads – she melts – she sighs – Love steals upon her –
> And then – Alas, poor Girl! – good night, poor Honour!

Countless warnings like this one by George Colman exposed the imputed giddy fantasy life of those high on reading, that solitary vice, in particular (according to the stereotypes) 'the young, the ignorant, and the idle' (Johnson's phrase), sucked down into the maelstrom of print. 'She ran over those most delightful substitutes for bodily dissipation, novels,' reflected Mary Wollstonecraft on her heroine's meretricious mother in *Mary* (1788) – ironically one of her own fictions. Charlotte Lennox's popular *The Female Quixote* (1752), an obvious reworking of Cervantes, was a classic account of an impressionable young woman disoriented by reading fiction. Thinking 'romances were real Pictures of Life', its heroine Arabella drew from them 'all her Notions and Expectations'.

Above all, the project of modelling one's life on fictional characters was exposed time and again as inane and pernicious – often in novels. Witness the comic villain Sir Edward Denham in Jane Austen's *Sanditon*, who

had read more sentimental Novels than agreed with him. His fancy had been early caught by all the impassioned, & most exceptionable parts of

Richardson; & such Authors as have since appeared to tread in Richardson's steps, so far as Man's determined pursuit of Woman in defiance of every opposition of feeling & convenience is concerned, had since occupied the greater part of his literary hours, & formed his Character.

Were not common readers being seduced by fiction, biting their nails and wetting their hankies over the fates of Richardson's heroines? And this dubious identification of the reader with the fictional – this 'novelization of life' – brought a further enigma: the elision of the *authorial voice* with his or her characters, a disorientation, was heightened by the appearance from 1759 of a startling first-person novel of interiority, Laurence Sterne's *Tristram Shandy*. Its vogue – as will be further explored in the next chapter – in large measure stemmed from the slippage of authorial persona between Tristram himself, first person (highly) singular, and his author, Sterne; as also between Sterne and Parson Yorick, subsequently cast as the hero of *A Sentimental Journey* (1768). Gaily and daringly, Sterne smudged the distinction between character and author, while readers were invited to condone the hero's self-revelatory impulses: 'Ask my pen, – it governs me, – I govern not it.'

Whereas *Tristram Shandy* was comically sentimental, later novels harped on the romantic, melodramatic and sexual, notably in the Gothic vogue launched by Horace Walpole's *The Castle of Otranto* (1765). Fascination with the subterranean depths of the emotions attended the dawn of Romantic self-expression; Wordsworth, whose *The Prelude* was a meditation on 'the growth of my own mind', and Coleridge exhaustively analysed their own poetic processes, initially through the enlightened psychologies of Locke and Hartley. The mysteries of consciousness were psychologized and philosophized in fiction no less than in autobiographies and diaries – indeed fiction permitted more daring explorations.

A striking instance of fiction, philosophy and life folding into each other and becoming indistinguishable is offered by *Emma Courtney* (1796), an intensely autobiographical epistolary novel by the petty-bourgeois London Dissenting intellectual Mary Hays. Its eponymous heroine falls for Augustus Harley, a man whose very name harks back to the hero of Henry Mackenzie's *The Man of Feeling*. Her passion unrequited, Emma pursues Harley obsessively, pounding him with love and self-pity, and even proposing sexual surrender ('my friend – I would give myself to you') since her affection 'transcended mere custom'. All to no avail. Tragedy then follows tragedy to a tear-jerking finale.

Striking is the portrayal of the identity of the heroine in terms lifted from contemporary philosophy and psychology. Hays drew extensively upon the determinism taught in her friend William Godwin's *An Enquiry concerning Political Justice*, as well as on Hartley's associationist psychology. Emma is thus driven 'irresistibly' by her passion; what was to blame, she insists in self-vindication, was that flawed sentimental childrearing, especially for girls, which Mary Wollstonecraft had lately condemned: being 'the offspring of sensibility', her infatuation and its consequences were thus utterly beyond her control. 'Enslaved by passion', she had fallen 'victim' to her own 'mistaken tenderness'. 'Is it virtue then', she asks, 'to combat, or to yield to, my passions?' The answer was obvious.

While Hays's heroine was ostensibly presented as a Wollstone-craftian '*warning*' of the mischiefs of 'indulged passion', she was equally evidently glamorized. Aware of these mixed messages, and pre-empting charges of immorality, Hays pitched her appeal to the 'feeling and thinking few', those enlightened readers soaring above 'common rules'. Her *Bildungsroman* was remarkable, but far from unique, in the portrait it offered of late-Enlightenment selfhood in all its deliciously dangerous ambiguities. Her heroine is simultaneously the upholder of earnest philosophical principles regarding sincerity, and a raging emotional inferno; she is fiercely independent, yet a child of circumstances; she is strong-willed, while the product of her environment, driven by forces beyond her control.

Above all, and most shockingly, the core was all autobiography. Emma's fictional miseries precisely embodied Mary Hays's own passion for her first love, John Eccles, and then for William Frend – a considerable Enlightenment figure who had been expelled from

Cambridge University for his Jacobinism. Emma's correspondence in the novel is almost a carbon-copy of some of Mary Hays's love-letters to Frend and also her exchanges with Godwin. Fact and fiction thus merged in the making of late-Enlightenment subjectivity.

The ultimate self-lacerating and, as it were, masochistic example of these rising tendencies to self-dramatization and self-exposure is William Hazlitt's remarkable *Liber Amoris*, published in 1823, the story of his tormented erotic desires for his landlady's daughter, Sarah Walker. *Liber Amoris* drips with self-disgust and self-hatred; the hero is revealed to be mean, jealous, obsessed and unmanly. The various strands of autobiography and autobiographical fiction had moved from the sinner's salvation typical of the spiritual autobiography to the ultimate self-revelation and abasement of its secular successor.

When Hobbes noted that a person was a player, it was in the service of a desperate attempt to restore stability by setting up an artificial ruler and carving out artificial rules and roles. Traditional notions of the self allowed considerable scope for role-playing – all the world was indeed a stage, so long as distinctions were kept crystal-clear between the divine, the natural and the theatrical – or, to put it another way, just so long as the scripts used were those of God's theatre.

In the eighteenth century this ceased to be the case. Pre-allotted parts were rejected. The distinctions between being oneself and playing a part broke down – or were deliberately smudged, and, fired in part by imaginative fiction, the desire arose to play a new part or a multiplicity of them. The scripts of life ceased to be God's: they were of man's own choosing.

17

AND WHO ARE YOU?

Autobiographies and first-person novels, being such personal genres, are often preoccupied with the relations between the body and the consciousness belonging to it. Their protagonists are commonly desperately striving to surmount the frailty and vulnerability of the flesh, to affirm the self in face of danger or desire. The very production of such a piece of writing may represent the attempt to give the musings of the mind some embodied form – the incarnation of print – which possesses an enduring existence of its own, beyond the unreliable and impermanent flesh. *The Narrative of the Life of Mrs. Charlotte Charke* (1755), for instance, reflected at length upon embodiment, being the life story, somewhat larger than life, of an actress notorious for cross-dressing both off and on the stage.

A classic of that kind, however, was Laurence Sterne's immortal comic inquiry into what it was to be a homunculus. *The Life and Opinions of Tristram Shandy, Gent.* was itself the testament of a dying man whose 'leaky bellows' had long before fallen victim to consumption (tuberculosis). Sterne had his first 'bed full' of blood while still a Cambridge undergraduate in the 1730s (he almost overlapped at Jesus College with David Hartley). By the late 1750s, when he embarked on his masterpiece, his condition was worsening, and he was eventually to suffer 'the most violent spitting of blood mortal man experienced'. Tortured by 'long and obstinate coughs and unaccountable haemorrhages', he fled from Yorkshire, where he was by now an Anglican clergyman, to France, in quest of health, hoping that air, mildness and asses' milk would preserve 'this weak taper of life'. France unavailing, he returned 'like a bale of cadaverous goods consigned to Pluto', finally succumbing to the disease in 1768.

Sterne's wasting constitution served as a *memento mori*. But reminders were hardly needed, for afflication and death pursued him constantly. All but one of his children were stillborn or died shortly after their birth, and his sole surviving daughter, Lydia, suffered from asthma and epilepsy. Moreover, his wife, Elizabeth, from whom he grew estranged, became disordered in her wits, probably spending some time in a private lunatic asylum. Small wonder that Sterne viewed life as a knot of fatalities ('Alas poor Yorick! *Remember thee!* pale ghost!', he wrote to his beloved mistress, Elizabeth Draper).

A man of griefs, Sterne took refuge, over many years, in writing *The Life and Opinions of Tristram Shandy, Gent.* Although his hero feared 'my OPINIONS will be the death of me', literary jesting was Sterne's prophylactic against calamity, his way (as he framed it in the dedication he penned to that great and gouty invalid, William Pitt the Elder) 'to fence against the infirmities of ill health, and other evils of life, by mirth'. Yet mishap and mayhem, disease and death scar the novel: the mirth is black of hue. As we obliquely discover, all the hero's family and familiars – his father and mother, brother and uncle, Aunt Dinah and Parson Yorick – have already been buried by the time Tristram, last of his line, comes to compose his life and those opinions which might be 'the death' of him too. 'Lean', with 'spider legs' and a 'vile cough', Tristram is himself the 'sport of small accidents'. He can 'scarce draw [breath] at all', due to a tubercular condition inherited from his father (himself a 'little phthisical'), and all is compounded by another kind of shortage of breath:

To this hour art thou not tormented with the vile asthma thou gattest . . . in Flanders? and is it but two months ago, that in a fit of laughter, on seeing a cardinal make water like a quirister (with both hands) thou brakest a vessel in thy lungs, whereby, in two hours, thou lost as many quarts of blood.

Although on a 'milk and vegetable diet' of the kind commended by Cheyne – the standard regimen for consumptives – the hero's health declines so alarmingly that, on reaching Book VII of his memoirs, 'DEATH himself knocked at my door': 'had I not better, Eugenius, fly for my life? 'Tis my advice, my dear Tristram, said Eugenius – Then my heaven! I will lead him a dance he little thinks of.'

Book VII then charts the hero's attempt to give death the slip. But, victim more than victor, his whole life has been a 'farce', one 'chapter of accidents' – which might explain this bizarre travesty of an autobiography in which the hero never progresses beyond his eighth year, and which regresses to conclude before his birth. Even his origin, he reveals, was misconceived in the toils of his parents' monthly 'little family concernments'. '*Pray, my dear*, quoth my mother, *have you not forgot to wind up the clock?*' – his mother is interrupting – '*Good G—!* cried my father, making an exclamation, but taking care to moderate his voice at the same time, —— *Did ever woman, since the creation of the world, interrupt a man with such a silly question?* Pray, what was your father saying? —— Nothing.' His father suffers an involuntary emission (one ejaculation brings on another), which 'scattered and dispersed the animal spirits, whose business it was to have escorted and gone hand-in-hand with the *HOMUNCULUS*, and conducted him safe to the place destined for his reception'. Our hero thus originated from a conception when 'the few animal spirits . . . with which memory, fancy, and quick parts should have been conveyed, —— — all dispersed, confused, confounded, scattered, and sent to the devil' – causing, according (as we have seen) to Thomas Willis and other best medical authorities, impairment of concentration, energy and virility. Further 'disgrazias' dog not just his conception but his entry into 'this scurvy and disastrous world'. Mrs Shandy's marriage articles guarantee her the right to be delivered in London, though that privilege is forfeit for this particular pregnancy, following a false alarm during the previous one. So she is brought to bed in rural Yorkshire, attended by the local midwife. The labour proving slow, that old worthy is pushed aside by Walter Shandy's accoucheur-crony, Dr Slop, who, incapacitated by a thumb cut to the bone in a previous mishap, extracts the hero clumsily with his patent forceps, with the result that his nose was 'squeezed as flat to my face, as if the destinies had actually spun me without one'. Though a certain Pamphagus, so Tristram volunteers in one of many ventures into misplaced erudition, judged '*Nihil me paenitet hujus nasi* . . . that is, my nose has been the making of me', his own nose's abridgment is the *marring* of Tristram – particularly galling as the maxim that to get ahead you needed a noble one was Walter Shandy's pet theory, backed up by his reading of scholarly authors' 'solution of noses' (' "Can noses be dissolved?", cried Uncle Toby, awakening').

'Begot and born to misfortunes', a 'child of . . . interruption', he was next misbaptized, losing his name and so symbolically his self. A critical fit which leaves him as black as the maid's shoe had necessitated that he be baptized without further ado. In transmission from Walter to the curate, his intended name, 'Trismegistus', gets abridged (like his nose) to 'Tristram', a melancholy misnomer, evoking as it does the Latin for 'sad', destined to blight its bearer still further, since Walter, slave to his system of names, was convinced that 'Tristram' must cast an evil spell.

Cursed in 'geniture nose and name', and robbed of his animal spirits, those superfine fluids essential for vitality and intelligence, Tristram then suffers further physical disaster, losing his foreskin (at least), and being circumcised – or perhaps castrated? – by the guillotine of a descending sash window:

The chamber-maid had left no ******* *** under the bed: – 'Cannot you contrive, master,' quoth Susannah, lifting up the sash with one hand, as she spoke, and helping me up into the window-seat with the other, – 'cannot you manage, my dear, for a single time to **** *** ** *** ******?'

Finally, in this fragmentary autobiography of loss and finitude ('nothing was well hung in our family'), Tristram loses his education. To remedy his son's afflictions, Walter had resolved to write for him the definitive education tract, the 'Tristrapaedia'. Unfortunately, the treatise grows more slowly than his son – foreshadowing *Tristram Shandy* itself: like father, like son, and, Walter being thus counterproductively engrossed, Tristram is left entirely to the devices of his bovine mother, who has 'no character at all'. Had he been able to go on to trace his life beyond his eighth year, well might Tristram have echoed Pope's complaint: 'this long disease my life':

from the first hour I drew my breath in it, to this, that I can now scarce draw it all, for an asthma I got in skating against the wind in Flanders; – I have been the continual sport of what the world calls fortune; . . . the ungracious Duchess has pelted me with a set of as pitiful misadventures and cross accidents as ever small HERO sustained.

This contagious morbidity infects not just Tristram but the entire body corporate of the Shandy household. Besides being 'phthisical' and racked with a 'sciatica', Walter is a crack-brain (the meaning of 'Shandy' in Yorkshire dialect), compulsively intellectualizing, and a dupe to the half-baked speculations of every sciolist from Descartes down to 'Coglionissimo Borri', and a pack of other dunces,* a man who, perennially prating, fuming and thwarted, will 'twist and torture everything in nature to support his hypothesis'.

Tristram's booby brother Bobby ('a lad of wonderful slow parts') expires in his youth. Their uncle Toby, blessed with preternatural modesty (he does not know 'the right end of a woman from the wrong'), has been wounded in the groin in service at the siege of Namur. Captain Shandy's willing servant Corporal Trim has likewise been 'disabled for the service' by a knee wound got at Landen. And few of the supporting characters escape unscathed. The midwife is widowed, as is, of course, Widow Wadman, whose husband, like Walter, had suffered from sciatica. Le Fever, whose wife was a war casualty at Breda, has a sentimental deathbed; the Abbess of Andouillets darkly suffers from a 'stiff joint'; the guileless grenadier in Mackay's regiment is mercilessly whipped; Amandus and Amanda, the lovers of Lyon,

calling out aloud,

$$\left. \begin{array}{l} \text{Is Amandus} \\ \text{Is my Amanda} \end{array} \right\} \text{ still alive?}$$

fly into each other's arms, and drop down dead for joy. Parson Yorick, another man racked by a tubercular cough, dies, and is

---

* Some are Sterne's inventions, some of the foreigners having obscenely comic names (an unconscious shaft against Walter). Thus Coglionissimo means Bigbollocked, and Hafen Slawkenbergius means Shithouse Shitheap.

commemorated by a black memorial (two black pages in the novel): 'Alas, poor YORICK!' Trim's brother Tom ('poor Tom'), married to a sausage-making Jewess whose husband had died of a 'strangury', is a prisoner of the Portuguese inquisition.

It is, in short, beyond question a 'dirty planet', with 'strange fatalities' raining down body blows against the 'delicate and fine-spun web' of life, all stage-managed, it seems, by a 'malignant spirit'; a world where, in anthropomorphic parody of human disasters, window sashes lack counter-weights, knives sever thumbs not string, parlour doors creak on their hinges, medical bags, mimicking their owners, get tied up fast in knots, and parsons' horses are forever 'clapped, or spavined, or greazed ... twitter-boned, or broken-winded': trains of 'vexatious disappointments' – literally

VEXATION

upon

VEXATION

– curse Tristram the archetypal human homunculus – 'skin, hair, fat, flesh, veins, arteries, ligaments, nerves, cartilages, bones' and so forth. Indeed, rather like Gulliver in Brobdingnag, Sterne's characters, to a man, shrink to mere homunculi, dwarfed and defenceless manikins, ill-starred and impotent, overgrown children strong only in the never-never land of their wishes – wishes upon which Tristram promises us an unwritten chapter (wishful thinking). Born under a 'retrograde planet', all the Shandy males are mutilated in some way, doomed to frustration. Toby is psychologically if not physically unmanned. Fortified by syllogisms and questing 'the North-west passage to the intellectual world', Walter has high hopes of turning knowledge into the power to fend off destiny, but falls victim to his hubris. Tristram himself is childless, his 'virility worn down to a thread', and even the Shandy family bull disgraces himself.

Combating this battery of infirmity and injury is a Sisyphean labour. Uncle Toby spends four years recuperating from his war wound, and all for what? Only to end 'wounded ... to his heart', 'love-sick' for Widow Wadman. The lusty widow herself agonizes over the location of Toby's groin wound, anxiously boning up on anatomical tomes on the organs of generation. For his part, Walter is a tireless medical theorist, seeking the elixir of life, and stung by Hippocrates' mocking aphorism, *ars longa, vita brevis* (life is short, but the labour is tedious). Tristram offers regular health bulletins on himself, promising – or threatening – one volume a year for forty years should his 'vile cough' spare him. And even the reader is implicated in this deluge of diseases and hypochondria:

– BONJOUR! – good morrow! – so you have got your cloak on betimes! – but 'tis a cold morning, and you judge the matter rightly – 'tis better to be well mounted, than go o' foot – and obstructions in the glands are dangerous – And how goes it with thy concubine – thy wife – and thy little ones o' both sides? and when did you hear from the old gentleman and lady – your sister, aunt, uncle, and cousins – I hope they have got better of their colds, coughs, claps, tooth-aches, fevers, stranguries, sciaticas, swellings, and sore eyes.

Of course, traditional medicine lent itself to humour. Gross slapstick centres on the squat Dr Slop, with his 'sesquipedality of belly' – Sterne's malicious caricature of the real Dr John Burton of York – who waddles in, all caked in mud, proceeds to reduce Toby's knuckles 'to a jelly' in demonstrating his obstetric instruments, and ends up duelling with the maid Susannah, slinging insults and cataplasms. It is a farce rooted in the Rabelaisian and Swiftian traditions of learned wit and Menippean satire. Dr Slop and Walter Shandy, a man 'given to much close reasoning upon the smallest matters', are both oblivious to reality through being possessed by their own pet medical theories, canting on in the old, exploded scholastic manner, about '*consubstantials, impriments,* and *occludents*': 'You puzzle me to death,' bewails Uncle Toby, on the receiving end one of Walter's lectures.

Walter views life's journey as one prolonged health hazard. Even the urge to reproduce can seem to him a sickness, which, with his habitual prudery, he declines to discuss: 'Nor is it to be imagined, for the same reason, I should stop to enquire, whether love is a disease, – or embroil myself with Rhasis and Dioscorides, whether the seat of it is in the brain or liver.' But he does, nevertheless, do so, countered by repeated doses of anti-aphrodisiac herbs to cool the blood. Once Venus has exercised her sway, the next health risk is birth. The normal birth position – head-first presentation – is, according to Walter, lethal; the laws of mechanics and hydraulics convince him that the pressures of head-first delivery are damaging to the intellec-tual parts, as was evidently true in Bobby's case:

the lax and pliable state of a child's head in parturition, the bones of the cranium having no sutures at that time, was such, – that by force of the woman's efforts, which, in strong labour-pains, was equal, upon an average, to a weight of 470 pounds averdupoise acting perpendicularly upon it; – it so happened that, in 49 instances out of 50, the said head was compressed and moulded into the shape of an oblong conical piece of dough, such as a pastry-cook generally rolls up in order to make a pie of.

That explained Walter's hankering after Caesarian section (was not that, together with the name, the clue to Hermes Trismegistus's greatness?) – at which Mrs Shandy blanched 'as pale as ashes'. Or, failing that, Dr Slop's pet hobby-horse, 'podalic version', bringing the child into the world 'topsy-turvy' or feet first. Next, once – if! – birth had been successfully negotiated, the soul needed protecting; though where its seat lay perplexed Walter: 'from the best accounts he had been able to get of this matter, he was satisfied it could not be where Des Cartes had fixed it, upon the top of the *pineal* gland of the brain' – yet another dissenter. But perhaps more crucial even than the soul was the duty of safeguarding the noble asset of a great nose – of that such learned authorities as Prignitz and Slawkenbergius convinced Walter. Walter's medical diagnoses and therapeutic endeavours knew no bounds.

Indeed, most of the Shandys' other hobby-horsical foibles were also ultimately addressed to infirmities of the flesh. To speed his convalescence, indicate to well-wishers where he got his wound, and satisfy himself whether the offending rock afflicted him by its projectile force or by gravity merely, Uncle Toby took up the science of fortifications, soon becoming engulfed to the point of monomania:

— stop! my dear uncle Toby, — stop! – go not one foot further into this thorny and bewildered track, – intricate are the steps! intricate are the mases of this labyrinth! intricate are the troubles which the pursuit of this bewitching phantom, KNOWLEDGE, will bring upon thee. – O my uncle! – fly – fly – fly from it as from a serpent. – Is it fit, good-natured man! thou should'st sit up, with the wound upon thy groin, whole nights baking thy blood with hectic watchings? – Alas! 'twill exasperate thy symptoms, – check thy perspirations, – evaporate thy spirits, – waste thy animal strength, – dry up thy radical moisture, — bring thee into a costive habit of body, impair thy health, – and hasten all the infirmities of thy old age. – O my uncle! my uncle Toby!

Sterne delights in this absurd paradox of man: such a tender piece of flesh, harbouring such fantasies of omniscience, self-knowledge (*nosce teipsum*) and physical wholeness; and he burlesques the delusion of medical Prometheanism – mirages of health themselves become pathological. Time and again, he calls into question the quest for ultimate physical truth. 'The whole secret of health' – Walter yet again is button-holing – depends on the equipoise of 'radical heat' and 'radical moisture', plunging into the thickets of these medical arcana, only to be punctured by the humble homespun wisdom of Corporal Trim (ever 'corporeal'), who had seen the light at the siege of Limerick: 'I infer, an' please your worship, replied Trim, that the radical moisture is nothing in the world but ditch-water – and that the radical heat, of those who can go to the expence of it, is burnt brandy.'

Sterne goes well beyond satire against prating doctors and medical pedantry. He was uncommonly sensitive to the conundrum of embodiment. In flesh and blood lay the self and its articulations. With its own elaborate sign-language of gesture and feeling, the body was the inseparable dancing-partner of the mind or soul – now in step, now a tangle of limbs and intentions, mixed emotions. Organism and consciousness, *soma* and psyche, heart and head, the outer and the inner – all merged, and all needed to be minutely observed, if the human enigma were ever to be appreciated:

ZOUNDS! . . . cried Phutatorius, partly to himself – and yet high enough to be heard – and what seemed odd, 'twas uttered in a construction of look, and in a tone of voice, somewhat between that of a man in amazement, and of one in bodily pain.

That blameless clergyman had been sitting harmlessly at the Visitation dinner. Whatever has happened? He has no idea – except that his linguistic reflexes tell him it is more *wounds*: 'Phutatorius was not able to dive into the secret of what was going forwards below, nor could he make any kind of conjecture, what the devil was the matter with it.' Sterne unveils the mystery, revealing the physiological circuits, culminating in *Zounds!*, which have been triggered by a hot chestnut plopping down through his fly:

The genial warmth which the chestnut imparted, was not undetectable for the first twenty or five-and-twenty seconds, – and did no more than gently solicit Phutatorius's attention towards the part: — But the heat gradually increasing, and in a few seconds more getting beyond the point of all sober pleasure, and then advancing with all speed into the regions of pain, — the soul of Phutatorius, together with all his ideas, his thoughts, his attention, his imagination, judgment, resolution, deliberation, ratiocination, memory, fancy, with ten battalions of animal spirits, all tumultuously crowded down, through different defiles and circuits, to the place in danger, leaving all his upper regions, as you may imagine, as empty as my purse.

Adopting a mock-scientific detachment, Sterne contrasts Phutatorius's instant ejaculation (matching the reader's intuitive flash of recognition) with the psycho-physiological drama, tantalizingly protracted in the minute and delaying fullness of physical detail. It is yet more pillorying of that noble piece of work, another roasting for the genitals. But the incident is not isolated.

For the intricate life-world of the novel ceaselessly parades, parodies, yet engages our sympathies with the incongruities of the homunculus, the embodied self, probing the secret (and often meaningfully hidden) interplay of match and mismatch, a mishmash ironically mirrored in the obliquities of words and things. And Sterne makes the reader his accomplice in these disjunctions by raising anticipations: when Toby promises Widow Wadman he will reveal where he got his wound, *she* expects he will unbutton his breeches, *he* sends for a map of Namur. But Sterne no less frequently discomfits – nay, embarrasses – the reader, by slyly inveigling him in complicity with the unwelcome vulgar connotations of scatology and sexual *double entendre*, daring him to see the dirty meaning, until the entire novel becomes a sewer of fiddlesticks, sausages, noses, whiskers, buttered buns, yards, spouts, asses, cabbage-planters, whim-whams, pipes, organs, holes, crevices, breaches, wind, battering-rams and horn-works (' "high! ho!", sighed my father').

Nudging, bawdy, smutty allusions and free-associative punning are only the tip of an iceberg of innuendo and imbroglios, leading us invariably back to a body which never lets the mind forget its presence. One word leads to another: words stir associations, associations disturb our bodies, and before we know it – Sterne might have it, before we *refuse* to know it – we are reacting and responding in ways proud reason would disown. Hearts throb, cheeks blush, pulses race, tears well, blood boils. The fuming Walter snaps his pipe – his body-wisdom's way of enacting anger while releasing 'heat'; Toby whistles *Lillabullero*, embarrassedly trying to drown unwanted sounds, the *Argumentum Fistulatorium* (argument of the windpipe) being the channel through which *his* passions 'got vent'. Time and again, Sterne, that grand frontiersman of the unconscious, demands by his wordplay that we rediscover, and own up to, those obscure, unwanted and frequently suppressed liaisons which animate the body and incorporate the soul.

Sometimes his characters are themselves all too little aware of the tricks of fate in a physical world beyond conscious control. Pious Toby, for example, launches into a dissertation denying the empire of chance, at the very instant that he lands Walter a blow on the shin with his crutch. Yet they also have their own oblique and sometimes scandalized presentiments of these demeaning sympathies of the flesh. The Abbess of Andouillets recognizes that only by uttering the obscenities 'bou-ger' and 'fou-ter' will her mule (her what?) be made to budge. Walter for his part knows the truth of physiognomy: the nose has it. And he at least comes clean on the magic of names. You may all mock and snigger but, Walter ripostes, 'your BILLY, Sir! would you, for the world, have called him JUDAS?' Walter keeps the Anglo-Saxon cleric Ernulphus's dread curse against the body handy on his parlour shelf, for emergency use. All this is of course ludicrous, partly because it backfires. After all, at Walter's encouragement, Dr Slop gives the coachman Obadiah the full works of the Ernulphusian anathema:

May he be cursed in eating and drinking, in being hungry, in being thirsty, in fasting, in sleeping, in slumbering, in walking, in standing, in sitting, in lying, in working, in resting, in pissing, in shitting, and in blood-letting! May he (Obadiah) be cursed in all the faculties of his body! . . . May he be damned in his mouth, in his breast, in his heart and purtenance, down to the very stomach. May he be cursed in his reins, and in his groin, (God in heaven forbid, quoth my uncle Toby) — in his thighs, in his genitals, (my father shook his head) and in his hips, and in his knees, his legs, and feet, and toe-nails.

Yet, cursed genitals and all, it is only this servant who seems capable of procreating.

Try as they might, Sterne's characters cannot escape being made aware that man is incorporated, even if the body often seems at cuffs with the will. They also know that, as Walter notes, the *separation* of the soul from the body is death. Yet the implications of this carnal knowledge are forever being blotted out. They do not want to feel polluted by the flesh, they want to know no more about it than their 'backsides'. Fearful and puritanical, seeking to be stoical, and desperately dousing himself against the flames of passion, Walter struggles to keep the flesh under his thumb. His advice to Toby, inflamed by 'the backslidings of Venus', is that he must master his flesh, his passions, or what he was pleased to call 'his ass': 'It was not only a laconic way of expressing – but of libelling, at the same time, the desires and appetites of the lower part of us; so that for many years of my father's life, 'twas his constant mode of expression – he never used the word *passions* once – but *ass* always instead of them.' A chip off the old block in this as in so many other matters, Tristram applauds the self-control of the Stoics and admires 'the Pythagoreans (much more than ever I dare tell my dear Jenny) for their . . . "*getting out of the body in order to think well.*" No man thinks right, whilst he is in it.'

And of course the novel proves him right: people *don't* think right in their bodies – though they don't think right in any other way. And yet, however much he trumpets the Stoics, Tristram cannot believe that mind can declare unilateral independence from the body. They are but two faces of the same coin; or rather 'a man's body and his mind, with the utmost reverence to both I speak it, are exactly like a jerkin, and a jerkin's lining; rumple the one – you rumple the other.' 'The soul and body, in short, are joint-sharers in everything they get: A man cannot dress, but his ideas get cloathed at the same time.' The human animal needs to be accepted, not denied: Sterne writes not as a stern moralist but in the comic vein.

Tristram sets himself the task of understanding the understanding. Attempts to reason about consciousness were, as we have seen, basic to the scientific movement and to the Enlightenment goal of a science of man. Yet such inquiries could also readily be regarded – Swift and Johnson hint as much – as symptomatic of the itch of Unreason. Introspection had always been regarded as a mark of the melancholic, and the Augustan fear of uncontrolled imagination could be so intense as to question the very wisdom of probing the mechanisms of mind. If, as Locke argued, right thinking hinged on something so potentially tenuous as habitual associations of ideas composed of atomized sensations, then wrong thinking lay but a step away, in their mismatch. Sterne's playful literary experiment sets Tristram's sanity in question precisely through documenting his attempts to probe this great issue.

Sterne of course makes his hero hyper-aware – at times at least – of the intimacy of mind and body, intention and action: 'I said, "we were not stocks and stones" – 'tis very well. I should have added, nor are we angels, I wish we were – but men cloathed with bodies, and governed by our imaginations.' Tristram flatters himself he can take such intricacies in his stride: after all, has he not pored over the best literature on the subject?

These little and hourly vexations which may seem trifling and of no account to the man who has not read Hippocrates, yet, whoever has read Hippocrates, or Dr James Mackenzie, and has considered well the effects which the passions and affections of the mind have upon the digestion, – (Why not of a wound as well as of a dinner?) – may easily conceive what sharp paroxysms and exacerbations of his wound my uncle Toby must have undergone upon that score only.

But there's the rub. If the filiations are indeed so convoluted, how can we really map life's twists and turns, that 'junketting piece of work ... betwixt [our bodies] and our seven senses'? Isn't it all 'something more inexpressible upon the fancy, than words can either convey – or sometimes get rid of'? Herein lies the core of both the comedy, yet also the agony, of the enterprise, the yawning gulf between the plethora of academic furniture available to Walter, Dr Slop and Tristram for unravelling the human condition, and their pitiful limitations when actually applied to the job in hand. The protagonists, Walter in particular, are forever tying themselves in knots with those very ideas they hope will unsnarl the tangled skein of life:

we live amongst riddles and mysteries – the most obvious things, which come in our way, have dark sides, which the quickest sight cannot penetrate into; and even the clearest and most exalted understandings amongst us find ourselves puzzled and at a loss in almost every cranny of nature's works.

If only we had Momus's glass, affording us a window into men's souls! It would then be child's play, as Tristram recognizes, to take a man's character:

nothing more would have been wanting, in order to have taken a man's character, but to have taken a chair and gone softly, as you would to a dioptrical bee-hive, and looked in, – viewed the soul stark naked; – observed all her motions, – her machinations; – traced all her maggots from their first engendering to their crawling forth; – watched her loose in her frisks, her gambols, her capricios.

But, he ruefully concludes, 'this is an advantage not to be had by the biographer in this planet', for 'our minds shine not through the body'. Hence we must advance by stealth, by roundabout means – there are, so Tristram insists, no straight lines to wisdom; biographizing is not like cabbage-planting. The clues to truth are at a remove; they need to be reconnoitred, subjected to 'translation'. Drawing on physiognomy, musical and acting theory and Hogarth's analysis of the line of beauty, Tristram tries to read the sign-language of move-ment and posture, gesticulation and response, adumbrating a semi-ology of pose, composition and attitude, both moral and physical. He seeks keys to resolve the glitches of fractured communication. Noting how, when expounding an abstruse point to Uncle Toby, his father adopts the same stance as Socrates in Raphael's *School of Athens*, he seizes this hermeneutic clue to the outer garb of man, and recognizes Wisdom.

A deeper puzzle still endlessly nags away at his consciousness, however, that of identity: 'And who are you, said he – Don't puzzle me; said I.' And behind that lurks the question: *why?* Tristram needs an *explanation* of his tormented life, of the 'thousand weaknesses both of body and mind, which no skill of the physician or the philosopher could ever afterwards have set thoroughly to rights'. Tristram knows *he* is not responsible; the cause does not lie within himself. The reason must be biological, physiological and ultimately embryological: the culprits are his parents:

I wish either my father or my mother, or indeed both of them, as they were in duty both equally bound to it, had minded what they were about when they begot me; had they duly considered how much depended upon what they were then doing . . . Had they duly weighed and considered all this and proceeded accordingly, — I am verily persuaded I should have made a quite different figure in the world, from that, in which the reader is likely to see me.

And, returning to the womb, the key (as by now we might guess) is in Locke and his theory of the (mis)association of ideas. It was misconceptions in his mother's head at the moment of conception, precipitating spillage of the animal spirits, which spelt his misconception and blighted his life.

Locke's theory, Tristram is confident, further explains the familial chaos and domestic turmoil into which he was born. Why are Walter's and Toby's heads abuzz with such obsessional schemes, obliterating more pressing matters? Why, in the household, are there such crossed wires and cross purposes? Why do his family constantly misread each other's words, gestures, meanings? Why is it that when Obadiah announces Bobby's decease ('My young master . . . is dead!'), the maid Susannah becomes possessed of a quite disgraceful idea: 'A green satin night-gown of my mother's, which had been twice scoured, was the first idea which Obadiah's exclamation brought into Susannah's head. – Well might Locke write a chapter upon the imperfections of words.'

Worse still, Walter's head at this point gets filled, to Toby's utter befuddlement, with Cicero. The reason, explains Tristram, lies in Locke's epistemology of mental (mis)association, the way sensations and ideas, first casually bobbing about, establish their own rutted paths of connection and come to programme consciousness. The mind, tells Tristram, getting into his stride, receives, retains, or loses impressions like sealing wax:

Call down Dolly your chamber-maid, and I will give you my cap and bell along with it, if I make not this matter so plain that Dolly herself should understand it as well as Malebranch. — When Dolly has indited her epistle to Robin, and has thrust her arm into the bottom of her pocket hanging by her right side; – take that opportunity to recollect that the organs and faculties of perception, can, by nothing in this world, be so aptly typified and explained as by that one thing which Dolly's hand is in search of. –

Your organs are not so dull that I should inform you – 'tis an inch, Sir, of red seal-wax.

When this is melted and dropped upon the letter, if Dolly fumbles too long for her thimble, till the wax is over hardened, it will not receive the mark of her thimble from the usual impulse which was wont to imprint it. Very well: If Dolly's wax, for want of better, is bees-wax, or of a temper too soft – though it may receive, – it will not hold the impression, how hard soever Dolly thrusts against it: and last of all, supposing the wax good, and eke the thimble, but applied thereto in careless haste, as her Mistress rings the bell: — in any one of these three cases, the print, left by the thimble, will be as unlike the prototype as a brass-jack.

Thus, Locke has impressed himself indelibly upon Tristram's (generally too soft) sealing-wax, as he did his father's before him: 'Pray, Sir, in all the reading which you have ever read, did you ever read such a book as Locke's *Essay upon the Human Understanding?*' This literary hero-worship is not surprising, perhaps, because Tristram sees the solution to his personal psychological dilemma in Locke's 'history': '– A history! of who? what? where? when? Don't hurry yourself. — It is a history-book, Sir, (which may possibly recommend it to the world) of what passes in a man's own mind'; for Locke's history resolves his tragedy:

the effects of which I fear I shall carry with me to my grave; namely, that from an unhappy association of ideas which have no connection in nature, it so fell out at length, that my poor mother could never hear the said clock wound up, — but the thoughts of some other things unavoidably popped into her head – & *vice versa:* — which strange combination of ideas, the sagacious Locke, who certainly understood the nature of these things better than most men, affirms to have produced more wry actions than all other sources of prejudice whatsoever.

But this by the bye.

And yet the joke, of course, is also on Tristram. Little can he see that he, in turn, just like his father, is trapped within his own pet explanations, a dupe of regression. Trapped in a jumble of blame, opinionated confidence, solipsism and digressions, his *apologia* does not truly unravel the knots of his existence, but spins further 'negations', still more *explicanda*. Perversely, the work proliferates. Resembling his tragic double, Hamlet the procrastinator, Tristram discovers he is taking far longer to explain his life than to live it; he has more and more to explain:

I am this month one whole year older than I was this time twelve-month; and having got, as you perceive, almost into the middle of my fourth volume – and no farther than to my first day's life – 'tis demonstrative that I have three hundred and sixty-four days more life to write just now, than when I first set out; so that instead of advancing, as a common writer, in my work with what I have been doing at it – on the contrary, I am just thrown so many volumes back – was every day of my life to be as busy a day as this . . . I should just live 364 times faster than I should write. – It must follow, an' please your worships, that the more I write, the more I shall have to write – and consequently, the more your worships read, the more your worships will have to read.

The medical consequences, as always, are dire: 'Will this be good for your worships' eyes?'

The point is, there is no way out, no solution, no biomedical panacea to settle the traffic of mind and body. Yet, we need not despair, the jest is a happy one. Sterne's characters are in search of their own 'North-west passage' to illumination, some resolution to their anxieties, yet it lies under their noses all the time; they are living it out, silently co-operating with the cunning of nature.

Sterne's characters are, no doubt, laughable, but they are not grotesque like Swift's dehumanized Cartesian machines. Sterne feels sympathy, not Swiftian misanthropy or Johnsonian despair. Sterne's characters ache and agonize with desire and suffering, even if these are usually expressed in fraught and unsatisfactory ways, or not at all. Sterne was a great man of feeling. He was, moreover, in touch with many of the new currents in the biomedical sciences. He was aware of a fresh emphasis upon nature as living and active, and of the new physiological importance of the nerves, organization, sensitivity and sexuality. The naturalists of his day were speaking less in terms of the machine models discussed in Chapter 3 and more in respect of process, change, 'animated nature'.

Tristram Shandy is a remarkable document. It is the first novel to bear the weight of a major philosophical shift. Its comedy made the new interiority of Lockean and Humean man – a creature of confused subjectivity – seem normal, and even sympathetic. The old regime of the self – that ordered hierarchy which housed the separate soul – was rendered a thing of the past. *Tristram Shandy* was a book whose moment had come, it caught on. 'Nothing odd will do long,' dogmatized Johnson: '*Tristram Shandy* did not last.' But he was so wrong. Thereafter, what lasted was what Johnson would have damned as odd.

18

UNREASON

Late in the eighteenth century the British mad-doctor William Pargeter thus conjured up an image of the maniac:

Let us then figure to ourselves the situation of a fellow creature destitute of the guidance of that governing principle, reason – which chiefly distinguishes us from the inferior animals around us. . . . View man deprived of that noble endowment, and see in how melancholy a posture he appears.

Implicit in this moving depiction is, of course, the noble ideal from which the madman had fallen: the paragon of *homo rationalis* now reduced to one of the 'inferior animals'. In one way or another, all accounts of the self formulated in the transition to modernity took it for granted that man was a rational being, even if, as for Swift, the race was only *homo capax rationis*. But there was always, waiting in the wings, the negation of that ideal: irrational man, the madman or lunatic, the dread warning of what was in store were man to divest himself of the use of his noblest gift – or, in the hands of satirists and print-makers, the mortifying critique of the abuses actually wrought by *soi-disant* rational man himself. So how did the age of reason explain the man without reason?

The eighteenth century inherited various models of madness, medical, philosophical and religious. In the Reformation era, insanity had often been diagnosed as preternatural in origin, whether divine or diabolical. Madness thus revealed an affliction of the soul or possession of the Devil; loss of reason and free will implied that salvation was jeopardized.

A major thrust of enlightened thinking lay in the questioning and condemnation of traditional beliefs about witchcraft and other supposed interventions of the Devil in human affairs. All that was

305

now dismissed as superstition and priestcraft, and in this new thinking new theories of madness played a major part. If the supposed manifestations of diabolical possession – trances, shrieking, coma and convulsions – were neither fraudulent nor truly the work of supernatural spirits, then what else could they be but sickness and therefore the responsibility of the doctors?

From the mid-seventeenth century, criticism mounted of the self-styled saints and prophets accused of creating civil chaos. Such religious fanaticism was, it was now widely claimed by physicians and by critics such as Hobbes, symptomatic of mental disorder: self-styled saints and puffed-up prophets were literally brain-sick. Medical men would point to clear affinities between the manifestations of the religious lunatic fringe and lunatics proper: convulsions, seizures, glossolalia, visions and hallucinations, psychopathic violence (as with regicides), weepings and wailings. Hence charismatic individuals and entire religious sects might now be demonized on medical authority: 'enthusiasm' and 'zeal' could be psycho-pathologized. In France, Jansenist convulsionaries were singled out, while in Britain such doctrines were used against the significantly named Quakers, Shakers and Ranters and then, in the eighteenth century, against Methodists – 'Methodistically mad' became a favourite insult.

While in some parts of Europe demonological debate continued among academic physicians well into the eighteenth century, in Britain all prominent physicians dealing with madness from 1700 onwards interpreted religious melancholy wholly naturalistically, indeed somatically. Referring to the 'visions' of early Quakers, the Newtonian Robinson insisted they were 'nothing but the effects of mere madness, and arose from the stronger impulses of a warm brain'. Richard Mead's *Medica Sacra* (1749), a commentary on diseases occurring in the Bible, provided rational explanations for cases of possession and other scriptural diseases traditionally regarded as proofs of possession. Such beliefs were 'vulgar errors . . . the bugbears of children and women'.

With the rise of enlightened outlooks, the old religious models were replaced by secular and medical doctrines. The orderly, mechanical, law-governed universe presupposed by the new mechanical philosophy discounted Satanic possession of sufferers' minds and bodies. After the bloodshed of the witch-craze and the Thirty Years War, respectable opinion turned against 'Convulsionaries', 'Ranters', and the religious 'lunatic fringe', declaring rather that the 'possessed' were afflicted by the spleen, hysteria or other morbid conditions. Religious madness, once even an eligible state, was thus psychopathologized, being reduced to a somatic disease. Its teeth were thus drawn.

New theories of insanity filled the explanatory vacuum. Mania and melancholy, physicians now argued, originated not from transcendental powers but from the body; the aetiology of insanity was organic, its source not Satan but the *soma*. Moreover, among the medical community, the old humoral readings of mental disorder, which had highlighted the role of blood or yellow bile ('choler') in precipitating mania, and of black bile in melancholia, lost credit as the 'new science' pictured the body in mechanistic terms, stressing not the fluids but the solids. The upshot was that, in the medical writings of the first half of the eighteenth century, the idea of 'mental disease' in its strict sense was turned almost into a misnomer or a contradiction in terms; the possibility of a diseased mind or soul was virtually ruled out by the ideological and rhetorical strategies of the day. In talking about strange disorders, doctors diplomatically referred to diseases of the body; within what may loosely be described as a dualist or Cartesian framework, the presumption was that the mind or the soul remained absolutely inviolable. Here also lay success for physicians in a turf war: in future it would be they, rather than the clergy, who would have responsibility for the malady.

The comforting conclusion that a lunatic's soul was not jeopardized by his deranged condition – and that his mad talk was truly not inspired – left the onus upon physicians to explain the real causes, nature and seat of madness. They typically contended that impairment of the mental faculties and operations arose from bodily defects. Prominent was the model advanced by a number of British iatro-mathematicians and iatro-mechanists in the early decades of the eighteenth century, building upon modified Cartesian models. Archibald Pitcairn, a Scot who taught at the University of Leiden in the Dutch Republic, and his protégé, Richard Mead, grafted onto Descartes's belief that madness was illusion another Cartesian concept, namely involuntary or reflex muscular motion. A lunatic, Mead thus argued, suffered from the abnormal representation of false ideas induced by the impact of the animal spirits flowing in a chaotic manner; in turn, through some feedback loop, these induced the muscular fibres to produce bizarre and uncontrolled motions in the limbs and extremities.

Authors influenced by the latest in physical science thus portrayed the deranged individual as a hydraulic machine in a state of disorder: irregularities in the circulation of animal spirits would give rise to false sensations and disordered locomotion. Delirium, Mead held, was 'not a distemper of the mind but of the body', for, 'it is very manifest that in reality the defect is not in the rational but corporeal part'. Here lay a plausible and attractive somatic explanation of a terrifying and mysterious disease, one designed to reduce fear and stigma.

This eagerness to ascribe madness to the body was most systematically codified in the teachings of Hermann Boerhaave, the highly influential Leiden medical professor. In true Cartesian manner, Boerhaave and his numerous disciples, in England as well as on the Continent, maintained that the mark of mental illness lay in the production of false images, that is, ideas lacking external reality. At the same time, perfectly aware that such illusion alone was not madness *per se*, they attempted to formulate a more sophisticated variant of the Cartesian doctrine. For the Swiss-born Albrecht von Haller, something other than mere physical sensation must be involved in the perception of external objects; for a mind to become positively crazy, it also had to be convinced of the *reality* of false images.

As anatomical investigations advanced, the workings of the nerves – another somatic answer – were increasingly invoked to explain the production of illusions or delusion. Followers of Pitcairn, in particular his fellow Scot, George Cheyne, in *The English Malady*, speculated about the interaction of the vascular and nervous systems with the brain. Contested notions of the nerves as hollow pipes (Willis and Boerhaave) or as filaments conveying waves or impulses (Hartley) led to rival theories as to how disordered thought, moods and behaviour arose from some organic defect which caused excessive tension, slackness or obstructions in the nervous system.

Cheyne's attribution of disorders to the nerves gave expression to an astute patient-management strategy, not least because it dissociated sufferers from any imputation either of downright lunacy on the one hand, or of self-indulgent and perverted malingering on the other. Catering for wealthy and influential patients, Cheyne was aware that couching a diagnosis in tactful terms was not only an essential but a delicate business. Physicians were commonly put on the spot by 'nervous cases', because such conditions were easily dismissed by the 'vulgar' as tell-tale marks of 'peevishness' or, when ladies were afflicted, of 'fantasticalness' or 'coquetry'. Recourse to somatic categories, by contrast, was music to the ears of patients and their families, craving as they did diagnoses which confirmed the reality of their disorders. Foolish people (Cheyne explained) might suppose that the spectrum of maladies which included hysteria and the spleen were 'nothing but the effect of Fancy, and a delusive Imagination'; such charges were ill-founded, however, because 'the consequent Sufferings are without doubt real and unfeigned'. Even so, hitting upon *le mot juste* required great tact. 'Often when I have been consulted in a Case . . . and found it to be what is commonly call'd Nervous,' Cheyne mused, 'I have been in the utmost Difficulty, when desir'd to define or name the Distemper, for fear of affronting them or fixing a Reproach on a Family or Person. . . . If I said it was Vapours, Hysterick or Hypochondriacal Disorders, they thought me mad or Fantastical.'

His colleague Richard Blackmore chewed over similar difficulties. 'This Disease, called Vapours in Women, and the Spleen in Men, is what neither Sex are pleased to own', he emphasized,

for a doctor cannot ordinarily make his Court worse, than by suggesting to such patients the true Nature and Name of their Distemper. . . . One great Reason why these patients are unwilling their Disease should go by its right Name, is, I imagine, this, that the Spleen and Vapours are, by those that never felt their Symptoms, looked upon as an imaginary and fantastick sickness of the Brain, filled with odd and irregular Ideas. . . . This Distemper, by a great Mistake, becoming thus an Object of Derision and Contempt: the persons who feel it are unwilling to own a Disease that will expose them to Dishonour and Reproach.

Any such imputations of shamming would be scotched, insisted Dr Nicholas Robinson, once it was made clear that such disorders were not 'imaginary Whims and Fancies, but real Affections of the Mind, arising from the real, mechanical Affections of Matter and Motion'; for 'neither the Fancy, nor Imagination, nor even Reason itself . . . can feign . . . a Disease that has no Foundation in Nature'. After all, he stressed, one could not 'conceive the Idea of an Indisposition, that has no Existence in the Body'. So if madness were somatic, the explanations offered rang true and they rendered a shocking condition reassuringly commonplace.

As has just been hinted, Sir Isaac Newton's achievements provided a further model attractive to physiologists and physicians. The fervent Newtonian Nicholas Robinson maintained in his *A New System of the Spleen* (1729) that it was the nerve fibres which controlled behaviour; a pathological laxity or relaxed state in them was the primary cause of melancholia. 'Every change of the Mind,' he thus maintained, 'therefore, indicates a Change in the Bodily Organs.' Insanity was assuredly a genuine disorder, he insisted, not a mere matter of 'imaginary Whims and Fancies'; it arose from 'the real, mechanical Affections of Matter and Motion'.

These and similar organic interpretations of madness remained highly popular up to mid-century. But thereafter a major theoretical transformation came about. This was in large measure due to the growing acceptance of associationist theories of mind pioneered by Locke and further developed in France by the sensationalism of Condillac.

In his *Essay concerning Human Understanding*, Locke had suggested that madness was due to some fault in the process of the association of ideas. Locke argued that madmen, unlike imbeciles, had not 'lost the Faculty of Reasoning'. In fact, madmen, 'having joined together some *Ideas* very wrongly . . . mistake them for Truths; and they err as Men do, that argue right from wrong Principles'. One madman, for instance, wrongly fancied himself a king, but he correctly reasoned from that that he should have 'suitable Attendance, Respect and Obedience'. Another believed that he was made out of glass and drew the correct inference that he should take suitable precautions to prevent his brittle body from breaking. Locke's doctrine that the madman's reason was wholly intact had been clearly formulated in the 1677 *Journals*, where he had remarked that 'Madnesse seems to be noething but a disorder in the imagination, and not in the discursive faculty'. Locke's view that insanity was essentially 'deluded imagination' was decisively to shape British thinking about madness in the second half of the eighteenth century.

William Cullen (1710–90), the most prominent professor in Edinburgh University's flourishing medical school, produced a more medical version of this psychological model of madness. Cullen basically ascribed madness to the brain; hallucinations for their part were disorders of the senses, while false appetites stemmed from the organs governing the respective passions. As a mark of the centrality of the nervous system to his theory, intensity of cerebral excitement was identified as the key to both the cause and the cure of madness.

Overall, Cullen defined insanity ('vesania') as a nervous disorder. Aetiologically, it arose in the 'common origin of the nerves', that is, the cortex, and occurred neuro-physiologically when there was 'some inequality in the excitement of the brain'. Yet insanity was also, in his view, an 'unusual and commonly hurried association of ideas' leading to 'false judgement' and producing 'disproportionate emotions'. This allowed him to view insanity in a Lockean manner as a mental disorder, grounded in dynamic neuro-physiology.

While Cullen thus did not banish the body from his understanding of insanity, he certainly did not understand madness wholly in neuro-anatomical terms. He had a philosophical and psychological inspiration in David Hume, whose influence is plain in his account of judgement and its disorders. For Cullen, the keys to judgement were custom and the association of ideas, which Hume reckoned the basis of all intellectual operations.

Since judgement depended on customary associations of ideas, Cullen viewed madness as involving deviations from such habits: 'delirium is where we do not follow our ordinary train [of thought], but, on the contrary, pursue one inconsistent with all our former established principles or notions.' Together with an emphasis on the physiology of the nervous system and the pathology of the brain, Cullen's model of madness called for close scrutiny of the patient's mental disposition. The significance of his thinking lay in reintroducing the mental element into medical discourse on madness.

The break with the essentially somatic understanding of madness was widespread by around 1780. Applying Cullen's physiology in conjunction with a philosophy of mind, Edinburgh graduates were actively promoting the new model. In his *Observations on the Nature, Kinds, Causes and Prevention of Insanity, Lunacy or Madness* (1782–6), Thomas Arnold, who had studied under Cullen before taking over a madhouse in Leicester, constructed a nosology of insanity explicitly on the basis of the Lockean philosophy of mind, distinguishing 'ideal insanity' (hallucination: seeing what was not there) from 'notional insanity' (delusion: mistaking what was present).

Many other physicians advanced rather psychological models of madness. *An Inquiry into the Nature and Origin of Mental Derangement* (1798) by Alexander Crichton – also trained in Edinburgh – held that the philosophy of mind formed an essential component of understanding madness: 'It is evidently required that he who undertakes to examine this branch of science,' he wrote concerning psychiatry, 'should be acquainted with the human mind in its sane state.' In this respect, he acknowledged his debt to 'our British Psychologists, such as Locke, Hartley, Reid, Priestley, Stewart, Kames'. The great French psychiatrist Philippe Pinel (see below) similarly wrote that he had 'felt the necessity of commencing my studies with examining the numerous and important facts which have been discovered and detailed by modern pneumatologists', that is, 'Locke, Harris, Condillac, Smith, Stewart, etc.'

The coming conception of madness as a psychological disorder brought radical changes in the scope and structure of psychiatric knowledge. A physician henceforth had to pay close attention to the patient's mind. An indication of this change lies in the proliferation of detailed case histories taken and published in the late eighteenth and early nineteenth centuries: in sharp contrast to earlier works, some of the books appearing at this time consisted entirely in the accumulation of case histories.

These new concepts of madness transformed the old craft of caring for the insane into the practice of systematic psychological and psychiatric observation. From around 1780, especially in England, there was a rapid growth of psychiatric publications by private madhouse proprietors: William Perfect's *Methods of Cure, in Some Particular Cases of Insanity* (1778) was followed by the work of Joseph Mason Cox, William Hallaran and many others in the early decades of the nineteenth century. While private madhouses had been spreading since the late seventeenth century, initially they had hardly been sites for the generation and publication of medical knowledge. All this changed, as the new theories privileged and demanded the observation of the individual patients.

The somatic theories of madness popular early in the eighteenth century promised therapeutic interventions. After all, if insanity arose from organic disease, would it not – like other organic maladies – be responsive to physical treatments? Hence various drug 'cures', like camphor, came into vogue, some designed to sedate maniacs, others to invigorate melancholics; opium was freely prescribed for both purposes! There were also physical treatments like blood-lettings, emetics and violent purges to discharge toxins; shock treatments like cold showers, baths and douches; new technological fixes like electric shocks, rotatory chairs and mechanical swings, designed to disrupt *idées fixes*; and, when all else failed, mechanical restraints like chains and straitjackets, designed to quieten maniacs. William Perfect, keeper of a private madhouse in Kent, deployed upon his patients a battery of physical techniques, designed to tranquillize the delirious. He had recourse to opiates, solitary confinement in darkened rooms, cold baths, a 'lowering' diet, blood-letting, purgatives and so on. These would pacify the body, so as to render the mind more receptive to reason.

In the latter part of the century, hope came to be vested in the therapeutic potential of the madhouse itself. The asylum's segregative environment was tailor-made for the new psychiatric techniques of mastering madness, aimed at overpowering the delinquent will and passions. Moreover, as the inadequacies of drugs became plain, and with humane critics condemning use of manacles and whips as cruel and counter-productive, the well-run asylum commended itself as the ideal site of therapy for an enlightened age.

Europe's oldest madhouse, Bethlem Hospital, founded in 1247, made trifling attempts to put its house in order. But inertia was the bone of contention in the skirmish between John Monro, its physician, and William Battie, the founder of St Luke's, a new London charitable asylum. In 1758 Battie's *Treatise on Madness* blamed Bethlem for its backwardness: it was insular, it failed to teach students, it used discredited remedies. His honour impugned, Monro retaliated in the same year with *Remarks on Dr. Battie's Treatise on Madness.*

In his book, Battie stressed the value of early confinement in asylums where the accent should lie upon *management*. Management would achieve more than medicine, he stressed, in a phrase which became the shibboleth of progressive psychiatry in Britain. His division of madness into 'original' (congenital) and 'consequential' (acquired) was also attractive. Following Locke, he believed that 'deluded imagination' was the essential feature of consequential madness and that it could be cured by timely confinement.

The new outlooks arising after 1750 in which madness was increasingly viewed as a psychological condition, the result of bad habits and misfortunes, required a new psycho-therapeutics. The solution evidently lay in managing the mind. Dr William Pargeter, for instance, placed his faith in a kind of psychodrama between mad-doctor and patients. 'When I was a pupil at St. Bartholomew's Hospital employed on the subject of Insanity,' he reported of one of his cases,

I was requested . . . to visit a poor man . . . disordered in his mind . . . The maniac was locked in a room, raving and exceedingly turbulent. I took two men with me, and learning that he had no offensive weapons, I planted them at the door, with direction to be silent, and to keep out of sight, unless I should want their assistance. I then suddenly unlocked the door – rushed into the room and caught his eye in an instant. The business was then done – he became peaceable in a moment – trembled with fear, and was as governable as it was possible for a furious madman to be.

What Pargeter describes seems a little like a secular version of exorcism. Not every late-eighteenth-century mad-doctor, of course, exercised charisma in such a theatrical, almost Mesmeric, manner. But common to most was the belief that madness was curable, to be treated through person-to-person encounters and psychological expertise.

The contemporary term for this new psychological strategy was 'moral management' – 'moral' in the sense of addressing itself to the patient's mind, rather than merely to the body, establishing a consciousness-to-consciousness rapport; 'management' because the mad-doctor had to prove dynamically resourceful and inventive in initiatives designed to impose discipline. The Manchester physician John Ferriar stressed that humanity must replace brutality, and moral treatment had to supplant physical. 'The management of the mind', he explained, 'is an object of great consequence, in the treatment of insane persons, and has been much misunderstood. It was formerly supposed that lunatics could only be worked upon by terror; shackles and whips, therefore, became part of the medical apparatus.' 'The chief reliance in the cure of insanity must be rather on management than medicine,' explained Pargeter for his part. 'The government of maniacs is an art, not to be acquired without long experience, and frequent and attentive observation.' The new psychiatrists condemned a 'dark age' when lazy approaches to madness – whether soporific draughts or chains – had prevailed. No eighteenth-century 'moral manager' dogmatically dismissed physical coercion and constraint. But such methods came to be regarded as, at best, necessary evils, commonly over-used and abused. 'Here', enthused Benjamin Faulkner about his own private madhouse, 'all unnecessary confinement is avoided.'

Moral management radically altered treatment of the insane, and thereby changed the shape of discourse about madness. Traditionally, writings concerning insanity had been philosophical, religious, anatomico-medical or classificatory. In a new genre rising to prominence towards 1800, close observation of the everyday behaviour of the insane became the great priority, and the course of the disorder under treatment was charted. For the first time, the criterion for proper knowledge about madness became the close encounter with patients under confinement.

How was the mad person to be regarded? Mental disorders sparked much public debate during the 'age of reason': why had the progress of civilization apparently led to the increase of mental instability and suicide? Under a variety of terms – hypochondriasis, the vapours, the spleen, melancholy and low spirits – what later came to be known as the 'neuroses' – were said to be particularly prevalent among the English, whose climate, affluence and fashionable lifestyles supposedly produced what George Cheyne styled the 'English malady'. 'Refined sensibilities' were said to be most susceptible and, in the new 'age of feeling', members of polite society might pride themselves upon 'hypochondriack' or 'hysterick' disorders, as signs of their superiority. Hysteria became a fashionable diagnosis among doctors faced with bizarre and unpredictable symptoms in their female patients – pains in the genitals and abdomen, shooting from top to toe, or rising into the thorax and producing constrictions around the throat (the '*globus hystericus*'), twitchings, tics and spasms, seizures and paralyses. According to the neurological pioneer Thomas Willis, 'when at any time a sickness happens in a Woman's Body, of an unusual manner, or more occult original, so that its causes lie hid, and a Curatory indication is altogether uncertain . . . we declare it to be something hysterical . . . which oftentimes is only the subterfuge of ignorance'. Enlightened physicians too professed bafflement at the Sphinxian-riddles of psyche–*soma* affinities. The notable clinician William Heberden was hesitant to seem dogmatic as to the root-causes of such conditions, for 'hypochondriac and hysteric complaints seem to belong wholly to these unknown parts of the human composition'. In a society in which 'distinction' counted, illness, as we saw in Chapter 13, could be a treasured resource and, at least in the form of 'the hyp' and hysteria, mental illness could stake a claim to attention or even fame. '*We Hypochondriacks*', declared Boswell, 'console ourselves in the hour of gloomy distress, by thinking that our sufferings mark our superiority.'

George III's 'madness' dramatically drew attention to mental disorders; and the fact that the 'mad king' recovered from his incapacitating attack of 1788–9 bred optimism. Together with the 'convulsion' of the French Revolution, the madness of King George points to enigmatic connexions between the age of reason and the prevalence and comprehension of insanity. The close of the century nevertheless brought a remarkable synthesis between new psychological thinking and reformist practice. This was 'moral therapy', a movement associated with the humane management of asylum patients.

One pioneer was the Florentine physician Vincenzo Chiarugi, whose ideas were set out in a major three-volume treatise, *Della Pazzia* (On Madness: 1793–4). In France, the physician Philippe Pinel was the leading advocate of the new approach, condemning harsh therapies and recommending close observation of the patient. In 1793 he was placed in charge of the Bicêtre, the main public madhouse in Paris for men, becoming head of its female equivalent, the Salpêtrière, two years later. His celebrated striking off the chains from his patients is probably mythical. Nevertheless, the cumulative impact of his careful work at the Bicêtre and Salpêtrière was considerable, and his *Traité médico-philosophique sur l'aliénation mental ou la manie* (1801) described the path by which he came to his ideas on the moral causation and moral treatment of insanity.

Such developments were paralleled in England by the founding of the York Retreat in 1796, set up after the mysterious death of a Quaker patient in the York Asylum. Partly by religious conviction, partly by practical trial and error, it was to evolve a distinctive therapeutics grounded on quiet, comfort and a supportive family atmosphere in which the insane were to be treated like ill-behaved children. Its success was publicized by Samuel Tuke's *Description of the Retreat* (1813), which offered a shining model for early nineteenth-century reformers.

As with Pinel, in England moral therapy was justified on the twin grounds of humanity and efficacy. The Retreat was modelled on the ideal of family life, and restraint was minimized. Patients and staff lived, worked and dined together in an environment where recovery was encouraged through praise and blame, rewards and punishment, the goal being the restoration of self-control. The root cause of insanity, be it physical or mental, mattered little. Though far from hostile to doctors, Tuke, a tea-merchant by profession, stated that experience proved that nothing medicine had to offer did any good.

What do these changing models of madness tell us about attitudes to reason and the irrational in the move to modernity? If images of the insane may be read as projected negations of cherished ideals of humanity, it is clear that, back in the seventeenth century, anxieties ran deep that the Christian must be decisively demarcated over and against the brute kingdom ('inferior animals') on the one hand and the damned on the other. In an age of secularization, when those particular fears waned, the attributions of madness to bodily disorders subsequently proved a strategy for preserving the mind free from the taint of madness, an important dignifying and exculpatory strategy. In time, however, the prevalence of Lockean outlooks undermined the rigid polarity between the sane and the mad (the difference lay only in proper and false associations of ideas). This strategy no longer caused terror because first the fashionable cults of individualism and sensibility and then later Romanticism permitted a new pluralism and permissiveness in the sane while enlightened optimism held out hope that the insane were genuinely curable, perhaps in those new lunatic asylums which were promoted as resembling the new bourgeois vision of heaven.

PART IV

THE SCIENCE OF MAN
FOR A NEW SOCIETY

19

SCOTTISH SELVES

> There is no question of importance, whose decision is not
> compriz'd in the science of man; and there is none, which
> can be decided with any certainty, before we become
> acquainted with that science.
>
> DAVID HUME

The Enlightenment gave birth or favour to many sorts of 'men'. There was, for example, *homo faber*, man the maker, the harbinger of technological man; and his cousin, *homo faber suae fortunae*, man the maker of his own fortune, that Baconian model of the progressive individual, the Robinson Crusoe figure. Perhaps the most famous, however, is *homo economicus*, economic man, indelibly associated with Adam Smith's *Wealth of Nations*.

All these, however, were subordinate to the 'Man' who was the object of that science of human nature so energetically pursued by the enlightened. In an essay of 1741, David Hume proposed that politics should be reduced to a science. Something of the sort had been a goal at least since Newton, in the Queries appended at the end of his *Opticks*, had indicated the road ahead: 'And if natural Philosophy in all its Parts, by pursuing this Method, shall at length be perfected, the Bounds of Moral Philosophy will be also enlarged.' Sir Isaac thus entertained the prospect of the elucidation of human nature grounded upon natural science, and that was a goal especially pursued by the Scots but by none more so than by David Hume, who aspired to become the Newton of the 'moral' – that is, human – sciences. What Hume meant by 'the science of man' was a public and principled search for human nature, a science independent of received authority and the *ex cathedra* pronouncements of the Churches. But it was also the outgrowth of his own personal odyssey.

Born in Edinburgh in 1711, Hume inherited a patrimony which guaranteed him modest financial independence. During the course of half-hearted attempts to launch a career in trade and then the law, both of which he found unpalatable, the young Hume developed the aspiration to be *homo philosophicus*. Was this not a noble ambition? After all, had not the very act of philosophizing, in the great Stoic tradition, been the declaration of rational autonomy, the quest for true philosophical 'apathy', that is, aloofness from the trivia of the workaday world? What a disaster, then, for a philosopher to fall sick and thus not to liberate, but to disorient, the mind? That was precisely Hume's fate.

Abandoning his legal studies and launching onto the murky waters of philosophy, Hume plunged into a personal crisis in his late twenties. For a while he studied with great enthusiasm at fever-pitch, but he then succumbed to languor and ennui: 'I could no longer raise my Mind to that pitch, which formerly gave me such excessive Pleasure.' He endeavoured to work, but by the spring of 1730 he was experiencing marked disturbance. He grew rawboned, looked consumptive, and developed 'scurvy', a disordered condition of the skin. He was inclined to blame his studies for his sickness, for he had thrown himself into the philosophy of the ancients, which, being abstract and metaphysical, had engulfed him in the suggestive fantasies of the imagination. Not least, those brave 'Reflections against Death, & Poverty, & Shame & Pain' which he read, among such Stoics as Cicero and Marcus Aurelius, had the contrary effect upon him: far from enabling him to transcend his malaise, they merely accentuated his perception of sickness, and of falling short of the ideals of his heroes.

All this time, driven by an exacting and sceptical honesty, he was wrestling with his daringly innovative experimental science of the self, abandoning the rather Cartesian philosophy of sublime *a priori* reason touted by such figures as Samuel Clarke and William Wollaston for an unremitting examination of every scratch of sensation upon the consciousness – studies which were to lead to the bold *A Treatise of Human Nature.*

Hume grew disordered. He was unwilling to accept that his condition was wholly in the head – due, say, to hypochrondria or the 'vapours' – for that would have implied a disturbing loss of self-command. He surmised, or preferred to believe, that something organic was amiss, and a physician obligingly 'prescribed anti-scorbutic juices'. These palliatives for the scurvy, however, were only partly successful, and the doctor was not deceived: 'he laughed at me, & told me I was now a Brother, for that I had fairly got the Disease of the Learned.' For this the patient was next prescribed 'a Course of Bitters, & Anti-hysteric Pills', claret and riding, for his nerves and spirits needed reinvigorating.

Over the course of eighteen months, Hume's health went up and down. 'I now began to take some Indulgence to myself,' he later reflected, upon finding that a regime requiring moderation and balance seemed beneficial:

[I] studied moderately, & only when I found my Spirits at their highest Pitch, leaving off before I was weary, & trifling away the rest of my Time in the best manner I could. In this way, I liv'd with Satisfaction enough; and on my return to Town next Winter found my Spirits very much recruited . . . For these Reasons, I expected when I return'd to the Countrey, & cou'd renew my Exercise with less Interruption, that I wou'd perfectly recover.

But he was wrong. The next May he began to suffer palpitations; he found concentration difficult and lacked stamina; conscious of fatigue, he could not work without frequent diversions. Still, he wished to believe it was no mere personality disorder – we might say 'nervous breakdown' – for that would have implied either hypochondria, incipient madness or the public stigma of malingering. It was, he held, rather due to organic 'weakness' than to 'lowness of spirits'. This was a comforting excuse, yet he could not shut his eyes to the fact that his condition had some psychological tinge. The closest parallel, Hume noted with some trepidation and much self-irony, lay

in the strange sicknesses suffered by religious mystics, as recorded in
their pious outpourings or spiritual autobiographies. 'I have notic'd
in the Writings of the French Mysticks, & in those of our Fanatics
here,' he reflected,

that, when they give a History of the Situation of their Souls, they mention
a Coldness and Desertion of the Spirit, which frequently returns, & some
of them, at the beginning, have been tormented with it many Years. As this
kind of Devotion depends entirely on the Force of Passion, & consequently
of the Animal Spirits, I have often thought that their Case & mine were
pretty parallel, & that their rapturous Admirations might discompose the
Fabric of the Nerves & Brain, as much as profound Reflections, & that
warmth or Enthusiasm, which is inseparable from them.

Hume thus painted a devastatingly sardonic and self-deprecating
self-portrait of the philosopher as a young 'enthusiast' – hardly a
flattering fate for one who was already experiencing deep religious
doubts.

He was in a cleft stick. Study prostrated him, but an easy life left
him empty and frustrated. After four years of intermittent depression,
he had had enough. 'I began to rouze up myself; & being encourag'd
by Instances of Recovery from worse degrees of this Distemper, as
well as by the Assurances of my Physicians, I began to think of
something more effectual, than I had hitherto try'd.' His recourse
was to lay bare the history of his complaints in a long and revealing
letter addressed to a physician, probably George Cheyne, the great
expert on such maladies, or perhaps John Arbuthnot, both London-
domiciled Scotsmen whom we have already encountered.

It is at least possible that the very act of composing this epistle
composed his malady – indeed, that he *expected* it to do so – enabling
Hume, through taking his own 'history' in the guise of his own
physician, finally to master his condition. Thus, he may have effected
a self-cure, using the actual doctor as a surrogate, and at last discovering in the process the true power of mind over matter – not in
the Stoic sense of detached superiority ('apathy'), but through an
insightful self-analytical psychology. Hume apparently 'found him-

self', and thereafter he managed his temper perfectly, enjoying sunny equanimity through the remainder of his prosperous career. Admittedly, *A Treatise of Human Nature*, published in 1739 and 1740, 'fell dead-born from the press', but later works enjoyed better success. In 1741 and 1742 he published the *Essays Moral and Political*, which was better received. Concluding that the failure of the *Treatise* 'had proceeded more from the manner than the matter', Hume then recast the first part of it as the *Enquiry Concerning Human Understanding* (1748), and later parts as the *Enquiry Concerning the Principles of Morals* (1751). In the following year he published *Political Discourses*, which had a warm reception. He was appointed librarian to the Faculty of Advocates in Edinburgh, and began work on the *History of England under the House of Tudor* (1759), as well as two volumes of a *History of Great Britain* under the Stuarts (1754, 1757), while *The Natural History of Religion* appeared in 1757. In the late 1760s he held various diplomatic posts, and saw his reputation rise, principally as a historian and man of letters. The *Dialogues Concerning Natural Religion* was completed shortly before he died in 1776.

This early and acutely self-monitored sickness episode was a critical episode in shaping Hume's philosophical temper and credo. For it was living proof of the desperate frailty of pure reason, a demonstration of the inescapably psychosomatic and somato-psychic nature of consciousness: thinking could not divorce itself from sensation, and sensation was rooted in the senses, in the body. His nervous collapse surely indicated that his own special philosophical project – which included delving into sensations so as to resolve the problem of identity – risked and required the kind of morbid introspection that made him sick. Philosophy was inseparable from autobiography.

Yet out of his sickness Hume emerged as the advocate of a new breed of philosopher, in a way notably paralleled a century later by the outcome of John Stuart Mill's nervous breakdown, which transformed the young scientific utilitarian into a libertarian individualist. Those who wallowed in morbid introspection remained religious enthusiasts; to understand and overcome the condition led to Humean philosophy.

Largely on the basis of such personal psychological experience, Hume advanced radical notions of the self in his *Treatise*, with its call for a new science of human nature, the foundation of the edifice of the human sciences. Man was to be understood scientifically, that is, naturalistically, independently of vulgar anthropocentric prejudices and of the dictates of faith. For by then Hume had become a religious sceptic who, over the years, would advance a profound critique of belief in miracles and propose the illegibility of any ultimate order, meaning or purpose to the cosmos. There was no rational basis upon which to make inferences from creation as 'effect' to any fundamental 'cause' or Creator, and hence no natural religion – a conclusion intriguingly anticipating William Blake's, though from a totally different perspective.

Hume's critique of the orthodox natural-theological claim that a knowledge of God could be derived from facts about nature hinged on the ingenious critique of causality advanced in his *Treatise*. The concept of causation was doubtless the basis of all knowledge, but it was not itself capable of demonstration. Experience showed the succession of events, but did not reveal any necessity in that succession – it was habit which created the expectation that one event would invariably follow from another. Custom was not knowledge, however, and did not strictly justify projections from past to future, from the known to the unknown. Causality was thus not a principle derived from the order of things but a mental postulate. Belief in a rational order of nature was only a premise, and so no God could reasonably be inferred from nature. The thrust of Hume's later religious thinking was that religion was irredeemably anthropomorphic and animistic, the projection of human attributes upon God, or the gods.

Hume thus lived and died an unbeliever, much to the consternation of James Boswell, who hovered around his deathbed, desperate for a last-minute confession (as did Catholic priests at Voltaire's). None was forthcoming, and Hume died faithful to his lifelong scepticism. In consequence, he entertained no belief in a non-material Christian or Platonic soul, or, for that matter, in life after death, and his religious writings offer shrewd reflections upon the self-delusions which engendered 'superstition' among Roman Catholics and 'enthusiasm' among Protestants, bodying forth fantasies of existence beyond the grave. In this way, Hume pulled the rug away from under Christianity by proposing a naturalistic psychology of faith. What then was left of religion? 'The whole is a riddle, an enigma, an inexplicable mystery. Doubt, uncertainty, suspense of judgement, appear the only result of our most accurate scrutiny concerning this subject.'

Religion could thus provide no privileged account of man – in this Hume was advancing views far more radical than those of Locke and his immediate followers. Hence the need for a science of human nature. Man was properly an object of scientific enquiry, based upon experience, in line with the fact-based natural science of Newton and the philosophical empiricism of Locke. The *Treatise* was subtitled 'An Attempt to Introduce the Experimental Method of Reasoning into Moral Subjects'.

Such a 'science of man' was necessarily critical and subversive in tendency: it asked 'Where am I, or what? From what causes do I derive my existence, and to what condition shall I return?' Through such questioning, Hume explored and exploded the grounds of traditional ideas of the subject: received 'truth' turned out to be wishful thinking for the most part, betraying a deplorable readiness to be deceived for the sake of reassurance. In the process he criticized sloppy metaphysicians and theologians for the illegitimate thought-leaps they made from 'is' to 'ought', from mere matters of fact to supposed duties and eternal fitnesses. Hume sought a rigorous account of the self derived from 'careful and exact experiments', the 'only solid foundation' for which lay in 'experience and observation'. All neo-Cartesian apriorism was out: 'any hypothesis, that pretends to discover the ultimate original qualities of human nature, ought at first to be rejected as presumptuous and chimerical.'

Hume, indeed, drove empiricism much further than Locke, dissolving his rather confident category of 'demonstration' (knowledge) into 'belief'. It was not that Hume was bent upon showing that all was random or unintelligible, only that man's mental equipment for understanding it was circumscribed and imperfect. 'When I reflect on the natural fallibility of my judgment, I have less confidence in my opinions than when I only consider the objects concerning which I reason.' He was, however, prepared to fall back upon the general experience of the uniformity of human responses: 'Would you know', he famously asked, 'the sentiments, inclinations, and course of life of the Greeks and Romans? Study well the temper and actions of the French and English. . . . Mankind are so much the same, in all times and places.' On that basis, he was confident of the feasibility of a science meant to 'discover the constant and universal principles of human nature'.

The *Treatise* opened by addressing the capacity of the mental faculties to generate knowledge about the self and the world beyond. Eliminating all concepts not derived from experience and observation, Hume explained that our knowledge was limited to 'impressions' (perceptions) derived from observation and introspection. All complex ideas were to be traced back to such elementary sense 'impressions' or to internal impressions or feelings, and to associations derived therefrom. The hoary scholastic doctrine of 'substance' was slain, once again, as vacuous verbiage, nor could true causal powers be discovered – one must live with 'constant conjunctions' reliant upon belief in the uniformity of nature.

For these reasons, no fixed and stable self was knowable (or, for all we could be sure, present at all). Resuming Locke's discussion of identity (conscious selfhood), Hume drove it to sceptical conclusions: since experience was made up of 'impressions', and these – for Hume, as for Locke's radical disciple Anthony Collins – were irredeemably atomized and discrete, there was, in truth, no such demonstrably constant unity as a 'person', merely *pointilliste* impressions of continuity, dots on a page which we might be disposed to join up. Personal identity was thus necessarily contingent and wreathed in doubt. Truths still self-evident to the theist Locke could not survive Hume's sceptical scrutiny. Peering into himself, he discovered (he reported) no coherent, unitary, sovereign self, master in its own house, only a flux of perceptions. During sleep, existence in effect ceased. Given the inability to meld disparate perceptions, identity was thus 'merely a quality which we attribute to them, because of the union of their ideas in the imagination . . . Our notions of personal identity proceed entirely from the smooth and uninterrupted progress of the thought along a train of connected ideas'.

If the first book of the *Treatise* was thus shockingly sceptical, the last two books, on the passions and morals respectively, struck a more conciliatory note. Analysis of such desires as pride, love and hate uncovered internal feelings or sentiments which Hume called the 'moral sense'. In thus delineating propensities integral to human existence, Hume noted that Christian theologians and Platonic philosophers alike had condemned such appetites, for being sinful or mutinous. For Hume, by contrast, feelings, albeit egoistic, were the true springs of such vital and cohesive social traits as love of family, attachment to property and the desire for reputation. Rather as for Mandeville, pride and other pilloried passions were the very cement of society. Dubbing its denigrators 'monkish', Hume defended pride when it was well-regulated; indeed, magnanimity, or greatness of mind (that quality of all the greatest heroes), was 'nothing but a steady and well-establish'd pride and self-esteem'. Pride was needed for a person to acquit himself well in his station – indiscriminate humility would reduce social life to a standstill. Much that was traditionally reproved from the pulpit as egoistic and immoral was reinstated by Hume as beneficial.

Charging man that he 'ought' to struggle against his nature was, in any case, about as useful as ordering falling apples to resist gravity. Unlike the cynical Mandeville, however, the complacent Hume wanted not to outrage his readers but to reconcile them to the realities of human emotions, beliefs and conduct, and guide them to social usefulness. What mattered in that respect was that desirable social conduct arose not from reason but from feelings. Hence Hume's celebrated paradox that reason was and ought to be 'the slave of the passions' – since the emotions, like the force of gravity, constituted motives and hence controlled what people were actually moved to do. Reason *per se* could not prompt action, it was not of itself a *motive*.

' 'Tis not contrary to reason', he reflected outrageously, 'to prefer the destruction of the whole world to the scratching of my finger.' Strictly speaking, there was no such thing as that civil war between reason and the passions pretended by Plato: 'Reason . . . can never pretend to any other office than to serve and obey them.'

Personal identity, in short, was something in flux, discontinuous, confusing and complicated. Hume never broached 'multiple personality' as such, but, echoing Locke, he clearly thought people were different awake and sleeping and in various moods. Identity was not a given but a variable, a construct upheld by memory, habit and custom, and by the bonds of society. Memory was a powerful instrument but it was also imperfect, and Hume was always emphatic about how much people forgot – he challenged readers to remember exactly what they were doing, or what they were thinking, in previous months.

In a celebrated group of essays about different philosophies, Hume made clear his stance towards the relation between philosophy and life. In 'The Platonist' and 'The Stoic', he implied that such philosophical ideals were wholly divorced from the realities of living. In 'The Epicurean', he argued that the achievement of pleasure and the elimination of pain alone were good. Pleasure might be bodily, such as that cultivated in physical health; the superior forms of pleasure were mental, however, obtained in freedom from anxiety. The wise, who had nothing to fear from those around them, could ultimately find their pleasure in friendship.

Epicurus – for whom read Hume – further employed atomism as a weapon against superstitious fears of gods and demons, thereby countering both the unhappiness which superstitions caused, and the dread of death. Since the atoms of which the soul was composed dispersed upon death, humans need not fear.

For Hume, the Stoic sage exemplified virtue, not merely by living rationally in harmony with nature, but also by understanding that rationality, and consciously assenting to it. Believing that unruly passions posed a threat to virtue, the sage used his reason to master them, engendering an apathy or indifference towards them. Hume's assertion that the 'true philosopher . . . subdues his passions, and has learned, from reason, to set a just value on every pursuit' expressed the gist of Stoicism, but lay in ironic tension to the *Treatise*'s assertion that 'reason is, and ought only to be the slave of passion'.

Here we glimpse the yawning gulf between Hume and William Godwin. Hume held that so tenuous and intangible was our sense of the continuity of self that it needed to be buttressed by a fabric of familiar associations – family, home, place, location, habits and customs. His was a scepticism – in some ways deeply corrosive – the remedy for which was conservatism, cementing things together to create an artificial sense of identity, association and affiliation, so as to counter the tendency to breakdown, Hume's early nightmare.

Hume's staunchest friend and closest intellectual ally was Adam Smith. Born in 1723 – twelve years after Hume – at Kirkcaldy in Fifeshire, Smith obtained a sound classical education at the University of Glasgow, being particularly influenced by Francis Hutcheson, the Professor of Moral Philosophy. Hutcheson's teachings were based upon the notion of an innate moral sense and postulated the promotion of the greatest happiness for the greatest number as the ultimate ethical goal. For a Scot of his time, Hutcheson's outlook was remarkably optimistic and free from the Calvinism of the Kirk.

Smith spent some time at Balliol College, Oxford – an unhappy experience. His academic break came when he was invited to give a series of public lectures in Edinburgh on *belles lettres*. These proving highly popular, he was appointed in 1751 to the chair of logic at his old university at Glasgow, and the year following he transferred to moral philosophy, commencing a period of twelve years which he afterwards proclaimed to have been 'by far the most useful, and therefore by far the happiest and most honourable period' of his life. The publication in 1759 of *The Theory of Moral Sentiments* won him a European reputation.

Smith passed a couple of years from 1764 travelling abroad as tutor to the young Duke of Buccleuch. In Paris he met the physiocrats, the leading economic thinkers of the day. Returning to London, he spent his time in the reading-room of the recently opened British

Museum, gathering materials for a major economic text. In 1767 he went back to Kirkcaldy to reside with his now aged mother, dictating every morning to a secretary: *An Inquiry into the Nature and Causes of the Wealth of Nations* was finally published in the spring of 1776. The last years of his life were spent in Edinburgh, and he died in 1790, regretting that 'he had done so little'. While not a Humean sceptic in religion, he seems to have been more of a Deist than a Christian.

The *Wealth of Nations* did not create, but it unambiguously validated, the model of *homo economicus*, that economic player who pursued enlightened rational self-interest, buying cheap, selling dear and maximizing profits. Smith was able to think in this way because he comprehensively rejected established economic theorizing (bullionism, mercantilism, physiocracy and so on) as short-sighted, unscientific and subservient to vested interests, above all those of merchants, farmers and politicians. An economy would work best, he argued, when each individual (*homo economicus*) was left free to follow his own business or to deploy his labour as he pleased. Let the laws of supply and demand operate freely, without privileges, monopolies or government busybodying, and everything would find its own level, rather as in the Newtonian physics to which Smith looked for intellectual support. Efficiency would be optimal, and thirst for profit would ensure that demand – that is, the consumer's interests – was best met, indeed, it would spur technological and business innovation (the division of labour). Self-interest would optimize the system thanks to the operation, he occasionally wrote, of an 'invisible hand', or what Christian followers sometimes called Providence.

Like traditional 'anti-luxury' theorists, though reversing their condemnations, Smith stressed the importance of the imagination (rather than mere day-to-day needs) in energizing the economy. Fantasized objects of desire (the 'luxuries' so denounced by traditional moralists) were indirectly productive of benefit to society at large. There was, admittedly, a deception in this process – luxuries could not be guaranteed to bring the conveniences, glory and status-gains anticipated – but it is well that nature imposes upon us in this manner. It is this deception which rouses and keeps in continual motion the industry of mankind. It is this which first prompted them to cultivate the ground, to build houses, to found cities and commonwealths, and to invent and improve all the sciences and arts, which ennoble and embellish human life; which have entirely changed the whole face of the globe.

Homo economicus was remarkable because he was in so many ways the very bogey figure – the greedy, acquisitive opportunist consumed by gain – universally condemned by classical moralists and Christian theologians alike. Smith, however, accepted the type without moral opprobrium and, indeed, could cast him as a public benefactor, not because of any altruism on the player's part, but because his activities were wealth-producing. Within a competitive system, profit-oriented activities would prove socially valuable, generating what his teacher Hutcheson, and later Jeremy Bentham, would style the greatest happiness for the greatest number. Wealth production was, in turn, productive of better sorts of people – more peaceful, sociable, cultured and better integrated. The advance of wealth was the creation of a more civilized society.

There has been much discussion as to the legitimation of entrepreneurial economic man at this time, viewed as part of the wider advance of 'possessive individualism'. Max Weber and R. H. Tawney classically found the root rationale for such individualism in Puritanism, the Christian's need to prove his justification, before God, by works in a Calvinist world in which the Pope no longer possessed the keys to heaven and purgatory had been abolished: if the Churches could not save, the individual had to, through pursuit of this-worldly asceticism. Robinson Crusoe, the castaway forced to re-create civilization by his own hands, marks the transition between the Puritan's calling and Smithian profit-driven *homo economicus*.

More important, surely, as a stimulus to Smith was his acute awareness of the economic plight, but also opportunities, of contemporary Scotland – a backward nation catching up fast – and the intellectual value-system of the Scottish Enlightenment. He followed his great friend Hume in arguing that in the economic development of commercial society lay the key not just to material well-being but to the forging of a social order which would be more peaceful, orderly and progressive, and of personalities better adapted to the modern world.

Smith's moral teachings spell out his ideal of the modern self. As Professor of Moral Philosophy at Glasgow, he imparted to his students a moral system that was essentially non-Christian, following in the footsteps of Hutcheson. His mentor's moral system had been based upon innate faculties – benevolence, sympathy, pride – implanted in the mind by God. Smith agreed that such faculties existed, notably pity and sympathy. The self was a construct of various force-fields of sympathy between individuals, grounded upon an innate capacity for pity: 'How selfish soever man may be supposed, there are evidently some principles in his nature, which interest him in the fortune of others, and render their happiness necessary to him, though he derives nothing from it, except the pleasure of seeing it,' Smith explained:

Of this kind is pity or compassion, the emotion which we feel for the misery of others, when we either see it, or are made to conceive it in a very lively manner. That we often derive sorrow from the sorrow of others, is a matter of fact too obvious to require any instances to prove it.

Even among 'ruffians', he argued, 'fellow-feelings' for others are present; there is honour among thieves.

When others are in danger, it moves us; if they are happy, we feel joy with them. Why is this? It is through the capacity to stand in another's shoes, or by 'changing places in fancy with the sufferer':

When we see a stroke aimed, and just ready to fall upon the leg or arm of another person, we naturally shrink and draw back our own leg or our own arm; and when it does fall, we feel it in some measure, and are hurt by it as well as the sufferer. The mob, when they are gazing at a dancer on the slack rope, naturally writhe and twist and balance their own bodies as they see him do, and as they feel that they themselves must do if in his situation.

Sympathy between people is mediated, as this example shows, through the body, its instinctual movements, its facial expressions. It is also ultimately determined by physiology; those with more sensitive, or morbid, nervous systems in some ways sympathize the more:

Persons of delicate fibres and a weak constitution of body complain, that in looking on the sores and ulcers which are exposed by beggars in the streets, they are apt to feel an itching or uneasy sensation in the corresponding part of their own bodies. The horror which they conceive at the misery of those wretches affects that particular part in themselves more than any other; because that horror arises from conceiving what they themselves would suffer, if they really were the wretches whom they are looking upon, and if that particular part in themselves was actually affected in the same miserable manner. The very force of this conception is sufficient, in their feeble frames, to produce that itching or uneasy sensation complained of.

In the moral economy of vice and virtue, public judgements as to the good and the bad are based upon empirically grounded expectations that people will as a matter of fact sympathize with the plight of others. The capacity to sympathize is thus the basis of practical moral responses. As moral actors we experience approval or disapprobation because we are able to put ourselves under others' skins, project how *we* would wish or hope to behave in those situations, and how we would want our fellows to respond to *our* conduct. 'Nature, when she formed man for society,' Smith explained, 'endowed him with an original desire to please, and an original aversion to offend his brethren. She taught him to feel pleasure in their favourable, and pain in their unfavourable regard.'

In other words, we want our actions to be not merely directly gratifying to ourselves but to bring the gratification of others' esteem. We seek praise, and therefore aim to do that which is praiseworthy. Society operates a value system of moral approbation and condemnation predicated upon the natural capacity to sympathize or pity.

Some of Smith's sharpest observations highlight the dialogue between body and sensibility. The body evidently affects the mind – our health determines our spirits. But, equally, the mind affects the body, for example, in blushing. Various inflections of bodily conduct win or lose approbation. Physical grossness – gluttony, farting, belching – is dis-esteemed: 'Such is our aversion for all the appetites which take their origin from the body: all strong expressions of them are loathsome and disagreeable.' That applies particularly to physical actions shared with the 'brutes'. And context is all: 'To talk to a woman as we should to a man is improper: it is expected that their company should inspire us with more gaiety, more pleasantry, and more attention' – and there is a sting in the tail. 'an entire insensibility to the fair sex renders a man contemptible in some measure even to the men.'

In all these responses, the workings of the imagination are critical. Imagination determines the limits of sympathetic projection. 'The true cause of the peculiar disgust which we conceive for the appetites of the body when we see them in other men,' explained Smith, 'is, that we cannot enter into them. To the person himself who feels them, as soon as they are gratified, the object that excited them ceases to be agreeable.' Thus, he went on, 'when we have dined, we order the covers to be removed; and we should treat in the same manner the objects of the most ardent and passionate desires, if they were the objects of no other passions but those which take their origin from the body.' Here Smith may have had in mind the succeeding of sexual elevation by sexual disgust.

Acknowledging the role of imagination in the formation of moral judgements, Smith proposed (with an obvious reference back to Addison and Steele) the device of the 'impartial spectator'. This was many things for him. It could be the identity of a real person ('the attentive spectator') in concrete situations, whose approval was valued. More pertinently, this 'impartial spectator' lay more within the imagination than in the real world – the fiction was the 'supposed spectator of our conduct'. At the most sophisticated level, the figure was thoroughly internalized as 'the abstract and ideal spectator', or, in other words, conscience. This internal tribunal – 'the demi-god within the breast' – was thus a monitor, an alter ego, conjured up to negotiate social intricacies. 'When I endeavour to examine my own conduct,' Smith meditated, when I endeavour to pass sentence upon it, and either to approve or condemn it, it is evident that, in all such cases, I divide myself, as it were, into two persons; and that I, the examiner and judge, represent in a different character from that other I, the person whose conduct is examined into and judged of.

Smith's theory of the building of a social personality deriving from sympathies – putting ourselves in others' shoes – should be read in the context of the practical morality already advanced by Addison and Steele and Hume, with their recognition that society was complex and required astute skills in difficult social situations to help people lead effective, happy and virtuous lives and avail themselves of expanding opportunities. Overall, Smith was a sensitive observer of learnt responses to psycho-social situations, an analyst (anticipating, we might say, Norbert Elias) of the adaptive social constraints regulating attitudes towards the embodied self and its functions.

He was an acute observer of the deep ambiguities in social attitudes towards bodies. We sympathize with pain experienced by others – but only up to a point. For pain reminds us of the physical, and too much concentration on and absorption in the physical is disgusting. Yet pain in others, when accompanied by danger, engages our sympathies:

We sympathize with the fear, though not with the agony, of the sufferer. Fear, however, is a passion derived altogether from the imagination, which represents, with an uncertainty and fluctuation that increases our anxiety, not what we really feel, but what we may hereafter possibly suffer. The gout or the toothache, though exquisitely painful, excite very little sympathy; more dangerous diseases, though accompanied with very little pain, excite the highest. . . . Some people faint and grow sick at the sight of a chirurgical operation; and that bodily pain which is occasioned by tearing the flesh, seems, in them, to excite the most excessive sympathy. We conceive in a much more lively and distinct manner the pain which proceeds from an external cause, than we do that which arises from an internal disorder. I can scarce form an idea of the agonies of my neighbour when he is tortured with the gout, or the stone; but I have the clearest conception of what he must suffer from an incision, a wound, or a fracture. The chief cause, however, why such objects produce such violent effects upon us, is their novelty. One who has been witness to a dozen dissections, and as many amputations, sees, ever after, all operations of this kind with great indifference, and often with perfect insensibility. Though we have read, or seen represented, more than five hundred tragedies, we shall seldom feel so entire an abatement of our sensibility to the objects which they represent to us.

Such psycho-physiological responses had significant consequences:

The little sympathy which we feel with bodily pain is the foundation of the propriety of constancy and patience in enduring it. The man who under the severest tortures, allows no weakness to escape him, vents no groan, gives way to no passion which we do not entirely enter into, commands out highest admiration. . . . We approve of his behaviour, and from our experience of the common weakness of human nature, we are surprised, and wonder how he should be able to act so as to deserve approbation.

Smith was characteristic of the Scottish Enlightenment in his alert charting of changing norms of body socialization. Despite certain caveats, both Hume and Smith believed that economic development and the resulting sophisticated commercial and urban society were working to improve the personality, bringing into being more sensitive, responsive, advanced subjects. Hume believed that the customary bonds of society, and Smith that the hidden ties of economics, would create the social glue which critics feared analytical or possessive individualism would corrode. Critics of Hume in particular were fearful that his rejection of religious commandments, his scepticism as to absolute truths, and his stress upon the atomistic nature of consciousness would prove corrosive. Indeed, individualism undoubtedly opened the doors to new forms of introspective *anomie*, to the possibility of individuals experiencing themselves as solitary, disconnected outsiders. Some, like Hume, had nervous breakdowns, some went mad, while new movements, including Romanticism and William Godwin's anarchism, developed more extreme forms of individualism. Hume and Smith, however, were broadly optimistic, subscribing as they did to the progressive vision of historical change so prevalent among the thinkers of the Scottish Enlightenment.

Notably in post-Union (1707) Scotland, the starkness of the contrast between the traditional society of the Highlands and Islands on the one hand, and the rapidly developing midlands valley from Glasgow to Edinburgh on the other, made it especially tempting to juxtapose the savage and the civilized, past and present, and reflect upon how much had been shed – for better or for worse – in the creation of civilization. It was very common to picture the savage mind as barely rational, gripped by terror of the unknown, unpredictable and overpowering events of nature – volcanoes, earthquakes, tidal waves, droughts, floods, lightning, eclipses, comets. Fear and the desire to appease destructive forces beyond led mankind to invent deities to be worshipped and placated. Hume held that all religion whatsoever had its origins in such fear and ignorance. In this he echoed earlier sceptics, for example Mandeville, who held that primitive man assumed that an 'invisible enemy' lurked behind

every Mischief and every Disaster that happens to him, of which the Cause is not very plain and obvious; excessive Heat and Cold; Wet and Drought, that are offensive; Thunder and Lightning, even when they do no visible Hurt; Noises in the dark, Obscurity itself, and every thing that is frightful and unknown.

In time, Hume argued, the progress of the mind drew monotheism out of polytheism, clarity out of confusion. Similarly, according to Adam Smith, psychological processes gradually transcended these primitive responses to the terrifying world, and saw order – through study of the cycles of the seasons and so on. The collective mind advanced from wonder to understanding, and reason replaced panic reaction.

The psychological and aesthetic dynamics of fathoming nature were pondered by Smith in a remarkable meditation on the history of astronomy. Addressing Plato's claim that philosophy begins in wonder, he proposed that it was the mind's uneasiness with the strange which provided the driving force for attempts to eliminate perplexity through theories, models and formulas. The roots of scientific thinking lay in the psychological – surprise at the unexpected would be followed by relief upon assimilating irregularities into the familiar. A scientific theory gave satisfaction when it overcame disquiet at anomalies: 'philosophy is the science of the connecting principles of nature,' he summarized,

Nature, after the largest experience that common observation can acquire, seems to abound with events which appear solitary and incoherent with all that go before them, which therefore disturb the easy movement of the imagination; which makes its ideas succeed each other, if one may say so, by irregular starts and sallies; and which thus tend, in some measure to introduce . . . confusions and distractions. . . . Philosophy, by representing the invisible chains which bind together all those disjointed objects, endeavours to introduce order into this chaos of jarring and discordant appearances.

The savage mind thus experienced disorder everywhere, and the progress of science marked the mind's quest for regularity. Uniformity and order were desiderata of the striving, restless progressive intellect at least as much as they were present in nature. Smith thus inlaid the rise of science into the wider evolutionary history of the mind advanced in conjectural histories of civilization. No more a Christian than Hume, he acclaimed science as 'the great antidote to the poison of enthusiasm and superstition'.

In respect of science, Smith and others judged this progress unalloyed. In other domains of life, this transformation of the psyche from primitive sensation to civilized reason was a mixed blessing, for primitive responses to Nature had also involved the immediacy of the imagination which fired the finest poetry and epics. That explains why Adam Ferguson and others looked back to earlier mentalities for the peaks of poetry. The old bardic authors, including, Ferguson believed, Ossian, were unsurpassed in imaginative power.* The

* Ossian, of course, turned out to be a forgery.

advent of civilization had resulted in a shift in poetric mentality which gave rise to more sophisticated, regular and civilized expressions of poetic craft, but these had the drawback of being dilute, tepid and conventional. The poetic psyche gave way to that of prose, rhapsody and possession yielded to logic.

This loss of poetic voice or soul was a problem which transcended the divided identities of the Scots: it also preoccupied many late-eighteenth-century English intellectuals, anxious about psychological wholeness and alienation. Briefly in the *Lyrical Ballads* and explicitly in *The Prelude*, William Wordsworth pondered the position of the poet in the history of consciousness. For Wordsworth, civilized Augustan versifying, as practised by such popular authors as Erasmus Darwin, was meretricious. He had no illusions about a return to the bardic verse of a bygone era, but he did entertain hopes that the peasantry still possessed some core of their native instinctual responses – paralleled perhaps by the natural sensibility of children – which he, as a Lake District poet, would be able to share and voice. 'Low and rustic life was generally chosen', he explained in a famous passage in the Preface to *Lyrical Ballads*,

because in that situation the essential passions of the heart find a better soil in which they can attain their maturity, are less under restraint, and speak a plainer and more emphatic language; because in that situation our elementary feelings exist in a state of greater simplicity and consequently may be more accurately contemplated and more forcibly communicated.

The boldest attempt to vindicate the status of the modern mind came from Wordsworth's older contemporary, the Professor of Philosophy at Edinburgh, Dugald Stewart, who may be taken as the successor of Adam Smith in his embodiment of the aspirations of Scottish Enlightenment thinking. Stewart linked the march of mind with the emergence of modern Scotland and, more specifically, with the role of Edinburgh University as the educator of the new élite. In his discussion of Smith's *Dissertation on the Origin of Languages*, he summarized his project as being to grasp 'by what gradual steps the transition has been made from the first simple efforts of uncultivated nature, to a state of things so wonderfully artificial and complicated'. He sought to document the introspective psychology of the operations of the mind: it was the office of the enlightened to create a proper, analytical, clear-headed understanding of how the mind worked.

Heightened self-awareness would distinguish the intellectual over the herd. Natural philosophy became science, Stewart held, when enquiry, freed from exploded metaphysical conjecture, was directed towards discovering, by observation and experiment, the laws governing the connection of physical phenomena. The transformation of the philosophy of mind was to be similar. The phenomena of consciousness must be approached without conjecture, and the laws of their connection established inductively. The aim of a science of mind was to arrive at a knowledge of the 'general laws of our constitution' which would correspond to Newtonian principles in physics, and, like them, make possible the deductive explanation of a great range of phenomena.

Stewart had a bone to pick with aspects of commonsense philosophy, especially as expressed by some of his Scottish contemporaries who (he believed) had sacrificed true analytic philosophy to support for social convention and Kirk orthodoxy, by simply using their philosophy to endorse commonplace beliefs. Instead of 'the principles of common sense', Stewart preferred to speak of 'the fundamental laws of human belief'. Nevertheless, he broadly sided with commonsense philosophy against the subversives – the sceptical Hume and such materialists as Hartley and Priestley (see the following chapter), whose views he condemned as speculative, unsubstantiated by evidence and, therefore, the relics of a former, pre-inductive age of metaphysics.

Stewart was the philosophical champion of the soul. The soul is not something of which we are introspectively conscious: our knowledge of it is wholly 'relative', derived from the phenomena of consciousness at large. His polemics against materialism are couched in a form which is methodological rather than religious or moralistic; any proposal to substitute a physiological for an introspective psychology struck, he thought, at the philosophical integrity of the science of mind. He did, however, maintain that the immateriality of the mind was important among the considerations leading us to expect life after death. It established a presumption of immortality, permitting the countering of objections to the possibility of an existence apart from the body. Other considerations turned on the principle that, as experience showed, our nature was adapted to the nature of things. Tendencies deeply rooted within our nature required a future life for their realization.

Stewart's argument for the continuation of the soul after death seems to echo the thinking of Shaftesbury and the *Spectator*: an adequate sense of self as a human hinged upon the idea of prolongation and futurity, and would be frustrated and cheated by extinction. Would the psychological need for the soul to be immortal have been implanted by a benign Deity had it not corresponded with reality?

Stewart represents a principled critique of unreflective Christian faith recuperated onto a higher level, with expectations both of intellectual progress on this earth and of some consummation in a world to come. Overall, he was the culmination of Scottish academic attempts to discover in history the progressive manifestation of Mind. Central to enlightened thinking was the goal of extending scientific thinking to human nature and society. Living in a rapidly changing society with a strong academic tradition, Scots were prominent in that movement, contributing particularly coherent philosophies of progress.

These typically Scottish ideas filtered into the wider consciousness, partly through the *Edinburgh Review*, founded in 1802, which trumpeted the 'march of mind'. In their vulgarized form they were later deliciously parodied in Thomas Love Peacock's novel *Crotchet Castle* (1831):

'God bless my soul, sir!' exclaimed the Reverend Doctor Folliott, bursting one fine May morning, into the breakfast-room at Crotchet Castle, 'I am out of all patience with this march of mind. Here has my house been nearly burned down, by my cook taking it into her head to study hydrostatics, in a sixpenny tract, published by the Steam Intellect Society, and written by a learned friend who is for doing all the world's business as well as his own, and is equally well qualified to handle every branch of human knowledge.'

20

PSYCHOLOGIZING THE SELF

Teachings about the soul long dominated the everyday faith preached on Sundays from Anglican pulpits. God had made a double creation, the immaterial and the material, the permanent and the passing. The body temporarily housed an immaterial spirit which was a unity, self-conscious and endowed with free will. The office of reason was to govern the flesh, which had no sway over a healthy mind – fury, madness and sickness were exceptions which proved the rule. A human was thus what Dr Johnson called an incorporated mind, defined by a soul accountable to its Maker. Deeds done during that soul's earthly sojourn decided its fate beyond the grave. Altogether, it was a schedule of beliefs that was meant to provide moral and social glue: if, as that frantic Restoration libertine the Earl of Rochester declared, 'After Death, nothing is', what was to stop a wild plunge into vice and crime?

Pillars of the Church and of learning upheld such teachings. In discussing our 'future state', Joseph Butler, the much-respected Bishop of Durham, asserted that all the evidence pointed to 'the simplicity and absolute Oneness of a living Agent', that is, the accountable soul, and that 'we may exist out of our Bodies' as well as in them. Half a century later, Thomas Reid, Professor of Moral Philosophy at Glasgow University, echoed him: 'A person is something indivisible.' Such views were designed to scotch those who raised doubts about the traditional Christian 'incorporated mind'.

As we have already seen, coffee-house wits and freethinkers like Anthony Collins had run with the notion, floated by Locke, of 'thinking matter', consciousness reduced to some bodily emission – inanities nervously mocked by Swift. Unlike in France, however, the majority of nay-sayers in Britain were not scoffing unbelievers but

347

heterodox Christians, earnestly pursuing what they saw as religious truth. Among those, the most penetrating and influential rethinker of the self, both temporal and celestial, was David Hartley.

This extraordinary psychologist (with him the term is barely an anachronism) has been neglected or misunderstood, largely because his writings defy modern academic categories. The title accorded him by some modern psychologists as 'father of modern behaviourism' offers praise at the cost of screening out the religious and eschatological dimensions of his thinking, elements which seem quaint and obsolete today but which were integral to his world view. Hartley the monist has been ironically split in two: he must be put back together again.

David Hartley was born in 1705, the son of a poor Anglican clergyman. Orphaned early, he attended Bradford Grammar School and went on to Jesus College, Cambridge, at precisely the moment when a synthesis of Newtonian natural philosophy and Lockean philosophy was modernizing the undergraduate curriculum. Graduating in 1726, he held a college fellowship until marriage four years later compelled him to quit it.

There had been an expectation that Hartley would be ordained into the Church of England and become a country clergyman, but he could not square it with his conscience to subscribe to all of the Thirty-Nine Articles (he did not believe in the eternity of hellfire torments). Such scruples were becoming more common among liberal-minded Cambridge graduates, leading to a bitter 'subscription controversy' some forty years later: should graduates be forced to swear to Articles which they regarded as muddled, unsound or obsolete? As later with his admirer Joseph Priestley (who edited his work), the idea that Christianity was riddled with mysteries to be accepted in blind faith was for Hartley a travesty of religion. Hence, though without any degree or licence, he started to practice medicine: if not in holy mysteries, truth evidently lay in the body. Thereafter Hartley devoted himself to showing how the flesh revealed God's way with the soul.

After the death of his wife in childbirth, Hartley remarried in 1735, and his second wife's fortune enabled him to settle close by London's fashionable Leicester Square, then the physicians' quarter, before her ill-health induced them to move to Bath, where he built up a successful practice. He evidently impressed. He became a fellow of the Royal Society and moved in superior circles, his friends including the top physician Sir Hans Sloane, who became president of the Royal Society, the Revd Stephen Hales, famous for his pioneering physiological experiments, and Joseph Butler, whose doctrines of the soul buttressed orthodoxy. He also played his part in key philanthropic causes, championing smallpox inoculation and writing pamphlets to secure parliamentary aid for Mrs Joanna Stephens's nostrum against kidney- and bladder-stones – he had personally suffered from that agonizing disorder while still a young man.

Hartley's great work was his two-volume *Observations on Man, His Frame, His Duty, and His Expectations*, published in 1749, a book which further developed and systematized views earlier set out in his *The Progress of Happiness Deduced From Reason* (1734) and *Conjecturae Quaedam de Sensu, Motu, et Idearum Generatione* (Some Conjectures on Sense, Motion and the Generation of Ideas: 1746). The *Observations on Man* unfolded a comprehensive philosophy of man, considered both as an earthly being and in regard to a future state. It unreservedly embraced Locke's empiricist theory of the mind, his 'way of ideas'. Nothing was innate to the consciousness – that would have been yet another mystery, like the Trinity, and therefore incomprehensible – a card up the sleeve or a *deus ex machina*. All ideas and values within the mind derived from experience, from visible and tangible external reality: that was what made it intelligible and so allowed man to understand God's ways, as surely He intended.

Hartley had also absorbed the novel utilitarianism of the Revd John Gay's *Preliminary Dissertation Concerning the Fundamental Principle of Virtue or Morality* (1731), which made pleasure and pain psychology the key to moral development and hence to ethics. Together with Locke and Gay, Hartley dismissed all innatist theories of cognition and morality as arbitrary and anti-scientific – mere mystifying hocus-pocus. Complex ideas and attitudes could best be explained by showing how they were built up, by association, in a regular, gradual (hence *understandable*) manner, from simple inputs through repeated combinations of 'sensations of the soul'. The mind was thus not some impenetrable enigma, but was open to inquiry.

Going beyond his mentors, however, Hartley sought to ground these epistemological and psychological operations in solid corporeal foundations: the anatomy of the nervous system and the physiology of 'motions excited in the brain'. For this he drew upon the theory of sensation broached in the 'Queries' to Isaac Newton's *Opticks*. Newton had shown how light vibrated in a medium, and how such vibrations impacted upon the retina. Having struck the eye, these corpuscular motions (according to Hartley's reading of Newton) activated further vibrating waves which passed along the nerves to the brain. Associations of ideas were thus visualized and materialized by Hartley in terms of repeated vibrations in the white medullary matter of the spinal cord and brain, which were productive of the lasting traces which he styled 'vibratiuncles' (little vibrations). These vestiges served as the physical substrate of complex ideas, memory and attitudes. The mechanisms of the nerves and brain generated consciousness: in these 'good vibrations' lay Locke's 'thinking matter' incarnate.

Unlike such atheist *philosophes* as La Mettrie, the author of the scandalous *L'Homme machine* (1748), Hartley piously framed his materialist physiological psychology in terms of the grand Christian narrative. How could materialism be the slippery slope to atheism? For it had been the Christian God who had endowed matter with all its active powers and potentialities in the first place. The necessarianism entailed by materialism was, indeed, the perfect guarantee of the universal operation of cause and effect, hence of the uniformity of nature, and so of the boundless power and wisdom of the Creator. Arguments about the law-governed workings of the natural world, familiar since Newton and blessed by natural theology, Hartley applied to the moral order.

As befitted a medical man, the first volume of *Observations on Man* thus addressed neuro-physiology, discussing the senses, sensations and thought in terms of the consolidation of complex ideas and habits out of elementary, organically grounded impressions. In so arguing, Hartley had to take a stand on the quarrels over nerves and fibres raging since Descartes, and engage with the popular theories of the Leiden medical professor Hermann Boerhaave, who regarded the nerves as hollow tubes. This was the crux of the issue in the dispute between mechanists and animists over the soul's relation to the body. As we saw in Chapter 3, Thomas Willis had held that the theatre of the soul was limited to the brain. It could experience sensations from, and initiate actions in, the rest of the body, through the nerves; these, he believed, were hollow conduits for the animal spirits produced by the brain to flow along. Following Willis, mechanists, Boerhaave included, also maintained that the nerves were hollow ducts. Their vitalist opponents, by contrast, most notably the German Georg Ernst Stahl, argued for the existence of 'a rational agent presiding over the fabric of the body, and producing effects that are not subject to the laws of mechanism' – a pervading *anima* or soul. They sought to vindicate their position by demonstrating that nerves were solid fibres – hence no such channel, as needed by the mechanists, existed to explain the brain's command over the body.

Hartley esteemed the Dutch professor's thinking concerning the structure and functions of the brain, yet he insisted, *pace* Boerhaave, that the brain was not a gland, neither were the nerves hollow. Boerhaave's 'tubular' hypothesis had been disproved experimentally: attempts to inject fluids into the nerves or brain had failed. Clearly no fluid or animal spirits flowed through the nerves: rather they were made up of tiny particles, which Hartley termed 'the component molecules of the brain'. Thus, it was Newton to the rescue! For Hartley, it was the vibrations of solid nerves which provided the physiological confirmation of Locke's sensationalist epistemology and association of ideas.

Hartley set a learning model at the very heart of his psychology of human nature: all was to be explained by development. His theory of how sensations become ideas is made clear in his paradigmatic account of the development of habits, so essential in the forming of the personality. Take, for instance, the motions of the hands in learning a musical instrument. First of all they pass 'through the several degrees of voluntariness', but in time and with practice their action becomes on many occasions automatic, though still perfectly voluntary on others, namely, 'whensoever an express act of the will is exerted'.

As they become perfect, Hartley explained, many types of actions, just like those of the hands, become secondary and automatic, dependent 'upon the most diminutive sensations, ideas, and motions, such as the mind scarce regards'. The more automatic a complex action becomes, the less the agent has to mind it, and consequently the more attention can be freed from direct concerns and fixed upon more demanding ones.

Hartley's interest in habit-formation was doubtless linked to the fact that he was an acute observer of children. (Freud's wife, we are told, insisted that psychoanalysis stopped at the nursery door: Hartley stepped boldly in and observed how his own offspring grew.) In particular, he divined the key role in psychological development of the transference of emotion. Through association, primary sensations become compounded, through complex combinations, into the pleasurable and the painful. These come in six different classes: imagination, ambition, self-interest (subdivided into gross and refined), sympathy, theopathy and the moral sense. Each manifestation of pleasure is factitious, that is, a learnt response.

Man being a divinely designed machine programmed for ultimate happiness, the teleology of spiritual improvement (blessedness or salvation) which Hartley found at the heart of the Christian gospel is validated by experience itself. 'Some Degree of Spirituality', he declared, 'is the necessary Consequence of passing through Life. The sensible [that is, of the senses] Pleasures and Pains must be transferred by Association more and more every day, upon things that afford neither sensible Pleasure nor sensible Pain in themselves, and so beget the intellectual Pleasures and Pains.' Experience, in other words, teaches us to value higher things, the intellectual over the sensual. And the divine plan is beyond dispute, since on balance pleasures do actually outweigh pains, the result being that 'Association . . . has a Tendency to reduce the State of those who have eaten of the Tree of the Knowledge of Good and Evil, back again to a paradisiacal one.'

Human nature has been designed by God in such a way that experience and association invariably lead, by trial and error, to higher pursuits and nobler feelings. A baby, for instance, initially associates its parents with the *pleasures* which it derives from them: babies are selfish. In due course, forgetting the original motive (gaining gratification), the infant learns to *respect* and *love* them: a purely self-centred motive thus matures into a benevolent one. Conversely, someone who initially links money with the satisfaction it can buy might forget, over time, the original association (money buys pleasure) and experience naked greed pure and simple – and thus turn into a miser. Affects and attitudes are thus all artifacts, arising out of psychological and mental activity. It is therefore up to parents and teachers to structure education and environmental influences so as to secure the association of pleasure with socially and morally desirable objects. Man may rarely rise to pure altruism, but he is certainly capable of benevolence. And that, held Hartley,

has also a high Degree of Honour and Esteem annexed to it . . . and is most closely connected with the Hope of Reward in a future State, and with the Pleasures of Religion, and of Self-approbation, or the Moral Sense. . . . It is easy therefore to see, how such Associations may be formed in us, as to engage us to forego great Pleasure, or endure great Pain, for the sake of others.

Such transference and transformation of emotion through associations was, in Hartley's system, what explained the evolution of the personality, grounded in material reality but operating within frameworks of cultural conventions and expectations. Consider his perceptive account of laughter. Newborns, he observed, do not laugh. When they begin to do so, 'the first occasion of doing this seems to be a surprize, which brings on a momentary fear first, and then a momentary joy in consequence of the removal of that fear'. Laughter is thus at first a purely physical response (shock, surprise) to some specific stimulus, occasioned by a moment of fear followed at once by relief. It is the product of breaking the ambiguous pleasure–pain barrier: 'if the same surprize', noted this acute observer, 'which makes young children laugh, be a very little increased, they will cry' – tickling being a good case in point. When tickled, a child experiences 'a momentary pain and apprehension of pain, with an immediately succeeding removal of these'.

Originating thus in the discharge of fear and the attainment of relief, laughter shifts its nature in course of development, from immediate and physical occasions (like tickling) to more social situations, in which learnt cultural factors come to play their part: 'The progress in each particular is much accelerated and the occasions multiplied, by imitation.' Children, he noted, 'learn to laugh, as they learn to talk and walk; and are more apt to laugh profusely, when they see others laugh'. As with all other emotions, laughter is thus not a given or a constant, it is the product of psycho-social growth and thus 'a principal source' of the pleasures of sociability and benevolence, emergent at later stages of development.

With the ability to speak, the objects prompting laughter change: there is an enlargement from the physical to the cultural, symbolic and abstract. As with other expressions of emotions, laughter tends to become imaginative and vicarious. 'As children learn to use the language,' observed Hartley,

they learn also to laugh at sentences or stories, by which sudden alarming emotions and expectations are raised in them, and again dissipated instantaneously. And as they learnt before by degrees to laugh at sudden unexpected noises, or motions, where there was no fear, or no distinguishable one, so it is after some time in respect of words. Children, and young persons, are diverted by every little jingle, pun, contrast, or coincidence, which is level to their capacities. . . . And this is the origin of that laughter, which is level to that excited by wit, humour, buffoonery, etc.

The escape from fear to relief is still what causes laughter, but the fear and relief are now derived at several removes – for example, from frightening stories: a tale that arouses 'sudden alarming emotions and expectations' which are not dissipated in laughing might be stored away and might cause nightmares – evidence of further layers, chambers and motions of the psyche.

The complex learning processes thus outlined were, insisted Hartley, overall conducive to happiness. Why this confidence? It was because God had endowed the brain with such powers as to be self-adjusting and regulatory. People naturally attempt to do what will produce happiness and prevent pain. When they inadvertently act in ways inimical to those ends – for example, through gluttony – those contrary tendencies are automatically brought into line by self-rectifying mechanisms. Gross gratifications (for instance, binge-ing on a certain food) lose their relish, and bad habits which produce pain (drunkenness, for example, with its throbbing hangovers) will correct themselves.

All form part of the grand design of God. But Hartley felt obliged boldly to address a further issue, the very presence of 'the idea of God, as it is found in fact among men, particularly amongst Jews and Christians'. How do we have a knowledge of God? It was a question not usually posed by Christians. Hartley's view was that there is a series of stages – all was gradual in Hartley – in the process by which children, or the ignorant, come to possess an emergent idea of God. It is part of the culture at large, noted Hartley, that 'many actions and attributes belonging to men are . . . in common language, applied to God'. For that reason, 'in their first attempts to decypher the word', children would suppose 'God' to stand for 'a man whom they have never seen, and of whom consequently they form a com-pound fictitious idea'. They first imagine God as some *real* stranger; but the young soon realize that adults attribute things to God which are true of no actual person whom they personally know. This is puzzling:

When they hear or read, that god resides in heaven, (i.e. according to their conceptions, in the sky, amongst the stars,) that he made all things, that he sees, hears, and knows all things, can do all things, &c. . . . vivid ideas, which surprise and agitate the mind, (lying upon the confines of pain,) are raised in it; and if they are far advanced in understanding, as to be affected with apparent inconsistencies and impossibilities in their ideas, they must feel great perplexity of imagination, when they endeavour to conceive and form definite ideas agreeable to the language of this kind.

The child is at this point thrown into cognitive dissonance – he is expected to picture God as a person, but as a person who can do the impossible. The child's image of God thereby becomes unclear while, at the same time, the emotional charge carried by the notion of God intensifies – he is told this mysterious person is a loving father, whom he must revere. Thus, 'this perplexity will add to the vividness of the ideas, and all together will transfer upon the word *God* . . . such secondary ideas, as may be referred to the heads of magnificence, astonishment, and reverence'.

Bewilderment linked to emotional vividness will further increase when the child learns that God has qualities which it is *inconceivable* for any human to possess:

When children hear that God cannot be seen, having no visible shape, no parts; but that he is a spiritual infinite being; this adds much to their perplexity and astonishment, and by degrees destroys the association of the fictitious visible ideas before mentioned with the word *God*.

So, in course of time, the label 'God' ceases to be associated with the picture of a venerable white-bearded fellow, dwelling in the sky. 'However, it is probable', added Hartley, 'that some visible ideas, such as those of the heavens, a fictitious throne placed there, a multitude of angels, &c., still continue to be excited by the word *God* and its equivalents.' Thus, while the idea of that venerable gentleman may in time be obliterated by the more sophisticated teaching that God is a 'spiritual infinite being' with no limbs or face, certain anthropomorphic images, however, may not fade: the throne in the palace, the hovering angels.

As the visual imagery associated with God grows ever more vague, the emotions excited by the term become more vivid, in a process perhaps comparable to Edmund Burke's contemporary notion of the aesthetics of the sublime: obscurity makes things intense. This emotional charge is particularly heightened, he explained, 'when the child hears, that God is the rewarder of good actions, and the punisher of evil ones, and that the most exquisite future happiness and misery (described by a great variety of particulars and emblems) are prepared by him for the good and bad respectively'. By associating the concrete idea of an inescapable judge with such nebulous notions raised by 'spiritual infinite being', the child 'feels strong hopes and fears arise alternately in his mind'.

Summarizing these steps in the evolution of the idea of God and its emotional associations, Hartley concluded that

it will appear that, amongst Jews and Christians, children begin probably with a definite visible idea of God; but that by degrees this is quite obliterated, without anything of a stable precise nature succeeding in its room; and that, by farther degrees, a great variety of strong secondary ideas, *i.e.* mental affections, (Attended indeed by visible ideas, to which proper words are affixed, as of angels, general judgement, &c.) recur in their turns, when they think upon God.

Christians, in other words, do not have anything like what Descartes might have termed a 'clear and distinct' idea of God at all. They end up entertaining an imprecise visual picture, vaguely associated with clusters of abstractions – *infinite, almighty, all-knowing, eternal, spiritual*. Nevertheless, through association, they fix powerful feelings upon God – feelings deriving partly from their perplexities and, more importantly, from their sense that this Infinite Being minds deeply about their conduct, and will reward or punish them accordingly. God holds the key to 'the greatest happiness possible', and it is in their rational self-interest to be among those God counts as *good*.

Hartley's discussion of God is pregnant with many possibilities and may be read on several different levels. It was, for one thing, a perceptive psychological narrative (whether empirical or conjectural) of the emergence and transformation of the notion of God in someone undergoing education and emotional maturation. It was also meant by Hartley to be a vindication of the more sophisticated notions of the Deity held by such as himself – the anthropomorphic image of the old man with the beard was naïve or childish. Evidently he was also painfully aware how hard it was for ordinary people, stuck with their ignorant literal-mindedness, to grasp the truth. It was also further proof of the point, central to his philosophy, that no ideas were innate. Somewhat inconsistently, Locke had assumed that belief in God was somehow self-evident to reason: Hartley, by contrast, felt it incumbent upon him to show how, like everything else, God-talk would emerge. But that thought also unfolded the more subversive possibility, as broached by cynics and freethinkers: might the idea of God (perhaps like that of witches) be simply a phantom, a mere projection of the fears and errors of the confined and childish mind, confused by the tricks of words? This was not of course Hartley's intention – he believed the notion of God was a true product of authentic experience. But his psychological reconstruction had seemingly left the door open to anyone minded, like Hume, to claim that 'God' was no more than a word or an image, a product of the meanderings of the mind, not a faithful perception of reality.

Hartley's astute analysis of thinking about death and the hereafter seems to raise the same complexities. Using a psychological approach once again, he demonstrated how our understanding of death and futurity proceeds from mental processes, shaped by pleasure and pain associations. 'The frequent recurrency of these fears and anxieties' of death, he reflected, 'must embitter all guilty pleasures, and even the more innocent trifling amusements; . . . And thus men live in bondage all their lives through the fear of death; more so than they are aware of themselves . . . and still much more so than they own and express to others.' Recognition of the certainty of death causes uncertainty and fear. Thrust below the consciousness threshold, such fear then embitters pleasures.

So what *is* in store for man after death? By the 'light of Nature' alone, Hartley held that some sort of future existence is 'probable', citing the analogy of a dormant seed. The biblical Christian in

Hartley entertained no doubts about the afterlife and, as a liberal Arminian, he looked to a final universal salvation as a 'fundamental doctrine'. His heroes – Newton, Locke and Clarke – all discounted the possibility of eternal punishment of the damned: interminable hellfire did not square for Hartley with the proofs manifest throughout Creation of Divine beneficence.

Respecting the future destiny of the soul (never separate from its material embodiment), Hartley – not surprisingly, given his materialism – leant towards a mode of mortalism, of a kind common since the mid-seventeenth century. '*It seems probable, that the Soul will remain in a State of Inactivity, though perhaps not of Insensibility, from Death to the Resurrection*,' he suggested:

That the soul is reduced to a state of inactivity by the deposition of the gross body, may be conjectured from its entire dependence upon the gross body for its powers and faculties . . .

And, upon the whole, we may guess, that though the soul may not be in an insensible state, yet it will be in a passive one, somewhat resembling a dream; and not exert any great activity till the resurrection, being perhaps roused to this by the fire of the conflagration . . .

– a nice homely touch.

At the final reckoning, the soul would be reanimated by God. Hartley also suggested a spiritualization of matter after death – what he called an 'annihilation'; this would be a continuation of the psychological development in life from a self purely selfish to one which became progressively more benevolent, even altruistic and spiritual. The pious Hartley was emphatically no believer in the traditional heaven with trumpeting angels – that was for him a psychologically primitive way of conceptualizing the glory of God, strictly for the young or unenlightened.

Hartley vindicated the rather shocking and unsettling materialism pervading his system by arguing that it confirmed two truths. First, it chimed with the universality of divine law and causality. Just as matter in motion in the natural world was the basic postulate of Newtonian philosophy, so in the human and psychological realm, the material cornerstone of cause and effect eliminated the arbitrary and accidental. All this was the best refutation of infidelity – what would truly have given joy to advocates of atheism would have been a random universe of chance and contingency. Second, it was materialism which enabled man to adjust to the realities of this mundane world – it gave proof of God's benign intentions and laid bare the mechanism through which God would ensure happiness itself.

Because he died fairly soon after the publication of the *Observations on Man*, Hartley never developed his views further and, in the short run, his book had a limited impact. It was subsequently popularized by Joseph Priestley as *Hartley's Theory of the Human Mind, on the Principle of the Association of Ideas; with Essays relating to the Subject of it* (1775), although the physiology was omitted on the grounds that it was speculative and controversial. Priestley's edition, being more easily available, encouraged the separation of Hartleyan associationism psychology from his physiology of vibrations, and so fostered the later image of Hartley as a psychologist. The psychology was subsequently widely taken up by such utilitarian educators as James Mill, who prized his associationism but dismissed his theology. In this descent through philosophical radicals, Hartley's tenets provided the framework for the associationist heritage in psychology, in particular learning theory. He had launched a compelling vision of the self as a dynamic, interactive development of the human powers, the flesh bodying forth consciousness and consciousness turning the being from something low and self-regarding into a higher entity. Within God's providential plan, man thus made himself: self or personality was not a given but a potential, something which in every way developed.

Before that time, Hartley's writings proved influential among liberal intellectuals in the second half of the century. He was notably the inspiration for Erasmus Darwin (see the next chapter). The Hartleyan notion of the physiology of association as the vehicle of habit, reflex and automatic action was the *sine qua non* for Darwin's evolutionary tendency, that power in living beings to adapt to circumstances and learn, in ways which over the generations brought specific change and maximized happiness.

Hartley was a turning-point. Within a framework of biblical piety, he made it possible to ditch the separate soul (mystifying and muddled) and think of the self as a simple, undivided unity, scientifically intelligible. The old 'incorporated mind' was discredited as a divided self, which Hartley was proposing to reunite. All the old objections as to how man possessed faculties that were far too sophisticated to be the product of brute matter were swept aside in Hartley's conscientious and convincing demonstrations of how complex ideas, sophisticated behaviours and subtle moral attitudes could be acquired, by gradual processes of adaptation. Earlier Lockean notions that man was the child of experience and circumstance had been put on a sound material and scientific footing. A viable new model of man was available.

In considering changing thinking about what it was to be a 'person' (as defined by Hobbes, Locke and others), we have focused so far on humans, although, as noted, in their attempts to define man, writers have held up animals, machines or automata by way of contrast. For Descartes, a human was precisely unlike a beast, machine or automaton.

In many ways the most fundamental question surrounding the person was not, however, that of man but of the person of God. The God of Judaism was very sure of His Selfhood: 'I AM THAT I AM.' Christianity, of course, equally prided itself upon being founded upon monotheism, the unity of God – those who espoused polytheistic religions, like the Greeks and Romans, were derided for their trivial, frivolous, puerile deities. But from the early Fathers, orthodox Christianity was not monotheistic in the Hebrew, or Islamic, way, but Trinitarian. And if Catholicism, with its burgeoning cults of the Virgin, saints and martyrs, proved a particularly fertile seedbed for the proliferation of objects of veneration, then orthodox Lutheran and Calvinist Protestantism, while shunning Mariolatry and saint-worship, proved no less staunchly Trinitarian. The Anglican Prayer

Book and liturgy were Trinitarian through and through, and most leading Puritans, too, upheld that doctrine, as did eighteenth-century Presbyterians.

The exact nature of the Triune God – that is, the relationship between the Father, Son and Holy Ghost – was always surrounded in controversy. Many people advanced rational accounts (God was like a three-sided triangle, for example), while for others the glory of the doctrine was precisely that it was the mystery of mysteries, part and parcel of the other great sacramental secrets of the Church, above all the bread-turned-body of the Eucharist. Mysteries were a school of faith. (Unbelievers turned the *hoc est corpus meum* of the Eucharist into 'hocus pocus'.)

Yet rational voices in philosophy and divinity raised stubborn and taxing questions about the nature of the Trinity – and above all the status of Christ. How did the Bible depict Jesus? Would He somehow be more exalted if adored as integral to a Triune Godhead, or as a unique Messiah and holy man?

John Locke maintained an audible silence on Trinitarian issues. All that was demanded of a Christian, he said, was to believe that the Bible was God's truth and that Jesus was the Messiah. But it is not clear – and here Locke was perhaps idiosyncratic – whether he believed that the Messiah was divine like the Father. Not surprisingly, it was widely suspected, by friends and foes alike, that Locke was a closet Arian, that is, one who denied the consubstantiality of Christ with God the Father while upholding his divinity.

Questions of the Trinity and hence the personhood of Christ were inseparable from the wider status of Christianity as a rational creed. Debates as to the primacy of faith over reason, or vice versa, had run throughout Church history. Should a true Christian exclaim, with the fideistic Sir Thomas Browne, *credo quia absurdum* (I believe because it is absurd)? One line spun by Deists and freethinkers, notably John Toland, was that Christianity was 'not mysterious'; the cash value of that dictum was that any aspect of traditional teachings deemed enigmatic or irrational – for instance, the Trinity – was *ipso facto* spurious and to be discarded without further ado. Christian doctrine had to pass the rationality test, and the Trinity manifestly did not: how could anything be one and three all at once? It was nonsense.

In the first half of the eighteenth century, critical Deists used the yardstick of reason to put in the dock all the miraculous and mysterious elements of Christianity, in particular those connected with wonders respecting the flesh. The point was either to pare Christianity down to its bare minimum (doctrinal cleansing) or to demonstrate that the faith was a tissue of fantasy through and through. Had demons genuinely possessed the Gadarene swine? Had Christ miraculously given sight to the blind and caused the lame to walk? Had He really raised Lazarus from the dead? And, most crucially, had Christ Himself truly risen from the dead? Or had His corpse been stolen from the tomb; or had He simply just fallen into a deep swoon – was His 'resurrection' a not uncommon case of a person awakening from coma? Drawing upon the teachings of medicine and natural science, freethinking critics supplied mechanical, material, rational, natural or commonsensical explanations for events which occurred to bodies in biblical times and in the early Church which were claimed to be miraculous – or they dismissed them all as pious frauds cooked up by priests to hoodwink the credulous. Rationalists and Protestants were equally hawk-eyed about modern Catholic 'miracles' involving bizarre happenings to the flesh – such as miracle-healing by saints, or virgins who fasted for years, eating only the host.

Not surprisingly, certain Protestant Dissenters were to the fore in movements of this kind that scrutinized orthodox Christian teachings. Forced by the established Church to become outsiders and to teach in rather hand-to-mouth higher education academies, it was natural that Nonconformists should look to the searchlight of reason and the standard of free debate: unlike the privileged, port-swilling dons of Oxbridge, they had no stake in the authority of ancient tradition. And none did so more staunchly, consistently and candidly throughout a long career than Joseph Priestley.

Born into a Yorkshire Presbyterian family, Priestley became a conspicuous autodidact in his teenage years and gradually diverged more and more from the orthodox Calvinism in which he had been nurtured. Fearing in his youth that he would be doomed to go to hell because he had not experienced a 'new birth', he came to see those childhood teachings as 'darkness', imparting as they did a hateful vision of the Almighty; and he grew increasingly liberal in his divinity. In his early years as a Dissenting minister he adopted Arian beliefs. Later he parted still further from orthodoxy and became a full-blown Unitarian or Socinian – one who believed in the unity of God: while the Messiah and a supreme teacher, Jesus Christ was 'a man like ourselves' (though 'a man approved by God'), human rather than part of the Godhead. Since Jesus was 'as much a creature of God as a loaf of bread', to worship him was 'idolatrous'.

In a giant heap of learned, somewhat eccentric, and frequently tenaciously polemical tracts written over his long career – he died with a pen in his hand – Priestley strove to set Christology straight, on the basis of both the Bible and reason – or, perhaps more precisely, he documented in enormous detail the countless errors of others from the early Fathers to contemporary Anglican bishops. The key to his theology was his *History of the Corruptions of Christianity* (1782) and his *History of Early Opinions Concerning Jesus Christ* (1786), in which he argued that the Bible gave not the slightest scrap of support to the Trinity. Neither did reason – the three-in-one of the Trinity was frankly an insult to rationality. His strategy was to document how, largely out of pagan Greek metaphysics, the early Catholic Church had smuggled in this mysterious and, to Priestley, quite un-Christian and absurd doctrine, and all it entailed.

By way of further confirmation, he also aimed to demonstrate that the dogma of an immortal, immaterial separate soul likewise had no support from the Bible or from reason. The Old Testament Jews had not held such a doctrine. It was another illegitimate importation from Greek and 'Oriental' metaphysics (and the Eastern 'method of allegorizing') which similarly had no place within the scriptural Christianity that was the core of true Protestantism: it was a heathen stowaway, a cuckoo in the nest. Once the doctrines of the separate soul and the 'Logos' had been established, the way was paved for any number of illicit and incoherent theological fancies, including transubstantiation, the 'divinization' of Christ and his worship, the atonement, and so forth. One invention invited another.

Cunning Romanist priests had crafted the separate soul to feather their nests, notably through the fiction of purgatory. On the basis of that fabricated penal colony or way-station *en route* to heaven, the Vatican required offerings to redeem the souls of the departed – hence the abuse of chantries and the pensioning of countless monks and friars to pray for the souls of the departed. An edifice of gross corruption had been built upon a quite bogus philosophical principle.

With what did Priestley want to replace these papist falsehoods taken over, in large part, not only by Anglicanism but by moderate Nonconformity? As already noted, he believed in Christ the Messiah, a man like any other man, though one with a divine teaching mission. So what was a 'man like any other man' actually like?

Reason and intelligibility – in other words, the Hartleyan anti-mystification test – required that one should believe that God had created only one substance, which was matter or body. Corporeal matter was clear, tangible, concrete; why postulate two sorts of created stuff when one would do perfectly well? By contrast, traditional Platonic-cum-Cartesian dualism, with its polarity between body and soul, or extension and consciousness, created no end of philosophical confusion, not least the conundrum as to how those two poles would ever meet (the pineal gland problem). Intelligibility, simplicity and the Newtonian rule of economy demanded that Ockham's razor be wielded; one should believe in a single entity, created by God, and that was matter. Through natural-philosophical reasoning and extensive electrical and chemical experiments, Priestley demonstrated to his own satisfaction that matter itself was active, and hence had the potential to sustain life and be the medium of consciousness.

In particular, in debate with fellow Dissenting minister Richard Price, Priestley argued that the traditional doctrine of matter authorized by the mechanical philosophy, notably by Newton's *Mathematical Principles of Natural Philosophy*, was erroneous. The ensconced doctrine of the impenetrability of matter was shallow. Matter was active as well as passive, it could expand and contract, it was penetrable, it possessed resistance as well as gravity. Accept that matter was polyvalent – that it had many potentialities – and the idea that man was made up of matter alone – that matter, properly organized, could generate consciousness – made perfect sense.

As will be evident, Priestley leant very heavily upon the teachings of his great hero David Hartley, whose *Observations on Man* he republished in 1775 – as already noted, leaving out the physiology as being too speculative. Priestley thus reinstated Hartley's materialist doctrine of the brain as the organ of the mind, a view regarded by his many orthodox foes as dangerously radical, subversive and flatly anti-Christian. Priestley fairly countered that there was nothing in the Bible to mandate Cartesian or Platonic dualism.

Priestley had also been an early convert to the doctrine of necessity advanced, above all, by the freethinker Anthony Collins, another man he admired. (Prima facie, it might seem odd that Priestley had such respect for thinkers – another was Hobbes – who were clearly not Christian; it shows either his candour or his gullibility.) The doctrine of necessity or determinism might be read as a naturalized and rationalized version of the Calvinist predestination into which he had been indoctrinated – minus of course the ramifications about majority damnation and the implications that carried for divine benevolence. Calvinist predestination saw necessity as a proof and consequence of the Lord's omnipotence. Following Hartley, by contrast, Priestley regarded necessity as a guarantee of order and hence of the reign of natural laws. Determinism in the human world was merely an extension of the laws of cause and effect in the cosmos at large. The vulgar doctrine of human free will contravened our experience of the universe: it was evidently a symptom of crass human vanity.

Priestley never denied that, in some sense, people were free agents. But just as in the physical world motion was subject to the laws of cause and effect, so in human affairs what produced action was not caprice but sufficient motive: no action without an adequate predisposing motivation – just as in Newtonian mechanics. Motives could be studied, and motivation modified. By stressing the cause–effect chain of motive–action, Priestley believed he could show how human behaviour was intelligible and predictable. It could therefore be brought within science – indeed, within a utilitarian programme of the pursuit of pleasure towards the goal of happiness, not least in political science. Unlike Hartley, Priestley was a highly political animal – the more so the older he grew – and it was crucial for him to vindicate his radical liberalism and individualism with a scientific psychology of human nature and motivation, the laws of human action.

With his perennial energy, Priestley set about rebutting all and sundry defenders of vulgar free will and the immateriality of the separate soul. He took on, for instance, Andrew Baxter. In his *Enquiry into the Nature of the Human Soul* (1733), this influential Scottish divine had argued that dreaming and absent-mindedness were proofs that, even during temporal existence, the mind or soul could detach itself from the body. In any case, the spirit never tired – it was willing when the flesh was weak – further evidence that body and soul were essentially distinct. Priestley countered: the spirit might be willing, but the usual consequence was inactivity (though not, it seems, in the case of the tireless Priestley). During sleep, he argued further, reactivating an old controversy, the mind was as dormant as the body: dreaming (that 'imperfect manner' of thinking) was a pathological aberration, not the norm. No evidence existed of the continuation of consciousness beyond death in the form of ghosts. Belief in witches was naïve and exploded, the trash of a credulous age.

Priestley's positions are important because he pursued the rationalizing logic of Protestantism, so as to create, within a biblical piety, a model of man detached from the traditional ecclesiastical and liturgical supports or straitjackets – efficacious sacraments, sustaining Church, miracle-working saints or priests, a mysterious Godhead, a separate soul and all the other palaver. As a Protestant, he indeed embraced scriptural eschatology – the Last Judgement, the Resurrection of the Dead – but these doctrines were to be believed as the revealed word of God, the Revelation of His Will.

While on earth, it was for man to go about his business – the pursuit of happiness. The utilitarian in Priestley was in large measure a champion of commercial and industrial society, especially as contrasted to the aristocratic indolence and privilege he detested. Man also had an overriding duty to pursue truth through rational and scientific inquiry. Priestley thus replaced Church-centred doctrines with bourgeois man, thinking for himself, rational, individual, liberty-loving, self-improving, involved in a quest for truth and freedom, and requiring no Church to help him to salvation: material man in a material world.

Paramount in all this was mental autonomy: 'should free inquiry lead to the destruction of Christianity itself', he reflected, 'it ought not, on that account, to be discontinued; for we can only wish for the prevalence of Christianity on the supposition of its being true; and if it fall before the influence of free inquiry, it can only do so in consequence of its not being true.' Ironically, through the Scriptures and a quest for the real Christ, Priestley and his followers ushered into being, thanks to the cunning of reason, an essentially secularized, or at least non-ecclesiastical, image of middle-class, liberal, individual man.

As a dauntless pursuer of the naked truth, William Hazlitt (1778–1830) was a kindred spirit to Priestley who emerged out of similar circles. The son of a Unitarian minister, turbulent in character and inveterate and embittered by experience, his sense of being a perennial outsider ('born under Saturn') owed much to his Dissenting origins.

Hazlitt had hailed the French Revolution: 'a new world', he wrote, 'was opening to the astonished sight'. And he remained an unwavering Jacobin: 'The love of liberty consists in the hatred of tyrants.' A prose Byron, Hazlitt characterized his times as the age of betrayal. But if a ruthless critic of others, he was no less severe on himself, lacerating himself in private, in public and in print. His *Liber Amoris* (see Chapter 16), his story of his humiliating infatuation with his landlady's daughter, is perhaps the most searing autobiographical account of love-madness ever written.

Hazlitt's intellectual pedigree was similar to that of his intellectual heroes – men such as Hartley and Priestley. How then did he see the self? His first work, *An Essay on the Principles of Human Action*, published in 1805 when he was just 27, was the culmination of views on personal identity begun by Locke and developed by Collins, Hume, Law, Hartley, Priestley and Godwin. Broadly speaking, it claimed to establish moral philosophy on the idealist basis of 'disinterest'. Rather as for Godwin, the good man transcends self-interest for a rational vision of the good which escapes Hobbesian or Mandevillian egoism.

The distinctive insight of the *Essay* lay in an idea which, Hazlitt said, had come to him in a flash of inspiration back in 1794, when he was just 16. We are naturally connected to our past and present selves, physically (corporeal continuity) and through conscious memory. But (here is the new idea) we are only *imaginatively* connected to our future selves. Indeed, with respect to the future, our own selves-to-come are, as of now, no more real than are those of other people – all are imaginative projections. And so our future selves should carry precisely the same moral and prudential status as that of anyone else's future self. Hazlitt then derived certain conclusions from these insights. Emphasizing the distinction between memory and imagination, he construed memory along Lockean lines, as the replication in the present of past experience, coupled with the feeling that that experience is of something that happened in earlier times. But he stressed the crucial difference between our relations to our past and future selves: we are already affected by past stages of ourselves and not yet affected by future stages. At any given time, imagination plays a greater role in linking current to future stages of ourselves, than to our past.

Hazlitt's insight into the contingency of future identity was as disturbing to any notion of a solid and constant self as Locke's notion of conscious selfhood had been in its day. Locke had seemingly denied physical continuity, especially respecting the afterlife; Hume had undermined the sense of self-evident self-transparency still accepted by Locke – much was interrupted, a broken thread. Now Hazlitt further questioned our relationship to our future self – on earth and, by implication, beyond the grave. It was a philosophy appropriate to the Romantic perception of the impermanent and the ephemeral in our future hopes. It also, by implication, turned any future reality of a soul into a psychological projection.

The idea that *psychological development* was an inseparable aspect of the self was taking root from the mid-eighteenth century, stimulated by Hartley's associationist account of the mind and passions. Largely under his influence, Priestley placed emphasis upon the role of education in the acquisition of concepts of the self. Hazlitt added a psychological account of how people identify with their future selves. Their seeming identities with their future selves are fantasies. His observation was a further nail in the coffin of any traditional notion of a given, invariable, core self, in the Platonic or Cartesian mould.

Seventeenth-century philosophers, as we have seen, still tended to subscribe to a basically Platonic conception of the soul, integral to orthodox Christianity. That conception was challenged by Locke, yet he retained, or took over uncritically, some traditional commitments. One was the idea that we each have an intuitive knowledge of our own existence as a self; another was the reflexive nature of self-consciousness – being conscious of being conscious; and a third was a static account of the acquisition of self-concepts.

Locke's critics challenged and repudiated the simple memory-view of personal identity they assigned to him, and slighted his intimations about mental development. They held up as an objection to Locke the idea that the self as he conceived it was by implication a fictional construct – the notion extrapolated by the coffee-house wits. Samuel Clarke, Joseph Butler and many others protested that, if Locke's view were true, the self would be a mask; people would have no reason to take account of their future selves beyond the grave – and so everyone could do what they liked.

Among those willing to embrace Locke's view of the person as conscious selfhood was Hume, who developed the atomized idea of the self via the scepticism expressed in Book I of the *Treatise*: we lack an impression of a 'simple and continu'd self'.

It was Hazlitt who took such subversive implications to the limit.

He rejected Locke's belief that we all have intuitive knowledge of our own selfhood, and the consequent commitment to the reflexive nature of consciousness. Like Hume, Hazlitt embraced the idea that the self is a construct and – faithful student of Priestley that he was – he embedded this idea within a materialistic ontology. He advanced the idea, latent in the Lockean tradition and made explicit by Hartley, that people acquire their conceptions of their selves (and those of others) in developmental stages. Far from being destructive to theories of rationality and ethics, the notion of the self as a construct was actually their guarantee. Hazlitt was thus the culmination of the tradition of thinking about the nature of self and personal identity which began with Locke.

This tradition amounted to the creation of a new body of thinking: the psychologization of identity. It is significant that Hartley specifically wrote of a 'psychology, or theory of the human mind', locating that endeavour as part of 'natural philosophy'. In validating the experience of a thinking principle – the ego or self, understood independently of orthodox divinity – the intelligentsia was framing a new domain of knowledge, increasingly actually styled 'psychology'. According to Chambers' *Cyclopaedia* (1728) – a work hugely influential, since it served as a template for Diderot and d'Alembert's *Encyclopédie* – such 'psychology' – 'a Discourse concerning the Soul' – constituted a subdepartment *not* of 'theology' but rather of 'anthropology', that is, the study of man.

Chambers glossed soul and mind in terms of Lockean categories. By linking the soul with 'physiology' and 'logic', and by transferring study of the mind from the realm of pneumatology (that is, the traditional doctrine of 'incorporeal' substances, concerning God, angels, and so on) to 'psychology', his *Cyclopaedia* inscribed and relocated 'psychology' within science not divinity.

The endeavour to effect a scientific probing of consciousness subsequently threaded its way through Mesmerism to Victorian spiritualism and parapsychology. A different strand of the science of the soul led, on the other hand, towards modern reductionism, as exemplified by Francis Crick's *The Astonishing Hypothesis* (1994), subtitled *The Scientific Search for the Soul,* in which that old will-o'-the-wisp is finally hunted down to some obscure chamber of the brain, a modern pineal gland. Berating human pride *à la* Voltaire, Crick there asserts that, once upon a time, the soul was a theological entity, the chattel of the Church. At a later stage, thanks to Descartes, Locke and the Enlightenment, it was translated into the self, and so sovereignty over it fell to philosophy. From now on, however, it will not be intellectuals but neuroscientists who will be authorized to pronounce upon mind and its meanings. 'Many people used to believe that the "seat" of the soul was somewhere in the brain,' the anti-psychiatrist R. D. Laing expressed the matter, rather brutally: 'Since brains began to be opened up frequently, no one has seen "the soul". As a result of this and like revelations, many people do not now believe in the soul.'

More poignantly, such conclusions can be inserted into an evolutionary anthropology of the soul construed as the decline and fall of animism or perhaps the changing mind of Hartley's child as it grew up. Once upon a time, every atom of creation had a soul, observed the Victorian ethnologist Edward Tylor in a moving elegy; but this ghost-world was gradually whittled down:

Animism, indeed, seems to be drawing in its outposts, and concentrating itself on the first and main position, the doctrine of the human soul. This doctrine has undergone extreme modification in the course of culture. It has outlived the almost total loss of one great argument attached to it, – the objective reality of apparitional souls or ghosts seen in dreams and visions. The soul has given up its ethereal substance, and become an immaterial entity, 'the shadow of a shade'. . . . There has arisen an intellectual product whose very existence is of the deepest significance, a 'psychology' which has no longer anything to do with 'soul'. The soul's place in modern thought is in the metaphysics of religion.

In such transformations, the eighteenth century was evidently a watershed. The Christian soul ceased to be a given. The workings of the soul, or mind, became the subjec- matter of psychological inquiry, focused upon the learning habits of children and the instinctual wisdom of the body. What was next needed was an overarching theory of evolution. That came with Erasmus Darwin.

21

INDUSTRIAL BODIES

By firm immutable immortal laws
Impress'd on Nature by the GREAT FIRST CAUSE.
Say, MUSE! how rose from elemental strife
Organic forms, and kindled into life;
How Love and Sympathy with potent charm
Warm the cold heart, the lifted hand disarm;
Allure with pleasures, and alarm with pains,
And bind Society in golden chains.

ERASMUS DARWIN

Looking back, as he so often did, the dyspeptic Thomas Carlyle accused the Industrial Revolution of reducing men to machines. 'Were we required', he pronounced in 'Signs of the Times' (published in the *Edinburgh Review* in 1829),

to characterise this age of ours by any single epithet, we should be tempted to call it, not an Heroical, Devotional, Philosophical, or Moral Age, but, above all others, the Mechanical Age . . . which, with its whole undivided might, forwards, teaches and practises the great art of adapting means to ends. . . . Our true Deity is Mechanism. It has subdued external Nature for us, and we think it will do all other things.

The debates of the century after Milton – about the future of the soul, the autonomy of the mind, the power of environment and circumstances over the self, indeed the question of the actual constitution of identity – had been settled, concluded the gloomy Romantic Carlyle, less by argument than by accommodation: living in a world in which wealth and power were increasingly measured by machines, it was natural that humans, too, should be so defined. Man the machine had ceased to be a controversial claim and had been reduced to a fact of life in the emergent world of manufactures.

That society brought together intellectuals and artists in centres such as Manchester, Newcastle and Bristol whose outlooks were shaped by the presence of industry. One of those leading groupings was the Birmingham-based Lunar Society. From the late 1760s a group of friends – Matthew Boulton, Erasmus Darwin, Thomas Small, Josiah Wedgwood, Richard Lovell Edgeworth, James Watt and James Keir, joined by others later, notably Joseph Priestley, would occasionally meet up. The gatherings grew more regular, being held monthly at full moon, to help light their way home. A mix of entrepreneurs, engineers, men of science, technologists, doctors, educators, Dissenting ministers and gentlemen-intellectuals, the 'Lunatics' would discuss topics of common interest, generally relating to the development of the industrial society they were themselves forging.

It should be no surprise that the Lunar circle adopted a broadly materialist slant to its thinking – industry, after all, is concerned with making things out of matter. Matthew Boulton was minting coins of the realm, the potter Josiah Wedgwood was turning clay – that Old Testament symbol for the human – into wealth. His aim in running his works, he declared, was to 'make such *machines* of *Men* as cannot err'. The workforce clocked on in the morning: man was driven by mechanical time.

The old fantasy – or for others, nightmare – of making a fully fledged social person from mere raw materials or the logical consequence of the Lockean vision of the human being as a *tabula rasa*, capable of unlimited programming, was taken up by one of the Society's more idealistic intellectuals, Thomas Day, a follower of Rousseau who tried out the latter's educational project as outlined in *Émile*. Indeed, following the Pygmalion myth, Day specifically aimed to sculpt a female as a wife for himself. Declaring that 'he that undertakes the education of a child undertakes the most important duty of society', he put theory into practice by acquiring a living doll to transform into an angel schooled to despise fashion, live in domestic retirement and devote herself to her husband and offspring. Day selected for his experiment a blond girl of 12 from the Shrewsbury orphanage, whom he named Sabrina Sidney. He then went to the London Foundling Hospital where he chose her an 11-year-old brunette companion, Lucretia. To avoid scandal, he took his protégées to France, where he endeavoured to fire them with true Rousseauvian contempt for luxury, dress, title and frivolity. They quarrelled, however, irked him, and finally caught smallpox. After a year, Day returned to England, apprenticed the 'invincibly stupid' Lucretia to a milliner, and set Sabrina up in Lichfield. His experiments in training his intended's temper proved, however, deeply disillusioning. When he dropped melted sealing wax on Sabrina's arm to inure her to pain – a good Rousseauvian experiment – she actually flinched; worse, when he fired blanks at her skirts, she shrieked. Concluding she was a poor subject, he packed her off to boarding-school, decided she also had a weak mind, and abandoned her.

Day was regarded as quixotic even by his cronies. Indeed he died, a true enlightened martyr, in pursuit of another of his educational fads – breaking in a horse without cruelty: it threw him and he died. How that would have tickled Swift!

Day was an idealist. The Lunar Society boasted two thinkers, however, who were wedded to systematic materialism. We have already encountered Joseph Priestley's Christian materialism, with its conviction that reason and the Bible together advanced a vision of man comprised of homogeneous matter, endowed with the capacity for thinking and action. Materialism squared with his scientific findings in experimental physics and met the principles of simplicity (Ockham's razor) and intelligibility.

Priestley's almost exact contemporary, Erasmus Darwin, for his part came to materialism from similar scientific sources – but minus the eccentric Christianity. Born near Nottingham in 1731, young Erasmus went up to St John's College, Cambridge, subsequently, like so many others, crossing the Tweed to complete his medical training in Edinburgh. He then set up in medical practice in Lichfield, which remained his home for twenty-five years. He there conducted at least one dissection as part of a public lecture series – not, one imagines, an altogether uncontroversial undertaking:

October 23rd, 1762 – The body of the Malefactor, who is order'd to be executed at Lichfield on Monday the 25th instant, will be afterward conveyed to the House of Dr Darwin, who will begin a Course of Anatomical Lectures, at Four o'clock on Tuesday evening, and continue them every Day as long as the Body can be preserved, and shall be glad to be favoured with the Company of any who profess Medicine or Surgery, or whom the Love of Science may induce.

A physician first and foremost, Darwin practised for some forty years, and his *magnum opus*, *Zoonomia* (1794–6) was a work of medical theory, heavily influenced by Hartleyan materialist neuro-physiology. Despite his busy practice, however, Darwin poured his ample energies into a multiplicity of projects. In 1771 he was dabbling with a mechanical voicebox. Symptomatic of his taste for sailing close to the wind of blasphemy, the speaking-machine was meant to recite 'the Lord's prayer, the creed, and ten Commandments in the vulgar tongue'. Religion was thus reduced to blasts of air, calling to mind Swift's satires against the 'Aeolists' in *A Tale of a Tub*: what had been objects of fanciful ridicule for Swift were now being realized in the Midlands.

Many of Darwin's ventures were more grounded. With Wedgwood and the engineer James Brindley, he was involved in extending the Grand Trunk Canal; aided by his friend Brooke Boothby, he founded the Lichfield Botanic Society, which brought out translations of Linnaeus. On a site west of Lichfield he established a botanic garden, the inspiration for his later poem of that name. Uniting arts and sciences, medicine, physics and technology, Darwin was not only a man of the broadest interests but the very embodiment of enlightened values. Not least, he was an unabashed materialist.

Darwin had abandoned the Christian faith quite early. 'That there exists a superior ENS ENTIUM, which formed these wonderful creatures, is a mathematical demonstration,' he proclaimed while still a teenager, but reason gave him no warrant for believing that the First Cause was a Jehovah or the Christian loving father: 'That HE influences things by a particular providence, is not so evident. . . . The light of Nature affords us not a single argument for a future state.' Indeed, the doctor in Darwin found the Christian Almighty quite repellent: how could a loving patriarch visit such terrible diseases upon innocent children? And the notion of a jealous Lord was quite perverse. Darwin detested the Churches' fixation upon guilt, punishment and suffering; and his *Zoonomia* pathologized religious enthusiasm and superstition, diagnosing such religiosity as symptomatic of mental imbalance.

Although they were both materialists, Darwin thus differed fundamentally from Priestley in respect of Christianity and materialism. For Priestley, these were mutually reinforcing: God had created a universe of matter, the chain of material events led up to God. For Darwin, materialism sabotaged that faith. Yet their materialism shared common roots. Both were passionate supporters and developers of David Hartley's progressive psycho-physiological materialism. 'Give to my ear the progress of Mind,' Darwin expressed it in *The Temple of Nature*:

> How loves, and tastes, and sympathies commence
> From evanescent notices of sense?
> How from the yielding touch and rolling eyes
> The piles immense of human science rise?

For both thinkers, the brain was the organ of mind, and hence mind – the product of education and experience – was progressive, programmed to learn and develop. As with Hartley but unlike Priestley, Darwin's materialism derived from strong biomedical interests.

Indeed, medically trained in Cambridge and Edinburgh when its medical school was at its peak, Darwin's whole bent was shaped by medical theories, including that of John Brown, the maverick but highly influential follower of the great Edinburgh professor William Cullen. Brunonianism (as his system came to be called) held that illness was a consequence of excessive, or deficient, excitation, and was hence to be treated, respectively, by the application of lesser or greater stimulus: it was a medical analogue of the Lockean *tabula rasa*. The living being needed continual external stimulus (for instance, from heat and food) in order to survive and thrive. Questions of health and disease were thus reduced to variations of 'excitability'. Life was hence to be understood not as a spontaneous state but as a 'forced condition', the product of the action of external stimuli.

Darwin, too, had enormous faith in stimulants. He advised opium for many complaints: for instance, for sleepwalking, 'Opium in large doses'. His generous prescriptions may well have been responsible for the addiction of his friend and patient, Josiah Wedgwood's son, Tom Wedgwood. Treating James Watt's daughter, wasting away with what was evidently tuberculosis, Darwin energetically tried strong drugs. 'The principal thing, which can be done in these cases,' he explained, 'is by some stimulus a *little* greater than natural, and *uniformly* taken for months or years, to invigorate the digestive power.'

Viewing life through the daily practice of medicine, seeing how illness affected the spirits and the mind and medicines like opium produced counter-effects, Darwin was a materialist through and through. 'Dr Darwin often used to say', remembered the pious Quaker Mrs Schimmelpenninck, a close acquaintance who admired his skills yet mistrusted his brisk irreverence:

Man is an eating animal, a drinking animal, and a sleeping animal, and one placed in a material world, which alone furnishes all the human animal can desire. He is gifted besides with knowing faculties, practically to explore and to apply the resources of this world to his use. These are realities. All else is nothing; conscience and sentiment are mere figments of the imagination.

(Surely, in male company, Darwin used a saltier, or less euphemistic, phrase than 'a sleeping animal'?)

Darwin's early writings show him an advocate of classic medical moderation. But, as a Brunonian, he came round to recommending the consumption of large quantities of rich and stimulating food. 'Eat or be eaten!' he declared, thereby hinting at the biological truth of

the Hobbesian view of mankind. Like his fellow Lichfieldian Samuel
Johnson, he was fond of cream and sugar, and so became exceedingly
fat. He grew, however, extremely suspicious of alcohol: it brought
on his gout, and he feared the ill-effects of drunkenness. In short,
man was, for Darwin, not principally *homo rationalis* or *homo rationis
capax*, not primarily a thinking creature, still less a disembodied soul:
he was flesh and blood.

Darwin probed the interaction of body and mind. Mental disturbances were consequences of physical disease. Following earlier critical
Deists, Darwin treated what he considered morbid religious beliefs
as illnesses. Sections of *Zoonomia* dealt with such conditions as self-
starvation, masochistic tendencies, self-destructiveness, suicide, morbid fears and anxieties, all largely put down to physiological
dysfunctions mediated through the distorting lens of religion, as
in his analysis of 'superstitious hope': 'In India devotees consign
themselves by vows to most painful and unceasing tortures . . . while
in our part of the globe fasting and mortification, as flagellation, has
been believed to please a merciful deity!' Of that he documented an
example close to home:

Mr —, a clergyman, formerly of this neighbourhood, began to bruise and
wound himself for the sake of religious mortification, and passed much time
in prayer, and continued whole nights alone in the church. As he had a
wife and family of small children, I believed the case to be incurable; as
otherwise the affection and employment in his family connections would
have opposed the beginning of this insanity. He was taken to a madhouse
without effect, and after he returned home, continued to beat and bruise
himself, and by this kind of mortification, and by sometimes long fasting,
he at length became emaciated and died.

The influence was not all one way: consciousness in turn affected
the body. Stammering – a matter dear to him because he himself
had a notorious stammer – was not simply a physical malfunction
but a psychological consequence of anxiety. Darwin likewise pointed
to the psychological roots of impotence.

A disposition to reduce the lofty to the material, the mysterious to the intelligible, pervades Darwin's thought. Discussing the aesthetics of nature he explained, in a manner owing much to Hartley – and, as it were, prefiguring Freud – how our enjoyment of the soft contours of hills derives from the infant's experience of fingering the breast and sucking the nipple. The idea of beauty arises as a result of associating the 'female bosom' with generosity and fertility – an association which in time becomes insensible or subliminal: 'Hence at our maturer years, when any object of vision is presented to us, which by its waving or spiral lines bears any similitude to the form of the female bosom . . . we feel a general glow of delight, which seems to influence all our senses. . . . This animal attraction is love.' Early tactile experiences thus imprinted themselves on the developing imagination, built up associations, and were rendered permanent in the brain. Darwin thus showed the psycho-physiological basis of Hogarth's 'line of beauty'.

Like Blake, but for different reasons, Darwin the materialist championed sexual expression. Panegyrizing love as 'the purest source of human felicity, the cordial drop in the otherwise vapid cup of life', he sired fourteen children, twelve of them legitimate. *The Temple of Nature* was a paean to the 'Deities of Sexual Love', for they it was who propelled evolutionary progress through the superfecundity of the generative powers. The arc of life itself rose from asexual to sexual reproduction, which was 'the chef d'œuvre, the master-piece of nature', not only improving and diversifying the stock, but creating more cosmic happiness as well.

In thus hailing these deities, Darwin conscripted pagan mythology to the cause of his scientific botany, invoking a cast of nymphs and sylphs in fables of botanical and zoological processes. The familiar Greek myths, Darwin explained, were anthropomorphic and figurative representations of natural truths: pagan mythology was preoccupied by love precisely because natural man – before the wretched triumph of Christian asceticism! – had an intuitive awareness of how nature was driven by sexual impulses. Like Blake, Darwin offered creation myths of his own, supplanting the Bible.

Numerous contemporary radical doctors adopted materialist

slants upon the human condition, notably Darwin's friend, Thomas Beddoes, discussed in the following chapter. What makes Darwin unique is that he translated his materialism into a comprehensive theory of biological evolution. In a total reconceptualization of the Chain of Being as upheld by Ralph Cudworth and by Pope's *Essay on Man*, Darwin reasoned that life had not been created in the Garden of Eden but had arisen naturally and gradually, by stages, from the most elemental microscopic stuff. Everything contained some basic potential or energy. By continual exercise of that life force – which, in the case of higher creatures, eventually burgeoned into conscious will – existence became ever more intricate and full of capabilities. A struggle for survival resulted from the superfecundity of nature: the strong defeated the weak, the sophisticated the simple.

Evolution exhibited an imperceptible rise from mere sensation to irritability, will (volition) and finally consciousness. Consciousness in turn produced complex associations and ideas; by a mechanism we would nowadays tend to call 'Lamarckian', such culture could be inherited. This inheritance of acquired characteristics shows that, while Darwin was a committed materialist, he fully valued the (materially based) mind and its role in the transgenerational transmission of culture. Nature, as the Greek atomists had contended, is everywhere in motion, and creatures are ever adapting themselves to their environment – 'the hares and partridges of the latitudes which are long buried in snow, become white during the winter months'. Domestication, moreover, brings 'great changes', transmitted from generation to generation, as in the breeding of pedigree pets and livestock.

The face of nature is thus undergoing ceaseless change. The starting-point for understanding its dynamics lay for Darwin in the inherent motility possessed by organized matter: 'In every contraction of the fibre there is an expenditure of the sensorial power, or spirit of animation.' Living beings do not react solely in a mechanical billiard-ball manner to external pressures but possess an inherent responsiveness of their own, a capacity to interact with the environment.

Fibres contract, producing 'irritation'; irritation leads to 'sensation', and in their turn, the tribunals of pleasure and pain generate desire and aversion, giving rise to the superior plane of volition, that is, a creature's capacity to act in the light of pleasure and pain sensations. Volition, Darwin insisted, drawing on Hartley and Priestley, should not be confused with the discredited theological conception of free will, which was tantamount to an arbitrary whim.

Probing the functions of the mind, Darwin addressed the links between volition and habit. 'The ingenious Dr Hartley in his work on man,' he stated, 'and some other philosophers, have been of the opinion, that our immortal part acquires during this life certain habits of action or of sentiment, which become for ever indissoluble, continuing after death in a future state of existence.' Darwin naturalized this insight: 'I would apply this ingenious idea to the generation or production of the embryon, or new animal, which partakes so much of the form and propensities of the parent.' Frequent repetition of an action, he explained, patterns behaviour; once habits are established, subsequent performance demands less conscious play of mind. At the keyboard the tyro thus has to give all his concentration, whereas the seasoned pianist can, while playing expertly, attend to other things as well. As for Hartley, habit does not supersede volition, it frees it to operate on a higher plateau, forming a better adaptation to the complex demands on creatures needing to do more than one thing at once.

This capacity to advance from isolated acts to behaviour patterns supplied Darwin with a comprehensive model for organic progress. Animals – humans included – are not born inherently endowed with repertoires of know-how and skills – schooled in Locke, Darwin had no truck with 'innate ideas' or their Scottish 'commonsense' variant. Rather, he noted, with repetition of particular actions, habits form which, undergoing modification over time, tailor behaviour to environmental opportunities and niches. The sanctions of pleasures and pains force organisms to learn and, through learning, to progress. Sense responses translate, via habit, into the volition which gives creatures – some more than others – the capacity to be progressive.

Intelligent materialist thinking resolved the needless mysteries of nature.

What enables such adaptive behaviour to assume truly complex forms, especially in humans, is a further power of the organism: the association of ideas as classically formulated by Locke. Many higher creatures act intelligently, but only humans have the capacity to form complex ideas. Building on Hartley, Darwin held that the expression of emotion – anger, fear, laughter – comprises the learnt product of chains of responses, transmitted from parents to offspring over the generations by the power of imitation.

Association was crucial to Darwin's concept of evolution and progress. It is through that mechanism that behaviour achieves ever more complex expression, generating, for instance, the sense of beauty and feelings of sympathy which create mutual affection among sociable animals. Through imagination, the brain-based mind becomes the storehouse of experience. And in turn, the imagination plays a crucial role in reproduction, in shaping the future.

Controversy had long raged over the mechanics of generation and heredity. Darwin repudiated the 'preformationism' popular with the early mechanical philosophers – for him, foetal growth amounted to far more than the mechanistic enlargement of microscopic parts (like a balloon being blown up) that were 'given' from the dawn of time. Offspring did not remain carbon copies down the generations: in all its manifestations innatism was mistaken. Most importantly, he was convinced that mind, as an integral part of the organism, had a part to play in hereditary transmission to the offspring. Such views were not uncommon, for folklore and certain medical theorists alike credited to the mother's imagination a pathological power to impress its contents upon the embryo at conception – 'monstrous' births had long been explained that way. This view was rejected by Darwin, but he did propose an analogous (and equally sexist) doctrine – that it is the *male* imagination which impresses itself upon the conceptus. A mechanism was thus provided whereby 'improvements' – products of experience over time – could be passed on to offspring: as with his contemporary Lamarck, Darwin's evolutionary theory programmed in the idea of the inheritance of acquired characteristics. It might thus be called a secular version of the 'traducian' theory of the implantation of the soul.

Darwin held sexual reproduction to be optimal: simpler, pre-sexual modes of reproduction led to deterioration over the generations, as was evident in the case of bulbs. In any case, sexual coupling provided the opportunity for 'joy', and it carried a further advantage: by supplying the means whereby 'ideas' could be conveyed to the next generation, sexual breeding could be evolutionarily progressive, the adaptations of one generation being passed down to the next.

Analysis of living beings showed that life contained the capacity for repeated, continued, gradual modifications: 'Would it be too bold to imagine', he appealed,

that . . . all warm-blooded animals have arisen from one living filament, which THE GREAT FIRST CAUSE endued with animality, with the power of acquiring new parts, attended with new propensities, directed by irritations, sensations, volitions, and associations; and thus possessing the faculty of continuing to improve by its own inherent activity, and of delivering down those improvements by generation to its posterity, world without end?

As a radical alternative to Genesis, evolution was thus first established as a biomedical theory and creation myth in Darwin's *Zoonomia*. Its implications specifically for man and society were further spelt out in *The Temple of Nature*, posthumously published in 1803. A sublime panorama of change was unfolded in that didactic poem, from the coagulation of nebulae up to the steam engine, from mushrooms to machines. Irritation was the initial trigger of the life forces, unlocking the potentialities of animated powers, leading to the awakening of feelings:

> Next the long nerves unite their silver train,
> And young SENSATION permeates the brain;
> Through each new sense the keen emotions dart,
> Flush the young cheek, and swell the throbbing heart.

Sensation in turn quickened the perceptions of pleasure and pain and triggered volition:

> From pain and pleasure quick VOLITIONS rise,
> Lift the strong arm, or point the inquiring eyes . . .

These then produced the awakening of mind:

> Last in thick swarms ASSOCIATIONS spring,
> Thoughts join to thoughts, to motions motions cling;
> Whence in long trains of catenation flow
> Imagined joy, and voluntary woe.

And, thanks to the association of ideas, there followed habit, imitation, imagination and the higher mental powers, generating language, the arts and sciences, the love of beauty, and the moral and social powers engendered by sympathy. Through such evolutionary processes man had become the lord of creation – a pre-eminence stemming not from a divine mission or from any innate Cartesian endowments, but because of basic physical advantages: highly sensitive hands, for instance, had permitted the development of superior powers of volition and understanding.

'All nature', he proclaimed, 'exists in a state of perpetual improvement.' Doubtless, endless competition of organic forms also resulted in death, destruction and even extinction:

> From Hunger's arm the shafts of Death are hurl'd,
> And one great Slaughter-house the warring world!

Nevertheless, rather as for Adam Smith, competition spelt improvement, and population rise brought not Malthusian misery but Darwinian delight:

> Shout round the globe, how Reproduction strives
> With vanquish'd Death, – and Happiness survives;
> How Life increasing peoples every clime,
> And young renascent Nature conquers Time.

Contrast Darwin's epic of progress with such earlier visions as *Paradise Lost* and the *Essay on Man*. For Milton, what was fundamental was the spoilt relationship between man and God: endowed with reason and free will, Adam's offence lay in violation of God's command; man's destiny was couched in divine revelation. Pope for his part presented the human condition as a divided self, fixed on a divinely ordained scale:

> Plac'd on this isthmus of a middle state,
> A being darkly wise, and rudely great;
> With too much knowledge for the Sceptic side,
> With too much weakness for the Stoic's pride;
> He hangs between; in doubt to act or rest;
> In doubt to deem himself a God or Beast;
> In doubt his Mind or Body to prefer . . .

The static Chain of Being in mind, Pope viewed humans suspended between angels and animals, a predicament at once laughable and lamentable,

> Created half to rise, and half to fall;
> Great lord of all things, yet a prey to all.

Man was thus 'the glory, jest and riddle of the world'.

Darwin, by contrast, painted a more naturalistic, this-worldly and optimistic picture, grounded on evolution. Human capacities were products of biological and physiological developments which guaranteed 'the progress of the Mind'. There was no Lucifer, and no Fall. Neither was there any fundamental Popean mind–body dichotomy. Evolutionary tendencies bridged the gap. What in Hartley had been a monism of individual development became in Darwin a monism of evolutionary improvement.

Viewing humanity from Nature's perspective not God's, Darwin granted mankind a more elevated position: man alone had consciousness of the natural order. The human animal which Pope satirized, Darwin celebrated – though he couldn't resist tagging on a warning against hubris, in respect of the pride engendered by Christianity:

> Imperious man, who rules the bestial crowd,
> Of language, reason, and reflection proud,
> With brow erect who scorns this earthy sod,
> And styles himself the image of his God;
> Arose from rudiments of form and sense,
> An embryon point, or microscopic ens!

While *Paradise Lost* related mankind's fate in terms of disobedience, sin and punishment and perhaps redemption – to justify the ways of God to man, and the *Essay on Man* offered man as a riddle, even if, in principle at least, he was capable of self-knowledge, Darwin presented a materialist view of man making himself, a Promethean vision of infinite possibilities. God was now nothing more than a distant cause of causes; what mattered was matter, and man acting in nature. The theodicy, the master-narrative, had become secularized.

It is illuminating to differentiate Erasmus Darwin's materialism from that of his contemporary William Godwin. The latter (see Chapter 23) held that progress lay in mind controlling, and (he hoped) ultimately superseding, the biological: the triumph of reason would render physical bodies redundant. No such vision was entertained by Erasmus Darwin, who would doubtless have chortled at Godwin's view for being vain, pretentious and impractical – on a par with theological nonsense! Darwin had no faith in pure reason – as a physician he saw disease, decay and death all too often destroying human hopes. When his own son died after a dissecting accident as a medical student, Darwin warned that too much trust should not be placed in rationality: 'Reason but skins the wound, which is perpetually liable to fester again.' The frailties of the flesh could be rationalized, not transcended.

Neither was the Godwinian triumph of reason over the flesh something that Darwin would remotely have *wanted*. The utilitarian physician had huge faith in physical, material happiness – it was that which drove evolution. Happiness ultimately came from bodily energies. Darwin's vision was the triumph of Eros over Thanatos. Industrial development was an extension of such life-enhancing powers; agricultural and industrial improvement would provide the food and wealth which would support the increased number of mouths the sexual drive would bring about. He was thus a fan of the flesh, by contrast to Godwin's zeal for disembodied reason and Malthus's pessimism about baser instincts. *Nosce teipsum* still applied, but it was essentially human biology which was to be known, as human kind emancipated itself from ignorance:

Ignorance and credulity have ever been companions, and have misled and enslaved mankind; philosophy has in all ages endeavoured to oppose their progress, and to loosen the shackles they had imposed; philosophers have on this account been called unbelievers; unbelievers of what? of the fictions of fancy, of witchcraft, hobgoblins, apparitions, vampires, fairies; of the influence of stars on human actions, miracles wrought by the bones of saints, the flights of ominous birds, the predictions from the bowels of dying animals, expounders of dreams, fortune-tellers, conjurors, modern prophets, necromancy, cheiromancy, animal magnetism, metallic tractors, with endless variety of folly? These they have disbelieved and despised, but have ever bowed their hoary heads to Truth and Nature. . . .

In regard to religious matters, there is an intellectual cowardice instilled into the minds of the people from their infancy; which prevents their inquiry: credulity is made an indispensable virtue; to inquire or exert their reason in religious matters is denounced as sinful; and in the catholic church is punished with more severe penances than moral crimes.

*

Carlyle's pessimism notwithstanding, Erasmus Darwin should not be seen as offering a crude model of man for his times. In the light of Wedgwood's desire to turn his workforce into such machines 'as do not err', it might be anticipated that the poet-doctor's vision would be of *l'homme machine*, in which man was reduced to a robot, responding mechanically to external sticks and carrots.

There is, it must be admitted, something curious about the view of human agency in industrial society conveyed by Darwin's writings: the poetic tropes of *The Temple of Nature* are mystifying, for all the actual work is depicted as being done either by heroic machines or by even more heroic inventors:

So ARKWRIGHT taught from Cotton-pods to cull,
And stretch in lines the vegetable wool . . .

The actual workforce in Arkwright's factories is conspicuously absent. Darwin certainly never advocated a model of industrial man as an automaton, to be drilled into discipline. In many ways he was concerned to *rescue* man from the aspersions of being just a machine. He constantly stressed inner energy and drives – both the capacity and the need to learn, the inventiveness and adaptiveness of *homo faber*, the man who makes himself. His was a prophecy of Promethean man for the machine age, but it was not a vision of man the machine.

For something approaching that one must look forward to Robert Owen, the most remarkable entrepreneur-philosopher of the industrial era (at least until Friedrich Engels), a truly astonishing instance of the self-made man. His was a rags-to-riches story of the kind soon to be celebrated by Samuel Smiles. The experience of being a self-made individual, however, led Owen to recognize that nothing whatever was *given*, nothing had been *created* just-so, for all time, in a fixed place, by a Creator. All was made – be it self-made or made by others. God therefore dropped out of the picture, and the entrepreneur-philosopher stepped into his shoes, the classic self-made man who worshipped his maker.

Born in 1771 in Newtown, Montgomeryshire, the son of a saddler, Owen had only a bare elementary education before becoming a draper's assistant first in Stamford and then London. Little is known of his early years, but he tells us that, as early as the age of 10, it had dawned on him that there was something wrong with religions, because of the contradictions between them. One day, at the counter, he realized that these different faiths 'emanated . . . from the same false imaginations of our early ancestors': contemporary faiths were thus relics of primitive errors. Man, he concluded, was not responsible to God for his behaviour, for he was entirely 'the child of Nature and Society'.

In 1788, at the age of 17, this precocious lad went to seek his fortune in Manchester, and a few years later he moved north to Scotland, where he built up the Lanark textile mills at Paisley, just outside Glasgow. There he became not just a highly successful entrepreneur, but a passionate advocate of the crucial role of industry – understood both as a mode of production and as disciplined hard work – in generating progress. Industry was the principle of improvement; it would turn wastelands into wealth. 'Those who were engaged in the trade, manufactures, and commerce of this country thirty or forty years ago formed but a very insignificant portion of the knowledge, wealth, influence or population of the Empire,' he reflected. Since then things had been quite transformed, mainly thanks to the 'mechanical inventions which introduced the cotton trade into this country'. But their effect had been deeply equivocal. They brought riches – but they also created poverty and all its problems:

The general diffusion of manufactures throughout a country generates a new character in its inhabitants; and as this character is formed upon a principle quite unfavourable to individual or general happiness, it will produce the most lamentable and permanent evils, unless its tendency be counteracted by legislative interference and direction.

Mechanical efficiency had the capacity, however, to create the blessings of order and satisfaction, without which it could not itself thrive. Optimal human functioning would, obviously, service the factory to best effect, but, more broadly, it would make happiness prevail. The creation of such ideal workplace conditions was the responsibility of the paternalistic factory-owner. He must develop model factory villages equipped with schools, good housing, libraries, meeting halls and so forth, so as to produce a healthy, well-balanced workforce. 'After breakfast we walked to New Lanark . . .,' wrote Robert Southey, no great friend to the industrial system, either in his early incarnation as a Jacobin radical or later, as here, as a pillar of Toryism:

In the course of going thro' these buildings, [Owen] took us into an apartment where one of his plans . . . was spread upon the floor. And with a long wand in his hand he explained the plan. . . . Meantime the word had been given: we were conducted into one of the dancing rooms; half a dozen fine boys, about nine or ten years old, led the way, playing of fifes, and some 200 children, from four years of age till ten, entered the room and arranged themselves on three sides of it.

Southey was rather impressed by the appearance of successful, caring paternalism, but insistent that Owen himself was a phoney:

He is part-owner and sole Director of a large establishment, differing more in accidents than in essence from a plantation: the persons under him happen to be white, and are at liberty by law to quit his service, but while they remain in it they are as much under his absolute management as so many negro-slaves. His humour, his vanity, his kindliness of nature (all these have their share) lead him to make these *human machines* as he calls them (and literally believes them to be) as happy as he can, and to make a display of their happiness.

Turning visionary, Owen had come to believe that the founding of model villages or factory colonies, inhabited by these *human machines*, would put an end to the gross miseries caused by beggar-my-neighbour competitive capitalism of the kind encouraged by classical free-market economics. 'The governing principle of trade, manufacturers, and commerce is immediate pecuniary gain,' he reflected:

All are sedulously trained to buy cheap and to sell dear: and to succeed in this art, the parties must be taught to acquire strong powers of deception; and thus a spirit is generated . . . destructive of that open, honest, sincerity, without which man cannot make others happy, nor enjoy happiness himself.

In such circumstances, the workforce was treated as 'mere instruments of gain' and, partly as a consequence, they retaliated by acquiring 'a gross ferocity of character'. This, warned Owen, 'will sooner or later plunge the country into a formidable and perhaps inextricable state of danger'.

Fortunately, the solution was to hand: co-operation would create the harmony which wise counsels dictated. William Godwin, a man with much philosophically in common with Owen, loathed co-operation as destructive of individuality; Owen craved it for its capacity to create the harmony which was the *sine qua non* of happiness.

A true man of the Enlightenment, like Godwin, Owen championed reason with fanatical passion. 'Expose [error] but for an instant to the clear light of intellectual day,' he declared, 'and, as though conscious of its own deformity, it will instantaneously vanish, never to reappear.' Here was the Socratic creed that evil was error, awaiting refutation – a belief taken over by Godwin – being expressed again with great warmth: great is truth and will prevail.

In the tradition launched by Locke, Owen looked to education to dispel such error – or, better, to prevent it in the first place. In particular, he took up the ideas on education of Helvétius, who had developed Locke's ideas as filtered through the medium of his fellow Frenchman, Condillac. More overtly than Locke, Helvétius held human beings to be radically conditionable, putty in one's hands, a position which Owen enthusiastically endorsed. Central to his philosophical programme was the 'formation of character': 'the members of any community may by degrees be trained to live *without idleness, without poverty, without crime, and without punishment*; for each of these is the effect of error in the various systems prevalent throughout the world. *They are all the necessary consequences of ignorance.*' Why could he be so optimistic? It was because

human nature, save the minute differences which are ever found in all the compounds of the creation, is one and the same in all; it is without exception universally plastic, and, by judicious training, THE INFANTS OF ANY ONE CLASS IN THE WORLD MAY BE READILY FORMED INTO MEN OF ANY OTHER CLASS.

Here, with a vengeance, was the absolute malleability of man. Owen's new view of the power of education to condition men's minds depended heavily upon radical notions of necessity, notably the thinking of Godwin. And precisely how could bad conditioning be turned into good? The personality of the workforce must be moulded by intellectual superiors who had embraced rational views of progress. Since 'the end of government is to make the governed and the governors happy,' he declared, further nailing his utilitarian colours to the mast, 'that government then is the best, which in practice produces the greatest happiness to the greatest number.'

Owen early became, as we have seen, a religious sceptic, and he turned into a militant secularist who found a scapegoat for the world's ills in organized religion. He deplored the dire influence of Churches which degraded and defamed the true potential and latent goodness of human beings – such creeds 'have created, and still create, a great proportion of the miseries which exist in the world'. Yet he left the door open for the creation of a new and pure faith: 'a knowledge of truth on the subject of religion would permanently establish the happiness of man.' Owen was convinced of the value of public religion in promoting the cause of harmony. His was, to all intents and purposes, a new religion of mankind, a gospel of industrial work, co-operation and communitarianism, in which men would be happiest when best organized.

Ironically, if hardly surprisingly, Owen's vision for the future may be seen as secularized Christianity. He naturalized and fused two related religious traditions, eschatology and utopianism. The Christian apocalyptic tradition was discussed in Chapter 2, and we shall see the enduring circulation of antinomianism in Blake in Chapter 24. Attempts to render biblical prophecy and eschatology spiritual, and thus to give them a renewed currency with different inflections, were numerous in the exhilarating French Revolutionary decades. Wordsworth proclaimed that the theme of his poetic autobiography *The Prelude* concerned godlike powers and actions internalized as processes of his own mind –

> of Genius, Power,
> Creation and Divinity itself,
> I have been speaking.

And in the verse 'Prospectus' to *The Excursion*, he announced that his poetic journey must ascend beyond 'the heaven of heavens', past 'Jehovah – with his thunder, and the choir/Of shouting Angels', and also sink deeper than the lowest hell, without ever leaving the confines of 'the Mind of Man –/My haunt, and the main region of my song'. The conclusion he drew was the recovery of a lost Paradise – a paradise within all of us – to be achieved in a consummation viewed as an apocalyptic marriage between mind and nature: 'Paradise, and groves/Elysian, Fortunate Fields.'

Blake, Wordsworth, Coleridge, Southey and others responded to the great events of the 1790s by writing visionary epics which depicted mankind's dark and turbulent past and present but hailed the Revolution as the critical turning-point ushering in a new world which would combine the pagan golden age with the biblical paradise or Last Judgement. In the conclusion of the 'Argument' for *Religious Musings*, written in 1794, Coleridge laconically reviewed this prophetic reading of contemporary events: 'The present State of Society. The French Revolution. Millennium. Universal Redemption. Conclusion.'

Owen the unbeliever also thought in secularized eschatological terms. Unlike the Romantics, however, whose hopes for a glorious transformation collapsed with the failure of the French Revolution to deliver universal liberty and the rights of man – leading them to turn reactionary – Owen's hopes remained buoyed up by the prospects of a grand industrial future. In 1837, in a famous debate with the Revd J. H. Roebuck, he issued an impassioned apostrophe to the coming 'moral world', with direct echoes of the prophet Isaiah:

Oh . . . that the time may now commence when men shall become rational, and, in consequence, turn their spears into pruning hooks, and their swords into ploughshares; when each man shall sit under any vine, or any fig tree, and there shall be none to make him afraid.

He there set out his vision of the perfectibility of man, and of the role of the enlightened in bringing it about:

Until the characters of men can be new-created by society, from their birth, so as to form them into rational beings who will act wisely and consistently through life, *an intermediate or preparatory government* must be made to govern those townships, while the new characters are in progress of formation from birth.

Did this plant in Marx's mind the germ of the 'dictatorship of the proletariat'?

Owen fused this secular eschatology with utopianism owing much to Plato's *Republic* and More's *Utopia*. A just society required central direction to eliminate poverty, war, inequality, repression and so forth, and create an order in which people willingly participated for the good of the whole. For Owen, utopian thinking was truly a vision of a new harmony, be it at the Lanark mills, or at 'New Harmony' in the United States, the utopian colony he later set up in the New World.

The Book of the New Moral World (1836) contains his mature thought on 'a NEW MORAL WORLD, in which, evil, except as it will be recorded in the past sufferings of mankind, will be unknown'. All was now revealed: 'truth is nature, and nature God' – that is, God had become a God within, the old idea of the divine had been transferred to Nature. Owen once more set out his pleasure–pain psychology in the service of an early version of behaviourism. Human beings were shaped by their training; with correct educational arrangements, they would turn into superior beings. What had been mistaken for an innate strain of evil was really the product of bad education, creating false incentives for the child.

Owen thus looked to a benign paternalism, through which the world was perfectible – the millennium was literally at our doors. 'The rubicon between the Old Immoral and the New Moral Worlds is finally passed,' he proclaimed:

and Truth, Knowledge, Union, Industry, and Moral Good now take the field, and openly advance against the united powers of Falsehood, Ignorance, Dis-Union, and Moral Evil. . . . The time is therefore arrived when the foretold millennium is about to commence, when the slave and the prisoner, the bond-man and the bond-woman, and the child and the servant, shall be set free for ever, and oppression of body and mind shall be known no more.

Thus, militant secularism became a faith in itself.

Perhaps ironically, perhaps predictably, this truculent unbeliever turned late in life to the new craze for spiritualism – that Victorian attempt to surmount the gap between the living and the dead (created in part by the Protestant abolition of purgatory) and to prove an afterlife. Was this a turnabout – the foible of an old man facing death? Or was it the further extension of rational, secular, industrial principles to one of religion's remaining outposts?

Although his thought was hardly subtle, Owen's historical significance is immense. He was the first in the industrial age to formulate a secular doctrine which both explained the place of men within the economic order – how industry shaped human nature – and promised to change it, to forge new men in a new economic and social order. Like Erasmus Darwin, he came to terms with the machine. He accepted mechanization as an irrevocable fact, and welcomed the wealth it brought, as long as it was properly distributed. But he saw the danger of the machine subverting the morality upon which society ought to rest; and in proposing certain practical solutions he attempted to surmount them. Many of the radical thinkers who preceded him seem to belong to another era – William Godwin, for example, confident that man's rationality must inevitably prompt him towards the good and that this would result in the abolition of government and authority. Such individualism heralded a dignity for the lone individual, unsupported by God, the soul, the Chain of Being or the Church; but it abstracted that individual from society. Owen recognized how man was necessarily – for good or ill – a product of the society in which he lived – in this case a mechanized society dedicated to making products. Marx was but a step away.

22

DEPENDENT BODIES

Enlightenment philosophical, scientific and medical radicalism asserted that man could be understood in natural terms, by a ready extension of that law-seeking method which the mechanical philosophy had espoused and the Newtonian synthesis vindicated. Through this search an end would be put to the obscurantist mystery-mongering which had always proved so useful a tool for the powers-that-be.

Hume may have confused matters by exposing causality as nothing other than constant conjunction, but his friend Adam Smith reassuringly demonstrated that the progress of the mind brought the supersession of primitive wonder by a more satisfying grasp of the underlying regularities governing nature. The revolution which students of the self were seeking was an equivalent for man: an understanding of motivation in terms of the laws of mechanism – the inner clockwork of the self, the springs, balances, pulleys, levers and hinges by means of which the organism functioned.

Radicals grounded human science in a metaphysics of determinism. As formulated by Hartley, necessity became the clarion call for William Godwin and for Benthamite philosophical radicals. If determinism was not shouted from the rooftops by all comers, it was nevertheless, at a practical level, implicit in utilitarian and economic thinking at large: everyone accepted, tacitly at least, that people invariably sought pleasure and shunned pain, followed self-interest and pursued profit – and that they could predictably be assumed, or trained, to behave on that basis.

Emergent psychology thus broadly traded in assumptions about the constant drives, proclivities and passions of individuals, notably a fundamental selfishness. Similarly, medical thinking took a broad determinism for granted: at bottom, the laws of the organism determined life and consciousness: fevers would produce delirium, madness probably had physical roots, a good digestion aided a happy and contented mind – or, contrariwise, bad dreams followed from eating too much old cheese, or raw pork, for supper; and, alongside taxes, death was certain.

The body's hold over the mind was not, however, to be encouraged. A man had the power, and duty, to guard his health and look after his constitution, by self-regulation, by tending his body and mastering his passions. Traditional Christian humanists saw this primarily as an exercise of will; progressives like Hartley viewed it more as a matter of harmonizing with the dictates of nature. Loss of such rational control became a matter of growing concern to philosophers of the self.

The eighteenth century brought the birth of the 'consumer society'. Among the items consumed in greater range and larger quantities were food and drink; this brought growing anxiety about the harmful consequences of abuse, notably drunkenness. Alcohol had traditionally been viewed as a good thing: drinking was convivial, wine nutritious, invigorating and medicinal. But, as with everything, excess was bad. Drunkenness had traditionally been viewed, like fornication or swearing, as a failure of self-control on the part of the individual which it was his duty to correct. This viewpoint was somewhat challenged by the gin craze of the 1730s and 1740s – the product of dirt-cheap rot-gut – which forced public opinion to confront the phenomenon of mass and lethal intoxication.

Partly in the light of that craze, the suggestion gathered support that habitual drunkenness was not simply a personal weakness of will: it needed to be understood in terms of a tyranny of habits which, reinforced by the chemistry of alcohol, became ever more ingrained and difficult to combat – indeed, engulfed the personality.

The Scottish doctor George Cheyne for one ventured to explain · how old soaks succumbed to 'cravings':

They begin with the weaker wines; These, by Use and Habit, will not do; They leave the Stomach sick and mawkish; they fly to stronger Wines, and stronger still, and run the Climax from Brandy to Barbados Waters, and double-distill'd Spirits, till at last they find nothing hot enough for them.

Thus, the penal servitude of 'Necessity upon Necessity' set in, whereby 'Drams beget more Drams . . . so that at last the miserable Creature suffers a true Martyrdom'.

Somewhat later, the Quaker physician John Coakley Lettsom adumbrated the nature of progressive dependence. He displayed the fatal cycle leading from tippling for stimulus, relief or exhilaration; to low spirits, which were the inevitable after-effects; which in turn could be expunged only by further bouts of yet heavier drinking. 'Those of delicate habits, who have endeavoured to overcome their nervous debility by the aid of spirits,' he cited as an example:

many of these have begun the use of these poisons from persuasion of their utility, rather than from love of them: the relief, however, being temporary, to keep up their effects, frequent access is had to the same delusion, till at length what was taken by compulsion, gains attachment, and a little drop of brandy, or gin and water, becomes as necessary as food; the female sex, from natural delicacy, acquire this custom by small degrees, and the poison being admitted in small doses, is slow in its operations, but not less painful in its effects.

Eventually, such dependence would set in that 'neither threats nor persuasions are powerful enough to overcome it and the miserable sufferer is so infatuated, as in spite of locks and keys, to bribe by high rewards the dependent nurse, privately to procure the fatal draught'.

By 1804 it was possible to cast habitual drunkenness as a 'disease'. In his *Essay Medical Philosophical and Chemical on Drunkenness*, published in this year, Thomas Trotter – perhaps blessed with unrivalled experience with drunks, having served as physician to the Navy – stated point-blank that the 'habit of drunkenness' was indeed a 'disease' – indeed, he went on, it was a 'disease of the mind', 'like delirium'. Moralists and parsons, he condescendingly added, had been well-meaning in their exposés of drunkenness as vice or sin, but now, at last, 'it had been set within its rightful domain', medicine, to be managed by 'the discerning physician'. By mid-century the precise notion of 'alcoholism' had been formulated.

Other morbid personality traits commanded growing attention. *A Treatise of the Hypochondriack and Hysterick Diseases* (1730) penned by the fabulist of the bees, Bernard de Mandeville, pondered the fictional case of the liberally educated 'Misomedon', who had sufficient leisure to dwell upon his pains, and enough book-learning to be expert at fantasizing the workings of disease and drugs. Partly thanks to unscrupulous physicians, his life became a battle with 'diseases' which, though imaginary, materialized in time, as needless physicking took its toll.

Blasé doctors blamed the rise of such hypochondria upon the democratization of information which, they alleged, encouraged the laity to meddle in a matter, health, that was too hot for them to handle. Self-dosing, mocked the Bath physician Dr James Adair, had become the fad among those 'who are sick by way of amusement and melancholy to keep up their spirits'. Yet 'no disease is more troublesome,' he added, 'either to the Patient or Physician, than hypochondriac Disorders; and it often happens, that, thro' the Fault of both, the Cure is either unnecessarily protracted, or totally frustrated; for the Patients are so delighted, not only with a Variety of Medicines, but also of Physicians.' Therein lay the catch, for the paradox of hypochondria was that the doctor's intervention would, all too easily, merely reinforce that dependency from which the hypochondriac needed to escape. Hypochondria thus represented the faddish enculturation of sickly sensibility.

Hysteria developed similarly – indeed, the two were often represented as brother and sister. By the eighteenth century, hysteria, which had earlier been judged a somatic malady of women – a disease of the womb – was typically deployed to identify the volatile physical symptoms associated with hypersensitivity, a lability thought especially common in 'the sex', but – significantly, in a culture in which enlightened politeness was blamed for making men 'effeminate' – not exclusively so. The diagnosis signalled superiority in status, while also marking a mysterious *je ne sais quoi*, a malady that was intermittent and unpredictable, lacking tangible physical causes.

This 'coming-out' of the hypochondriac and hysteric constitutes an important symptom, the pathological downside of Enlightenment individualism. Polite society encouraged cultural narcissism: within the permitted degrees of conventional polish, the *literati* were expected to become *glitterati*. Yet such a licence had its price. The tension between the invitation to shine and the need for polite conformity bred anxieties, in turn somatized into physical complaints, which, through the conscious or insensible manipulation of the sick-role, could be variously owned and disowned. Sickliness provided a social alibi, while suffering might purchase the privilege of being different.

The new prominence of hypochondria also registers a health culture disrupted by commercialization. Sick people were consulting more doctors, more often, and paying them fatter fees, while still seeking out quacks and irregulars, and obtaining cascades of medication, stimulants and sedatives from apothecaries, nostrum-mongers and druggists. They were also devouring piles of books claiming to make *Every Man his Own Physician*, and investing in well-stocked proprietary medicine-chests. The profession deplored these perversions, while actually profiting nicely from them. Many medical bigwigs, it was observed, prostituted their art by pandering to the whims of the worried well, the pseudo-sick and valetudinarians, thereby appropriating for themselves the 'lucrative part' of the '*sick-trade*'.

The commercialization of health brought a further turn of the screw: commodification. As discussed earlier (Chapter 13), people had always eaten and drunk themselves to destruction. Critics now complained that sufferers – many of whom had read books which might just as well have been titled *Every Man his Own Poisoner* or *Every Man his Own Hypochondriac* – were *medicating* themselves to death – or at least indiscriminately swallowing stimulants and painkillers to relieve their (often imaginary) distempers, only to become dangerously habituated to their use. Drug-dependency was beginning to take shape.

The late Georgian age is seminal for encouraging addiction and conceptualizing the phenomenon. Trotter put his finger on it in noting that modern man was simultaneously 'the *creator* of his own *temperament*' and thereby 'the *creature of habit*'. Producer and product, man was the sum of all the stimuli encircling and determining him: here was the insight of Locke extended to items of consumption. Moreover, with the mobilization of market society, man the consumer assumed importance. There was an escalation in consumption of tea, coffee, tobacco, sugar, ardent spirits, fortified liquors (above all, port and brandy), bitters, tonics, narcotics, sedatives, quack, patent and proprietary medicines – most being widely regarded as deleterious, habit-forming and even poisonous and destructive. Opium use, for instance, rose staggeringly. 'I think amazing quantities are consumed every year,' it was remarked in 1796, 'and am of opinion, that there is twenty times more opium use now in England only, than there was fifteen or twenty years since.' The explanation was simple: opiates were far the most effective painkillers, and the 'age of feeling' was arguably lowering the pain threshold. Certainly the Georgians seized upon opiates for their remarkable analgesic properties, George Cheyne praising the poppy as 'a certain *Relief*, if not a Remedy, even to our most *intense Pains* and *extreme Miseries*' – indeed 'a standing and *constant Miracle*'. Doctors made light of the suspected harmful consequences – Sir Richard Blackmore specifically denied that opium was addictive – and hence prescribed freely. Not surprisingly, dozens succumbed to narcotic addiction – not merely such notorious cases as Coleridge and Thomas De Quincey, but also Robert Clive, Samuel Johnson's wife Tetty, his bosom friend Topham Beauclerk, William Wilberforce, and somewhat later, most of Tennyson's brothers.

Leading physicians deprecated drug-dependency as one of the evils of the age. The irony is that, precisely because of their advanced involvement with experimental chemistry, and their ardent humanitarianism, progressive physicians must shoulder much of the responsibility for drug-induced human tragedies. The circles around Thomas Beddoes were, for instance, eager to experiment, as we shall see, with narcotics, from nitrous oxide (laughing gas) to opiates. 'Do bring down some of the Hyoscyamine pills,' his friend and patient Coleridge on one occasion begged Tom Wedgwood, 'and I will give a fair trial of Opium, Henbane, and Nepenthe.' As we saw in the last chapter, the entrepreneur's son grew hooked: 'I cannot do it – my spirits become dreadful – the dullness of my life is absolutely unsupportable without it.'

Fears of a dependency society were percipiently analysed by Trotter. His *View of the Nervous Temperament* (1811) paraded a kind of 'Addict's Progress'. High-stress living weakened the nerves; the enfeebled constitution then needed the crutch or solace of drugs and stimulants, thereby precipitating a downward spiral of deteriorating health. Trotter pessimistically surveyed a 'nervous society' in the making – a drug-culture in which the habits of civilization themselves became disease: 'All nervous persons are uncommonly fond of drugs . . . Among some well-meaning people, this inordinate desire for medicine has frequently become of itself a disease.'

Under such circumstances, the putatively clear distinction between disease and medicine broke down. Medicating habits caused pain, and the craving for artificial stimulants was viewed, by Trotter and others, as a 'disease of the mind'. It was no accident that Coleridge defined addiction as 'the desire of a desire'. Enlightened introspectiveness about consciousness – the urge to create a new science of mind for a new society – led to the formulation of a category of disorders rooted in mental disturbances. Madness, as we saw in Chapter 18, was refigured as a mental disorder, and masturbation, alcoholism, nymphomania and drug-addiction all came to be seen as maladies of the mind. The championing of mind as an engine of liberation revealed its shadow side: mind's self-imprisoning potential.

Classic among such cases of an identity in thrall to dependency is Samuel Taylor Coleridge. Fired by revolutionary fervour and hounded by creditors, this Anglican clergyman's son quit Jesus College, Cambridge, without a degree in 1793, gravitating to the company of fellow radicals in Bristol, notably Robert Southey, and throwing himself into poetry, preaching and pamphleteering. The youthful friends projected a New World utopian community on the banks of the Susquehannah in Pennsylvania, untainted by the Old.

Although their plans predictably fell through, young Coleridge, on angel wings, continued to serve the cause of enlightenment. With its Baconian masthead 'KNOWLEDGE IS POWER', his *Watchman* periodical declared in 1796: 'A PEOPLE ARE FREE IN PROPORTION AS THEY FORM THEIR OWN OPINIONS.' Having made 'a diligent, I *may* say, an intense study of Locke, Hartley and others', he had espoused the progressive creed of Unitarianism, determinism and materialism, enthusing to Southey about the 'corporeality of *thought*'. Radical intellectuals like Godwin, Darwin and Priestley had, as he saw it, paved the way for revolution both political and mental: moral improvement was inevitable; and, guided by a 'small but glorious band . . . of thinking and disinterested Patriots', society was to make the world paradisiacal again. His *Religious Musings* (1794) presented a 'Vision' of human destiny moving to a 'blest future'.

His views, of course, underwent a turn-about with the new direction taken by the French Revolution. 'I have snapped my squeaking baby-trumpet of Sedition,' he announced in 1798. Tellingly, having named his first son Hartley, Coleridge christened his second Berkeley, to signal in the clearest possible way his rejection of his erstwhile materialism in favour of idealism. He had 'overthrown the doctrine of Association, as taught by Hartley,' he assured his friend Tom Poole in 1801, 'and with it all the irreligious metaphysics of modern Infidels – especially, the doctrine of Necessity.'

Increasingly (like Southey, a Church-and-King Tory), Coleridge abandoned Lockean empiricism for German transcendentalist idealism. Looking back to earlier religious traditions, notably Cambridge Platonism, and sideways to Kantian metaphysics, he trashed Locke in favour of a theory of mind which emphasized its innate activity and wisdom; developed a doctrine of the organic ('esemplastic') imagination, over and against the passive and mechanical faculty of 'fancy'; and contended that man was inherently religious. Regarding shallow empiricism as a sorry chapter in 'the long and ominous eclipse of philosophy', he would rescue and revive the Neoplatonism ditched by the Lockeans.

Coleridge's animus against his former creed of materialism grew ever more blazing. 'Newton was a mere materialist,' he scoffed in 1801, 'Mind, in his system, is always *passive*, – a lazy *Looker-on* on an external world.' Hence the bitterness in later years when he surveyed the aftermath of enlightened philosophy:

State of nature, or the Ourang Outang theology of the origin of the human race, substituted for the Book of Genesis, Ch. I–X. Rights of nature for the duties and privileges of citizens. Idea-less facts, misnamed proofs from history, grounds of experience, etc., substituted for principles and the insight derived from them. . . . Government by journeymen clubs; by reviews, magazines, and above all by newspapers.

No wonder that barbed satirist Thomas Love Peacock guyed this oracle: 'there is too much commonplace light in our moral and political literature,' pronounces Mr Flosky, a Coleridge twin, in *Nightmare Abbey*, 'and light is a great enemy to mystery.'

All this time Coleridge was blighting his life through his opium habit and the deviousness and despair consequent upon the growing discrepancy between his high ideals and promise on the one hand, and the realities of his tormented, incapacitated existence. Gradually enslaving himself to the poppy, this prophet of mental autonomy thus became the walking falsification of his own new-found philosophy of free will. His life was a somatic shadow of the Christian process of spiritual perdition – and, perhaps, salvation. His opium habits were no secret, and for many he became a bogey figure, a symbol of moral weakness: 'If Coleridge should be remembered, it will be as a warning,' wrote Harriet Martineau.

Coleridge, with his budding superfine sensibility seeking sensation, may have first made medicinal use of opium while still at school; he certainly took large quantities for rheumatic fever in 1791 while at Cambridge and graduated to using it recreationally during the 1790s, unaware of, or oblivious to, its side-effects. He recorded sweet dreams and feelings of release. Yet the young poet was soon to feel the pains of opium, too. He began substantial consumption on a regular basis from around 1801, soon after he discovered a potent, opium-based, proprietary medicine called 'Kendal Black Drop'. Initially he dosed himself to quell neuralgia associated with 'gout' and nervous shooting pains in the limbs and head, unable to bear the agonies these complaints produced on what Humphry Davy would call his 'excessive sensibility'.

Self-dosing brought emotional and physical sequelae of its own. Letters from the early 1800s testify to appalling insomnia – he feared sleep, since his nightmares were unendurable. Above all, he was seized by a paralysing dread of death. Organically, the habit led to 'the weakly Bowels of Disease' – the chronic constipation typical of opium. Many stimulants, including ginger, camphor and rhubarb, were required to counter this. Drugging also ruined his digestion; he could keep the opium down only by first settling his stomach with tumblers of brandy.

While affirming that 'my state of Health is a Riddle', Coleridge continued to tell himself and all and sundry that his maladies were straightforwardly organic, and he insisted to his wife that he used opium purely medicinally, to counter 'the exquisite Affectibility of my Skin' and assuring her that 'to a person, with such a Stomach & Bowels as mine, if any stimulus is needful, Opium in the small quantities, I now take it, is incomparably better in every respect better than Beer, Wine, Spirits, or any *fermented* Liquor – nay, far less pernicious than even Tea'. His convoluted vindication concluded with a pathetic coda giving instructions respecting the health of his sons: '*It is my particular Wish, that Hartley & Derwent should have as little Tea as possible – & always very weak, with more than half milk.*'

During his thirties, Coleridge continued his self-exonerations: his opium was purely a medicament. But, wracked by 'loneliness, continued Pain, accessory Irritations, and a sense of morbid Despondency', he became the man of sorrows, victim and martyr – indeed, the Ancient Mariner – destined for 'self suffering'. Eventually his agonies grew unbearable: 'For many weeks with only two Intervals, and those but day-long, I have been ill – very ill – confined mostly to my Bed, altogether to my bedroom. In my pain I earnestly wish to die.'

The poet remained acutely self-aware, and, no less importantly, guilt-ridden, about the self-indulgence of the suffering soul who had trespassed so extensively upon the goodwill of friends and family alike. From about 1808 he fitfully forced himself to confront a self that was sick, and at last he openly acknowledged the damaging effects of 'that accursed drug', into which he had been 'seduced' by 'the Horrors of Sleep' and 'the Dread of sudden Death'. He continued, nevertheless, to insist that he had taken it up purely for medicinal reasons: 'I was seduced into the use of narcotics . . . & saw not the truth, till my *Body* had contracted a habit & a necessity.' And how had this happened? As ever, Coleridge presented himself as victim: he had allowed himself to become habituated because of his '*Terror & Cowardice* of PAIN & Sudden Death, not (so help me God!) by any temptation of Pleasure, or expectation or desire of exciting pleasurable Sensations'. Nevertheless, the effects had been catastrophic, for addiction had produced a bondage of the will, a mental disease. The true evil of opium was that it produced alienation of mind:

By the long long Habit of the accursed Poison my Volition (by which I mean the faculty *instrumental* to the Will, and by which alone the Will can realize itself – it's Hands, Legs, & Feet, as it were) was compleatly deranged, at times frenzied, dissevered itself from the Will, & become an independent faculty: so that I was perpetually in the state, in which you may have seen paralytic Persons, who attempting to push a step forward in one direction are violently forced round to the opposite.

Bereft of free will, Coleridge thus saw himself, rhetorically at least, as reduced to 'a species of madness . . . You bid me rouse myself – go, bid a man paralytic in both arms rub them briskly together, & that will cure him. Alas! (he would reply) that I cannot move my arms is my Complaint & my misery.'

Here is a remarkable perception – a man acknowledging he has been possessed, to the point of paralysis, by a sickness, which in his guilty moments he sees to be self-induced, indeed, an expression of the self: 'In truth, I have been for years almost a paralytic in mind from self-dissatisfaction.' Thus enslaved to this '*free-agency-annihilating Poison*', the poet-philosopher underwent 'a continued act of thirty years' Self-poisoning thro' cowardice of pain'. For the 'tyranny of habit', the 'slavery to opium' – at rock bottom he had been consuming some five ounces of laudanum a day – wrought self-destruction.

Eventually, from the depths, Coleridge solicited the advice of physicians – something, he said, he had long wished to do but from which he had shrunk: 'I have however done it at last – and tho' the result after a severe Trial proved what I had anticipated, yet such is the Blessedness of walking altogether in Light, that my Health & Spirits are better [than] I have known them for years.' A slave to self, Coleridge could not effect a self-cure, and could be restored only through the agency of a physician, Dr James Gilman, who boarded him at his Highgate home for the remaining sixteen years of his life.

Despite his self-serving protestations, Coleridge's maladies were not principally external afflictions, but expressions of a self pained and traumatized by inability to act. Illness was a somatization of inner frailty which deflected spiritual conflicts while expressing them: 'I am a starling self-incaged . . . and my whole Note is, Tomorrow, & Tomorrow, & Tomorrow.'

Young Coleridge, we noted, was a philosophical and political Godwinian:

> Nor will I not thy holy guidance bless,
> And hymn thee, GODWIN! with an ardent lay,
> For that thy Voice, in Passion's stormy Day,
> When wild I roam'd the bleak Heath of Distress,
> Bade the bright Form of JUSTICE meet my Way,
> And told me, that her name was HAPPINESS!

The last thirty years of his life were spent, however, by way of self-reinvention, repudiating the materialism about which he had been so enthusiastic and which, in a sense, actually explained the opium addiction which he denied. Religion replaced rationalism. On the last day of 1796, he tells us, 'I retired to a cottage in Somersetshire, at the foot of the Quantocks, and devoted my thoughts and studies to the foundations of religion and morals'. His ensuing friendship with Wordsworth led him to a deeper reverence for Nature: 'Henceforth I shall know/That Nature ne'er deserts the wise and pure.' Already in 1801 he noted, while reading the medieval theologian Duns Scotus, 'I am burning Locke, Hume and Hobbes under his nose. They stink worse than feather or assafoetida. . . . I am confident that I can prove that the reputation of these three men has been wholly unmerited.'

The mature Coleridge diagnosed what had gone wrong with the enlightened thinking to which he himself had fallen a dupe. He recast the sorry saga of eighteenth-century empirical thought as 'the long and ominous eclipse of philosophy; the usurpation of that venerable name by physical and psychological empiricism'. Empirical science, he admitted, had been attended by enormous achievements, and so it had come to dominate thought; life had been reduced to formulas, and mind to the empirical basement of Locke's psychology. What emerged was a false view of man as an atomized individual, unrelated to past or future, living in isolation and lacking spirituality – roughly Burke's view. To counter this, Coleridge urged a return to that great Neoplatonic tradition: 'Dante, Petrarch, Spenser, Philip and Algernon Sidney, Milton and Barrow were Platonists.'

In a series of public lectures, delivered in London in 1818, Coleridge returned to the master: 'Plato! I really feel, unaffectedly, an awe when I mention his name.' The essence of Plato's philosophy, he declared, was that

he taught the idea, namely the possibility, and the duty of all who would arrive at the greatest perfection of the human mind, of striving to contemplate things not in the phenomenon . . . but lastly and chiefly as they exist in the Supreme Mind, independent of all material division, distinct and yet indivisible.

Behind the evanescence of appearances there lay an inner reality, from which it followed that 'there is a moral government in the world – that things neither happen by chance nor yet by any blind agency of necessity'. Not just through the senses, knowledge might also be arrived at by a kind of revelation 'which neither our senses, nor our understanding, nor our reason, could give us the least conception of'. This led him to conclude

that without a congenial philosophy there can be no general religion, that a philosophy among the higher classes is an essential condition to the true state of religion among all classes, and that religion is the great centre of gravity in all countries and in all ages, and according as it is good or bad, whether religion or irreligion, so all the other powers of the state necessarily accommodate themselves to it.

Transcendental idealism would thus shore up the system.

One baleful consequence of empirical science had been the triumph of materialism. The logical upshot of scientific materialism, Coleridge warned, would be the exclusion of religion. He returned to what was always for him the heart of the matter. For materialism

destroys the possibility of free agency, it destroys the great distinction between the mere human and the mere animals of nature, namely the powers of originating an act. All things are brought, even the powers of life are brought, into a common link of causes and effects that we observe in a machine, and all the powers of thought into those of life, being all reasoned away into modes of sensation, and the will itself into nothing but a current, a fancy determined by the accidental copulations of certain internal stimuli. . . . It is by [man's] bold denial of this, by an inward assertion, 'I am not the creature of nature merely, nor a subject of nature, but I detach myself from her. I oppose myself as man to nature, and my destination is to conquer and subdue her, to be lord of light and fire and the elements; and what my mind can comprehend that I will make my eye to see. . . . And why? Because I am a free being.'

One might sense a subtext of Coleridge blaming materialism for seducing himself into a weakness which had destroyed his will.

Fortified thus by Christianity and Plato – and the laudanum bottle – Coleridge reasserted man as a spiritual being, the Lord of Nature but for ever distinct from it because he was a moral creature, with powers of free choice.

Private events have public consequences. Many philosophical

radicals embraced the enlightened package of Locke, Hartley and so forth – man as a product of circumstances, as infinitely malleable and educable, hence indefinitely progressive. Some abandoned such thinking when the French Revolution turned to terror. Coleridge was one. But his volte-face was particularly vehement. That was because he had been reduced to agony and abjection by an opium habit which left him unable to face himself. The adoption, in the depths, of the most stringent Christian Platonic idealism, with its doctrine of reason, free will and the separate soul, was his only recourse. It was, at one level, a heroic deception, a gigantic pretence. Yet at another it was the belief which truly gave him hope: one day he might actually, once more, be able to live out the reality of that creed. Out of Coleridge's crisis emerged a body of thinking about the soul and self which then became inspirational for nineteenth-century culture – as John Stuart Mill acknowledged when he divided the thinkers of his day into the rival camps of Benthamites and Coleridgeans.

While resident in Bristol in the 1790s, Coleridge's physician was Thomas Beddoes, a mere bit player in Britain's cultural history, yet one whose symbolic role confirms the deep ambiguities in this story. Beddoes exposed, and was a fierce critic of, dependency as a disease of society: as we saw in Chapter 13, he abhorred the new chic lifestyles and the cant that accompanied them. Yet he was himself an ardent experimenter with new chemicals and gases, testing their medical and psychotropic effects. He distrusted doctors, yet commended them as the hope of the future. Another disciple of Lockean sensationalism, associationism, Hartleyan materialism and Brunonian medicine, he embraced sublime hopes for the perfectibility of man, yet his life ended in despair.

Born into a prosperous Shropshire tradesman's family in 1760, Thomas Beddoes typified the West Midlands character: thrusting, businesslike and ambitious. Trusting to his own energies and resenting tradition and privilege, he grew up a tenacious liberal individualist, dreaming of a society with room at the top. He pro-

ceeded in 1776 to Oxford and, unusually for the time, cultivated
scientific interests. Opting for medicine, on obtaining his BA he
migrated to London, the premier centre for practical medicine,
moving on in 1784 to Edinburgh to complete his medical education.
There he forged a lasting friendship with the chemist Joseph Black,
friend of Erasmus Darwin and the Lunar circle.

In 1786 he returned to Oxford, throwing himself into chemical
research. Bursting with energy, Beddoes widened his horizons and
started to publish. His scientific contacts grew; warm friendships
burgeoned with Erasmus Darwin, James Watt and other Lunar
Society members. And in a bold move, in 1787 he took a summer jaunt
to France, which led to his embracing the new French chemistry.

Breasting 30, he was at the peak of his potential. The young
scientist naturally welcomed the French Revolution with open arms.
Down with tyranny, oppression, priestcraft! A new age was at hand
– of liberty, the rights of man, and government by the people.

Beddoes became a political activist: his letters to his old college
friend Davies Giddy reveal him sporting a tricolour, singing revolutionary songs and cheering universal liberty. The sunny libertarian
skies soon turned stormy, however. With an anti-revolutionary
groundswell growing in his Alma Mater, his radicalism attracted
enemies. The Birmingham Riots of July 1791, in which loyalist
Church and King mobs torched the library and laboratory of Joseph
Priestley, shocked him, for Beddoes surely identified himself as Priestley junior. The Home Office was having him watched.

Jumping before he was pushed, Beddoes quit Oxford in 1793,
migrating to the Bristol suburb of Clifton, where he set up in medical
practice and, shortly afterwards, married Anna, the daughter of
his Lunar Society friend Richard Lovell Edgeworth. Bristol was a
congenial hotbed of intellectual radicalism, and the years from 1794
to 1797 brought ardent involvement in political campaigning, journalism and pamphleteering, above all, with the young Robert Southey
and with Coleridge.

These were at first heady and then also terrible times. Beddoes
grew uneasy about the Revolution itself. Unlike Coleridge and

Southey, his radicalism remained but it inevitably turned defensive, defending supporters of the rights of man even as he deplored the politics of the guillotine. He denounced government policy at home, especially its suspension of Habeas Corpus in 1793 and the 'Gagging Acts' of 1795 that restricted freedom of speech and assembly and, through a flurry of anti-Pitt pamphlets, he won his spurs as a polemicist.

For a few years, Beddoes spearheaded democratic resistance in a radical city. Thereafter the stuffing went out of protest, and he grew politically quieter and perhaps demoralized, though his anti-Establishment sentiments never wavered. Meanwhile he had other fish to fry, for a new age was dawning, not just in politics but in science. Exhilarating breakthroughs in gas chemistry, above all the discovery of oxygen, were sure to transform science and also produce astonishing medical advances. Works like *Considerations on the Medicinal Use of Factitious Airs* (1794) published his researches into a range of diseases.

Touting the applicability of the new gas chemistry to respiratory disorders, Beddoes predicted in 1793 that 'from chemistry, which is daily unfolding the profoundest secrets of nature', hopes could be entertained for 'a safe and efficacious remedy for one of the most frequent painful and hopeless of diseases', that is, consumption (tuberculosis) – a disease called by Erasmus Darwin a 'giant malady'. Inspired by late-Enlightenment optimism, he foresaw that 'however remote medicine may at present be from such perfection', there was no reason to doubt that 'the same power will be acquired over living, as is at present exercised over some inanimate bodies'. Chemistry thus portended a medical millennium. 'In a future letter', he informed his Lunar Society friend Erasmus Darwin,

I hope to present you with a catalogue of diseases in which I have effected a cure. . . . And if you do not, as I am almost sure you do not, think it absurd to suppose the organization of man equally susceptible of improvement from culture with that of various animals and vegetables, you will agree with me in entertaining hopes not only of a beneficial change in the practice of medicine, but in the constitution of human nature itself.

The gases upon which Beddoes pinned his medical millennium were oxygen and nitrous oxide. Oxygen was believed to be beneficial in scrofula, ulcers, dyspepsia, opium poisoning and so forth. As for nitrous oxide, its story began with Joseph Priestley, another man confident of the practical value of pneumatic chemistry. 'I cannot help flattering myself', he wrote, 'that, in time, very great medicinal use will be made of the application of these different kinds of air to the animal system.' In the mid-1790s, Priestley's friend James Watt administered gases both to himself and others in Birmingham. 'My asthma seems to have entirely left me as well as the spasm in my breast, I believe the former was cured by some small doses of H. C. [hydrocarbonate].'

Support grew. Back in 1794 Tom Wedgwood had agreed to help Beddoes to the tune of a thousand pounds. A wealthy patient, Lord Lambton, also assisted Beddoes financially, as did Erasmus Darwin. And soon after, Humphry Davy burst on the scene.

Born in Penzance in December 1778, the oldest son of a woodcarver, in 1794 young Davy was apprenticed to John Bingham Borlase, a local apothecary-surgeon. While an apprentice he began an ambitious plan of self-education that included physics and chemistry. In the winter of 1797 another of Watt's sons, Gregory, visited Cornwall seeking relief for tuberculosis and boarded with the Davy family. At about the same time Davy met and impressed Davies Giddy, Beddoes' old Oxford friend. When Beddoes sought a laboratory assistant for the Pneumatic Institution, Davy was highly recommended. On 2 October 1798 he left Penzance, and nine days later he was reporting 'new and wonderful events' to his mother:

. . . Dr Beddoes, who between you and me, is one of the most original men I ever saw – uncommonly short and fat, with little elegance of manners, and nothing characteristic externally of genius or science; extremely silent, and, in a few words, a very bad companion. Mrs Beddoes is the reverse of Dr Beddoes – extremely cheerful, gay, and witty; she is one of the most pleasing women I ever met with. We are already very great friends. She has taken me to see all the fine scenery about Clifton; for the Doctor, from his occupations and his bulk, is unable to walk much.

The nitrous oxide experiments Davy began at the Pneumatic Institution in spring 1799 were daring indeed, especially as the American experimenter Samuel Latham Mitchill had contended that this gas (then called gaseous oxyd of azote or 'septon') was the cause of most infectious diseases, perhaps even bubonic plague. The bold Bristol pair were prepared to test this theory, on themselves and others.

Davy worked incessantly for ten months and his findings were written up as *Researches, Chemical and Philosophical; Chiefly Concerning Nitrous Oxide, or Dephlogisticated Nitrous Air, and Its Respiration* (1800). His first experiments were made with impure nitrous oxide which he breathed mixed with air and oxygen, and he found the effect depressing, with a tendency towards giddiness and a slowing of the pulse. By April he had obtained the pure gas. On 16 April he inhaled three quarts, which produced 'a fullness of the heart accompanied by loss of distinct sensation and of voluntary power, a feeling analogous to that produced in the first stage of intoxication'. On the following day, he breathed four quarts from and into a silk bag with his nose closed, and in half a minute the sensations of the previous day 'were succeeded by a sensation analogous to gentle pressure on all the muscles, attended by a highly pleasurable thrilling, particularly in the chest and extremities . . . towards the last inspirations the thrilling increased, the sense of muscular power became greater, and at last an irresistible propensity to action was indulged in'. The gas left no hangover. Later, Davy reported another experiment:

By degrees as the pleasurable sensations increased, I lost all connection with external things; trains of vivid visible images rapidly passed through my mind and were connected with words in such a manner, as to produce perceptions perfectly novel. I existed in a world of newly connected and newly modified ideas. I theorised; I imagined that I made discoveries. When I was awakened from this semi-delirious trance by Dr Kinglake . . . I endeavoured to recall the ideas, they were feeble and indistinct; one collection of terms, however, presented itself: and with the most intense belief and prophetic manner, I exclaimed to Dr Kinglake, '*Nothing exists but thoughts! – the universe is composed of impressions, ideas, pleasures and pains!*'

The experiments created a great stir. On 5 June Southey told Grosvenor Bedford, an old boyhood friend: 'I am going to breathe some wonder-working gas, which excites all possible mental and muscular energy, and induces almost a delirium of pleasurable sensations without any subsequent dejection.' Next month he rhapsodized to his brother:

Oh, Tom! such a gas has Davy discovered, the gaseous oxyd. Oh, Tom! I have had some; it made me laugh and tingle in every toe and finger-tip. Davy has actually invented a new pleasure, for which language has no name. . . . Tom, I am sure the air in heaven must be this wonder-working gas of delight!

As high as heaven.

Beddoes persuaded a brave young lady to breathe the gas:

to the astonishment of everybody, [she] dashed out of the room and house, when, racing down Hope-square, she leaped over a great dog in her way, but being hotly pursued by the fleetest of her friends, the fair fugitive, or rather the temporary maniac, was at length overtaken and secured, without further damage.

Coleridge himself finally breathed the gas after his return from Germany in July 1799. On his first bagful, 'the only motion which I felt inclined to make, was that of laughing at those who were looking at me'. After the third time, when 'the mouthpiece was removed, I remained for a few seconds motionless, in great extacy'. The final try produced 'more unmingled pleasure than I had ever before experienced'. 'I felt as if composed of finely vibrating strings,' proclaimed Beddoes on one occasion.

The rest is history. In March 1801 Humphry Davy, at the invitation of Count Rumford, accepted an appointment as Professor of Chemistry at the Royal Institution in London. Seven years later Beddoes died, worn out at the age of 48, sad and despondent, 'as one who has scattered abroad the *avena fatua* [wild oats] of knowledge, from which neither branch nor blossom nor fruit has resulted'. It is sobering to ponder those two erstwhile allies, Coleridge and Beddoes, in their later days. Coleridge was in the throes of an addiction crisis which steered him into reactionary doctrines. Beddoes was experimenting with more mind-influencing drugs – self-experimentation, it has been suggested, contributed to the heart and lungs complaints which shortened his life. Neither seems to have resolved very happily the problems of private and public identities.

Meanwhile conservative satirists made merry with these visions of mankind given a new 'constitution' through gas – was radicalism not all a load of air? In a satire of 1798 on Erasmus Darwin's *The Loves of the Plants*, the *Anti-Jacobin Review* mocked fatuous views of the progress of humanity which were based on a risible natural philosophy which expected to raise man 'to a rank in which he would be, as it were, *all* MIND; would enjoy unclouded perspicacity and perpetual vitality; feed on *oxygene*, and never die, but *by his own consent*'. The *Anti-Jacobin* hardly needed to exaggerate.

The enlightened aspiration of a science of man, grounded in natural law, necessity and determinism, thus opened up novel prospects. There was the affecting picture of man the victim of social circumstances, exploited by political radicals and milked in sentimental novels. There was the image of the addictive personality, consumed by drink and drugs. There was also the Promethean medical vision of new drugs to cure old diseases – although these might turn, by a tragic twist, into diseases themselves. Whichever way, the ancient Christian humanist doctrine of free will was under threat, being exposed as mere rhetoric, wilfully ignoring all the circumstances of human life. The new determinism, by contrast, seemed to lack a logic of autonomous action, and Johnson remained to be answered: 'All theory is against the freedom of the will; all experience for it.'

23

WILLIAM GODWIN:
AWAKENING THE MIND

Intellect has a perpetual tendency to proceed.

Man is in a state of perpetual mutation.

The Greatest of all human benefits, that at least without which no other benefit can be truly enjoyed, is independence

WILLIAM GODWIN

As we saw in Chapter 20, Joseph Priestley developed a theology which incorporated the determinism of the freethinker Anthony Collins and the Christian materialism of David Hartley (thought the product of the brain). Prizing truth and candour – he had a horror of mystification and hypocrisy, identifying falsehood with the self-serving power-mongering of Anglicanism and its ivory-towered outposts – Priestley concluded that official dualism was neither Christian nor scientific.

Up to a point, William Godwin followed a parallel path. The early life and thinking of Godwin displays some similarities to Priestley's. Born in 1756 the son of a Calvinist minister, Godwin studied from 1775 at the Dissenting Academy at Hoxton on the north-east outskirts of London, a hotbed of critical thinking, and in 1778 was appointed minister to a Nonconformist congregation at Ware in Hertfordshire. His faith was soon shaken, however, first by his readings of Rousseau, d'Holbach, Helvétius and other *philosophes*, and then by the teachings of Priestley himself. Unlike that Dissenter, however, Godwin could not halt at Unitarianism – what Erasmus Darwin jeeringly called a 'feather bed to catch a falling Christian'; in 1783 he quit the ministry and soon lapsed into complete religious scepticism. Moving to London at the age of 27, Godwin found his *métier* among Grub Street journalists and metropolitan intellectual circles, beginning what would prove to be half a century of literary activity. Fame came when the French Revolution politicized him.

Appearing in 1793, *An Enquiry concerning Political Justice* won its author instant celebrity for its clarion statement of radical individualism. For some years Godwin shone as one of London's most celebrated men of letters, and his personal life doubled his notoriety, thanks to his liaison with Mary Wollstonecraft. Both held enlightened views on marriage – *Political Justice* deemed matrimony a stifling monopoly, while her word for it was 'legal prostitution'. 'It is my wish that Mr Godwin shall visit and dine out as formerly,' she wrote, early in their relationship, 'and I shall do the same; in short, I still mean to be independent.' The liberated couple, embodiments of 'modern philosophy', maintained separate homes and met for meals. They did, however, finally bow to convention when Mary became pregnant and they were married in March 1797. A child, Mary Godwin, was born on 30 August 1797. Ten days later Mary was dead.

Godwin never recovered from that private disaster or from the public collapse of revolutionary fervour, but he went on doggedly writing. *Caleb Williams* turned the themes of *Political Justice* into fiction; *The Enquirer* (1797) restated the political points of his earlier work; and he took to writing more novels, plays, children's books and dictionaries.

Crucial to Godwin's vision of man was his loss of Christian faith. Like Gibbon, he found he could not stomach the biblical God: 'Books have been handed down from generation to generation, as the true teachers of piety and the love of God, that represent him as so merciless and tyrannical a despot, that, if they were considered otherwise than through the medium of prejudice, they could inspire nothing but hatred.' Holding up for worship, as it did, a Lord of vengeance, nothing perhaps had contributed more to the growth of bigotry in the world than the doctrines of the Christian religion: 'It caused the spirit of intolerance to strike a deep root.' Committed, like Priestley, to candour, Godwin was proud to stand up and be counted: 'I am an unbeliever. I am thoroughly satisfied that no book in existence contains a record and history of the revelation of the will of an invisible being, the master of us all, to his creatures.'

Influenced in this respect probably by Hartley, Godwin suggested that the 'truths' of religion were best understood as products of the slipperiness of speech. 'Heaven', he pronounced, 'in reality is not so properly a place as a state of the mind' – which may explain a reported exchange at his wife's deathbed: 'Oh Godwin, I am in heaven,' exclaimed Mary, a pious Anglican; 'You mean, my dear,' replied the philosopher, 'that your physical sensations are somewhat easier.'

Political Justice imagines a world without God, where man shall have no 'master'. The old Christian tyranny and terror, as mediated through Throne and Altar, have disappeared; and men grow godlike, that is to say, autonomous rational beings, beholden to none. The book may thus be read as a foundational text of anarchism, declaring as it does the illegitimacy and 'euthanasia' of monarchy, aristocracy, armies, police, indeed the whole state apparatus and all its subaltern institutions. The existing distribution of wealth is also counter-utilitarian: capitalism is a system designed not for the creation of prosperity but for the manufacture of surplus (but unjustly distributed) wealth, hence of unnecessary labour, and thus of extremes of pro-fusion and poverty. These are, as will be obvious, anti-Mandevillian views, and much of Godwin may be read as a critical commentary upon that cynic.

Deeming government 'in all cases, an evil', and calling for the dissolution – though not by violence – of the existing juridical, political and social edifice, Godwin pinned future hopes entirely on the individual. His preferred society, such as it was, would comprise loose voluntary clusters of individuals, essentially self-sufficient, coming together only occasionally for mutual support – a devolved and decentralized utopia. 'Man is a species of being whose excellence depends on his individuality; and who can be neither great nor wise, but in proportion as he is independent.' Central to Godwin's vision for human regeneration was self-sufficiency: 'individuals are every-thing, and society . . . nothing.' The sovereignty of individual judge-ment – thinking for oneself – was a *sine qua non* for the advance of knowledge, and that in turn was the dynamo of improvement at large: 'The extent of our progress in the cultivation of knowledge is unlimited.' This was Locke taken to the limits.

Everyone must optimize his talents as a rational individual and avoid kowtowing to conventional beliefs and practices, as tradition-ally dictated by Church and State, and by the straitjacket of public opinion. Individual questing was paramount, permanent self-criticism crucial: 'The wise man is satisfied with nothing. . . . The wise man is not satisfied with his own attainments, or even with his principles and opinions. He is continually detecting errors in them; he suspects more; there is no end to his revisals and enquiries.' Like Socrates, Godwin rejected the unexamined life.

Discussion between equals expedited enquiry, but truth must never be imposed – force was no argument and was always wrong. Indi-viduals might legitimately seek to persuade each other, but even collaboration as generally understood was misguided, since it compromised originality: 'Everything that is usually understood by the term co-operation', he declared, astonishingly, 'is in some degree an evil.' For that reason, Godwin not only opposed the yoke of marriage, but cohabitation too, this being

also hostile to that fortitude which should accustom a man, in his actions, as well as his opinions, to judge for himself. . . . Add to this, that it is absurd to expect the inclinations and wishes of two human beings to coincide, through any long period of time. To oblige them to act and to live together is to subject them to some inevitable portion of thwarting, bickering and unhappiness.

Other forms of collective action were also questionable: 'shall we have concerts of music? . . . Will it not be practicable hereafter for one man to perform the whole?' Similarly, stage plays were inimical to 'individuality', for 'all formal repetition of other men's ideas seems to be a scheme for imprisoning, for so long a time, the operations of our own mind'. All in all, 'we ought to be able to do without one another,' judged Godwin, in a declaration as courageous as it was chilling.

Like Bunyan's pilgrim but without God, individuals must wend their way through the world alone, self-aware and self-reliant, except for candid and critical friends. The only extraneous prop would be lawful possessions, for Godwin had no doubts that private judgement and mental development presupposed private property, 'the palladium of all that ought to be dear to us'. In short: 'Property is sacred' – 'sacred' in this unbeliever's value-system pertaining to the sanctity of the individual.

Godwin's predilections, both personal and political – the personal *was* the political – reflected his revolt against Calvinism (total dependency upon God) and incorporated his fervent hatred of the *status quo*. Moreover, they also had weighty philosophical underpinnings. Analysing the human animal naturalistically and dispassionately rather than through religious or moral rhetorics, the prime device he deployed was Hartley's doctrine of necessity. It made a splash: 'throw aside your books of chemistry,' declared Wordsworth, initially enthusiastic, 'and read Godwin on necessity.'

Building on Hartley, Godwin developed the 'material system', which he touted as the key to the 'mechanism of the human mind'. Just as, in the natural world, Newton's laws are supreme – they are what make nature intelligible – so, in the human world, necessity (cause and effect) is equally the basis of any understanding of what makes human beings tick – and hence comprehensible. Moreover, only in a necessarian order is it possible to change what moves people, by correcting their motivation. Human behaviour is determined – people act as they do out of necessity. But that is precisely the reason why it should be possible, through education and persuasion, to change their incentives, and hence reform them.

Like Hartley's, Godwin's optimistic necessarianism drew on Locke's *tabula rasa* model of the mind: 'Children are a sort of raw material put into our hands, a ductile and yielding substance.' The understanding is wholly conditioned by sense inputs, man is entirely a creature of his environment, and individual differences arise from educational and external influences. Denying innate ideas and instincts, Godwin went as far as to doubt whether man can truly be said to have a mind as such; he used the word only provisionally as a shorthand to signify the lattices of thought which produce the complex of personal identity. It was in these natural facts – which created controversy because they seemed so blatantly to threaten free will and accountability – that Godwin found the intelligibility of human agency and the hope of improving it through education. 'The Characters of Men Originate in their External Circumstances', boldly declared the title of Book I, chapter iv of *Political Justice*, the next chapter being headed 'The Voluntary Actions of Men Originate in their Opinions'. At first sight this may seem the yoking of opposites, but it was central to Godwin's thinking and for him quite consistent, because 'the great stream of our voluntary actions essentially depends, not upon the direct and immediate impulses of sense, but upon the decisions of the understanding'.

Man could be led by reason to live in ways conducive to the greater happiness – as a convinced utilitarian, Godwin insisted that pain was in all circumstances an evil. The maximization of happiness was to be achieved through man's *duty* of exercising his reason. Reason should discern optimum personal and social arrangements and point to the correct – that is, the just – course of action. Of prime importance was the cultivation of the responsible individual mind – 'Of Awakening the Mind' is, significantly, the title of the leading essay in *The Enquirer*.

Rational action must triumph over the passions and the despotism of convention. It is in this light that, in *Caleb Williams*, Godwin contrasts his hero Caleb with the highborn Falkland who, while in his own fashion a decent man, is entirely the slave of inherited class prejudices. Countering *aristocratic* codes of honour, Godwin insists upon a basic, elemental *human* equality: 'superior' and 'inferior' are not laid down at birth – all privilege is detestable – but hinge on exercise of judgement: some people behave more rationally than others.

And rationally is the way one is duty-bound to behave. In what became a notorious thought-experiment, Godwin maintained that, in a blaze in which it is possible to save from the flames either the philosopher Fénélon or his valet, it is indubitably right to rescue the philosopher, because it is he who will further the happiness of the race. Only when the rational supersedes the emotional or sentimental will truth, justice and happiness prevail.

Progress consists in the gradual and invincible triumph of reason, held this latter-day Platonist who, although a principled materialist, was nevertheless confident that happiness would best be secured by the withering away of the inferior, or imagined, pleasures of the flesh – in favour not, of course, of those of the fictitious transcendental soul, but rather of the understanding.

Due recognition of the sovereignty of Mind is the key to man's destiny. Like Hartley and Erasmus Darwin, but with a different thrust, Godwin held that even such actions as walking, which might seem automatic and innate, are at bottom *voluntary*:

An attentive observer will perceive various symptoms calculated to persuade him that every step he takes, during the longest journey, is the production of thought. Walking is, in all cases, originally a voluntary motion. In a child, when he learns to walk, in a rope-dancer, when he begins to practise that particular exercise, the distinct determination of mind, preceding each step, is sufficiently perceptible.

In time, of course, certain acts (like walking) become mechanical habits or second nature, but that is not the point, for 'a species of motion which began in express design may, though it ceases to be the subject of conscious attention, owe its continuance to a continued series of thoughts flowing in that direction'. The proof? We get lost in thoughts: walking and talking, 'we actually find that, when our thoughts in a train are more than commonly earnest, our pace slackens, and sometimes our going forward is wholly suspended, particularly in any less common species of walking, such as that of descending a flight of stairs'. In citing absent-mindedness as testimony of the superiority of the mind Godwin was arguing along similar lines (although within a secular frame) to those defenders of the Christian soul – for example, Samuel Clarke – who had held that reverie and daydreaming attest the separate soul. What was at stake was not, of course, some separate soul but the possibility that mind could assert ever greater control over matter.

Godwin drove this line of speculation further, pondering whether thought plays a role in regulating blood circulation and heartbeat. 'When thought begins, these motions also begin,' he ventured, 'and, when it ceases, they are at an end.' Overall, 'there are probably no motions of the animal economy which we do not find it in the power of volition, and still more of our involuntary sensations, to hasten or retard', leading to the possibility: no thought, no motion. Mind is constantly and necessarily impinging upon operations that are apparently instinctual, physical and mechanical.

Following Hartley, and paralleling his older contemporary Erasmus Darwin, Godwin thus held that though initially conscious acts of will and attention (like learning to play the piano) turn into habits, they remain acts of mind. Darwin for his part studied habit for reasons of his own: by helping to bridge the apparent gap between man and beast (both were creatures of habit), habit lent support to his evolutionary theory (continuity). Godwin had very different fish to fry. He was interested in confirming the realm of reason, that is, the maintenance of perfect mental control over the flesh, including over what we would call 'autonomic' functions like breathing and digestion. He could rest content with nothing which imperilled mental autonomy.

The more reason extended its ascendancy over the flesh, the more it would be possible to prevent or overcome disease: through the adoption of rational diet, moderation, temperance and exercise, the body machine would be kept in perfect shape. Superficially, Godwin's teachings did not differ greatly from the commonsense medical regimens advocated by popular health champions from Cornaro to Cheyne. But there was one key difference. For Godwin, rational living held out some semblance of this-worldly immortality: reason could conquer death. Whereas Christians looked forward to the ultimate resurrection of the body, the Promethean in Godwin expected that reason could pre-empt decay of the flesh in the first place: 'In a word, *why* may not man be one day immortal?'

Giving Swift's Struldbrugs a wholly optimistic spin – he took much from Swift, if turning him upside down – Godwin positively looked forward to a future geriatric paradise. Such would be an extremely eligible state of affairs, because maturity brought wisdom, independence and hence happiness.

In pursuing such thoughts, Godwin drew upon the conjecture of the 'celebrated' Benjamin Franklin, that 'mind would one day become omnipotent over matter'. Finding this idea beguiling, he elaborated upon it. Experience proved the psychosomatic: 'Listlessness of thought is the brother of death. But cheerfulness gives new elasticity to our limbs, and circulation to our juices.' Our bodies work well when reason is captain, but 'when reason resigns the helm, and our ideas fluctuate without order or direction, we sleep. Delirium and insanity are of the same nature. Fainting appears principally to consist in a relaxation of intellect.' In short, he concluded, 'disease seems perhaps in all instances to be the concomitant of confusion'.

Godwin adduced further psychosomatic evidence. Did not unhappiness produce a 'broken heart' and trigger organic disease, while good news set physical complaints to rights? The energetic and busy had the power to resist setbacks sufficient to reduce the idle to illness. 'I walk twenty miles, full of ardour, and with a motive that engrosses my soul,' he declared:

and I arrive as fresh and alert as when I began my journey. Emotion, excited by some unexpected word, by a letter that is delivered to us, occasions the most extraordinary revolutions in our frame. . . . There is nothing of which the physician is more frequently aware, than of the power of the mind in assisting or retarding convalescence.

Having shown that 'our involuntary motions' are 'gradually to become subject to the power of volition', what were the limits? 'Is it not then highly probable, in the process of human improvement, that we may finally obtain an empire over every articulation of our frame?' These were astonishing speculations indeed. The progressive power of human reason would overcome the doom of death. But first, Godwin noted, sleep, death's image, must be banished, for 'sleep is one of the most conspicuous infirmities of the human frame'.

If sceptics and reactionaries baulked at these vainglorious thoughts, and declared such rational control 'beyond the limits of the human mind', Godwin countered that it was 'our vanity' which prompted us 'to suppose that we have reached the goal of human capacity' – they it was, not he, who were being presumptuous.

In short, Godwin the visionary predicted that 'the term of human life may be prolonged, and that by the immediate operation of intellect, beyond any limits which we are able to assign'. If, admittedly, 'it would be idle to talk of the absolute immortality of man', that was only because 'eternity and immortality are phrases to which it is impossible for us to annex any distinct ideas'.

But would not such prolongevism bring catastrophic overpopulation? No, because once reason triumphed over the flesh, people would cease to reproduce, since their sexual cravings would dissolve away. Libido – *pace* Mandeville – was no biological constant but all in the mind, and so capable of control. Anyway, what pleasure there was in the sexual act hardly derived from physical drives – it was largely a product of fantasies attending our current, unreconstructed condition. Even nowadays, 'strip the commerce of the sexes of all its attendant circumstances' and desire would droop. 'Tell a man that all women, so far as sense is concerned, are nearly alike,' suggested Godwin in a thought-experiment,

Bid him therefore take a partner without any attention to the symmetry of her person, her vivacity, the voluptuous softness of her temper, the affectionate kindness of her feelings, her imagination or her wit. You would probably instantly convince him that the commerce itself, which by superficial observers is put for the whole, is the least important branch of the complicated consideration to which it belongs.

Copulation *per se* was hardly worth the candle – its pleasures largely came from fantasies and these in truth were pretty small beer. Everyone knew how arousal was prey to suggestion:

Let us suppose a man to be engaged in the progressive voluptuousness of the most sensual scene. . . . he resigns himself, without power of resistance, to his predominant idea. Alas, in this situation, nothing is so easy as to extinguish his sensuality! Tell him at this moment that his father is dead, that he has lost or gained a considerable sum of money, or even that his favourite horse is stolen from the meadow, and his whole passion shall be instantly annihilated.

Perfect proof, concluded Godwin, of the 'precariousness of the fascination of the senses'! And if stray thoughts induced impotence in this manner, all the more should *noble ideals* subdue, and, he hoped supersede, the lusts of the flesh. Reason should thus mastermind the future: 'if the power of intellect can be established over all other matter, are we not inevitably led to ask, why not over the matter of our own bodies?'

Godwin's Prometheanism was mocked as visionary, and this victim of his own fantasies became a prime butt of satire: 'Come kick me – is his eternal language,' guffawed Southey. In 'The Loves of the Triangles' – chiefly a skit on Erasmus Darwin's *The Loves of the Plants* – the *Anti-Jacobin Review* parodied Godwinian perfectibilism, especially the notion that reason could assume command of creation. 'We contend', its Godwin puppet insisted, that man could be raised 'to a rank more worthy of his endowments and aspirations; to a rank in which he would be, as it were, *all* MIND . . . and never die, but *by his own consent*'.

It is no accident that Godwin fell into conflict with Thomas Robert Malthus, the population theorist. Malthus's father, Daniel, a personal friend of Rousseau, had been a torchbearer of the Enlightenment and had his son educated by the most advanced teachers. Schooled in Locke and Hartley, the young Malthus had been groomed to become a philosophical radical – before he exploded into what must be called his Oedipal revolt.

The champagne fizz of revolution had naturally created noble expectations of improvement, but were they rationally justified? asked Malthus in his *Essay on the Principle of Population* (1798). Was mankind truly about to realize such Promethean dreams? Malthus concluded that the radical programme of boundless progress was intrinsically self-defeating – knowledge would produce economic growth, this would increase wealth, wealth would then fire a population explosion. He had thus, he believed, exposed the visionaries' Achilles heel. The implications of such an increase had never been evaluated by such prophets of progress as Godwin and Condorcet in France. Fantasy had outrun thought: 'I have certainly no right to say that they purposely shut their eyes,' Malthus commented ironically, yet 'we are all of us too prone to err'.

Countering the day-dreamers, Malthus posed as the sober realist, scorning rhetoric and 'mere conjectures' in favour of facts. Radical plans were ravishing – Godwin's philosophy was 'by far the most beautiful and engaging of any that has yet appeared' – but utopian bubbles were pricked by hard facts. Zealots ascribed all evils to the *ancien régime*; abolish the old order and, hey presto, everything was possible. But 'the great error under which Mr. Godwin labours throughout his whole work, is, the attributing almost all the vices and misery that are seen in civil society to human institutions'. The real stumbling block was not the vices of the politicians but the nature of things.

How then did nature balance production and reproduction? 'I think', Malthus proposed, 'I may fairly make two postulata', namely that 'food is necessary to the existence of man', and that 'the passion between the sexes is necessary, and will remain nearly in its present state' ('These two laws . . . appear to have been fixed laws of our nature'). Population would thus inevitably tend to outrun resources and precipitate crisis: famine, epidemics and war. That was the great problem the radicals had never squarely faced – they had merely come up with frivolities, notably Godwin's silly suggestions 'that the passion between the sexes may in time be extinguished'. Nature herself, in other words, foiled dreams of social equality.

Godwin, as just shown, boldly held that such 'progress' would not, in actuality, be harmful, because of the future waning of sexual urges. Malthus, demographer, scientist, statistician, political economist and

Church of England divine, plumped for what to high-minded radicals like Godwin and William Hazlitt was the grossest of sexual materialisms, in which human propensities were unreformable, by inference because of Original Sin: man could not be trusted to curb his urges.

The godless Godwin countered Malthus by advancing a much more elevated view of mankind, one aspiring to transcend base urges in pursuit of the life of the mind. 'One tendency of a cultivated and virtuous mind is to diminish our eagerness for the gratification of the senses,' he declared:

They please at present by their novelty, that is, because we know not how to estimate them. . . . The gratifications of sense please at present by their imposture. We soon learn to despise the mere animal function, which, apart from the delusions of intellect, would be nearly the same in all cases; and to value it only as it happens to be relieved by personal charms of mental excellence.

The men therefore whom we are supposing to exist, when the earth shall refuse itself to a more extended population, will probably cease to propagate. The whole will be a people of men, and not of children. Generation will not succeed generation, nor truth have, in a certain degree, to recommence her career every thirty years.

Nor was that all, predicted Godwin, warming to his vision of heaven on earth:

There will be no war, no crimes, no administration of justice, as it is called, and no government. Beside this, there will be neither disease, anguish, melancholy, nor resentment. Every man will seek, with ineffable ardour, the good of all. Mind will be active and eager, yet never disappointed.

*

The Godwin–Malthus conflict highlights with great clarity the perhaps surprising alliance which has surfaced at various points in this book between Christian doctrine and a materialist view of human nature that accentuated the body. Contrariwise, it reveals the commitment of the liberal and progressive intelligentsia to a new view of mankind, elevated above the gross and fallen Christian flesh in pursuit of a millennium in which what counted was the march of mind, sanctity of intellect, freedom of the spirit, commitment to enquiry and the adventure of the life critically examined.

It was for its vulgar materialism that Godwin despised Christianity. 'Man is not a vegetable to be governed by sensations of heat and cold, dryness and moisture,' he expostulated. 'He is a reasonable creature, capable of perceiving what is eligible and right, of fixing indelibly certain principles upon his mind, and adhering inflexibly to the resolutions he has made.' By the nineteenth-century clerisy – by poets, bohemians and intellectuals emerging from the Romantic tradition – Christianity itself, yoked to material civilization, came to be questioned as gross and vulgar. A new, secular, imaginative, rational spirituality was emerging, based on the life of the mind and the holiness of the imagination. Godwin passionately championed the intellect and the intellectual: 'Intellect has a perpetual tendency to proceed. It cannot be held back, but by a power that counteracts its genuine tendency, through every moment of its existence.'

24

WILLIAM BLAKE: THE BODY MYSTICAL

Spirits are Lawful, but not Ghosts; especially Royal Gin is Lawful Spirit.

Vision or Imagination is a Representation of what Eternally Exists Really and Unchangeably

WILLIAM BLAKE

To say that idiosyncrasy was conventional in eighteenth-century England may seem paradoxical, but it was a nation rightly remarkable for what Edmund Burke snarlingly styled the 'dissidence of dissent'. Dissenters from the established Church in turn dissented from their chosen Nonconformist confessions, until dissenting ('I did it my way') became, in the eyes of conservative critics, an obligation, obsession or almost the *summum bonum*. Such elements, as we have just seen, permeate the philosophy of William Godwin, who pressed individualism to the point where 'co-operation' was regarded as an evil.

As exemplified by Johnson, Reynolds and Burke, the Christian humanist tradition warned against the presumption of singularity, stressing the 'uniformity of human nature' and the soundness of old truths. Conformity and submission were urged in view of human weakness and even depravity. But such figures were fighting a losing battle in an increasingly literate society marked by religious toleration, educational diversity and a lack of censorship. The old values of self-denial and self-repression were increasingly overwhelmed by calls for self-expression.

No one ploughed his own furrow more enthusiastically than Godwin's contemporary, William Blake ('The cut worm forgives the plough'). He would be a slave to no man – 'I must Create a System,' he declared, 'or be enslav'd by another Mans.' Growing up in London's rich radical artisan culture and apprenticed as an engraver, Blake became exposed to a multitude of marginal and subterranean religious, social, moral, political and mystical traditions, some derived from the antinomianism of the Commonwealth interlude and others from Continental religious groups, including the Moravians (Lutheran pietists). For a while Blake was a supporter of the Swedish visionary Swedenborg, before shifting allegiance to the seventeenth century mystic Jakob Boehme. In his ideas, which mainly found expression in verse, and in his line-engravings and water-colours, Blake was a law unto himself, his output a testament to a unique and supercharged imagination.

Blake plunged into debates about the nature of body and soul under God. He was inveterately hostile to the scepticism of the enlightened, preferring a religion of faith:

> Mock on, Mock on Voltaire, Rousseau:
> Mock on, Mock on: 'tis all in vain!

'Voltaire was immersed in matter,' scolds a character in Blake's early unfinished satire 'An Island in the Moon', '& seems to have understood very little but what he saw before his eyes.' And Blake himself derided the reductionist mechanistic materialism he associated with that tradition which, as we have seen, inspired Hartley and Priestley, Erasmus Darwin and Godwin, all striving for a natural scientific understanding of mankind. They understood nothing:

> The Atoms of Democritus
> And Newton's Particles of light
> Are sands upon the Red sea shore,
> Where Israel's tents do shine so bright.

It was unusual, at this time, for Newton to be thus consigned to the party of the infidel, for mainstream natural theology had confidently fused divine Creation and natural science. But for Blake, natural theology itself was blasphemy, indeed an oxymoron. He demonized the black trinity of Francis Bacon, John Locke and Isaac Newton, whose thinking jointly reduced 'that which is Soul & Life into a Mill or Machine':

> I turn my eyes to the Schools & Universities of Europe
> And there behold the Loom of Locke, whose Woof rages dire,
> Wash'd by the Water-wheels of Newton: black the cloth
> In heavy wreathes folds over every Nation: cruel Works
> Of many Wheels I view, wheel without wheel, with cogs tyrannic
> Moving by compulsion each other, not as those in Eden, which,
> Wheel within Wheel, in freedom revolve in harmony & peace.

Here as elsewhere, mechanistic thinking and mechanical models of the mind are (with good reason, as we saw in Chapter 21) linked by Blake to the technology of the Industrial Revolution and its new oppressions.

Touting a philosophy which read Nature as mechanistic and the mind as passive, the deadly trio had enthroned in place of the soul (accused Blake) the five material senses regarded as mere windows through which Nature impressed itself upon the sensorium, rather as in Locke's *tabula rasa*, in which the mind, blank at birth, is then inscribed by the outer world.

It certainly had not been the aim of Locke's empirical 'way of ideas' to preach the passivity of mind, but Locke had indeed denied the reality of innate and distinctive genius. All people were born much of a muchness, innate genius no more existed than innate ideas, and differentials in mind and character were products of experience: 'of all the men we meet with,' maintained Locke's *Some Thoughts Concerning Education*, 'nine parts of ten are what they are, good or evil, useful or not, by their education. It is that which makes the great difference in mankind.' Such ideas proved influential. 'Dr. Johnson denied that any child was better than another, but by difference of instruction,' recorded Boswell. Priestley for his part denied that there was anything special about Newton's mind; Adam Smith concurred: 'The difference of natural talents in different men is, in reality, much less than we are aware of'; and so did Godwin:

'Genius . . . is not born with us, but generated subsequent to birth.'

Such Lockean views reinforced classical teachings about artistic and literary production. For pundits like Pope, artistry was neither a gift nor supernaturally inspired but at bottom a matter of craftsmanship:

> True wit is nature to advantage dressed;
> What oft was thought, but ne'er so well expressed.

Sir Joshua Reynolds judged likewise: his aesthetics had no truck with divine illumination or spontaneous creativity. He found not merely pretentious but 'pernicious' all talk of 'waiting the call and inspiration of Genius'. Neither a 'divine gift' nor a 'mechanical trade', painting was a skill, demanding training, knowledge and practice. Imagination was of course prized – Addison celebrated the 'pleasures of the imagination', a phrase incorporated into Mark Akenside's poem of that title. But it had to be tempered with learning, wit and judgement, so as to nip in the bud what Johnson called that 'dangerous prevalence of imagination', which could lead to madness.

All this was challenged by new thinking that emerged in the generation before Blake, which refigured genius into a celebration of uniqueness and thought in terms not of composition but of creation. Mechanistic models of mental operations, notably the association of ideas, became supplanted by organic images of creative processes modelled on vegetative growth. In his *Conjectures on Original Composition* (1759), the Anglican clergyman-poet Edward Young saluted originality and creativity – Nature 'brings us into the world all *Originals:* No two faces, no two minds, are just alike'. 'The common judgment of humanity' and all the other old critical nostrums were now denounced as insipidly jejune: rather like youth, individuality deserved its head. Instead of the consensus the Augustans courted, singularity was to be valued: 'Born *Originals*, how comes it to pass that we die *Copies?*', bemoaned Young: 'That medling Ape *Imitation* . . . destroys all mental Individuality.' The greatest geniuses were those who went to Nature's school, and knew no other teacher, and the artist's first rule must be to have none: 'Thyself so reverence as to prefer the native growth of thy own mind to the richest import from abroad.' As we shall see, Blake would have found these defences pusillanimous: he set out to effect a complete rehabilitation of genius.

In 'An Island in the Moon', Blake mocks the reductionist tendencies of modern science, toying with the name of Locke (who became 'John Lookye Gent.', author of 'An Easy of Huming Understanding') and satirizing the folly and pretensions of chemists in a send-up targeted primarily against Priestley. Renamed 'Inflammable Gass', the materialist chemist it is who challenges the other prating philosophers with the cry 'Your reason – Your reason?', which Blake later converted into the accursed God Urizen.

Blake thus updated Jonathan Swift's view that in reducing nature to a passive concourse of atoms – the billiard-ball universe – scientists reduce themselves to myopic obsessives capable of figuring the universe only through their own microscopic projections. How could mechanical reason measure the infinite? To seek to know the reason of everything (the sin of Priestley or Urizen) was heresy: belief was what counted. The universe was a mystery to be celebrated by the artist, not a puzzle to be solved by the scientist.

Blake certainly regarded himself as first and foremost a Christian: all he knew 'was in the Bible', he told Henry Crabbe Robinson. He was, however, no common Christian defending orthodoxies (against such radicals as Priestley). Christianity, as taught by the Church that was established by law and upheld by pluralist placemen – Bishop Richard Watson was the one who came in for a particular drubbing* – was, in his view, a travesty of truth. 'It is an easy matter for a Bishop to triumph over Paine's attack, but it is not so easy for one who loves the Bible,' he comments in his marginal annotations to Watson's *An Apology for The Bible in a Series of Letters addressed to Thomas Paine*, insisting that 'it appears to me Now that Tom Paine is a better Christian than the Bishop'. That was a Blakean paradox, because the radical and perhaps revolutionary Paine, though born a Quaker, had explicitly

---

* Watson is an interesting figure. He was perhaps the most liberal of the bench of bishops in the 1790s, one of the very few who felt at all sympathetic to the French Revolution. But he was also a notorious placeman and pluralist, and his writings would readily communicate to Blake the complacency of rationalist divines.

repudiated Christianity. Brimming with indignation against the Old Testament's cruel and arbitrary God, his *The Age of Reason* (1794–6) ridiculed the 'riddles' and attacked the obscenities of the Scriptures, and praised natural religion: 'Every religion is good that teaches man to be good.' 'I do not believe', ran Paine's anti-creed, 'in the creed professed by the Jewish Church, by the Roman Church, by the Greek Church, by the Turkish Church, by the Protestant Church, nor by any church that I know of. My own mind is my own church.' As soon as the destruction of priestcraft put an end to mystery-mongering, 'the present age will hereafter merit to be called the Age of Reason'. Blake had no investment whatever in 'natural religion' or an age of reason, however, and his remark was clearly intended to say more about Watson than about Paine. 'To defend the Bible in this year 1798', he further declared, 'would cost a man his life': clearly Church of Englandism had nothing to do with the Bible which was the source of all the artist-visionary knew.

What Blake did share with Paine was the conviction that Christianity as established by law was a punitive and puritanical regime – the law oppressing true spirit. (Here, had he been less incensed, he might have seen he had common ground with Priestley.) Blake hated the preachings of Churches which spied only evil in the flesh, were obsessed with discipline, and made 'thou shalt not' their credo. Their persecuting bent created, authorized and policed a world of misery:

> I wander thro' each charter'd street,
> Near where the charter'd Thames does flow,
> And mark in every face I meet
> Marks of weakness, marks of woe.
>
> In every cry of every Man,
> In every Infant's cry of fear,
> In every voice, in every ban,
> The mind-forg'd manacles I hear.

The role of the Churches in upholding a sanctimonious, pharisaical puritanism which makes misery the will of a God of wrath – elsewhere termed by Blake 'Nobodaddy', the ultimate name of the father – is underlined in 'The Garden of Love' from the *Songs of Experience* (1794):

> I went to the Garden of Love,
> And I saw what I never had seen:
> A Chapel was built in the midst,
> Where I used to play on the green.
>
> And the gates of this Chapel were shut,
> And 'Thou shalt not' writ over the door;
> So I turn'd to the Garden of Love
> That so many sweet flowers bore;
>
> And I saw it was filled with graves,
> And tomb-stones where flowers should be;
> And Priests in black gowns were walking their rounds,
> And binding with briars my joys & desires.

Orthodoxy is thus exposed as systematic moral perversion, divorced from the true gospel ('God is love'). Such sick religion causes the very abominations it deplores and censures: 'Prisons are built with stones of Law, Brothels with bricks of Religion', he delivered as one of his 'Proverbs of Hell'. Blake as ever assails the Old Testament repressive regime of the 'Law', which creates the evils it pretends to combat. Warped value-systems which father misery, perversion and cruelty on God (making them thus ineluctable) rather than upon holier-than-thou pillars of orthodoxy have to be exposed for what they are, as in his ironically titled 'A Divine Image'.

> Cruelty has a Human Heart,
> And Jealousy a Human Face;
> Terror the Human Form Divine,
> And Secrecy the Human Dress.

The true gospel as preached by Christ prizes the innocent spiritual playfulness of the child. Such energies are expressions of the divine made flesh, themes prominent in his *Songs of Innocence* (1789).

Blake the philosopher abhorred the tendency of orthodox

Christian theology, as distorted by Cartesianism, to figure body and soul, flesh and spirit, as polar opposites within a bad–good hierarchy. Masquerading in *The Marriage of Heaven and Hell*, a print series engraved between 1789 and 1793, as 'the voice of the Devil', he declares what was evidently his own view:

All Bibles or sacred codes have been the causes of the following Errors:

1. That Man has two real existing principles: Viz: a Body & a Soul.

2. That Energy, call'd Evil, is alone from the Body; & that Reason, call'd Good, is alone from the Soul.

3. That God will torment Man in Eternity for following his Energies.

To Blake's mind such conventional pieties are, properly speaking, not divine truths but travesties of the faith. *The Marriage of Heaven and Hell* advances counter-commandments, in the guise of a Devil's charter: the truly divine lies in creative energy, however transgressive of respectable morality. In his provocative transvaluing way, Blake asserts, ventriloquizing through the Devil, that 'the following Contraries' are true:

1. Man has no Body distinct from his Soul; for that call'd Body is a portion of Soul discern'd by the five Senses, the chief inlets of Soul in this age.

2. Energy is the only life, and is from the Body; and Reason is the bound or outward circumference of Energy.

3. Energy is Eternal Delight.

And he asserts in the same work that 'Without Contraries is no progression. Attraction and Repulsion, Reason and Energy, Love and Hate, are necessary to Human existence.' Contraries are opposites in a dynamic, creative tension.

'Tyger' exemplifies the philosophy of holy energy:

> Tyger! Tyger! burning bright
> In the forests of the night,
> What immortal hand or eye
> Could frame thy fearful symmetry?

The beauty of ferocity transcends the prosaic mundane law of peace. 'One Law for the Lion & Ox is Oppression', declared Blake, among further 'Proverbs of Hell':

The tygers of wrath are wiser than the horses of instruction.

Expect poison from the standing water . . .

When thou seest an Eagle, thou seest a portion of Genius; lift up thy head! . . .

Damn braces: Bless relaxes.

Here may be seen the mind of one who had assimilated various mystical writers but above all perhaps also the antinomian tradition, for whom the spirit had superseded the law and so to the pure all things were pure. Blake set out the antinomian concept of Jesus as the supplanter of the Ten Commandments and the law. 'Jesus was all virtue, and acted from impulse, not from rules.'

Blake's denial of the depravity of the flesh and his celebration of 'Energy [which] is the only life, and is from the Body' distance him dramatically from the mainstream eighteenth-century desire to refine and discipline the body in the name of higher values (reason, politeness, progress). In endorsing physical desire and pleasure Blake may bear the most superficial resemblance to libertines for whom nothing was real but the (albeit transitory) joys of the flesh, and to utilitarians like Bentham for whom pleasure (whatever its source) was the sole criterion. Indeed, he overtly celebrated sexual fulfilment:

> In a wife I would desire
> What in whores is always found –
> The lineaments of Gratified desire.
>
> Abstinence sows sand all over
> The ruddy limbs & flaming hair,
> But Desire Gratified
> Plants fruits of life & beauty there.

But, as is here evident, Blake's investment in the erotic utterly transcends the libertine or hedonistic; for the artist in him it establishes the link between sexual energy and a higher aesthetic: 'Exuberance is Beauty.' It is of a piece with the creative fires of life.

Blake sanctioned this erotic liberation by giving it a biblical framework. In their backyard in Lambeth, he and his wife Catherine would sit naked, in a re-creation of the paradise garden. 'At the end of the little garden in Hercules Buildings there was a summer-house,' recorded Blake's London patron, Thomas Butts. Calling one day he 'found Mr. and Mrs. Blake sitting in this summer-house, freed from "those troublesome disguises" which have prevailed since the Fall. "Come in!" cried Blake; "it's only Adam and Eve, you know!"' The Blakes had appropriately been reciting passages from *Paradise Lost*, and the garden represented Eden. To the pure, all was still as pure as in Eden.

Above all, Blake proclaimed the true spirituality and holiness of the flesh, as shone forth in such images as *Bright Day*, his rendering of Vitruvian man; we should compare also the image of Christ in 'Jerusalem':

> And did those feet in ancient time
> Walk upon England's mountains green?
> And was the holy Lamb of God
> On England's pleasant pastures seen?

Resurrection for Blake was the reunification of what had been one and whole in paradise but which had become divided, polarized into flesh and spirit, male and female and numerous other dichotomies. Reunification – restoration of the original androgynous oneness of Adam in Eden – was the essential meaning of resurrection, and the earnest of it was the pulse of the spirit within. The recurrent plot of Blake's prophetic poems, as described at the opening of *The Four Zoas*, concerns 'a Perfect Unity . . . of Eden', figured as a single Primal Man, followed by 'His fall into Division & his Resurrection to Unity'. This course of events was a spiral progress from simple innocence up and back to an 'organized innocence'.* Outer man should be the

---

* Blake made much of the tension (usually a creative one) between the male and the female principles. In paradise man was originally one, that is, androgynous. Then Eve was created. Blake had a vision that the gendered self would finally be reunited.

expression of the inner spiritual person, that complete primal man, undivided as before the divisions of the Fall: the inner and the outer fused. 'That the Poetic Genius is the true man,' Blake announced, 'and that the body or outward form of Man is derived from the Poetic Genius. Likewise that the forms of all things are derived from their Genius, which by the Ancients was call'd an Angel & Spirit & Demon.' Blake would have nothing of the mind–body or soul–body antithesis: that was false – indeed, fallen – philosophy. But he did give primacy to the internal or spiritual, as is illustrated by the moral of his poem on the little black boy, quoted in Chapter 14:

> My mother bore me in the southern wild,
> And I am black, but O! my soul is white.

And this was for the familiar antinomian reason: God was within: 'All deities reside in the human breast.'

For Blake, the Hartleyan or Priestleyan notion that man consists merely of matter was as false as the belief that the mind is a passive receptacle. Personal experience confuted such claims. He himself had visions. 'I am not ashamed, afraid, or averse to tell you what Ought to be Told,' he informed Thomas Butts: 'that I am under the direction of Messengers from Heaven, Daily & Nightly.' He believed in the prophetic power of dreams and in the holiness of the imagination (we might say 'creativity' or, as he called it, 'the Human Eternal Body in Every Man'). 'I know that This World Is a World of imagination & Vision,' he wrote to his friend Thomas Trusler:

I see Every thing I paint In This World, but Every body does not see alike. To the Eyes of a Miser a Guinea is more beautiful than the Sun. . . . Some Scarce see Nature at all. But to the Eyes of the Man of Imagination, Nature is Imagination itself. As a man is, So he Sees.

The senses were the active antennae of the soul rather than, as for Locke, pinholes through which data impacted upon a passive mind.

It was in respect of imagination that Blake took issue with his *bête noire* Sir Joshua Reynolds, representative both of the commercial artistic establishment, which Blake despised, and of conventional humanistic views about artistic values and the artist. Reynolds upheld tradition, traditional judgements, public taste, a view of art as formal craft and recognized skill. Blake dismissed all this as mere conventionality: 'This Man was Hired to Depress Art.' This mattered to Blake, as he believed in the sublime mission of the arts: 'The Arts & Sciences are the Destruction of Tyrannies or Bad Governments. . . . The Foundation of Empire is Art & Science. Remove them or Degrade them, & the Empire is No More. Empire follows Art & Not Vice Versa as Englishmen suppose.' Reynolds, in Blake's view, wanted to reduce art to 'rules'. He demurred: 'Genius begins where rules end.' Like Burke, Reynolds mocked 'Inspiration and Vision'.

Indeed, Blake had visions as such. 'Thirteen years ago,' he told the poet William Hayley, 'I lost a brother & with his spirit I converse daily & hourly in the Spirit & See him in my remembrance in the regions of my Imagination. I hear his advice & even now write from his Dictate. . . . I am the companion of Angels.' Perhaps he was also being literal when he wrote as follows: ' "What", it will be Question'd, "When the Sun rises, do you not see a round disk of fire somewhat like a Guinea?" O no, no, I see an Innumerable company of the Heavenly host crying "Holy, Holy, Holy is the Lord God Almighty".' Addressing this visionary faculty, he explained, 'I question not my Corporeal or Vegetative Eye any more than I would Question a Window concerning a Sight. I look thro' it & not with it.'

Blake recorded conversations with the Archangel Gabriel. He had been reading Edward Young's *Night Thoughts*, which he had agreed to illustrate, and came across the passage in which the poet asked 'Who can paint an angel?' Closing the book, he spoke aloud:

BLAKE: Aye! Who can paint an angel?
VOICE: Michael Angelo could.

Looking round the room, he saw nothing 'save a greater light than usual'.

BLAKE: And how do *you* know?
VOICE: I *know*, for I sat to him: I am the arch-angel Gabriel.

BLAKE: Oho! You are, are you? I must have better assurance than that of a wandering voice; you may be an evil spirit – there are such in the land.

VOICE: You shall have good assurance. Can an evil spirit do this?

Seeking the source of the voice, he became aware of a shining shape, with bright wings, radiating light:

As I looked, the shape dilated more and more: he waved his hands; the roof of my study opened; he ascended into heaven; he stood in the sun, and beckoning to me, moved the universe. An angel of evil could not have *done that* – it was the arch-angel Gabriel.

Such elements in Blake have, of course, been called delusional, and his putative clinical state has long attracted attention. But it is much more pertinent to treat his views as the natural outcome of certain mystical Christian responses to the empiricist Enlightenment philosophy of self.

In some ways, Blake was himself an example of enlightened individualistic anti-rationalism. Yet he tirelessly combated all such reductionist tendencies and espoused a primitive faith which gave pride of place to imagination as the emanation of the divine. He was also to the fore in those emergent aesthetic tendencies which translated what had once been primarily religious and transcendental into the artistic. He became the prototype for the wayward, wilful genius, entering into an ambiguous dance with the power or poison of the irrational.

Blake rejected the traditional self of Christian Platonic humanism, as philosophized by Cartesian dualism. Such views sanctioned alienation and oppression. But his rejection of these traditions did not follow the scientific path of the Enlightenment – quite the opposite. Blake saw Bacon, Locke and Newton as the problem not the solution: their philosophy could end up with nothing but a partial and straitjacketing model of natural man. Blake would have none of such reductionism. He longed to reunite body and soul, nature and spirit. The inner unity of man had to be recovered – through rethinking conventions, through transvaluation, through the holiness of art –

and that primarily meant through the untrammelled imagination. Whereas almost all the other thinkers discussed so far in this book expressed fears about the imagination – it would create phantoms, it would cocoon the individual from society – Blake was ardent. Imagination was 'the Human Eternal Body in Every Man' or 'the Divine Body of the Lord Jesus, blessed for ever'.

Not least, living at the dawn of the Romantic age, Blake asserted the sanctity of the individual. God was within, man was a visionary and to the pure all things were pure.

25

BYRON: SEXY SATIRE

I am no Platonist.

I have always believed that all things depended upon Fortune, and nothing upon ourselves. I am not aware of any one thought or action worthy of being called good to myself or others, which is not to be attributed to the Good Goddess, Fortune!

> So, we'll go no more a roving
>   So late into the night,
> Though the heart be still as loving,
>   And the moon be still as bright.
>
> For the sword outwears its sheath,
>   And the soul wears out the breast,
> And the heart must pause to breathe,
>   And love itself have rest.

BYRON

The Enlightenment called into question the pilgrim's progress, the Christian soul sojourning a while on earth before final translation at the Last Trump to a life glorious and eternal in heaven. The doctrine of the nerves, Locke's epistemological breakdown of the personality as conscious selfhood, studies of dreams and delusions, Shaftesbury's glorying in the role of imagination, and myriad other inquiries which made up the emergent human sciences – all tended to dissolve the pilgrim into the unsettled ambiguities of the ego.

At the close of the eighteenth century Romanticism grew out of such enlightened questings – 'grew out' in a dual sense, both drawing upon and casting aside. Most Romantics – Blake pre-eminently – despised the desiccated reductive materialism apparently championed by enlightened science and philosophy, replacing it with an imaginative self, more dynamic, creative, loftier and divine. Romanticism dramatized the struggles of the individual – typically male – portrayed as forming and forging himself over and against the oppressions of power and the stale conventions and numbing constraints of polite society. The Romantic psyche declared war upon the 'world' as colloquially understood, and also grappled with its own lower elements. Inner conflict, self-destructiveness even, were integral to the Romantic agony.

In Byron in particular, such Romantic struggles assumed a heroic and dramatic form, but one uniquely (for the Romantics) brought refreshingly to earth by a biting irony, a satirical wit which undercut poetic pretensions. Byron wrote in a destabilizing register; never at rest, never at home, never comfortable, his mind always evoked the might-have-been and the never-to-be: the arch-enemy of cant and hypocrisy, that was one Enlightenment heritage the rebel in Byron never renounced. He famously dubbed Gibbon 'the lord of irony'; the epithet fits Byron himself no less.

Byron was open about not being a Christian, with all that that entailed: 'I have lived a Deist, what I shall die I know not; however, come what may, *ridens moriar.*' 'In morality,' he declared, 'I prefer Confucius to the Ten Commandments, Socrates to St. Paul' – adding, with a sting in the tail, 'though the two latter agree in their opinion of marriage' – ever a sore point after Byron's own disastrous union with Annabella Milbanke. A restless, sceptical questing streak marked his temper:

> 'To be, or not to be?' – Ere I decide,
>> I should be glad to know that which *is being.*
> 'Tis true we speculate both far and wide,
>> And deem, because we *see*, we are *all-seeing*:

For my part, I'll enlist on neither side,
    Until I see both sides for once agreeing.
For me, I sometimes think that Life is Death,
Rather than Life a mere affair of breath.

'*Que sçais-je?*' was the motto of Montaigne,
    As also of the first academicians:
That all is dubious which man may attain,
    Was one of their most favourite positions.
There's no such thing as certainty, that's plain
    As any of Mortality's conditions;
So little do we know what we're about in
This world, I doubt if doubt itself be doubting.

Not least, he championed Alexander Pope against those solemnly pious Romantics, notably Wordsworth, who so resented the great Augustan's 'tingling, jingling' verse. Byron is the true descendant of the enlightened coffee-house scoffer, the shade of Rochester the libertine and the Restoration wits. So much is, of course, patently present in his notorious Don Juan philandering-mode but it is equally visible in his disdain for the credulity of those Christians – he was watching the Evangelical revival – who uncritically, if hubristically, embraced notions of immortality based upon literal (that is, naïve) readings of the Bible.

For Byron, the idea of bodily resurrection at the Last Trump was ridiculous, palpably the wish-fulfilment of miserable self-deceiving creatures unable honestly to face the plain facts of death and extinction. And who would want to believe in a Christian afterlife? 'A *material* resurrection seems strange and even absurd,' he declared,

except for purposes of punishment – and all punishment which is to *revenge* rather than *correct* – must be *morally wrong* – and *when* the *World is at an end* – what moral or warning purpose *can* eternal tortures answer? . . . the whole thing is inscrutable. – It is useless to tell one *not* to *reason* but to *believe* – you might as well tell a man not to wake but *sleep*.

Christian teachings were thus both unfathomable and detestable; their primitive, punitive God did not deserve veneration. It amused Byron to banter against the Churches' fantasy of life beyond the grave. 'We are miserable enough in this life, without the absurdity of speculating upon another,' he told his friend Francis Hodgson. 'If men are to live, why die at all? and if they die, why disturb the sweet and sound sleep that "knows no waking"? "Post Mortem nihil est, ipsaque Mors nihil".' The notion of neat and tidy piles of the saved and the damned beggared rational belief.

As to revealed religion, Christ came to save men; but a good Pagan will go to heaven, and a bad Nazarene to hell; 'Argal' (I argue like the gravedigger) why are not all men Christians? or why are any? If mankind may be saved who never heard or dreamt, at Timbuctoo, Otaheite, Terra Incognita, &c., of Galilee and its Prophet, Christianity is of no avail, if they cannot be saved without, why are not all orthodox? It is a little hard to send a man preaching to Judaea, and leave the rest of the world – Negers and what not – *dark* as their complexions, without a ray of light for so many years to lead them on high; and who will believe that God will damn men for not knowing what they were never taught?

The satirist in Byron, however, felt entitled once in a while to commandeer the Christian master-narrative for seditious purposes. In 1821 Robert Southey published a thumping piece of patriotism, dedicated to King George IV, entitled *A Vision of Judgement*. In it, the Poet Laureate praised the previous reign's glorious British military achievements, the 'perfect integrity of the whole administration of public affairs' under George III, the progress of religion, and so forth. The story-line teetered on the ludicrous: lulled by the death bell of old George III, the poet fell into a trance, and an angel revealed to him the dead king's spirit ascending to heaven, where the welcoming party included his illustrious royal predecessors, attended by Shakespeare and Milton.

Southey meant his poem as proof of how literature should serve public, pious purposes. Poetry had traditionally indeed been thus uplifting, but recently, he complained, a 'Satanic school' had emerged of poets whose 'diseased hearts and depraved imaginations' had rebelled against religion. The reference to Byron was glaring. Byron detested Southey as the arch-priest of cant, renegade from liberalism as he was; and the opportunity of a crushing retort to the turncoat was irresistible. He replied with a work with almost the same title. The opening lines of Byron's *The Vision of Judgment* (1822), established the tone of urbane scepticism:

> Saint Peter sat by the celestial gate:
>> His keys were rusty, and the lock was dull,
> So little trouble had been given of late;
>> Not that the place by any means was full.

Byron made fun of the Laureate's parade of religiosity. Southey had gloried in the exploits of war: Byron pictured the clerkly angels exhausted at inscribing the names of those slaughtered:

> Each day too slew its thousands six or seven,
>> Till at the crowning carnage, Waterloo,
> They threw their pens down in divine disgust –
> The page was so besmear'd with blood and dust.

Southey had apotheosized George III – the king was in heaven, his enemies in hell. Scarred by his ghastly childhood spent in Aberdeen under his orthodox Calvinist mother, Byron hated talk of damnation and the bigotry of public piety:

> I know this is unpopular; I know
>> 'Tis blasphemous; I know one may be damn'd
> For hoping no one else may e'er be so;
>> I know my catechism; I know we're cramm'd
> With the best doctrines till we quite o'erflow;
>> I know that all save England's church have shamm'd,
> And that the other twice two hundred churches
> And synagogues have made a *damn'd* bad purchase.

In Southey's poem the arrival of George III at heaven's gates was the occasion for a special fanfare. Byron pictured something quite different:

> 'George the Third is dead.'
> 'And who *is* George the Third?' replied the apostle:
> '*What George? what Third?*'

Was there not breathtaking blasphemy in Southey's suggestion that the Lord of Hosts himself must be impressed by the arrival of the British monarch? In a scene echoing Milton, Byron has the Archangel Michael appearing to conduct the trial of George III, and Satan turning up to claim his victim. The Devil delivers the indictment against the King: the influence of Lord Bute, the loss of America, the war against France, five million Catholics refused political equality, etc., etc.

> He ever warr'd with freedom and the free:
>   Nations as men, home subjects, foreign foes,
> So that they utter'd the word 'Liberty!'
>   Found George the Third their first opponent . . .

Finally, Southey arrived to read his poem in praise of the king, but at the sound of the first lines all the spirits howled and fled, and thus the trial was left incomplete:

> All I saw farther, in the last confusion,
>   Was, that King George slipp'd into heaven for one;
> And when the tumult dwindled to a calm,
>   I left him practising the hundredth psalm.

Just thinking of the Last Judgement was thus a sordid farce.

Not least for Byron, reincarnation was somewhat disgusting: was not temporal embodiment quite enough? Through the hundreds of stanzas of *Childe Harold*, *Don Juan* and the like, the greasy obesity of the aristocratic high life of the day, the podgy Prince of Wales and all the dowdy dowagers excited the deepest revulsion. The Christian threat of all that fat flesh further reincarnated did not merely offend Byron's reason; it turned his stomach.

Byron was wont to assume a lofty disdain for the flesh: he was above all that. Ever the scoffer, however, he equally mocked his own stoical pretensions, and brought himself down to earth. 'I once thought myself a Philosopher and talked nonsense with great Decorum,' he confessed, 'I defied pain, and preached up equanimity . . . At last, a fall from my horse convinced me, bodily suffering was an Evil, and the worst of an argument overset my maxims and my temper at the same moment.'

This self-criticism helps explain Byron's contempt for Joseph Priestley. The aristocratic poet looked down upon the petty-bourgeois Yorkshire Dissenter with his earnest but uncritical scriptural belief in progress. How absurd for such a busy little bee to be prating on about such lofty themes! In particular, Byron found the chemist's solemn theologico-philosophical materialism, which embraced the resurrection of the flesh, particularly galling: what a degrading faith to espouse! Christian or no, Byron certainly did not want the faith sullied by the likes of Priestley. 'I have often been inclined to Materialism in philosophy,' he admitted,

but could never bear it's introduction into *Christianity* – which appears to me essentially founded upon the *Soul*. – For this reason, Priestley's Christian Materialism – always struck me as deadly. – Believe the resurrection of the *body* – it you will – but *not without* a *Soul*. . . . I own my partiality for *Spirit*.

Such tosh as Priestley's 'Immortal Materiality' was too ludicrous for words. How insufferable for him to drag the rather noble idea of the spirit down to bourgeois bathos by insisting it was all a matter of atoms and points of force: what a grovelling lack of soul! The patrician opted for true spirit, even if its existence might be a bit of a *jeu d'esprit*.

In his deflating reductionism the satirist himself was perforce a materialist after his fashion. Pomposity, pretensions, high-flown nonsense, flatteries, the vanity of royalty, nobles and the fashionable beautiful people and *bien pensants* – all such are perpetually brought down by his scabrous wit to the most basic, gross material level: the greed, spite, malice, lust, and above all hypocrisy which were at the corrupt heart of their being. 'Went to my box at Covent-garden to-night,' he recorded one evening in 1813,

and my delicacy felt a little shocked at seeing S***'s mistress (who, to my certain knowledge, was actually educated, from her birth, for her profession) sitting with her mother, 'a three-piled b—d, b—d-Major to the army,' in a private box opposite. I felt rather indignant; but, casting my eyes round the house, in the next box to me, and the next, and the next, were the most distinguished old and young Babylonians of quality; – so I burst out a laughing. It was really odd; Lady ** *divorced* – Lady ** and her daughter, Lady **, both *divorceable* – Mrs. **, in the next the *like*, and still nearer ******! What an assemblage to *me*, who know all their histories. It was as if the house had been divided between your public and your *understood* courtesans; – but the Intriguantes much outnumbered the regular mercenaries. . . . How I do delight in observing life as it really is! – and myself, after all, the worst of any. But no matter – I must avoid egotism, which, just now, would be no vanity.

In such moods Byron could find the world too wicked, too absurd, to countenance even the idea of some presiding intelligence. 'I wonder how the deuce any body could make such a world,' he asked himself, rhetorically: 'for what purpose dandies, for instance, were ordained – and kings – and fellows of colleges – and women of "a certain age" – and many men of any age – and myself, most of all . . . Is there any thing beyond? – *who* knows?' Materialism was thus the bottom line, the acid-test dividing illusion, delusion and hypocrisy from reality. And the passionate Byron who prided himself upon being an honest sinner in an age of cant subscribed to a sardonic no-illusions materialism, the Mandevillian sexual egoist, as a frank take on the human condition.

He did of course rejoice in a certain macho materialism, that of firm and fit flesh. No mere literary lion, Byron sought admiration for his looks and animal magnetism; the 'action man' persona was meticulously groomed. In a dandyish era when youth and fitness counted (see Chapter 13), much attention was devoted to cultivating

a manly, handsome body. He was proud of having swum the Helles-
pont, an act self-consciously echoing ancient Leander. He dedicated
himself to the martial arts, in particular fencing and boxing. 'I have
been sparring with Jackson for exercise this morning,' he wrote in
March 1814 (he was then 25), 'and mean to continue and renew my
acquaintance with the muffles. My chest, and arms, and wind are in
very good plight, and I am not in flesh. . . . At any rate, exercise is
good and this the severest of all; fencing and the broadsword never
fatigued me half so much.' In physical exertion lay the antidote
against his tendency to be '*ennuyé*', his leanings towards 'spleen and
all uncharitableness, [being] a complete misanthrope': 'Today I have
been very sulky – but an hour's exercise with Mr. Jackson of pugilistic
memory – has given me spirits & fatigued me into that state of
languid laziness which I prefer to all other.' Animal spirits kept his
doomed and cursed sense of despondency at bay. An aristocrat born
lame with the handicap of a club foot, he was delighted to slum and
spar with the professional pugilists of the day.

Keeping trim, keeping his figure, was crucial. Slimming had
become a preoccupation while he was an undergraduate at Cambridge. 'You will be surprized to hear I am grown *very thin*,' he told
his friend John Hanson in April 1807:

I have lost 18 LB in my weight, that is one Stone & 4 pounds since
January . . . However dont be alarmed, I have taken every means to accom-
plish the end, by violent exercise, & Fasting, as I found myself too plump.
– I shall continue my Exertions, having no other amusement.

How had he done it? 'I wear *seven* Waistcoats, & a great Coat,' he
told his friend:

run, & play at cricket in this Dress, till quite exhausted by excessive
perspiration, use the hot Bath daily, eat only a quarter of [a] pound, [of]
Butcher's meat in 24 hours, no Suppers, or Breakfast, only one meal a Day,
drink no malt Liquor, [only?] a little Wine, & take Physic occasionally, by
these means my *Ribs* display a Skin of no great Thickness, & my Clothes,
have been taken in nearly *half a yard*.

By July of that year it was his boast he could 'vie with the *slim* beaux of modern times', and three months later, he declared to another friend: 'I weigh less by *three Stone*, & 9 *pounds*, than I did 6 months ago. – My weight was then *14* stone & 6 LB. It is now *10 Stone 11* LB!!!' There was not an ounce of flab upon him, he had learnt to master his flesh.

The profound ambiguities of the Romantic body shine through Byron's writings, to say nothing of his doings. He gloried in a firm, youthful physique, which meant that the frailties of the flesh needed to be endlessly disciplined. But he also went in for hedonistic dissipation, a self-indulgent, carefree wallowing in alcohol, that state of 'hiccup and happiness'. The tipsy rake formed no small part of Byron's image, and yet he hated the hangover, the bloated morning after, the unbearable heaviness of being. And over-indulgence at the dinner table disgusted him. 'I have dined regularly to-day, for the first time since Sunday last – this being Sabbath, too,' he wrote in his journal in 1813: 'I wish to God I had not dined now! – It kills me with heaviness, stupor, and horrible dreams; – and yet it was but a pint of bucellas, and fish. . . . The horrors of digestion!' For long spells Byron lived off dry biscuits and soda water. 'I wish I could leave off eating altogether,' he declared.

The irresolvability of the flesh – the desire to be fit, sexy, handsome and youthful, and yet the paradoxical temptation to wreck it all in bored self-indulgence – was central to the Byronic dilemma. It surfaced, perhaps, in such seemingly petty concerns as the state of his teeth: 'Went to Waite's [the dentist]. Teeth are all right and white.' But how could man respect himself when he was always being brought down to earth by the most banausic things? Suffering from a bout of food poisoning brought on by bad cockles, 'I remarked in my illness the complete inertion, inaction, and destruction of my chief mental faculties. I tried to rouse them, and yet could not – and this is the *Soul*!!! I should believe that it was married to the body, if they did not sympathise so much with each other.'

For Byron the romantic hero the conventional life of fashionable London or Venice spelt exhaustion. *Ennui* was to be resisted with rebellious energy – that it was which gave the spice of life – 'I like energy – even animal energy – of all kinds; and I have need of both mental and corporeal,' he declared in 1813. 'The great object of life', he insisted, 'is Sensation – to feel that we exist, even though in pain.' The energy of youth, however, was also doomed to succumb to age and decrepitude:

> We wither from our youth, we gasp away –
> Sick – sick; unfound the boon, unslaked the thirst.

From his mid-twenties, Byron grew quite obsessed with ageing: 'I shall soon be six-and-twenty,' he recorded on 22 January 1814:

Is there any thing in the future that can possibly console us for not being always *twenty-five?*

> 'Oh Gioventu!
> Oh Primavera! gioventu dell' anno.
> Oh Gioventu! primavera della vita.'

'My health is good,' now 28, he informed his half-sister Augusta Leigh,

but I have now & then fits of giddiness, & deafness, which make me think like Swift – that I shall be like him & the *withered* tree he saw – which occasioned the reflection and 'die at top' first. My hair is growing grey, & *not* thicker; & my teeth are sometimes *looseish* though still white & sound. Would not one think I was sixty instead of not quite nine and twenty?

By his thirties, he felt quite elderly:

It is three minutes past twelve. – ''Tis the middle of the night by the castle clock,' and I am now thirty-three!

> 'Eheu, fugaces, Posthume, Posthume,
> Labuntur anni' . . .

And at 35? 'Do not believe all the lies you may hear', he chafed Augusta: 'Hobhouse can tell you that I have *not* lost *any* of my *teeth hitherto*, – since I was 12 years old . . . and so far from being fatter –

at *present* I [am] much thinner than when I left England.' His fear was not of not having many years left; it was rather a despondency at having done so little with the good years.

On top of all this, compounding the complexities and confusions was, of course, Byron the poet. There was the autobiographical versifier who brilliantly recorded his exploits as a bundle of tormented desires and an object of freakish fascination. But there was also the poet-persona. The macho man, swimmer, boxer and warrior who died that Greece might still be free, was also a bard, a man of imagination and wit. It is qua poet that Byron resurrected the exploded and discarded immortal Christian soul by bodying it forth through the notion of soul conceived as poetic imagination.

Verse itself could assume immortality, could be a proof of the 'soul' in the sense of the transcendence of the gross and tawdry. Byron held out for a heroic immortality, the autonomy of the lone and courageous individual freed from hidebound convention and all that was detestable. It was an imperishability that was essentially subjective and personal. 'Matter is eternal – always changing – but reproduced and, as far as we can comprehend Eternity Eternal,' he mused, 'and why not Mind? Why should not the Mind act with and upon the Universe? – as portions of it act upon and with the congregated dust – called Mankind?' Mind, after all, was ceaselessly active:

Of the Immortality of the Soul – it appears to me that there can be little doubt – if we attend for a moment to the action of Mind. – It is in perpetual activity; – I used to doubt of it – but reflection has taught me better. – It acts also so very independent of body – in dreams for instance incoherently and madly – I grant you; – but still it is *Mind*, & much more *Mind* – than when we are awake.

The Byronic soul, however, was not Christian and orthodox but personal and idiosyncratic:

How far our future life will be *individual* – or rather – how far it will at all resemble our *present* existence, is another question but that the *Mind is eternal*

– seems as possible as that the body is not so. – Of course – I have venture[d] upon the question without recurring to Revelation.

Such belief, Byron admitted, was, more than anything else, a personal, psychological necessity: 'Every body clings to it – the stupidest, and dullest, and wickedest of human bipeds is still persuaded that he is immortal.'

Immortality might be achieved by fame, by the enduring life of his verse. Some semblance of it might also be gained through a triumph of the will, the conviction (perhaps similar to that expressed by the *Spectator*, but far more forcibly) that there *must* be something beyond, transcending the wretched failing frailties of the flesh. In an almost Nietzschean way, struggle would be the proof:

> 'Tis to create, and in creating live
> A being more intense, that we endow
> With form our fancy, gaining as we give
> The life we image, even as I do now,
> What am I? Nothing: but not so art thou,
> Soul of my thought!

And, through struggle, some kind of ultimate identification with nature, with the cosmos, could be achieved:

> But I have lived, and have not lived in vain:
> My mind may lose its force, my blood its fire,
> And my frame perish even in conquering pain;
> But there is that within me which shall tire
> Torture and Time, and breathe when I expire;
> Something unearthly, which they deem not of,
> Like the remember'd tone of a mute lyre,
> Shall on their soften'd spirits sink, and move
> In hearts all rocky now the late remorse of love.

Soul was thus the condition of being in sympathy with, at one with, the great, vast, impersonal forces of nature – those avalanches, earthquakes, volcanoes, snowstorms and blizzards Byron loved to describe:

> Are not the mountains, waves, and skies, a part
> Of me and of my soul, as I of them?
> Is not the love of these deep in my heart
> With a pure passion?

In losing himself in these lay Byron's hope that the tawdry, paltry limitations of the human condition could be transcended.

Of course, Byron knew full well that poetry in itself was no proof of soul or immortality. Like Swift, he could deflate the poet's pretensions, reducing them to bodily tics and psycho-pathology. What did he make of Keats's poetry, he was asked: 'such writing is a sort of mental masturbation – he is always f—gg—g his *Imagination*. – I don't mean that he is *indecent*, but viciously soliciting his own ideas into a state which is neither poetry nor any thing else but a Bedlam vision produced by raw pork and opium.' Thus did Byron reduce bad verse to bodily dysfunctions. In another satirical poem penned to his publisher John Murray, he suggested that a play written by his former friend Dr Polidori should be treated not as literature but rather, at best, as a work of medicine or, at worst, a manifestion of disease; while lacking artistic quality, the drama might serve as a purgative. Murray should turn it down in the following terms:

> Dear Doctor – I have read your play
> Which is a good one in it's way,
> Purges the eyes & moves the bowels
> And drenches handkerchiefs like towels
> With tears that in a flux of Grief
> Afford hysterical relief
> To shatter'd nerves & quicken'd pulses
> Which your catastrophe convulses. . . .
> My hands are full – my head so busy –
> I'm almost dead – & always dizzy –
> And so with endless truth & hurry –
> Dear Doctor – I am yours,
>
> John Murray.

Precisely as for Swift and Pope, bad art is inseparable from the disorders of the body. But great art, for Byron, may be the emancipation of the soul.

The sceptic or cynical deflater should have the last word. After the golden and silver ages, Byron commented, his was an 'age of rags', avalanched by paper. And in such a time, was there any vanity like the author's?

I was out of spirits – read the papers – thought what *fame* was, on reading, in a case of murder, that 'Mr. Wych, grocer, at Tunbridge, sold some bacon, flour, cheese, and, it is believed, some plums, to some gipsy woman accused. He had on his counter (I quote faithfully) a *book*, the Life of *Pamela*, which he was *tearing* for *waste* paper, &c., &c. In the cheese was found, &c., and a *leaf* of *Pamela wrapt round the bacon*.' What would Richardson, the vainest and luckiest of *living* authors (*i.e.* while alive) – he who, with Aaron Hill, used to prophesy and chuckle over the presumed fall of Fielding (the *prose* Homer of human nature) and of Pope (the most beautiful of poets) – what would he have said, could he have traced his pages from their place on the French prince's toilets (see Boswell's Johnson) to the grocer's counter and the gipsy-murderess's bacon!!!

What would he have said? What can any body say, save what Solomon said long before us? After all, it is but passing from one counter to another, from the bookseller's to the other tradesman's – grocer or pastry-cook. For my part, I have met with most poetry upon trunks; so that I am apt to consider the trunk-maker as the sexton of authorship.

26

CONCLUSION: THE MARCH OF MIND

The cultured and well-connected East India Office civil servant Thomas Love Peacock is best remembered for his sparkling series of satirical novels, beginning with *Headlong Hall* (1816). The commentary they offer on the exchanges about man's estate surveyed in this book aptly introduces this Conclusion.

Each of Peacock's novels centres upon a country-house gathering of gentlemen (garnished by a few token desirable damsels) representative of the leading currents of opinion and faddish sensibilities of the day. The debates conducted by these pundits over their pheasant and port constitute a wry intellectual symposium, a pot-pourri of different sounds – political, religious, social, philosophical and aesthetic – giving Peacock the opportunity to poke gentle fun, not just at each persuasion individually but at his age's infatuation with earnest intellectual chatter.

Like every satirist, Peacock delighted in the bizarre assortment of tenets tenaciously adopted (no foible or crotchet but had its impassioned defender) and in the preposterous lengths to which those mounted upon their curious hobby horses would canter with their doctrines. Comparison is obviously expected with the *Spectator* club a century earlier. Addison and Steele had aimed to show how in a polite urbane world diverse types – the landowner, the merchant, the soldier, the beau, the cleric – should be able to club harmoniously together; and the fact that a similar congregation manages to sit down at Peacock's tables and sink their differences as they sink their bumpers may, in effect, be taken as evidence of the success of the Spectatorial endeavour. Certain changes are also highly conspicuous. In the Spectator club, diversity is principally a function of social type and rank. By Peacock's time, what count are the intellectual and ideological, rather than the social, divides. A world of variegated and polarized opinion has emerged – a clear indication of the rise in the intervening century of a lay intelligentsia buoyed up by the printing revolution and the media. Peacock's talking heads do not so much express vested class and professional interests as offer rival readings of human personality, behaviour and destiny. Evidently, the business of defining the very nature of man had become a major source of unsettling controversy.

While they are indeed models of conviviality, Peacock's thinkers hold views as sharply polarized as those grotesquely parodied in *A Tale of a Tub*. Whereas for Swift, however, the disparate doctrines expressed were all primarily theological in complexion, in Peacock's world the intricacies of Christian doctrine had become utterly marginal to debates over the nature of man. Even his clergymen – for example, the Revd Dr Gaster in *Headlong Hall* – are, as his very name reveals, typically bon vivants, concerned more with gastronomy than God. At a comparable dining table in *Melincourt* (1817), the Revd Mr Portpipe (again, *nomen est omen*) expounds a theological pragmatism, obviously meant to remind readers of Archdeacon William Paley:

When I open the bottle, I shut the book of Numbers. There are two reasons for drinking: one is, when you are thirsty, to cure it; the other, when you are not thirsty, to prevent it. . . . Wine is the elixir of life. 'The soul,' says St. Augustine, 'cannot live in drought.' What is death? Dust and ashes. There is nothing so dry. What is life? Spirit. What is Spirit? Wine.

As is hinted by the honest divine's materialization of spirit, Peacock is depicting a world essentially secular. Admittedly, in *Nightmare Abbey* (1818), Mr Flosky, aka Samuel Taylor Coleridge, champions the supernatural: 'He dreamed with his eyes open, and saw ghosts dancing round him at noontide.' Indeed, his conversation is mainly spectral: 'It is seldom that ghosts appeal to two senses at once; but, when I was in Devonshire, the following story was well attested to me,' is one of his opening gambits. But another guest, Mr Hilary, will have none of this, proceeding to psycho-pathologize Flosky's spirits: 'All these anecdotes admit of solution on psychological principles,' he counters:

It is more easy for a soldier, a philosopher, or even a saint, to be frightened of his own shadow, than for a dead man to come out of his grave. Medical writers cite a thousand singular examples of the force of imagination. Persons of feeble, nervous, melancholy temperament, exhausted by fever, by labour, or by spare diet, will readily conjure up, in the magic ring of their own phantasy, spectres, gorgons, chimeras, and all the objects of their hatred and their love.

Peacock's caricatures encompass some of the leading doctrines then circulating about human nature and self-identity. Notable are the by-then standard perfectibilists like Mr Foster in *Headlong Hall*. 'Every thing we look on', he declares, 'attests the progress of mankind in all the arts of life, and demonstrates their gradual advancement towards a state of unlimited perfection.' Such progressives are counterbalanced by nostalgia-mongers, like Mr Escot in the same novel, who hanker after mankind in its state of primitive simplicity, holding that the human race began hale and hearty, and has subsequently degenerated. 'The natural and original man', he opines,

lived in the woods: the roots and fruits of the earth supplied his simple nutriment: he had few desires, and no diseases. [But since] man first applied fire to culinary purposes . . . the stature of mankind has been in a state of gradual diminution, and I have not the least doubt that it will continue to grow *small by degrees, and lamentably less*, till the whole race will vanish imperceptibly from the face of the earth.

Escot was the archetypal lambaster of luxury and *laudator temporis acti*.

Gaster, Foster, Escot and others – by contrast to Flosky – were not meant by Peacock to epitomize a single living individual: they were versions of types prominent in Georgian debates about health, diet, education and the vices and virtues of civilization.

As well as satirizing distinct models of man, Peacock gave his own renderings of some of the key intellectual debates of the day. One, for instance, was the furore over Malthus's *Essay on the Principle of Population* (see above, Chapter 23). In *Crotchet Castle* (1831), Mr Fax – such a brilliant moniker for the Revd Thomas Robert Malthus! – argues that reform of society and social progress are quite out of the question without a root-and-branch transformation of human nature, that is, the withering away of sexual instincts – or, in other words, are pie in the sky. By contrast, *in Nightmare Abbey* Scythrop – that is, Percy Bysshe Shelley – is endlessly hatching plans for effecting precisely that regeneration of mankind. 'He now became troubled with the *passion for reforming the world*,' discloses Peacock in a phrase he liked so much he used it repeatedly. 'He built many castles in the air, and peopled them with secret tribunals, and bands of illuminati, who were always the imaginary instruments of his projected regeneration of the human species.' In this parody of Shelley, Peacock was spot-on in drawing attention to the Hartleyan and Godwinian underpinnings of Scythrop's philosophical musings:

'Action,' thus he soliloquised, 'is the result of opinion, and to new-model opinion would be to new-model society. Knowledge is power; it is in the hands of a few, who employ it to mislead the many, for their own selfish purposes of aggrandisement and appropriation. What if it were in the hands of a few who should employ it to lead the many? What if it were universal, and the multitude were enlightened? No. The many must be always in leading-strings; but let them have wise and honest conductors.'

Here in a nutshell was a precise if cruel simplification of the thrust of Godwinian ideology, viewed as the culmination of the debate about the malleability of human nature (central to this study) which went back as far as Locke.

Still more radical, perhaps, as a satire on human nature, and harking back to many sources, including *Gulliver's Travels*, is the character introduced in *Melincourt* of Sir Oran Haut-Ton. This higher primate has been taught to dress in human clothes, and despite – or rather precisely because of – being utterly silent, Sir Oran makes an impeccable backbench Tory MP.* 'Sir Telegraph [Paxarett] looked earnestly at the stranger, but was too polite to laugh,' writes Peacock, framing this monster through the bemused eyes and mystified brain of another guest:

though he could not help thinking there was something very ludicrous in Sir Oran's physiognomy, notwithstanding the air of high fashion which characterized his whole deportment, and which was heightened by a pair of enormous whiskers, and the folds of his vast cravat. He therefore bowed to Sir Oran with becoming gravity, and Sir Oran returned the bow with very striking politeness.

. . . Sir Oran preserved an inflexible silence during the whole duration of dinner, but showed great proficiency in the dissection of game.

Over the dinner table, Sir Oran's unusual origins are finally revealed, in a sequence which displays Peacock's matchless ear for the nuances of inane upper-class dialogue:

MR. FORESTER. Sir Oran Haut-ton was caught very young in the woods of Angola.

SIR TELEGRAPH PAXARETT. Caught!

MR. FORESTER. Very young. He is a specimen of the natural and original man – the wild man of the woods; called, in the language of the more

---

* The book originated with Lord Monboddo's positive belief that the orang-utan was not an ape but a variety of the human species, and that its lack of speech was incidental. Peacock's idea was that this would furnish a central character who should be introduced to polite society, attend the opera, receive a baronetcy, be elected for a pocket-borough and take his seat in the House of Commons.

James Burnett, Lord Monboddo, was a Scottish judge, who put forward, as original, the views of Rousseau, which he expounded with no sense of the need for experiment or of the value of evidence. He was serious, confused and gullible, and occasionally, by pure chance, one of his absurdities came near to being the truth. Peacock delighted in him and handled him most tenderly, with his tongue just perceptibly in his cheek. This tenderness did not extend to the Tories. The Napoleonic wars had been won; the British people were impoverished, and the Government was using victory to stamp out liberty at home and abroad, muzzling freedom of speech and the liberty of the press. Its power was based on a mockery of the parliamentary representation and functioned partly by widespread bribery and corruption.

civilized and sophisticated natives of Angola, *Pongo,* and in that of the Indians of South America, *Oran Outang.*

SIR TELEGRAPH PAXARETT. The devil he is!

MR. FORESTER. Positively. Some presumptuous naturalists have refused his species the honours of humanity; but the most enlightened and illustrious philosophers agree in considering him in his true light as the natural and original man.

Here Peacock kills several birds with one stone. He satirizes the views of Lord Monboddo, who held that mankind had evolved from the higher primates which were themselves human although as yet lacking the power of speech. He also spikes the absurdity of the Tory Party, which evidently possessed the brains of apes and hadn't a word to say for itself. (By implication the political public was also derided, for being taken in by such speechless wonders.) Little did Peacock know it, but around the same time Charles Darwin was pencilling in one of his notebooks: 'He who understands baboon would do more toward metaphysics than Locke.' Evidently, he should have been one of the guests.

Sir Oran's physiognomy is found 'ludicrous', and it is noteworthy that other anthropological send-ups in Peacock's satires, trading upon the tendentious notion that the inner man can be fully ascertained by his exterior casing, include the after-dinner lectures given to the guests at Headlong Hall by an adept of the fashionable new science of phrenology. 'Mr. Cranium stood up and addressed the company,' opens Peacock's spoof upon Franz Gall:

Ardently desirous, to the extent of my feeble capacity, of disseminating, as much as possible, the inexhaustible treasures to which this golden key admits the humblest votary of philosophical truth, I invite you, when you have sufficiently restored, replenished, refreshed, and exhilarated that osteosarchæmatosplanchnochondroneuromuelous, or to employ a more intelligible term, osseocarnisanguineovisceri cartilaginonervomedullary, *compages,* or shell, the body, which at once envelops and develops that mysterious and inestimable kernel, the desiderative, determinative, ratiocinative, imaginative, inquisitive, appetitive, comparative, reminiscent, congeries of ideas and notions, simple and compound, comprised in the comprehensive denomination of mind, to take a peep with me into the mechanical arcana of the anatomico-metaphysical universe.

We are evidently back to Swift and his mechanical operation of the spirit: the mechanical-reductionist bug was still biting. As practised by Mr Cranium, phrenology repeated what Peacock presumably took to be the ancient error (earlier enshrined in physiognomy) of reducing the human to the mechanical or the animalistic. 'Here is the skull of a beaver, and that of Sir Christopher Wren,' declares the lecturer. 'You observe, in both these specimens, the prodigious development of the organ of constructiveness.'

As these novels reveal, by the early nineteenth century a cartload of contrasting philosophies of social and personal identity was on offer – one probably much more varied than a century earlier. In particular, such systems had become notably secular: by Peacock's day a lay intelligentsia was blithely expounding a comprehensive syllabus of conflicting scientific and ideological views (many would say *errors*) about human nature and destiny.

This book has surveyed – selectively rather than systematically – changing thinking about the self and the personality in modernizing Britain. No simple unilinear shift from point A to position Z can be discerned: there was no undeviating teleological development, no final solution. A variety of traditions of thinking about the self blossomed; controversies flared up and raged unresolved. Different parties, cliques and religious sects advanced favourite nostrums of their own; women's thinking dissented from male orthodoxies, and there were always stand-offs between radical alternatives and reactionary rebuttals. Indeed, the innovations in material culture brought by the commercial society and consumer culture – above all, growing literacy, the explosion of print, the rise of privacy, the emergence of such genres as the novel that created chambers of private thinking for the reader – invited questioning of old truths and the proliferation of new models for self-fashioning. All such developments spurred further diversification: by the early nineteenth century the creeds of the seventeenth century had divided out into that kaleidoscope of opinions so brilliantly captured not just by Peacock but also by Hazlitt's *The Spirit of the Age* and chewed over so earnestly by the *Edinburgh Review*, the *Quarterly Review* and the other new literary heavies.

It is, nevertheless, worth attempting to highlight some salient changes. Practically all seventeenth-century thinkers derived their ideas of the self from fundamental Christian doctrines. That is true even of those who were heterodox (like the mortalists) or idiosyncratic (for instance, John Asgill) or those who, like Thomas Hobbes, were outed as the Devil quoting Scripture. This authorized version, preached by the Churches, held man to be a compound of mortal earthly clay and an immaterial and immortal soul that was destined to outlive the dissolution of the flesh, until reunion at the Last Judgement. Psychologically satisfying for individual believers, this doctrine equally met the needs of Church and State for a regulatory, disciplinary and punitive model of accountability infinitely extended beyond life on earth. It had biblical sanction; it found incarnation as epic verse in *Paradise Lost*, Edward Young's *Night Thoughts*, and in myriad other poetic and painterly forms; and it had been given rational, philosophical sanction through Greek philosophies, with their championing of the separateness and superiority of the soul, as codified by the Schoolmen and reinforced by Descartes's dualism and the mechanical philosophy.

This standard model experienced various challenges, and became soft-pedalled, sidelined or superseded. Traditional theological teachings about life after death came under fire from freethinkers for being irrational, incoherent, incredible or, in the eyes of liberal Deists, repugnant and immoral. Biting critics dismissed such doctrines of the soul as the cankered fruits of superstitious fears, exploited by priestcraft. In particular, as religion in Britain became lay-driven, responsible more to the formulations of Addison and Steele than the pontifications of prelates, a more populist 'bourgeois' fantasy of life after death gained support. Heaven became pictured as a kind of retirement home, or an extension of domestic life, or even an idealized state which only the vulgar would view in the infantile terms of angels chanting hallelujahs. Once Protestantism had abandoned purgatory, the gulf between the living and the dead widened, indeed grew unbridgeable, and it became far more difficult for the Churches to keep control of believers' visions of the life beyond.

One consequence of all such developments was a naturalization or even secularization of the self in which, while life beyond the grave was rarely explicitly denied, the emphasis was increasingly set upon one's earthly existence as an end in itself. This entailed a kind of practical utilitarianism in ethics and lifestyle: worldly happiness could now, for the first time within Christendom, be presented as a worthy design.

Under the new banner of progress, such secular prophets as Erasmus Darwin, William Godwin and Robert Owen focused their sights on the perfection and prolongation of life on earth, independently of whatever otherworldly prospects might be in store. The fortune of the self became figured in terms of an enticing career on earth rather than the Christian *memento mori* – 'live to die and die to live'. Within enlightened ideology, paradise *now* in heaven *below* became the new call.

Another key theme of this book, sharply focused by these religious changes, has been, of course, the evaluation of the flesh itself. On the body and carnality, the 'authorized version' presented a plausible and coherent package. On the one hand, the flesh was vile, bodies sordid, desires concupiscent, carnal knowledge suspect: viewed thus, the flesh was endlessly flayed and punished by the Churches. Yet it was also given a key and honourable function, unique within world religions and philosophies. God had become incarnate in Jesus Christ who had died on the Cross; man was made in God's image, and he would be reunited with his flesh at the Last Judgement and translated, triumphantly re-embodied, to heaven. Christianity thus catered in subtle ways for deep personal psychological attachment to the body.

Enlightened élites found this Christian preoccupation with the flesh – in both punishment and salvation – naïve, vulgar, implausible and gross. Such reactions manifested themselves in many ways – for example, in the growing emphasis among progressives upon the benightedness of corporal and capital punishment. Making the body an object of retribution seemed wrong-minded – for reasons both of humanity and of superior efficiency, criminal justice must address the mind rather than the flesh, as only thereby would correction lead to true repentance and reform.

In many departments of life, emphasis was shifted from the physical to the psychological. The true object of the perfection of man became the cultivation of mind or sensibility. With the displacement of the expressly Christian idea of the soul, consciousness itself moved centre stage. Mind was enshrined as the principle of freedom of the will, the repository of memory. It should, proclaimed men and ladies of sensibility, be tinglingly excited, or, for others, the agent of progress. Empirical psychologists insisted that mind was a faculty which emerged, through natural, law-governed activities, from the oper-ations of the senses and education: mind was rooted in the mundane and the temporal. Indeed, for a powerful, if minority, tradition, grounded in Locke and associated with Hartley, Priestley and Godwin, mind was programmatically figured as mechanical, predi-cated upon the operations of the body, and thus completely indepen-dent of the 'authorized version' Christian soul.

That is not to say that thinkers of this Hartleyan materialist tendency consequently celebrated the superiority of the flesh, the corporeal over the conscious, nor that they became crass hedonists. Far from it. They set about creating new structures, paralleling those of the old-style Church belief they were replacing, which would set the psyche on the throne in place of the traditional immortal soul, figured as the captain of the self, exactly as the secular intellectual élite was replacing the clergy as the superior guiding force of society. The representatives of gross corporeality were the vulgar, the labour-ing poor; élites upheld their own superiority as creatures of mind rather than base matter.

Mind was meant to surpass matter in many ways. It could be engaged in disciplining the body through a stiff upper lip neo-

Stoicism, in a new reserve and control of the body prefiguring the Victorian culture of denial. It could be the preoccupation with delicate and superfine feeling that was displayed in the cult of sensibility. It might be the Romantic cult of the imagination, soaring above the moils and toils of the world that is too much with us. It could be the radical dictatorship of the body by the mind that was so provocatively advanced by William Godwin.

In other words, although there were tendencies towards naturalization, even secularization, in the long eighteenth century, this does not mean that the new self was identified with, reduced to, or seen as coterminous with the flesh. Rather it meant the moulding, disciplining and subordination of the flesh, the analysis and subordination of the *soma* which mind, imagination and education would bring.

This required uneasy and unstable compromises. In the nineteenth century powerful trends deplored what was regarded as the excessive prominence of or reliance upon the flesh spelt by commercial, industrialized and mechanized society. The reduction of workers to hands, the dissection of animals in laboratories – all these seemed, to many traditionalists, dangerous surrenders to a materialism whose explicit or implicit tendency was reductionism and the erosion of all moral and social order.

Equally, the Victorian era brought powerful psychological conflict. With new ambiguities about the immortal soul and growing stress upon the sovereignty of mind, death itself became all the more unthinkable and unspeakable. One consequence was the mawkish Victorian cult of death, with all its palaver and mystifications of belief masking a fundamental denial. The decline and fall of the traditional biblical and Christian story of the self did not result in the triumph of any single rival, but brought new and lonely agonies, evidenced for instance in Tennyson's *In Memoriam* (1850), with its hope of a future life, or, more positively, in John Henry Newman's *The Dream of Gerontius* (1865).*

---

* Both of these spelt out a doctrine of progressive salvation which was congenial to the Victorians. It was a kind of backdoor purgatory.

To reduce such changes to the grossest of functionalist terms, the mission of the emergent lay élites of the long eighteenth century was to elbow aside the traditional clergy, and so the old Christian soul became displaced; and to lord it over the plebs – hence its resistance to any embracing of or identification with the body as such. The new mental and cultural élites had a stalking-horse and shibboleth of their own: it was mind, and soon the march of mind, and for them progress became the secularization of salvation. The doctrine of mind over matter stood for power over the people.

BIBLIOGRAPHY

Mary Abbott, *Family Ties: English Families, 1540–1920* (London: Routledge, 1993).

Mary Abbott, *Life Cycles in England 1560–1720: Cradle to Grave* (London: Routledge, 1996).

R. M. Adams, *The Land and Literature of England: A Historical Account* (London: W. W. Norton, 1984).

Joseph Addison, *The Freeholder*, ed. James Leheny (Oxford: Oxford University Press, 1979).

John Addy, *Sin and Society in the Seventeenth Century* (London and New York: Routledge, 1989).

John Addy, *Death, Money and the Vultures: Inheritance and Avarice 1600–1750* (London: Routledge, 1992).

Jean-Christophe Agnew, *Worlds Apart: The Market and the Theater in Anglo-American Thought, 1550–1750* (Cambridge: Cambridge University Press, 1986).

William Albert, *The Turnpike Road System in England 1663–1840* (London: Cambridge University Press, 1972).

Geoffrey Alderman, *Modern Britain: 1700–1983: A Domestic History* (London: Croom Helm, 1986).

Geoffrey Alderman and Colin Holmes (eds.), *Outsiders and Outcasts: Essays in Honour of William J. Fishman* (London: Duckworth, 1991).

David Alexander, *Retailing in England during the Industrial Revolution* (London: Athlone Press, 1970).

Beverly Sprague Allen, *Tides in English Taste (1619–1800)* (New York: Pageant Books, 1958).

David Elliston Allen, *The Naturalist in Britain: A Social History* (London: Allen Lane, 1976).

Robert Joseph Allen, *The Clubs of Augustan London* (Cambridge, Mass.: Harvard University Press, 1933).

Richard D. Altick, *The Shows of London: A Panoramic History of Exhibitions, 1600–1862* (Cambridge, Mass.: Belknap Press, 1978).

Richard D. Altick, *Paintings from Books: Art and Literature in Britain, 1760–1900* (Columbus: Ohio State University Press, 1985).

Susan Dwyer Amussen, *An Ordered Society: Gender and Class in Early Modern England* (Oxford: Basil Blackwell, 1988).

Susan D. Amussen, 'Punishment, Discipline, and Power: The Social Meanings of Violence in Early Modern England', *Journal of British Studies*, 34 (1995), 1–34.

Susan D. Amussen and Mark A. Kishlansky (eds.), *Political Culture and Cultural Politics in Early Modern England: Essays Presented to David Underdown* (Manchester: Manchester University Press, 1995).

Michael Anderson, *Family Structure in Nineteenth Century Lancashire* (London: Cambridge University Press, 1971).

Michael Anderson, *Approaches to the History of the Western Family 1500–1914* (London: Macmillan, 1980).

Michael Anderson, *Population Change in North-*

Western Europe, 1750–1850 (London: Macmillan Education Ltd., 1988).

M. S. Anderson, *Historians and Eighteenth-Century Europe 1715–1789* (Oxford: Oxford University Press, 1979).

M. S. Anderson, *War and Society in Europe of the Old Regime, 1618–1789* (New York: St Martin's Press, 1988).

Patricia Anderson, *The Printed Image and the Transformation of Popular Culture 1790–1860* (Oxford: Clarendon Press, 1991).

R. D. Anderson, *Education and the Scottish People 1750–1918* (Oxford: Clarendon Press, 1995).

Donna T. Andrew, *Philanthropy and Police: London Charity in the Eighteenth Century* (Princeton: Princeton University Press, 1989).

Raymond A. Anselment, *'Betwixt Jest and Earnest': Marprelate, Milton, Marvell, Swift and the Decorum of Religious Ridicule* (Toronto: University of Toronto Press, 1979).

Raymond A. Anselment, *The Realms of Apollo: Literature and Healing in Seventeenth-Century England* (Newark, Del.: University of Delaware Press/Associated University Presses, 1995).

Joyce Oldham Appleby, 'Locke, Liberalism and the Natural Law of Money', *Past and Present*, 71 (1976), 43–69.

Joyce Oldham Appleby, 'Ideology and Theory: The Tension between Political and Economic Liberalism in Seventeenth Century England', *American Historical Review*, 81 (1976), 499–515.

Joyce Oldham Appleby, *Economic Thought and Ideology in Seventeenth-Century England* (Princeton: Princeton University Press, 1978).

Joyce Oldham Appleby, 'Modernization Theory and the Formation of Modern Social Theories in England and America', *Comparative Studies in Society and History*, 20 (1978), 259–85.

Joyce Oldham Appleby, 'Consumption in Early Modern Social Thought', in John Brewer and Roy Porter (eds.), *Consumption and the World of Goods* (London: Routledge, 1993), 162–75.

Anthony Arblaster, *The Rise and Decline of Western Liberalism* (Oxford: Basil Blackwell, 1984).

John Arbuthnot, *The History of John Bull* (Oxford: Oxford University Press, 1976).

Philippe Ariès, *Centuries of Childhood: A Social History of the Family* (Harmondsworth: Penguin Books, 1973).

Philippe Ariès, *Western Attitudes towards Death: From the Middle Ages to the Present* (London: Marion Boyars, 1976).

Philippe Ariès, *L'Homme devant la mort* (Paris: Seuil, 1977), trans. Helen Weaver as *The Hour of our Death* (London: Allen Lane, 1981).

David Armitage, Armand Himy and Quentin Skinner (eds.), *Milton and Republicanism* (Cambridge: Cambridge University Press, 1996).

Alan Armstrong, *Farmworkers in England and Wales: A Social and Economic History 1770–1980* (Ames: Iowa State University Press, 1988).

Nancy Armstrong and Leonard Tennenhouse, *The Imaginary Puritan: Literature, Intellectual Labor, and the Origins of Personal Life* (Berkeley: University of California Press, 1992).

W. H. G. Armytage, *Heavens Below: Utopian Experiments in England 1560–1960* (London: Routledge and Kegan Paul, 1961).

W. H. G. Armytage, *Yesterday's Tomorrows: A Historical Survey of Future Societies* (London: Routledge and Kegan Paul, 1968).

W. H. G. Armytage, *Four Hundred Years of English Education*, 2nd edn. (Cambridge: Cambridge University Press, 1970).

Ronald G. Asch (ed.), *Three Nations – A Common History? England, Scotland, Ireland and British History c. 1600–1920* (Bochum: Universitätsverlag Dr N. Brockmeyer, 1993).

Richard Ashcraft and Alan Roper, *Politics as Reflected in Literature* (Los Angeles: William Andrews Clark Memorial Library, University of California, 1989).

T. S. Ashton, *An Eighteenth-Century Industrialist: Peter Stubs of Warrington* (Manchester: Manchester University Press, 1939).

T. S. Ashton, *An Economic History of England: The Eighteenth Century* (London: Methuen, 1955).

T. S. Ashton, *Economic Fluctuations in England 1700–1800* (Oxford: Clarendon Press, 1959).

T. S. Ashton, *The Industrial Revolution 1760–1830* (Oxford: Oxford University Press, 1968).

P. S. Atiyah, *The Rise and Fall of Freedom of Contract* (Oxford: Clarendon Press, 1979).

John Aubrey, *Brief Lives*, ed. Richard Barber (Totowa, NJ: Barnes and Noble, 1983).

Nina Auerbach, *Romantic Imprisonment: Women and Other Glorified Outcasts* (New York: Columbia University Press, 1985).

Peter Aughton, *Endeavour: The Story of Captain Cook's First Great Epic Voyage* (Moreton-in-Marsh: Windrush Press, 1999).

Stanley Ayling, *John Wesley* (London: Collins, 1979).

Stanley Ayling, *Edmund Burke: His Life and Opinions* (London: John Murray, 1988).

James Ayres, *English Naive Painting, 1750–1900* (London and New York: Thames and Hudson, 1980).

Philip Ayres, *Classical Culture and the Idea of Rome in Eighteenth-Century England* (Cambridge: Cambridge University Press, 1997).

Robert W. Babcock, *The Genesis of Shakespeare Idolatry, 1766–1799: A Study in English Criticism of the Late Eighteenth Century* (Chapel Hill: University of North Carolina Press, 1931).

Paula R. Backscheider, *Daniel Defoe: His Life* (Baltimore: Johns Hopkins University Press, 1992).

Paula R. Backscheider, *Spectacular Politics:*

Theatrical Power and Mass Culture in Early Modern England (Baltimore: Johns Hopkins University Press, 1994).

Paula R. Backscheider and Timothy Dystal, *The Intersections of the Public and Private Spheres in Early Modern England* (London: Frank Cass, 1996).

D. W. R. Bahlman, *The Moral Revolution of 1688* (New Haven: Yale University Press, 1957).

Stephen Bailey, *Taste: The Secret Meaning of Things* (London and Boston: Faber, 1991).

Victor Bailey (ed.), *Policing and Punishment in Nineteenth-Century Britain* (London: Croom Helm, 1981).

J. H. Baker (ed.), *The Reports of Sir John Spelman*, vol. 2 (London: Selden Society, 1978).

Chris Baldick, *In Frankenstein's Shadow: Myth, Monstrosity, and Nineteenth-Century Writing* (Oxford: Clarendon Press, 1990).

Harry Ballam and Roy Lewis (eds.), *The Visitors' Book: England and the English as Others Have Seen Them A.D. 1500–1950* (London: Max Parrish, 1950).

Jacqueline Banerjee, *Through the Northern Gate: Childhood and Growing Up in British Fiction, 1719–1901* (New York: Peter Lang, 1996).

A. Barbeau, *Life and Letters at Bath in the Eighteenth Century*, ed. A. Dobson (London: Heinemann, 1904).

Felix Barker and Ralph Hyde, *London As It Might Have Been* (London: John Murray, 1982).

Hannah Barker, *Newspapers, Politics and Public Opinion in Late Eighteenth-Century England* (Oxford: Clarendon Press, 1998).

Rodney Barker, *Politics, Peoples and Government* (London: Macmillan, 1994).

T. C. Barker, J. C. McKenzie and J. Yudkin, *Our Changing Fare: Two Hundred Years of British Food Habits* (London: McGibbon and Kee, 1966).

Theo Barker (ed.), *The Long March of Everyman 1750–1960* (Harmondsworth: Penguin, 1978).

F. J. Barker-Benfield, *The Horrors of the Half-Known Life* (New York: Harper and Row, 1976).

F. J. Barker-Benfield, *The Culture of Sensibility: Sex and Society in Eighteenth-Century Britain* (Chicago: University of Chicago Press, 1992).

Tony Barnard and Jane Clarke (eds.), *Lord Burlington: Architecture, Art and Life* (London: Hambledon Press, 1995).

Anthony Barnett, *Iron Britannia* (London: Allison and Busby, 1982).

John Barrell, *The Idea of Landscape and the Sense of Place 1730–1840: An Approach to the Poetry of John Clare* (London: Cambridge University Press, 1972).

John Barrell, *The Dark Side of the Landscape: The Rural Poor in English Painting, 1730–1840* (Cambridge: Cambridge University Press, 1980).

John Barrell, *English Literature in History, 1730–80: An Equal, Wide Survey* (London: Hutchinson, 1983).

John Barrell, *The Political Theory of Painting from Reynolds to Hazlitt: The Body of the Public* (New Haven: Yale University Press, 1986).

John Barrell (ed.), *Painting and the Politics of Culture: New Essays on British Art 1700–1850* (Oxford: Oxford University Press, 1992).

A. Barrow, *The Flesh is Weak: An Intimate History of the Church of England* (London: Hamilton, 1980).

Jonathan Barry (ed.), *The Tudor and the Stuart Town, 1530–1688: A Reader in English Urban History* (London: Longman, 1990).

Jonathan Barry and Christopher Brooks (eds.), *The Middling Sort of People: Culture, Society and Politics in England, 1550–1800* (Basingstoke: Macmillan, 1994).

Jonathan Barry and Colin Jones (eds.), *Medicine and Charity before the Welfare State* (London: Routledge, 1994).

Jonathan Barry, Marianne Hester and Gareth Roberts (eds.), *Witchcraft in Early Modern Europe: Studies in Culture and Belief* (Cambridge: Cambridge University Press, 1996).

Anne Barton, *Ben Jonson: Dramatist* (Cambridge: Cambridge University Press, 1984).

Richard Bauman, *Let Your Words Be Few: Symbolism of Speaking and Silence among Seventeenth-Century Quakers* (Cambridge: Cambridge University Press, 1983).

Michael Baumber, *General-at-Sea: Robert Blake and the Seventeenth-Century Revolution in Naval Warfare* (London: John Murray, 1989).

J. M. Beattie, 'The Criminality of Women in Eighteenth-Century England', *Journal of Social History*, 8 (1975), 80–116.

J. M. Beattie, *Crime and the Courts in England, 1660–1800* (Oxford: Oxford University Press, 1986).

E. D. Bebb, *Nonconformity and Social and Economic Life, 1660–1800* (London: Epworth Press, 1935).

D. W. Bebbington, *Evangelicalism in Modern Britain: A History from the 1730s to the 1980s* (London: Unwin Hyman, 1989).

Marvin B. Becker, *The Emergence of Civil Society in the Eighteenth Century: A Privileged Moment in the History of England, Scotland, and France* (Bloomington: Indiana University Press, 1994).

J. V. Beckett, *The Aristocracy in England, 1660–1914* (Oxford: Blackwell, 1986).

Robert Beddard (ed.), *The Revolutions of 1688* (Oxford: Clarendon Press, 1991).

A. V. Beedell and A. D. Harvey (eds.), *The Prison Diary (16 May–22 November 1794) of John Horne Tooke* (Leeds: Leeds Philosophical and Literary Society, 1995).

A. L. Beier, *The Problem of the Poor in Tudor and Early Stuart England* (London: Methuen, 1983).

A. L. Beier, *Masterless Men: The Vagrancy Problem in England 1560–1640* (London: Methuen, 1985).

A. L. Beier, ' "Utter Strangers to Industry, Morality and Religion": John Locke on the Poor', *Eighteenth Century Life*, 12 (1988), 28–41.

A. L. Beier, D. Cannadine and J. M. Rosenheim (eds.), *The First Modern Society: Essays in English History in Honour of Lawrence Stone* (Cambridge: Cambridge University Press, 1989).

A. L. Beier and Roger Finlay (eds.), *London 1500–1700: The Making of the Metropolis* (London: Longman, 1986).

Lucinda McCray Beier, *Sufferers and Healers: The Experience of Illness in Seventeenth-Century England* (London: Routledge and Kegan Paul, 1987).

John Belcham, *Industrialization and the Working Class: The English Experience, 1750–1900* (Aldershot: Scolar Press, 1990).

Ian H. Bell, *Literature and Crime in Augustan England* (London: Routledge, 1991).

R. Bellamy (ed.), *Victorian Liberalism: Nineteenth-Century Political Thought and Practice* (London: Routledge, 1990).

Mark Bence-Jones, *Great Catholic Families* (London: Constable, 1992).

J. Miriam Benn, *Predicaments of Love* (London: Pluto Press, 1992).

Michael Bentley (ed.), *Public and Private Doctrine: Essays in British History Presented to Maurice Cowling* (Cambridge: Cambridge University Press, 1993).

Maxine Berg (ed.), *Markets and Manufacture in Early Industrial Europe* (London: Routledge, 1991).

Maxine Berg, 'What Difference did Women's Work Make to the Industrial Revolution?', *History Workshop*, 35 (1993), 22–44.

Maxine Berg, *The Age of Manufactures, 1700–1820: Industry, Innovation and Work in Britain* (London: Routledge, 1994).

Maxine Berg and Helen Clifford (eds.), *Consumers and Luxury: Consumer Culture in Europe 1650–1850* (Manchester: Manchester University Press, 1999).

Maxine Berg, Pat Hudson and Michael Sonenscher (eds.), *Manufacture in Town and County before the Factory* (Cambridge: Cambridge University Press, 1983).

Lenard R. Berlanstein (ed.), *The Industrial Revolution and Work in Nineteenth-Century Europe* (London: Routledge, 1992).

Ann Bermingham, *Landscape and Ideology: The English Rustic Tradition 1740–1860* (Berkeley: University of California Press, 1986).

Ann Bermingham and John Brewer (eds.), *The Consumption of Culture, 1600–1800: Image, Object, Text* (London: Routledge, 1995).

Christopher J. Berry, *The Idea of Luxury: A Conceptual and Historical Investigation* (Cambridge: Cambridge University Press, 1994).

Jonquil Bevan, *Izaak Walton's 'The Compleat Angler': The Art of Recreation* (New York: St Martin's Press, 1988).

Hans Binneveld and Rudolf Dekker (eds.), *Curing and Insuring – Essays on Illness in Past Times: The Netherlands, Belgium, England and Italy, 16th–20th Centuries* (Rotterdam: Verloren Publishers and Erasmus University, 1993).

Derek Birley, *Sport and the Making of Britain* (Manchester: Manchester University Press, 1993).

Urs Bitterli, *Cultures in Conflict: Encounters between European and Non-European Cultures, 1492–1800*, trans. Ritchie Robertson (Oxford: Polity Press, 1989).

J. B. Black, *The Art of History* (New York: Russell and Russell, 1965).

Jeremy Black (ed.), *Britain in the Age of Walpole* (London: Macmillan, 1984).

Jeremy Black, *British Foreign Policy in the Age of Walpole* (Edinburgh: John Donald, 1985).

Jeremy Black, *The English Press in the Eighteenth Century* (London: Croom Helm, 1986).

Jeremy Black, *Natural and Necessary Enemies: Anglo-French Relations in the Eighteenth Century* (London: Duckworth, 1986).

Jeremy Black, 'England's "Ancien Regime"?', *History Today*, 38 (1988), 43–50.

Jeremy Black (ed.), *Knights Errant and True Englishmen: British Foreign Policy, 1660–1800* (Edinburgh: John Donald, 1989).

Jeremy Black, 'Party Politics in Eighteenth-Century Britain', *Lamar Journal of the Humanities*, 15 (1989), 2–38.

Jeremy Black (ed.), *British Politics and Society from Walpole to Pitt 1742–89* (London: Macmillan, 1990).

Jeremy Black, 'The British Press and Eighteenth-Century Revolution: The French Case', in P. Dukes and J. Dunkley (eds.), *Culture and Revolution* (London: Pinter Publishers, 1990), 110–20.

Jeremy Black, *Culloden and the '45* (Stroud: Sutton, 1990).

Jeremy Black (ed.), *Eighteenth-Century Europe 1700–1789* (London: Macmillan, 1990).

Jeremy Black, *Robert Walpole and the Nature of Politics in Early Eighteenth-Century Britain* (London: Macmillan, 1990).

Jeremy Black, 'Tourism and Cultural Challenge: The Changing Scene of the Eighteenth Century', in J. McVeagh (ed.), *English Literature and the Wider World*, vol. 1, *1660–1780: All Before Them* (London: Ashfield, 1990), 185–202.

J. Black, 'A Stereotyped Response?: The Grand Tour and Continental Cuisine', *Durham University Journal*, 83 (1991), 147–53.

Jeremy Black, *A System of Ambition? British Foreign Policy 1660–1793* (London: Longman, 1991).

Jeremy Black, *Pitt the Elder* (Cambridge and New York: Cambridge University Press, 1993).

Jeremy Black, *The Politics of Britain, 1688–1800* (Manchester: Manchester University Press, 1993).

Jeremy Black, *British Foreign Policy in an Age of Revolutions, 1783–1793* (Cambridge: Cambridge University Press, 1994).

Jeremy Black, *Convergence or Divergence? Britain and the Continent* (Basingstoke: Macmillan Press, 1994).

Jeremy Black, *European Warfare, 1660–1815* (London: UCL Press, 1994).

Jeremy Black, *The Grand Tour: The British Abroad in the Eighteenth Century* (Stroud: Sutton Publishing, 1996).

Jeremy Black, 'Cultural History and the Eighteenth Century', *Bulletin de la société d'études anglo-américaines des XVIIe et XVIIIe siècles*, 42 (1996), 7–20.

Jeremy Black (ed.), *Culture and Society in Britain 1660–1800* (Manchester: Manchester University Press, 1997).

Jeremy Black, *Maps and Politics* (London: Reaktion Books, 1997).

Jeremy Black and Jeremy Gregory (eds.), *Culture, Politics and Society in Britain, 1660–1800* (Manchester: Manchester University Press, 1991).

Jeremy Black and Roy Porter (eds.), *A Dictionary of Eighteenth-Century World History* (Oxford: Blackwell, 1994).

Olivia Bland, *The Royal Way of Death* (London: Constable, 1986).

T. C. W. Blanning (ed.), *The Eighteenth Century: Europe 1688–1815* (Oxford: Clarendon Press, 2000).

T. C. W. Blanning (ed.), *The Nineteenth Century: Europe 1789–1914* (Oxford: Clarendon Press, 2000).

Norberto Bobbio, *Hobbes and the Natural Law Tradition*, trans. Daniela Gobetti (Chicago: University of Chicago Press, 1993).

John Bohstedt, *Riots and Community Politics in England and Wales 1790–1810* (London: Harvard University Press, 1983).

Alan Bold (ed.), *Drink to Me Only: The Prose (and Cons) of Drinking* (London: Robin Clark, 1982).

R. R. Bolgar (ed.), *Classical Influences on Western Thought A.D. 1650–1870* (Cambridge: Cambridge University Press, 1979).

Christine Bolt, *The Women's Movement in the United States and Britain from the 1790s to the 1920s* (Amherst: University of Massachusetts Press, 1993).

Peter Borsay, 'The Rise of the Promenade:

The Social and Cultural Use of Space in the English Provincial Town, c. 1660–1800', *British Journal for Eighteenth-Century Studies*, 9 (1986), 125–40.

Peter Borsay, *The English Urban Renaissance: Culture and Society in the Provincial Town 1660–1770* (Oxford: Clarendon Press, 1989).

Peter Borsay (ed.), *The Eighteenth-Century Town: A Reader in English Urban History 1688–1820* (London: Longman, 1990).

Peter Borsay, *The Image of Georgian Bath 1700–2000* (Oxford: Oxford University Press, 2000).

Peter Borsay and Angus McInnes, 'The Emergence of a Leisure Town: Or an Urban Renaissance?', *Past and Present*, 126 (1990), 189–202.

Lourens van den Bosch and Jan Bremmer (eds.), *Between Poverty and the Pyre – Moments in the History of Widowhood* (London: Routledge, 1995).

Robert S. Bosher, *The Making of the Restoration Settlement* (London: Dacre Press, 1951).

Ray Boston, *The Essential Fleet Street: Its History and Influence* (London: Blandford Press, 1990).

Ian Bostridge, *Witchcraft and its Transformation, c.1650–c.1750* (Oxford: Clarendon Press, 1997).

James T. Boulton, *The Language of Politics in the Age of Wilkes and Burke* (London: Routledge and Kegan Paul, 1963).

Jeremy Boulton, *Neighbourhood and Society: A London Suburb in the Seventeenth Century* (Cambridge: Cambridge University Press, 1987).

E. W. Bovill, *English Country Life 1780–1830* (London: Oxford University Press, 1962).

George R. Boyer, *An Economic History of the English Poor Law, 1750–1850* (Cambridge: Cambridge University Press, 1990).

Michael J. Braddick, *The Nerves of State: Taxation and the Financing of the English State, 1558–1714* (Manchester: Manchester University Press, 1996).

James E. Bradley, *Religion, Revolution and English Radicalism: Non-Conformity in Eighteenth-Century Politics and Society* (Cambridge: Cambridge University Press, 1990).

Brendan Bradshaw and Peter Roberts (eds.), *British Consciousness and Identity: The Making of Britain, 1533–1707* (Cambridge: Cambridge University Press, 1998).

Stephen E. Braidwood, *London's Blacks and the Foundation of the Sierra Leone Settlement 1786–1791* (Liverpool: Liverpool University Press, 1994).

Dennis Brailsford, *Bareknuckles: A Social History of Prize-Fighting* (Cambridge: Lutterworth, 1988).

Dennis Brailsford, *Sport, Time and Society* (London: Routledge, 1990).

Dennis Brailsford, *British Sport: A Social History* (Cambridge: Lutterworth, 1992).

Dennis Brailsford, *Sport and the Making of Britain* (Manchester: Manchester University Press, 1993).

Patrick Brantlinger, *Bread and Circuses: Theories of Mass Culture as Social Decay* (Ithaca, NY: Cornell University Press, 1985).

Patrick Brantlinger (ed.), *Energy and Entropy: Science and Culture in Victorian Britain* (Bloomington: Indiana University Press, 1989).

Fernand Braudel, *The Structures of Everyday Life: The Limits of the Possible* (London: Collins, 1981).

Fernand Braudel, *Civilization and Capitalism, 15th–18th Century*, 3 vols. (London: Collins, 1981–4).

Peter Brears et al., *A Taste of History: 10,000 Years of Food in Britain* (London: English Heritage, 1993).

Gregory W. Bredbeck, *Sodomy and Interpretation: Marlowe to Milton* (Ithaca, NY: Cornell University Press, 1991).

Mark Breitenberg, *Anxious Masculinity in Early Modern England* (Cambridge: Cambridge University Press, 1996).

John Brewer, 'Party and the Double Cabinet:

Two Facets of Burke's *Thoughts*', *Historical Journal*, 14 (1971), 479–501.

John Brewer, 'The Faces of Lord Bute: A Visual Contribution to Anglo-American Political Ideology', *Perspectives in American History*, 6 (1972), 95–116.

John Brewer, 'The Misfortunes of Lord Bute: A Case Study in Eighteenth-Century Political Argument and Public Opinion', *Historical Journal*, 16 (1973), 3–43.

John Brewer, 'Lord Bute', in H. Van Thal (ed.), *The British Prime Ministers*, vol. 1 (London: Allen and Unwin, 1974), 103–13.

John Brewer, 'Rockingham, Burke and Whig Political Argument', *Historical Journal*, 18 (1975), 188–201.

John Brewer, 'Ideas of Revolution', in Kenneth Pearson (ed.), *1776: The British Story of the American Revolution* (London: Times Books, 1976).

John Brewer, 'The Look of London', in Kenneth Pearson (ed.), *1776: The British Story of the American Revolution* (London: Times Books, 1976).

John Brewer, *Party Ideology and Popular Politics at the Accession of George III* (Cambridge: Cambridge University Press, 1976).

John Brewer, 'Theatre and Counter-Theatre in Georgian Politics: The Mock Elections at Garrett', *Radical History Review*, 22 (1979–80), 7–40.

John Brewer, 'An Ungovernable People: Law and Disorder in Seventeenth and Eighteenth Century England', *History Today*, 30 (1980), 18–27.

John Brewer, 'The No. 45: A Wilkite Political Symbol', in Stephen Baxter (ed.), *England's Rise to Greatness* (Berkeley: California University Press, 1983), 349–80.

John Brewer, *The Common People and Politics, 1750–1790s* (Cambridge: Chadwyck Healey, 1986).

John Brewer, *The Sinews of Power: War, Money and the English State 1688–1783* (London: Unwin Hyman, 1989).

John Brewer, 'This Monstrous Tragi-Comic Scene', in David Bindman (ed.), *In the Shadow of the Guillotine: British Reactions to the French Revolution* (London: British Museum, 1989), 9–25.

John Brewer, 'Cultural Production in Eighteenth-Century England: The View of the Reader', in Rudolf Vierhaus *et al.* (eds.), *Frühe Neuzeit – frühe Moderne? Forschungen zur Vielschichtigkeit von Übergangsprozessen* (Göttingen: Vandenhoeck & Ruprecht, 1992), 375–408.

John Brewer, 'Cultural Production, Consumption and the Place of the Artist in 18th Century England', in Brian Allen, Michael Kitson, David Solkin *et al.* (eds.), *Towards a Modern Art World: Art in Britain c.1715–1880* (New Haven: Yale University Press, 1995), 7–25.

John Brewer, 'This, That and the Other: Public, Social and Private in the Seventeenth and Eighteenth Centuries', in Dario Castiglione and Lesley Sharpe (eds.), *Shifting the Boundaries: Transformation of the Languages of Public and Private in the Eighteenth Century* (Exeter: University of Exeter Press, 1995), 1–22.

John Brewer, *The Pleasures of the Imagination: English Culture in the Eighteenth Century* (London: HarperCollins, 1997).

John Brewer, 'Readers and Reading in Eighteenth-Century Britain', *Cultura: Revista de Historia e Teoria das Ideas*, 9 (1997), 159–185.

John Brewer, 'John Marsh's History of My Private Life, 1752–1828', in Tim Blanning and David Cannadine (eds.), *History and Biography: Essays in Honour of Derek Beales* (Cambridge University Press, 1996) 72–87.

John Brewer and Laurence Fontaine, 'Homo Creditus et Construction de la Confiance au XVIIIe siècle', in Philippe Bernoux and Jean-Michael Servet (eds.), *La Construction sociale de la confiance* (Paris:

Association d'Économie Financière, Collection Finance-Éthique-Confiance, 1997).

John Brewer and Eckhart Hellmuth, (eds.), *Rethinking Leviathan: The British and German States in Comparative Perspective* (German Historical Institute Publications; Oxford: Oxford University Press, 1999).

John Brewer and Roy Porter (eds.), *Consumption and the World of Goods* (London: Routledge, 1993).

John Brewer and Susan Staves (eds.), *Early Modern Conceptions of Property* (London: Routledge, 1995).

Asa Briggs, *The Age of Improvement 1783–1867* (London: Longmans, 1959).

Asa Briggs, *How They Lived: An Anthology of Original Documents Written between 1700 and 1815* (Oxford: Basil Blackwell, 1969).

Asa Briggs, 'The Language of "Mass" and "Masses" in Nineteenth-Century England', in David E. Martin and David Rubinstein (eds.), *Ideology and the Labour Movement: Essays Presented to John Saville* (London: Croom Helm, 1979), 62–83.

Asa Briggs, *A Social History of England*, 2nd edn. (Harmondsworth: Penguin, 1987).

Asa Briggs and Daniel Snowman (eds.), *Fins de Siècle: How Centuries End 1400–2000* (New Haven: Yale University Press, 1996).

John Briggs, Christopher Harrison, Angus McInnes and David Vincent, *Crime and Punishment in England: An Introductory History* (London: UCL Press, 1996).

Jean R. Brink, *Privileging Gender in Early Modern England* (Kirksville, Mo.: Sixteenth Century Journal Publishers, 1993).

Edward J. Bristow, *Vice and Vigilance: Purity Movements in Britain since 1700* (Dublin: Gill and Macmillan, 1977; Totowa, NJ: Rowman and Littlefield, 1977)).

M. G. Brock and M. C. Curthoys (eds.), *The History of the University of Oxford*, vol. 6: *Nineteenth Century Oxford, Part 1* (Oxford: Clarendon Press, 1997).

W. H. Brock, *From Protyle to Proton: William Prout and the Nature of Matter, 1785–1985* (Boston: Adam Hilger, 1985).

Jacob Bronowski, *William Blake: A Man Without a Mask* (London: Secker and Warburg, 1944).

Jacob Bronowski, *William Blake and the Age of Revolution* (London: Routledge and Kegan Paul, 1972).

Iris Brooke, *A History of English Costume* (London: Eyre Methuen, 1979).

Derek R. Brookes (ed.), *Thomas Reid: An Inquiry into the Human Mind on the Principles of Common Sense* (Edinburgh: Edinburgh University Press, 1997).

David Brown, *Walter Scott and the Historical Imagination* (London: Routledge and Kegan Paul, 1979).

Ford K. Brown, *Fathers of the Victorians: The Age of Wilberforce* (Cambridge: Cambridge University Press, 1961).

Jonathan Brown, *The English Market Town: A Social and Economic History, 1750–1914* (Marlborough: Crowood Press, 1986).

Kenneth D. Brown, *The English Labour Movement: 1700–1951* (New York: St Martin's Press, 1982).

K. D. Brown, *A Social History of the Non-Conformist Ministry in England and Wales, 1800–1930* (Oxford: Clarendon Press, 1988).

Laura Brown, *Ends of Empire: Women and Ideology in Early Eighteenth-Century English Literature* (Ithaca, NY: Cornell University Press, 1993).

Philip Anthony Brown, *The French Revolution in English History* (London: Frank Cass, 1965).

Richard Brown, *Church and State in Modern Britain 1700–1850* (London: Routledge, 1991).

Richard Brown, *Society and Economy in Modern Britain 1700–1850* (London: Routledge, 1991).

Stewart J. Brown, *Thomas Chalmers and the Godly Commonwealth in Scotland* (Oxford: Oxford University Press, 1982).

Alice Browne, *The Eighteenth Century Feminist*

Mind (Brighton: Harvester Press; Detroit: Wayne State University Press, 1987).

Reed Browning, *Political and Constitutional Ideas of the Court Whigs* (Baton Rouge: Louisiana State University Press, 1982).

Henry Broxap, *The Later Non-Jurors* (Cambridge: Cambridge University Press, 1924).

Anthony Bruce, *The Purchase System in the British Army 1660–1871* (London: Royal Historical Society, 1980).

Sir Arthur Bryant and J. P. Kenyon, *A History of Britain and the British Peoples*, vol. 2: *Freedom's Own Island: The British Oceanic Expansion* (London: Collins, 1986).

Margaret Bryant, *The Unexpected Revolution: A Study in the Education of Women and Girls in the Nineteenth Century* (London: University of London Institute of Education, 1980; distributed by NFER Publication Co. Ltd., Windsor).

Bill Bryson, *Mother Tongue: The English Language* (London: Hamish Hamilton, 1990).

W. H. Bryson, *The Equity Side of the Exchequer* (Cambridge: Cambridge University Press, 1975).

R. A. Buchanan, *The Engineers: A History of the Engineering Profession in Britain 1750–1914* (London: Jessica Kingsley, 1989).

Robert O. Bucholz, *The Augustan Court: Queen Anne and the Decline of Court Culture* (Stanford, Calif.: Stanford University Press, 1993).

Anne Buck, *Dress in Eighteenth-Century England* (London: B. T. Batsford Ltd., 1979).

Jerome Hamilton Buckley, *The Triumph of Time: A Study of the Victorian Concepts of Time, History, Progress, and Decadence* (Cambridge, Mass.: Harvard University Press, 1966).

Jerome Hamilton Buckley, *The Turning Key: Autobiography and the Subjective Impulse since 1800* (Cambridge, Mass.: Harvard University Press, 1984).

M. J. Buckley, *At the Origins of Modern Atheism* (New Haven: Yale University Press, 1987).

Julia Buckroyd, *Church and State in Scotland, 1660–1681* (Edinburgh: John Donald, 1980).

R. F. Bud and G. K. Roberts, *Science Versus Practice: Chemistry in Victorian Britain* (Manchester: Manchester University Press, 1984).

J. B. Bullen (ed.), *The Sun is God: Painting, Literature, and Mythology in the Nineteenth Century* (Oxford: Clarendon Press, 1989).

J. B. Bullen, *The Myth of the Renaissance in Nineteenth-Century Writing* (Oxford: Clarendon Press, 1994).

J. M. Bumsted, *The People's Clearance 1770–1815* (Edinburgh: Edinburgh University Press, 1982).

E. J. Burford, *Wits, Wenchers and Wantons: London's Low Life: Covent Garden in the Eighteenth Century* (London: Robert Hale, 1992).

Glenn Burgess, *Absolute Monarchy and the Stuart Constitution* (New Haven: Yale University Press, 1996).

Andre Burguiere *et al.* (eds.), *A History of the Family: The Impact of Modernity* (Cambridge: Polity Press, 1996).

John Burnett, *Idle Hands: The Experience of Unemployment, 1790–1990* (London: Routledge, 1994).

John Burnett, David Vincent and David Mayall (eds.), *The Autobiography of the Working Class: An Annotated, Critical Bibliography*, vol. 3: *Supplement 1790–1945* (Hemel Hempstead: Harvester Wheatsheaf, 1989).

R. M. Burns, *The Great Debate on Miracles, from Joseph Glanvill to David Hume* (Lewisburg, Pa: Bucknell University Press, 1981).

J. W. Burrow, *A Liberal Descent: Victorian Historians and the English Past* (Cambridge: Cambridge University Press, 1981).

J. W. Burrow, *Gibbon* (Oxford: Oxford University Press, 1985).

J. W. Burrow, *Whigs and Liberals: Continuity and Change in English Political Thought* (Oxford: Clarendon Press, 1988).

Anthony Burton, *William Cobbett: Englishman. A Biography* (London: Aurum, 1997).

Matthias Buschkühl, *Great Britain and the Holy See 1746–1870* (Dublin: Irish Academic Press, 1982).

M. L. Bush, *The English Aristocracy: A Comparative Synthesis* (Manchester: Manchester University Press, 1984).

M. L. Bush (ed.), *Social Orders and Social Classes in Europe since 1500: Studies in Social Stratification* (London: Longman, 1992).

Bob Bushaway, *By Rite: Custom, Ceremony and Community in England, 1700–1880* (London: Junction Books, 1982).

David Butler, *Methodists and Papists: John Wesley and the Catholic Church in the Eighteenth Century* (London: Darton, Longman and Todd, 1995).

Marilyn Butler, *Maria Edgeworth: A Literary Biography* (Oxford: Clarendon Press, 1972).

Marilyn Butler, *Jane Austen and the War of Ideas* (Oxford: Clarendon Press, 1975).

Marilyn Butler, *Peacock Displayed: A Satirist in his Context* (London: Routledge and Kegan Paul, 1979).

Marilyn Butler, *Romantics, Rebels and Reactionaries: English Literature and its Background 1760–1830* (Oxford: Oxford University Press, 1981).

Marilyn Butler (ed.), *Burke, Paine, Godwin, and the Revolution Controversy* (Cambridge: Cambridge University Press, 1984).

M. Butler, *Theatre and Crisis: 1632–1642* (Cambridge: Cambridge University Press, 1984).

Marilyn Butler, 'Romanticism in England', in Roy Porter and Mikuláš Teich (eds.), *Romanticism in National Context* (Cambridge: Cambridge University Press, 1988), 37–67.

James Buzard, *The Beaten Track: European Tourism, Literature, and Ways to Culture, 1800–1918* (Oxford: Clarendon Press, 1993).

W. F. Bynum, *Science and the Practice of Medicine in the Nineteenth Century* (Cambridge: Cambridge University Press, 1994).

W. F. Bynum and Roy Porter (eds.), *William Hunter and the Eighteenth-Century Medical World* (Cambridge: Cambridge University Press, 1985).

W. F. Bynum and Roy Porter (eds.), *Medical Fringe and Medical Orthodoxy 1750–1850* (London: Croom Helm, 1986).

W. F. Bynum and Roy Porter (eds.), *The Anatomy of Madness: Essays in the History of Psychiatry*, vol. 3: *The Asylum and its Psychiatry* (London: Routledge, 1988).

Penelope Byrde, *The Male Image: Men's Fashion in Britain 1300–1970* (London: Batsford, 1979).

Lucy Caffyn, *Workers' Housing in West Yorkshire, 1750–1920* (London: HMSO; Lanham, Md: Bernan Associates, 1986).

R. A. Cage (ed.), *The Scots Abroad: Labour, Capital, Enterprise, 1750–1914* (London: Croom Helm, 1985).

R. A. Cage (ed.), *The Working Class in Glasgow 1750–1914* (London: Croom Helm, 1987).

Susan Cahn, *Industry of Devotion: The Transformation of Women's Work in England 1500–1660* (New York: Columbia University Press, 1987).

P. J. Cain, *Economic Foundations of British Overseas Expansion* (London: Macmillan, 1980).

P. J. Cain and A. G. Hopkins, *British Imperialism: Innovation and Expansion 1688–1914* (London: Longman, 1993).

Barbara Caine, *English Feminism, 1780–1980* (Oxford: Oxford University Press, 1997).

Craig Calhoun, *The Question of Class Struggle: Social Foundations of Popular Radicalism during the Industrial Revolution* (Oxford: Basil Blackwell, 1982).

Charles Camic, *Experience and Enlightenment: Socialization for Cultural Change in Eighteenth-Century Scotland* (Edinburgh: Edinburgh University Press, 1983).

Charles Camic, 'Experience and Ideas: Education for Universalism in Eighteenth Century Scotland', *Comparative Studies in Society and History*, 25 (1983), 51–82.

R. H. Campbell, *Scotland Since 1707: The Rise of an Industrial Society* (Oxford: Blackwell, 1965).

R. H. Campbell and Andrew S. Skinner (eds.), *The Origins and Nature of the Scottish Enlightenment* (Edinburgh: Edinburgh University Press, 1982).

David Cannadine, *Lords and Landlords: The Aristocracy and the Towns, 1774–1967* (Leicester: Leicester University Press, 1980).

David Cannadine (ed.), *Patricians, Power and Politics in Nineteenth-Century Towns* (Leicester: Leicester University Press, 1982).

David Cannadine, 'British History: Past, Present – and Future?', *Past and Present*, 116 (1987), 169–81.

David Cannadine, *The Pleasures of the Past* (London: Collins, 1989).

David Cannadine, *The Decline and Fall of the British Aristocracy* (New Haven: Yale University Press, 1990).

David Cannadine, *Aspects of Aristocracy: Grandeur and Decline in Modern Britain* (New Haven: Yale University Press, 1994).

David Cannadine and Simon Price (eds.), *Rituals of Royalty: Power and Ceremonial in Traditional Societies* (Cambridge: Cambridge University Press, 1993).

David Cannadine and David Reeder (eds.), *Exploring the Urban Past: Essays in Urban History by H. J. Dyos* (Cambridge: Cambridge University Press, 1982).

John Cannon, *Parliamentary Reform 1640–1832* (London: Cambridge University Press, 1972).

John Cannon (ed.), *The Whig Ascendancy: Colloquies on Hanoverian England* (London: Edward Arnold, 1981).

John Cannon, *Aristocratic Century: The Peerage of Eighteenth-Century England* (Cambridge: Cambridge University Press, 1984).

John Cannon, *Samuel Johnson and the Politics of Hanoverian England* (Oxford: Clarendon Press, 1994).

Nicholas Canny, *The Upstart Earl: A Study of the Social and Mental World of Richard Boyle, First Earl of Cork, 1566–1643* (Cambridge: Cambridge University Press, 1982).

Nicholas Canny, *Kingdom and Colony: Ireland in the Atlantic World, 1560–1800* (Baltimore: Johns Hopkins University Press, 1988).

Geoffrey Cantor, *Michael Faraday: Sandemanian and Scientist* (London: Macmillan, 1991).

Leonard Cantor, *The Changing English Countryside, 1400–1700* (London: Routledge and Kegan Paul, 1987).

Bernard Capp, *Astrology and the Popular Press: English Almanacs, 1500–1800* (London: Faber & Faber, 1979).

Bernard Capp, *English Almanacs, 1500–1800: Astrology and the Popular Press* (Ithaca, NY: Cornell University Press, 1979).

Bernard Capp, *Cromwell's Navy: The Fleet and the English Revolution, 1648–1660* (Oxford: Clarendon Press, 1989).

John Carey, *John Donne: Life, Mind and Art* (London: Faber and Faber, 1981).

Charles Carlton, *Charles the First: The Personal Monarch* (London: Ark Paperbacks, 1984).

Charles Carlton, *Going to Wars: The Experience of the British Civil Wars 1638–1651* (London: Routledge, 1992).

W. B. Carnochan, *Confinement and Flight: An Essay on English Literature of the Eighteenth Century* (Berkeley: University of California Press, 1977).

S. C. Carpenter, *Eighteenth Century Church and People* (London: Murray, 1959).

Vincent Carretta, *George III and the Satirists from Hogarth to Byron* (Athens, Ga.: University of Georgia Press, 1990).

Vincent Carretta (ed.), *Olaudah Equiano: The Interesting Narrative and Other Writings* (New York: Penguin Books, 1995).

Vincent Carretta (ed.), *Unchained Voices: An Anthology of Black Authors in the English-Speaking World of the Eighteenth Century* (Lexington: University Press of Kentucky, 1996).

Bruce G. Carruthers, *City of Captial: Politics and Markets in the English Financial Revolution* (Princeton: Princeton University Press, 1996).

John Carswell, *The South Sea Bubble* (London: Cresset Press, 1960).

John Carswell, *From Revolution to Revolution: England 1688–1776* (London: Routledge and Kegan Paul; New York: Scribner, 1973).

John Carswell, *The Porcupine: The Life of Algernon Sidney* (London: John Murray, 1989).

H. B. Carter, *Joseph Banks 1743–1820* (London: British Museum (Natural History), 1988).

Jennifer J. Carter and Joan H. Pittock (eds.), *Aberdeen and the Enlightenment* (Aberdeen: Aberdeen University Press, 1987).

Field Marshal Lord Carver, *The Seven Ages of the British Army* (London: Weidenfeld and Nicolson, 1984).

Richard Carwardine, *Transatlantic Revivalism: Popular Evangelicalism in Britain and America 1790–1865* (London: Greenwood Press, 1978).

Terry Castle, *Masquerade and Civilisation: The Carnivalesque in Eighteenth-Century English Culture and Fiction* (London: Methuen, 1986).

Terry Castle, *The Female Thermometer: Eighteenth-Century Culture and the Invention of the Uncanny* (Oxford: Oxford University Press, 1994).

Hiram Caton, *The Politics of Progress: The Origins and Development of the Commercial Republic, 1600–1835* (Gainesville: University of Florida Press, 1988).

Gulgielmo Cavallo and Roger Chartier (eds.), *A History of Reading in the West* (London: Polity Press, 2000).

W. O. Chadwick, *The Secularization of the European Mind in the Nineteenth Century* (Cambridge: Cambridge University Press, 1975).

Christopher Chalklin, *The Provincial Towns of Georgian England: A Study of the Building Process, 1740–1820* (London: Edward Arnold, 1974).

Christopher Chalklin, *English Counties and Public Building 1650–1830* (London: Hambledon, 1998).

Christopher Chalklin, *The Rise of the English Town, 1650–1850* (Cambridge: Cambridge University Press, 2001).

James Chambers, *The English House* (London: Thames Methuen, 1985).

J. D. Chambers and G. E. Mingay, *The Agricultural Revolution 1750–1880* (London: Batsford, 1966).

J. A. I. Champion, *The Pillars of Priestcraft Shaken: The Church of England and its Enemies, 1660–1730* (Cambridge: Cambridge University Press, 1992).

David G. Chandler, *Sedgemoor, 1685: An Account and an Anthology* (New York: St Martin's Press 1985).

Keith Chandler, *'Ribbons, Bells and Squeaking Fiddles': The Social History of Morris Dancing in the English South Midlands, 1660–1900* (Enfield Lock: Hisarlik Press, 1993).

S. D. Chapman, *The Early Factory Masters: The Transition to the Factory System in the Midlands Textile Industry* (Newton Abbot: David and Charles, 1967).

S. D. Chapman, 'Industrial Capital Before the Industrial Revolution, 1730–1750', in N. Harte and K. Ponting (eds.), *Textile History and Economic History* (Manchester: Manchester University Press, 1973), 113–37.

Stanley Chapman, *Merchant Enterprise in Britain: From the Industrial Revolution to World War I* (Cambridge: Cambridge University Press, 1992).

J. A. V. Chapple, *Science and Literature in the Nineteenth Century* (Basingstoke: Macmillan, 1986).

Lindsey Charles and Lorna Duffin (eds.), *Women and Work in Pre-Industrial England* (London: Croom Helm, 1985).

Andrew Charlesworth (ed.), *An Atlas of Rural Protest in Britain, 1548–1900* (London: Croom Helm, 1982).

Andrew Charlesworth et al., *An Atlas of Industrial Protest in Britain 1750–1990* (London: Macmillan, 1996).

John Chartres and David Hey (eds.), *English Rural Society, 1500–1800: Essays in Honour of Joan Thirsk* (Cambridge: Cambridge University Press, 1990).

Malcolm Chase, *The People's Farm: English Radical Agrarianism, 1775–1840* (Oxford: Clarendon Press, 1988).

Sydney Checkland, *British Public Policy 1776–1939: An Economic, Social and Political Perspective* (Cambridge: Cambridge University Press, 1983).

Warren L. Chernaik, *The Poet's Time: Politics and Religion in the Work of Andrew Marvell* (Cambridge: Cambridge University Press, 1983).

Sir Norman Chester, *The English Administrative System 1780–1870* (Oxford: Oxford University Press, 1981).

Carl Chinn, *Better Betting with a Decent Feller: Bookmaking, Betting and the British Working Class, 1750–1990* (Hemel Hempstead: Harvester Wheatsheaf, 1991).

Anand C. Chitnis, *The Scottish Enlightenment and Early Victorian English Society* (Beckenham: Croom Helm, 1986).

Gale E. Christianson, *In the Presence of the Creator: Isaac Newton and his Times* (London: Collier Macmillan, 1985).

I. R. Christie, *Wars and Revolutions: Britain 1760–1815* (London: Edward Arnold, 1982).

I. R. Christie, *Stress and Stability in Late Eighteenth-Century Britain: Reflections on the British Avoidance of Revolution* (Oxford: Oxford University Press, 1984).

Roy Church, 'Advertising Consumer Goods in Nineteenth-Century Britain: Reinterpretations', *Economic History Review*, 53 (2000), 621–45.

Gregory Claeys, *Thomas Paine: Social and Political Thought* (London: Unwin Hyman, 1989).

Gregory Claeys, 'The French Revolution Debate and British Political Thought', *History of Political Thought*, 1 (1990), 59–80.

Gregory Claeys (ed.), *Utopias of the British Enlightenment* (Cambridge: Cambridge University Press, 1994).

Gregory Claeys (ed.), *Political Writings of the 1790s* (London: William Pickering, 1995).

Gregory Claeys (ed.), *The Politics of English Jacobinism: Writings of John Thelwall* (University Park, Pa.: Pennsylvania State University Press, 1995).

B. W. Clapp, *An Environmental History of Britain since the Industrial Revolution* (London: Longman, 1994).

Anna Clark, *Women's Silence, Men's Violence: Sexual Assault in England, 1770–1845* (New York: Pandora, 1987).

Anna Clark, *The Struggle for the Breeches: Gender and the Making of the British Working Class* (Berkeley: University of California Press, 1995).

Anna Clark, 'The Chevalier d'Eon and Wilkes: Masculinity and Politics in the Eighteenth Century', *Eighteenth Century Studies*, 32 (1998), 19–48.

Aylwin Clark, *An Enlightened Scot: Hugh Cleghorn, 1752–1837* (Forfar: Black Ace Books, 1992).

G. Kitson Clark, *The Making of Victorian England* (London: Routledge, 1965).

J. C. D. Clark, 'The Decline of Party, 1740–1760', *English Historical Review*, 93 (1978), 499–527.

J. C. D. Clark, 'A General Theory of Party, Opposition and Government, 1688–1832', *Historical Journal*, 23 (1980), 295–325.

J. C. D. Clark, *The Dynamics of Change: The Crisis of the 1750s and English Party Systems* (Cambridge: Cambridge University Press, 1982).

J. C. D. Clark, 'Eighteenth Century Social

History', *Historical Journal*, 27 (1984), 773–88.

J. C. D. Clark, *Revolution and Rebellion : State and Society in England in the Seventeenth and Eighteenth Centuries* (Cambridge: Cambridge University Press, 1986).

J. C. D. Clark, 'English History's Forgotten Context: Scotland, Ireland, Wales', *Historical Journal*, 32 (1989), 211–28..

J. C. D. Clark, 'National Identity, State Formation and Patriotism: The Role of History in the Public Mind', *History Workshop Journal*, 29 (1990), 95–102..

J. C. D. Clark, 'Reconceptualising Eighteenth-Century England', *British Journal for Eighteenth Century Studies*, 15 (1992), 135–9..

J. C. D. Clark, *The Language of Liberty 1660–1832: Political Discourse and Social Dynamics in the Anglo-American World* (Cambridge: Cambridge University Press, 1994).

J. C. D. Clark, *Samuel Johnson: Literature, Religion and English Cultural Politics from the Restoration to Romanticism* (Cambridge: Cambridge University Press, 1994).

J. C. D. Clark, *English Society, 1688–1832: Ideology, Social Structure and Political Practice during the Ancien Régime* (Cambridge: Cambridge University Press, 1985; 2nd edn.: *English Society, 1660–1832: Religion, Ideology and Politics during the Ancien Régime*, Cambridge: Cambridge University Press, 2000).

Peter Clark, *English Provincial Society from the Reformation to the Revolution: Religion, Politics and Society in Kent 1500–1640* (Hassocks: Harvester Press, 1977).

Peter Clark (ed.), *Country Towns in Pre-Industrial England* (Leicester: Leicester University Press; New York: St Martin's Press, 1981).

Peter Clark, *The English Alehouse: A Social History, 1200–1830* (London: Longman, 1983).

Peter Clark (ed.), *The Transformation of English Provincial Towns, 1600–1800* (London: Hutchinson, 1984).

Peter Clark, *Sociability and Urbanity: Clubs and Societies in the Eighteenth Century* (Leicester: Leicester University Press, 1986).

Peter Clark, 'The "Mother Gin" Controversy in the Early Eighteenth Century', *Transactions of the Royal Historical Society*, 38 (1988), 63–84.

Peter Clark, *British Clubs and Societies 1580–1800: The Origins of an Associational World* (Oxford: Clarendon Press, 2000).

Peter Clark (ed.), *The Cambridge Urban History of Britain*, vol. 2: *1540–1840* (Cambridge: Cambridge University Press, 2001).

Peter Clark and Paul Slack, *English Towns in Transition, 1500–1700* (London: Oxford University Press, 1976).

Peter Clark, Alan G. R. Smith and Nicholas Tyacke (eds.), *The English Commonwealth 1547–1640: Essays in Politics and Society Presented to Joel Hurstfield* (Leicester: Leicester University Press, 1979).

Samuel Clark, *Social Origins of the Irish Land War* (Princeton: Princeton University Press, 1980).

Samuel Clark and James S. Donnelly Jr (eds.), *Irish Peasants: Violence and Political Unrest, 1780–1914* (Madison: University of Wisconsin Press, 1983).

A. E. Clark-Kennedy, *London Pride: The Story of a Voluntary Hospital* (London: Hutchinson Bentham, 1979).

Edwin Clarke and L. S. Jacyna, *Nineteenth-Century Origins of Neuroscientific Concepts* (Berkeley: University of California Press, 1987).

George Clarke (ed.), *John Bellars: His Life, Times and Writings* (London and New York: Routledge & Kegan Paul, 1987).

I. F. Clarke, *Voices Prophesying War 1763–1984* (Oxford: Oxford University Press, 1966).

I. F. Clarke, *The Pattern of Expectation 1644–2001* (London: Jonathan Cape, 1979).

John Clarke, Allan Cochrane and Carol Smart, *Ideologies of Welfare: From Dreams to Disillusion* (London: Hutchinson, 1987).

Leslie Clarkson, *The Pre-Industrial Economy in*

England 1500–1750 (London: Batsford, 1971).

Leslie Clarkson, *Death, Disease and Famine in Pre-Industrial England* (Dublin: Gill and Macmillan, 1975).

Leslie Clarkson, *Proto-Industrialization: The First Phase of Industrialization* (Basingstoke: Macmillan, for Economic History Society, 1985).

L. A. Clarkson (ed.), *The Industrial Revolution: A Compendium* (London: Macmillan, 1989; 1990).

Constance Classen, David Howes and Anthony Synnott, *Aroma: The Cultural History of Smell* (London: Routledge, 1994).

Christopher Clay, *Public Finance and Private Wealth: The Career of Sir Stephen Fox 1627–1716* (Oxford: Clarendon Press, 1978).

C. Clay, *Economic Expansion and Social Change in England, 1500–1700*, 2 vols. (Cambridge: Cambridge University Press, 1984).

Tony Claydon, *William III and the Godly Revolution* (Cambridge: Cambridge University Press, 1996).

Alasdair Clayre, *Work and Play: Ideas and Experience of Work and Leisure* (London: Weidenfeld and Nicolson, 1974).

Timothy Clayton, *The English Print 1688–1802* (New Haven: Yale University Press, 1997).

Alina Clej, *A Genealogy of the Modern Self: Thomas De Quincey and the Intoxication of Writing* (Stanford, Calif.: Stanford University Press, 1995).

Heather A. Clemenson, *English Country Houses and Landed Estates* (London: Croom Helm, 1982).

J. T. Cliffe, *Puritans in Conflict: The Puritan Gentry during and after the Civil Wars* (London: Routledge, 1988).

J. T. Cliffe, *The Puritan Gentry Besieged, 1650–1700* (London: Routledge, 1993).

Alan C. Clifford, *Atonement and Justification: English Evangelical Theology, 1640–1970* (Oxford: Clarendon Press, 1990).

Robin Clifton, *The Last Popular Rebellion: The Western Rising of 1685* (London: Temple Smith, 1984).

Gerald Cobb, *English Cathedrals: The Forgotten Centuries* (London: Thames and Hudson, 1980).

J. S. Cockburn (ed.), *Crime in England 1550–1800* (London: Methuen, 1977).

J. S. Cockburn and Thomas A. Green (eds.), *Twelve Good Men and True: The Criminal Trial Jury in England, 1200–1800* (Princeton: Princeton University Press, 1988).

Thomas Cogswell, *The Blessed Revolution: English Politics and the Coming of War, 1621–1624* (Cambridge: Cambridge University Press, 1989).

Thomas Cogswell, *Home Divisions: Aristocracy, the State and Provincial Conflict* (Stanford, Calif.: Stanford University Press, 1998).

Ed Cohen, *Talk on the Wilde Side: Toward a Genealogy of a Discourse on Male Sexualities* (New York: Routledge, 1993).

I. Bernard Cohen, *The Newtonian Revolution* (Norwalk, Conn.: Burndy Library, 1987).

Michael Cohen, *Engaging English Art: Entering the Work in Two Centuries of English Painting and Poetry* (Tuscaloosa: University of Alabama Press 1987).

Michèle Cohen, *Fashioning Masculinity: National Identity and Language in the Eighteenth Century* (London: Routledge, 1996).

D. C. Coleman, *Industry in Tudor and Stuart England* (London: Macmillan, 1975).

D. C. Coleman, *The Economy of England 1450–1750* (London: Oxford University Press, 1977).

D. C. Coleman, *Myth, History and the Industrial Revolution* (London: Hambledon, 1992).

D. C. Coleman and R. S. Schofield, *The State of Population Theory: Forward from Malthus* (Oxford: Basil Blackwell, 1986).

Linda Colley, *In Defiance of Oligarchy: The Tory Party, 1714–1760* (Cambridge: Cambridge University Press, 1982).

Linda Colley, 'The Apotheosis of George III: Loyalty, Royalty and the English Nation', *Past and Present*, 102 (1984), 94–129.

Linda Colley, 'Whose Nation? Class and National Consciousness in England, 1750–1830', *Past and Present*, 113 (1986), 96–117.

Linda Colley, 'Britishness and Otherness: An Argument', *Journal of British Studies*, 31 (1992), 309–29.

Linda Colley, *Britons: Forging the Nation 1707–1837* (New Haven: Yale University Press, 1992).

Stefan Collini, Richard Whatmore and Brian Young (eds.), *Economy, Polity, and Society: British Intellectual History 1750–1950* (Cambridge: Cambridge University Press, 2000).

Stefan Collini, Richard Whatmore and Brian Young (eds.), *History, Religion, and Culture: British Intellectual History 1750–1950* (Cambridge: Cambridge University Press, 2000).

A. S. Collins, *Authorship in the Days of Johnson: Being a Study of the Relationship between Author, Patron, Publisher and Public 1726–1780*, 2 vols. (London: R. Holden & Co. Ltd., 1927; London: George Routledge and Sons, 1928).

A. S. Collins, *The Profession of Letters: A Study of the Relation of Author to Patron, Publisher and Public, 1780–1832* (London: George Routledge & Sons Ltd., 1928; reprinted, Clifton, NJ: Augustus M. Kelley, 1973).

Irene Collins, *Jane Austen and the Clergy* (London: Hambledon Press, 1994).

Stephen L. Collins, *From Divine Cosmos to Sovereign State: An Intellectual History of Consciousness and the Idea of Order in Renaissance England* (New York and Oxford: Oxford University Press, 1989).

Patrick Collinson, *English Puritanism* (London: Historical Association, 1987).

Patrick Collinson, *The Birthpangs of Protestant England: Religious and Cultural Change in the Sixteenth and Seventeenth Centuries* (London: Macmillan, 1989).

Patrick Collinson, *Elizabethan Essays* (London: Hambledon Press, 1994).

Robert Colls, *The Pitmen of the Northern Coalfield: Work, Culture and Protest, 1790–1830* (Manchester: Manchester University Press, 1987).

Carl B. Cone, *The English Jacobins: Reformers in Late 18th Century England* (New York: Scribner, 1968).

Carl B. Cone, *Hounds in the Morning: Sundry Sports of Merrie England* (Lexington: University Press of Kentucky, 1981).

S. J. Connolly, *Priests and People in Pre-Famine Ireland 1780–1845* (Dublin: Gill and Macmillan, 1982).

Harold J. Cook, *Trials of an Ordinary Doctor: Joannes Groenvelt in Seventeenth-Century London* (Baltimore: Johns Hopkins University Press, 1994).

Judith Cook, *Close to the Earth: Living Social History of the British Isles* (New York: Routledge and Kegan Paul, 1984).

J. E. Cookson, *The Friends of Peace: Anti-War Liberalism in England 1793–1815* (Cambridge: Cambridge University Press, 1982).

Frederick Cooper and Ann Laura Stoler (eds.), *Tensions of Empire: Colonial Cultures in a Bourgeois World* (Berkeley: University of California Press, 1997).

Esther S. Cope, *Politics Without Parliaments 1629–1640* (London: Allen and Unwin, 1987).

Stephen Copley (ed.), *Literature and the Social Order in Eighteenth-Century England* (London: Croom Helm, 1984).

Stephen Copley (ed.), *The Politics of the Picturesque: Literature, Landscape and Aesthetics since 1770* (Cambridge: Cambridge University Press, 1994).

Stephen Copley, 'Commerce, Conversation and Politeness in the Early Eighteenth Century Periodical', *British Journal for Eighteenth Century Studies*, 18 (1995), 63–77.

Stephen Copley and Kathryn Sutherland (eds.), *Adam Smith's Wealth of Nations: New Interdisciplinary Essays* (Manchester: Manchester University Press, 1995).

Alain Corbin, *The Lure of the Sea: The Discovery of the Seaside in the Western World, 1750–1840* (Cambridge: Polity Press, 1994).

P. J. Corfield, 'A Provincial Capital in the Late Seventeenth Century: The Case of Norwich', in Peter Clark and Paul Slack (eds.), *Crisis and Order in English Towns 1500–1700: Essays in Urban History* (London: Routledge and Kegan Paul, 1972).

P. J. Corfield, *The Impact of English Towns 1700–1800* (Oxford: Oxford University Press, 1982).

P. J. Corfield, 'Class by Name and Number in Eighteenth Century Britain', *History*, 72 (1987), 38–61.

P. J. Corfield, 'Small Towns, Large Implications: Social and Cultural Roles of Small Towns in Eighteenth-Century England and Wales', *British Journal for Eighteenth-century Studies*, 10 (1987), 125–38.

P. J. Corfield, 'Georgian Bath: The Magical Meeting Place', *History Today*, 40 (1990), 26–33.

P. J. Corfield, 'Walking the City Streets: The Urban Odyssey in Eighteenth-Century England', *Journal of Urban History*, 16 (1990), 132–74.

P. J. Corfield (ed.), *Language, History and Class* (Oxford: Blackwell, 1991).

P. J. Corfield, 'Georgian England: One State, Many Faiths', *History Today*, 45 (1995).

P. J. Corfield, *Power and the Professions in Britain 1700–1850* (London: Routledge, 1995).

P. J. Corfield and N. B. Harte (eds.), *London and the English Economy* (London: Hambledon Press, 1990).

P. J. Corfield and Derek Keene (eds.), *Work in Towns, 850–1850* (Leicester: Leicester University Press, 1990).

P. Corrigan and D. Sayer, *The Great Arch: English State Formation as Cultural Revolution* (Oxford: Basil Blackwell, 1985).

Art Cosgrove and Donal McCartney (eds.), *Studies in Irish History Presented to R. Dudley Edwards* (Dublin: University College, 1979).

Denis Cosgrove and Stephen Daniels (eds.), *The Iconography of Landscape: Essays on the Symbolic Representation, Design and Use of Past Environments* (Cambridge: Cambridge University Press, 1988).

Tess Cosslett, *The 'Scientific Movement' and Victorian Literature* (Brighton: Harvester Press, 1982; New York: St Martin's Press, 1983).

Bernard Cottret, *Cromwell* (Paris: Fayard, 1992).

Bernard Cottret (ed.), *Bolingbroke's Political Writings: The Conservative Enlightenment* (London: Macmillan, 1997).

Franklin E. Court, *Institutionalizing English Literature: The Culture and Politics of Literary Study, 1750–1900* (Stanford, Calif.: Stanford University Press, 1992).

Barry Coward, *The Stuart Age: A History of England 1603–1714* (New York: Longman Press, 1980).

Barry Coward, *Cromwell* (London: Longman, 1991).

Virginia Cowles, *The Great Marlborough & His Duchess* (London: Weidenfeld and Nicolson, 1983).

Maurice Cowling, *Religion and Public Doctrine in Modern England*, vol. 2: *Assaults* (Cambridge: Cambridge University Press, 1985).

John Richard Cox (ed.), *Sexuality and Victorian Literature* (Knoxville: University of Tennessee Press, 1984).

S. D. Cox, *'The Stranger Within Thee': The Concept of the Self in Late Eighteenth Century Literature* (Pittsburgh: Pittsburgh University Press, 1980).

Patricia B. Craddock, *Edward Gibbon, Luminous Historian 1772–1794* (Baltimore: Johns Hopkins University Press, 1988).

N. F. R. Crafts, *British Economic Growth during the Industrial Revolution* (Oxford: Oxford University Press, 1985).

Gerald R. Cragg, *From Puritanism to the Age of Reason: A Study of Changes in Religious*

Thought within the Church of England, 1660–1700 (Cambridge: Cambridge University Press, 1950).

Gerald R. Cragg, The Church and the Age of Reason (Harmondsworth: Penguin, 1960).

Gerald Cragg, Reason and Authority in the Eighteenth Century (Cambridge: Cambridge University Press, 1964).

David Craig, Scottish Literature and the Scottish People 1680–1830 (London: Chatto and Windus, 1961).

Roger Craik, James Boswell (1740–1795): The Scottish Perspective (Edinburgh: HMSO, 1994).

Geoffrey Alan Cranfield, The Development of the Provincial Newspaper 1700–1760 (Oxford: Clarendon Press, 1962).

Geoffrey Alan Cranfield, The Press and Society: From Caxton to Northcliffe (London: Longman, 1978).

Matthew Craske, Art in Europe 1700–1830: A History of the Visual Arts in an Era of Unprecedented Urban Economic Growth (Oxford: Oxford University Press, 1997).

Patricia Crawford, Women and Religion in England, 1500–1720 (London: Routledge, 1993).

David Cressy, Literacy and the Social Order: Reading and Writing in Tudor and Stuart England (Cambridge: Cambridge University Press, 1980).

David Cressy, 'Books as Totems in Seventeenth-Century England and New England', Journal of Library History, 21 (1986), 92–106.

David Cressy, 'Kinship and Kin Interaction in Early Modern England', Past and Present, 113 (1986), 38–69.

David Cressy, Coming Over: Migration and Communication between England and New England in the Seventeenth Century (Cambridge: Cambridge University Press, 1987).

David Cressy, Bonfires and Bells (London: Weidenfeld and Nicolson, 1989).

David Cressy (ed.), Religion and Society in Early Modern England (London: Routledge, 1996).

David Cressy, Birth, Marriage, and Death: Ritual, Religion, and the Life-Cycle in Tudor and Stuart England (Oxford: Oxford University Press, 1997).

Alan Cromartie, Sir Matthew Hale, 1609–75 (Cambridge: Cambridge University Press, 1995).

A. G. Cross, 'By the Banks of the Thames': Russians in Eighteenth-Century Britain (Newtonville, Mass.: Oriental Research Partners, 1980).

Claire Cross, Church and People 1450–1660 (London: Fontana, 1976).

Gary Cross, Time and Money: The Making of Consumer Culture (London: Routledge, 1993).

Nigel Cross, The Common Writer: Life in Nineteenth-Century Grub Street (New York: Cambridge University Press, 1985).

François Crouzet, The First Industrialists: The Problem of Origins (Cambridge: Cambridge University Press, 1985).

François Crouzet, Britain Ascendant: Studies in British and Franco-British Economic History (Cambridge: Cambridge University Press, 1991).

Ian Crowe (ed.), Edmund Burke: His Life and Legacy (Dublin: Four Courts, 1997).

Dan Cruickshank and Neil Burton, Life in the Georgian City (New York: Viking, 1990).

Eveline Cruickshanks (ed.), Ideology and Conspiracy: Aspects of Jacobitism, 1689–1759 (Edinburgh: John Donald, 1982).

Eveline Cruikshanks (ed.), The Stuart Courts (Stroud: Sutton Books, 2000).

Eveline Cruickshanks and Jeremy Black (eds.), The Jacobite Challenge (Edinburgh: John Donald, 1988).

L. M. Cullen, The Emergence of Modern Ireland 1600–1900 (London: Batsford, 1981).

A. J. G. Cummings and T. M. Devine (eds.), Industry, Business and Society in Scotland since 1700: Essays Presented to John Butt (Edinburgh: John Donald, 1994).

Hugh Cunningham, *Leisure in the Industrial Revolution, c.1780–c.1880* (London: Croom Helm, 1980).

Hugh Cunningham, 'The Language of Patriotism, 1750–1914', *History Workshop Journal*, 12 (1981), 8–33.

Hugh Cunningham, 'The Employment and Unemployment of Children in England c.1680–1951', *Past and Present*, 126 (1990), 115–50.

Hugh Cunningham, *The Children of the Poor: Representations of Childhood since the Seventeenth Century* (Oxford: Basil Blackwell, 1991).

Hugh Cunningham, *Children and Childhood in Western Society since 1500* (London: Longman, 1995).

James Stevens Curl, *Georgian Architecture* (Newton Abbot: David and Charles, 1993).

Patrick Curry, *Prophecy and Power: Astrology in Early Modern England* (Cambridge: Polity Press, 1989).

David Dabydeen (ed.), *The Black Presence in English Literature* (Manchester: Manchester University Press, 1985).

David Dabydeen, *Hogarth's Blacks: Images of Blacks in Eighteenth Century English Art* (Kingston: Dangeroo Press, 1985).

David Dabydeen, *Hogarth, Walpole and Commercial Britain* (London: Hansib, 1987).

David Dabydeen, 'On Not Being Milton: Nigger Talk in Modern England', in C. Ricks and L. Michaels (eds.), *The State of the Language* (London: Faber and Faber, 1990), 3–14.

H. M. Daleski, *The Divided Heroine: A Recurrent Pattern in Six English Novels* (New York: Holmes and Meier, 1983).

James Daly, *Sir Robert Filmer and English Political Thought* (Toronto: University of Toronto Press, 1979).

J. Lasley Dameron and Pamela Palmer, with introductory essays by Kenneth J. Curry and J. Lasley Dameron, *An Index to the Critical Vocabulary of Blackwoods Edinburgh Magazine, 1830–1840* (West Cornwall: Locust Hill Press, 1993).

Stephen Daniels, *Fields of Vision: Landscape Imagery and National Identity in England and the United States* (Cambridge: Polity Press, 1993).

Stephen Daniels, *Humphry Repton: Landscape Gardening and the Geography of Georgian England* (New Haven: Yale University Press, 1999).

Ruth Danon, *Work in the English Novel: The Myth of Vocation* (Beckenham: Croom Helm, 1985).

Lorraine Daston, *Classical Probability in the Enlightenment* (Princeton: Princeton University Press, 1988).

M. J. Daunton, 'Towns and Economic Growth in Eighteenth Century England', in Philip Abrams and E. A. Wrigley (eds.), *Towns in Societies: Essays in Economic History and Historical Sociology* (Cambridge: Cambridge University Press, 1978), 245–77.

M. J. Daunton, *Progress and Poverty: An Economic and Social History of Britain 1700–1850* (Oxford: Oxford University Press, 1995).

M. J. Daunton (ed.), *Charity, Self-Interest and Welfare in the English Past* (London: University College London Press, 1996).

Edward Davenport, 'The Devils of Positivism', in Stuart Peterfreund (ed.), *Literature and Science: Theory and Practice* (Boston: Northeastern University Press, 1990), 17–31.

R. P. T. Davenport-Hines, *Sex, Death and Punishment: Attitudes to Sex and Sexuality in Britain since the Renaissance* (London: Collins, 1990).

Leonore Davidoff, *Worlds Between – Historical Perspectives on Gender and Class* (Cambridge: Polity Press, 1995).

Leonore Davidoff and Catherine Hall, *Family Fortunes: Men and Women of the English Middle Class, 1780–1850* (London: Hutchinson, 1987).

Caroline A. Davidson, *A Woman's Work is Never Done: A History of Housework in the*

British Isles, 1650–1950 (London: Chatto and Windus, 1982).

Edward H. Davidson and William J. Scheick, *Paine, Scripture, and Authority: 'The Age of Reason' as Religious and Political Idea* (Bethlehem, Pa.: Lehigh University Press; London: Associated University Presses, 1994).

Neil Davidson, *The Origins of Scottish Nationhood* (London: Pluto Press, 2000).

Donald Davie, *The Language of Science and the Language of Literature, 1700–1740* (London: Sheed and Ward, 1963).

Donald Davie, *The Eighteenth-Century Hymn in England* (Cambridge: Cambridge University Press, 1993).

Horton Davies, *Worship and Theology in England from Watts and Wesley to Martineau, 1690–1900* (Grand Rapids, Mich.: William B. Eerdmans Publishing Company, 1996).

John Davies, *History of Wales* (London: Allen Lane, 1993).

Norman Davies, *Europe: A History* (Oxford: Oxford University Press, 1996).

Norman Davies, *The Isles: A History* (London: Macmillan, 2000).

Stevie Davies, *Unbridled Spirits: Women of the English Revolution, 1640–1660* (London: Women's Press, 1998).

Dorothy Davis, *A History of Shopping* (London: Routledge; Toronto: Toronto University Press, 1966).

J. C. Davis, *Utopia and the Ideal Society: A Study of English Utopian Writing 1516–1700* (Cambridge: Cambridge University Press, 1981).

J. C. Davis, *Fear, Myth and History: The Ranters and the Historians* (New York: Cambridge University Press, 1986).

Natalie Zemon Davis, *Women on the Margins: Three Seventeenth Century Lives* (Cambridge, Mass.: Harvard University Press, 1995).

R. Davis, *The Industrial Revolution and British Overseas Trade* (Leicester: Leicester University Press, 1979).

Mitchell Dean, *The Constitution of Poverty: Toward a Genealogy of Liberal Governance* (London: Routledge, 1991).

Phyllis Deane, *The First Industrial Revolution* (Cambridge: Cambridge University Press, 1965).

Phyllis Deane, *The Evolution of Economic Ideas* (Cambridge: Cambridge University Press, 1978).

Phyllis Deane and W. A. Cole, *British Economic Growth, 1688–1959: Trends and Structure*, 2nd edn. (Cambridge: Cambridge University Press, 1969).

Phyllis Deane, *The State and the Economic System: An Introduction to the History of Political Economy* (Oxford: Oxford University Press, 1989).

Seamus Deane, *The French Revolution and Enlightenment in England 1789–1832* (Cambridge, Mass.: Harvard University Press, 1988).

Peter Dear, *Discipline and Experience: The Mathematical Way in the Scientific Revolution* (Chicago: University of Chicago Press, 1995).

Gary Stuart De Krey, *The Politics of London in the First Age of Party, 1688–1715* (Oxford: Oxford University Press, 1985).

Margaret DeLacy, *Prison Reform in Lancashire, 1700–1850* (Manchester: Chetham Society, 1986; Stanford, Calif.: Stanford University Press, 1986).

François and Alexandre de Liancourt, *Innocent Espionage: The La Rochefoucauld Brothers' Tour of England in 1785*, trans. Norman Scarfe (Suffolk: Boydell and Brewer, 1995).

Richard Dellamora, *Apocalyptic Overtures: Sexual Politics and the Sense of an Ending* (New Brunswick, NJ: Rutgers University Press, 1994).

Robert DeMaria Jr., *Johnson's Dictionary and the Language of Learning* (Oxford: Clarendon Press, 1986).

Norman Dennis and A. H. Halsey, *English Ethical Socialism: Thomas More to R. H. Tawney* (Oxford: Clarendon Press, 1988).

Richard Dennis, *English Industrial Cities of the*

Nineteenth Century: A Social Geography (Cambridge: Cambridge University Press, 1984).

Bernard Denvir, *The Eighteenth Century: Art, Design and Society 1689–1789* (London: Longman, 1983).

Bernard Denvir, *The Early Nineteenth Century: Art, Design and Society 1789–1852* (London: Longman, 1984).

John W. Derry, *Charles, Earl Grey: Aristocratic Reformer* (Oxford: Blackwell, 1992).

C. De Saussure, *A Foreign View of England in 1725–29: The Letters of Monsieur César de Saussure to his Family* (London: Caliban, 1995).

Adrian Desmond, *The Politics of Evolution: Morphology, Medicine and Reform in Radical London* (Chicago: University of Chicago Press, 1992).

Alexis De Tocqueville, *Journeys to England and Ireland* (London: Faber and Faber, 1958).

T. M. Devine (ed.), *Conflict and Stability in Scottish Society, 1700–1850* (Edinburgh: John Donald, 1990).

T. M. Devine, *Clanship to Crofters' War: The Social Transformation of the Scottish Highlands* (Manchester: Manchester University Press, 1994).

T. M. Devine (ed.), *Scottish Elites* (Edinburgh: John Donald, 1994).

T. M. Devine, *The Transformation of Rural Scotland: Social Change and the Agrarian Economy 1660–1815* (Edinburgh: Edinburgh University Press, 1994).

Jan de Vries, *European Urbanization 1500–1800* (London: Methuen, 1984).

H. T. Dickinson, *Bolingbroke* (London: Constable, 1970).

H. T. Dickinson, *Politics and Literature in the Eighteenth Century* (London: Dent, 1974).

H. T. Dickinson, *Liberty and Property: Political Ideology in Eighteenth-Century Britain* (London: Weidenfeld and Nicolson, 1977).

H. T. Dickinson, *British Radicalism and the French Revolution 1789–1815* (Oxford: Blackwell, 1985).

H. T. Dickinson, 'How Revolutionary was the "Glorious Revolution" of 1688?', *British Journal for Eighteenth-Century Studies*, 11 (1988), 125–42.

H. T. Dickinson (ed.), *Britain and the French Revolution 1789–1815* (London: Macmillan, 1989).

H. T. Dickinson, *The Politics of the People in Eighteenth-Century Britain* (London: Macmillan, 1995).

David Dickson, *New Foundations: Ireland, 1660–1800* (Dublin: Helicon, 1987).

P. G. M. Dickson, *The Financial Revolution in England: A Study of the Development of Public Credit 1688–1756* (Aldershot: Gregg Revivals, 1993).

Anne Digby, *British Welfare Policy: Workhouse to Workfare* (London: Faber, 1989).

N. Merrill Distad, *Guessing at Truth: The Life of Julius Charles Hare* (Shepherdstown, W. Va.: Patmos Press, 1979).

Russell P. Dobash, R. Emerson Dobash and Sue Gutteridge, *The Imprisonment of Women* (New York: Basil Blackwell, 1986).

Betty Jo Teeter Dobbs, *The Janus Faces of Genius: The Role of Alchemy in Newton's Thought* (Cambridge: Cambridge University Press, 1991).

C. R. Dobson, *Masters and Journeymen: A Prehistory of Industrial Relations, 1717–1800* (London: Croom Helm; Totowa, NJ: Rowman and Littlefield, 1980).

Michael Dobson, *The Making of the National Poet: Shakespeare, Adaptation and Authorship, 1660–1769* (Oxford: Clarendon Press, 1992).

Brian Dolan, *Exploring European Frontiers: British Travellers in the Age of Enlightenment* (Basingstoke: Macmillan, 1999).

Jonathan Dollimore, *Sexual Dissidence: Augustine to Wilde, Freud to Foucault* (New York: Oxford University Press, 1991).

Horst Dölvers, *Fables Less and Less Fabulous: English Fables and Parables of the Nineteenth Century and their Illustrations* (Newark: University of Delaware Press, 1997).

Diana Donald, *The Age of Caricature: Satirical Prints in the Reign of George III* (New Haven: Yale University Press, 1996).

William Donaldson, *Popular Literature in Victorian Scotland: Language, Fiction and the Press* (Aberdeen: Aberdeen University Press, 1986).

Wendy Doniger, *The Bed Trick: Tales of Sex and Masquerade* (Chicago: University of Chicago Press, 2000).

Martin Doughty (ed.), *Building the Industrial City* (Leicester: Leicester University Press, 1986).

Kerry Downes, *Sir John Vanbrugh: A Biography* (London: Sidgwick and Jackson, 1987).

J. A. Downie, *Robert Harley and the Press: Propaganda and Public Opinion in the Age of Swift and Defoe* (Cambridge: Cambridge University Press, 1979).

J. A. Downie, *Jonathan Swift: Political Writer* (London: Routledge and Kegan Paul, 1984).

J. A. Downie, *To Settle the Succession of the State: Literature and Politics, 1678–1750* (London: Macmillan, 1994).

Brian Doyle, *English and Englishness* (London: Routledge, 1989).

Richard Drayton, *Nature's Government: Science, Imperial Britain, and the 'Improvement' of the World* (New Haven: Yale University Press, 2000).

Alice Domurat Dreger, *Hermaphrodites and the Medical Invention of Sex* (Cambridge, Mass.: Harvard University Press, 1998).

Frederick A. Dreyer, *Burke's Politics: A Study in Whig Orthodoxy* (Waterloo, Ont.: Wilfrid Laurier University Press, 1979).

Kirsten Dromer, *English Children and their Magazines, 1751–1954* (New Haven: Yale University Press, 1988).

J. Drummond and A. Wilbraham, *The Englishman's Food: A History of Five Centuries of English Diet*, revised by Dorothy Hollingsworth (Jonathan Cape, 1957).

Daniel Duman, *The Judicial Bench in England, 1727–1875* (London: Royal Historical Society, 1982).

Louis Dumont, *From Mandeville to Marx: The Genesis and Triumph of Economic Ideology* (Chicago: University of Chicago Press, 1977).

Patrick A. Dunae, *Gentlemen Emigrants: From the British Public Schools to the Canadian Frontier* (Vancouver: Douglas and McIntrye, 1981).

John Dunn, *Locke* (New York: Oxford University Press, 1984).

Christopher Durston, *The Family in the English Revolution* (Oxford: Basil Blackwell, 1989).

Christopher Durston (ed.), *The Culture of English Puritanism, 1560–1700* (London: Macmillan, 1996).

Ian Dyck (ed.), *Citizen of the World: Essays on Thomas Paine* (New York: St Martin's Press, 1988).

Jacqueline Eales, *Women in Early Modern England, 1500–1700* (London: UCL Press, 1995).

Peter Earle, *The World of Defoe* (London: Weidenfeld and Nicolson, 1976).

Peter Earle, 'The Female Labour Market in London in the Late Seventeenth and Early Eighteenth Centuries', *Economic History Review*, 42 (1989), 328–53.

Peter Earle, *The Making of the English Middle Class: Business, Society and Family Life in London, 1660–1730* (London: Methuen, 1989).

Brian Easlea, *Witch-Hunting, Magic and the New Philosophy: An Introduction to the Debates of the Scientific Revolution, 1450–1750* (Brighton: Harvester Press, 1980).

Audrey Eccles, *Obstetrics and Gynaecology in Tudor and Stuart England* (London: Croom Helm, 1982).

Francis Edwards, *The Jesuits in England: From 1580 to the Present Day* (Tunbridge Wells: Burns and Oates, 1985).

Owen Dudley Edwards, *Burke and Hare* (Edinburgh: Polygon Books, 1980).

Owen Dudley Edwards, *Macaulay* (London: Weidenfeld and Nicolson, 1988).

Paul Edwards and James Walvin, *Black Personalities in the Era of the Slave Trade* (London: Palgrave, 1983).

Peter Edwards, *The Horse Trade of Tudor and Stuart England* (Cambridge: Cambridge University Press, 1988).

Cyril Ehrlich, *The Music Profession in Britain Since the Eighteenth Century: A Social History* (Oxford: Clarendon Press, 1985).

John Ehrman, *The Younger Pitt*, vol. 2: *The Reluctant Transition* (London: Constable, 1983).

John Ehrman, *The Younger Pitt*, vol. 3: *The Consuming Struggle* (London: Constable, 1996).

Elizabeth L. Eisenstein, *The Printing Press as an Agent of Change*, 2 vols. (Cambridge: Cambridge University Press, 1979).

A. Roger Ekirch, *Bound for America: The Transportation of British Convicts to the Colonies, 1718–1775* (New York: Oxford University Press, 1987).

Roger Elbourne, *Music and Tradition in Early Industrial Lancashire 1780–1840* (Woodbridge: Folklore Society, 1980).

Geoff Eley and William Hunt, *Reviving the English Revolution: Reflections and Elaborations on the Work of Christopher Hill* (London and New York: Verso, 1988).

Andrew Elfenbein, *Byron and the Victorians* (Cambridge: Cambridge University Press, 1995).

Norbert Elias, *The Civilizing Process*, vol. 1: *The History of Manners* (New York: Pantheon, 1978); vol. 2: *Power and Civility* (New York: Pantheon, 1982); vol. 3: *The Court Society* (New York: Pantheon, 1983).

Miriam Eliav-Feldon, *Realistic Utopias: The Ideal Imaginary Societies of the Renaissance, 1516–1630* (Oxford: Clarendon Press, 1982).

Blanche Beatrice Elliott, *A History of English Advertising* (London: Business Publications Limited in association with B. T. Batsford, 1962).

Marianne Elliott, *Partners in Revolution: The United Irishmen and France* (London: Yale University Press, 1982).

Marianne Elliott, *Wolfe Tone: Prophet of Irish Independence* (New Haven: Yale University Press, 1989).

Joyce M. Ellis, *The Georgian Town, 1680–1840* (Basingstoke: Palgrave, 2001).

Geoffrey Elton, *The English* (Oxford: Blackwell, 1992).

G. R. Elton, *Studies in Tudor and Stuart Politics and Goverment*, vol. 4: *Papers and Reviews 1982–1990* (Cambridge: Cambridge University Press, 1992).

R. L. Emerson, 'Peter Gay and the Heavenly City', *Journal of the History of Ideas*, 28 (1967), 383–402.

R. L. Emerson, 'Scottish Universities in the Eighteenth Century, 1690–1800', *Studies on Voltaire and the Eighteenth Century*, 167 (1977), 453–74.

R. L. Emerson, 'Science and the Origins and Concerns of the Scottish Enlightenment', *History of Science*, 26 (1988), 333.

R. L. Emerson, *Professors, Patronage and Politics: The Aberdeen Universities in the Eighteenth Century* (Aberdeen: Aberdeen University Press, 1992).

Clive Emsley, *British Society and the French Wars 1793–1815* (London: Macmillan, 1979).

Clive Emsley, *Policing and its Context, 1750–1870* (London: Macmillan, 1983).

Clive Emsley, *Crime and Society in England, 1750–1900* (London: Longman, 1987).

Clive Emsley and James Walvin (eds.), *Artisans, Peasants and Proletarians 1760–1860: Essays Presented to Gwyn A. Williams* (London: Croom Helm, 1985).

Todd M. Endelman, *The Jews of Georgian England 1714–1830: Tradition and Change in a Liberal Society* (Philadelphia: Jewish Publication Society of America, 1979).

Evelyne Ender, *Sexing the Mind; Nineteenth-Century Fictions of Hysteria* (Ithaca, NY: Cornell University Press, 1995).

Elliot Engel and Margaret F. King, *The Victorian Novel before Victoria: British Fiction during the Reign of William IV, 1830–37* (New York: St Martin's Press, 1984).

The English Satirical Print 1600–1832, 7 vols. (London: Chadwyck-Healey, 1986).

James A. Epstein, *Radical Expression: Political Language, Ritual and Symbol in England, 1790–1850* (Oxford: Oxford University Press, 1994).

David V. Erdman, *Blake, Prophet Against Empire: A Poet's Interpretation of the History of his own Times* (3rd edn., Princeton: Princeton University Press, 1977).

Alan Ereira, *The People's England* (London: Routledge and Kegan Paul, 1981).

Amy Louise Erickson, *Women and Property in Early Modern England* (London: Routledge, 1993).

Elizabeth Deeds Ermarth, *Realism and Consensus in the English Novel* (Princeton: Princeton University Press, 1983).

Howard Erskine-Hill, *The Augustan Idea in English Literature* (London: Edward Arnold, 1983).

Howard Erskine-Hill, *Poetry of Opposition and Revolution: Dryden to Wordsworth* (Oxford: Clarendon Press, 1996).

E. Evans, *The Forging of the Modern State: Early Industrial Britain, 1783–1870* (London: Longman, 1983, 1991).

John T. Evans, *Seventeenth-Century Norwich: Politics, Religion, and Government 1620–1690* (Oxford: Clarendon Press, 1980).

Nesta Evans, *The East Anglian Linen Industry: Rural Industry and Local Economy, 1500–1850* (Aldershot: Gower Publishing, 1985).

R. Evans, *The Fabrication of Virtue: English Prison Architecture 1750–1840* (Cambridge: Cambridge University Press, 1982).

Richard J. Evans, *Rituals of Retribution: Capital Punishment in Germany, 1600–1987* (Oxford: Oxford University Press, 1996).

Elisabeth Ewing, *Fashion in Underwear* (London: Batsford, 1971).

Elisabeth Ewing, *Dress and Undress: A History of Women's Underwear* (London: Batsford, 1978).

John M. Eyler, *Victorian Social Medicine: The Ideas and Methods of William Farr* (Baltimore: Johns Hopkins University Press, 1979).

Richard Faber, *Young England* (London: Faber and Faber, 1987).

M. Falkus, *Britain Transformed: An Economic and Social History, 1700–1914* (Ormskirk: Causeway, 1987).

Lincoln B. Faller, *Turned to Account: The Forms of Criminal Biography in Late Seventeenth- and Early Eighteenth-Century England* (Cambridge: Cambridge University Press, 1987).

Patricia Fara, *Sympathetic Attractions: Magnetic Practices, Beliefs, and Symbolism in Eighteenth-Century England* (Princeton: Princeton University Press, 1996).

Trevor Fawcett, *The Rise of English Provincial Art: Artists, Patrons and Institutions outside London, 1800–1830* (Oxford: Clarendon Press, 1974).

John Feather, *The English Provincial Book Trade Before 1850: A Checklist of Secondary Sources* (Oxford Bibliographical Society, Occasional Publication, 16; Oxford: Oxford Bibliographical Society, 1981).

John Feather, 'The Commerce of Letters: The Study of the Eighteenth-Century Book Trade', *Eighteenth-Century Studies*, 17 (1984), 405–24.

John Feather, *The Provincial Book Trade in Eighteenth-Century England* (Cambridge: Cambridge University Press, 1985).

John Feather, *A History of British Publishing* (London: Routledge, 1988).

John Feather, *Publishing, Piracy and Politics: An Historical Study of Copyright in Britain* (London: Mansell, 1994).

J. K. Fedorowicz, *England's Baltic Trade in the Early Seventeenth Century* (Cambridge: Cambridge University Press, 1980).

Mordechai Feingold (ed.), *Before Newton: The Life and Times of Isaac Browne* (Cambridge: Cambridge University Press, 1990).

David Feldman and Gareth Stedman Jones

(eds.), *Metropolis, London: Histories and Representations since 1800* (London: Routledge, 1989).

Frank Felsenstein, *Anti-Semitic Stereotypes: A Paradigm of Otherness in English Popular Culture, 1660–1830* (Baltimore: Johns Hopkins University Press, 1995).

K. Fenwick (ed.), *Ned Ward: The London Spy* (London: Folio Society, 1950).

Moira Ferguson, *First Feminists: British Women Writers, 1578–1799* (Bloomington: Indiana University Press; Old Westbury, NY: Feminist Press, 1985).

Eva Figes, *Sex and Subterfuge: Women Writers to 1850* (London: Macmillan, 1982).

Valerie A. Fildes (ed.), *Women as Mothers in Pre-Industrial England: Essays in Memory of Dorothy McLaren* (Wellcome Institute Series in the History of Medicine; London: Routledge, 1990).

Kenneth Fincham (ed.), *The Early Stuart Church, 1603–1642* (Basingstoke: Macmillan, 1993).

Robert Finlay, *Population and Metropolis: The Demography of London 1580–1650* (Cambridge: Cambridge University Press, 1981).

Richard B. Fisher, *Edward Jenner: 1749–1823* (London: André Deutsch, 1991).

Mark C. Fissell (ed.), *War and Government in Britain, 1598–1650* (Manchester: Manchester University Press, 1991).

Betty Fladeland, *Abolitionists and Working-Class Problems in the Age of Industrialization* (Baton Rouge: Louisiana State University Press, 1984).

M. Kay Flavell, 'The Enlightenment Reader and the New Industrial Towns: A Study of the Liverpool Library 1758–1790', *British Journal for Eighteenth-Century Studies*, 8 (1985), 17–35.

Anthony Fletcher, *The Outbreak of the English Civil War* (London: Edward Arnold, 1981).

Anthony Fletcher, *Reform in the Provinces: The Government of Stuart England* (London: Yale University Press, 1986).

Anthony Fletcher, *Gender, Sex and Subordination in England 1500–1800* (New Haven: Yale University Press, 1995).

Anthony Fletcher and Peter Roberts (eds.), *Religion, Culture and Society in Early Modern Britain* (Cambridge: Cambridge University Press, 1994).

Anthony Fletcher and John Stevenson (eds.), *Order and Disorder in Early Modern England* (Cambridge: Cambridge University Press, 1985).

M. W. Flinn, *Men of Iron: The Crowleys in the Early Iron Industry* (Edinburgh: Edinburgh University Press; 1962).

Michael W. Flinn, *The History of the British Coal Industry*, vol. 2: *1700–1830: The Industrial Revolution* (Oxford: Oxford University Press, 1984).

Roderick Floud, Annabel Gregory and Kenneth Wachter, *Height, Health and History: Nutritional Status in the United Kingdom, 1750–1980* (Cambridge: Cambridge University Press, 1990).

Roderick Floud and Donald McCloskey (eds.), *The Economic History of Britain since 1700*, 3 vols., 2nd edn. (Cambridge: Cambridge University Press, 1994).

Wyn Ford, 'The Problem of Literacy in Early Modern England', *History*, 78 (1993, 22–37.

Michael Fores, 'The Myth of a British Industrial Revolution', *History*, 66 (1981), 181–98).

Adrian Forty, *Objects of Desire: Design and Society since 1750* (New York: Pantheon Books, 1986).

Michael Foss, *Man of Wit to Man of Business: The Arts and Changing Patronage 1660–1750* (Bristol: Bristol Classical Press, 1988).

R. F. Foster, *Paddy and Mr Punch: Connections in Irish and English History* (Harmondsworth: Allen Lane, 1993).

Roy Foster (ed.), *The Oxford Illustrated History of Ireland* (New York: Oxford University Press, 1991).

Shirley Foster, *Victorian Women's Fiction:*

Marriage, Freedom and the Individual (Totowa, NJ: Barnes and Noble, 1985).

Alastair Fowler, *A History of English Literature* (Cambridge, Mass.: Harvard University Press, 1987).

Alan Fox, *History and Heritage: The Social Origins of the British Industrial Relations System* (London: Allen and Unwin, 1985).

Louise Olga Fradenburg (ed.), *Women and Sovereignty* (Edinburgh: Edinburgh University Press, 1992).

Genevieve Fraisse and Michelle Perrot (eds.), *A History of Women in the West*, vol. 4: *Emerging Feminism from Revolution to World War* (Cambridge Mass.: Harvard University Press, 1993).

Mark Francis and John Morrow, *A History of English Political Thought in the Nineteenth Century* (New York: St Martin's Press, 1994).

Joseph Frank, *The Beginnings of the English Newspaper, 1620–1660* (Cambridge, Mass.: Harvard University Press, 1961).

Robert G. Frank Jr., *Harvey and the Oxford Physiologists: A Study of Scientific Ideas and Social Interaction* (London: University of California Press, 1980).

A. W. Franks, *Nineteenth Century Collecting and the British Museum* (London: British Museum Press, 1997).

Antonia Fraser, *A History of Toys* (London: Weidenfeld and Nicolson, 1966).

Antonia Fraser, *King Charles II* (London: Weidenfeld and Nicolson, 1979).

Antonia Fraser, *The Weaker Vessel: Woman's Lot in Seventeenth-Century England* (London: Weidenfeld and Nicolson, 1984).

Derek Fraser (ed.), *The New Poor Law in the Nineteenth Century* (London: Macmillan, 1976).

Derek Fraser, *Power and Authority in the Victorian City* (Oxford: Basil Blackwell, 1979).

Derek Fraser (ed.), *Municipal Reform and the Industrial City* (Leicester: Leicester University Press; New York: St Martin's Press, 1982).

Derek Fraser, *The Evolution of the British Welfare State: A History of Social Policy since the Industrial Revolution* (London: Macmillan, 1984).

Derek Fraser (ed.), *Cities, Class and Communication: Essays in Honour of Asa Briggs* (Hemel Hempstead: Harvester, 1991).

Derek Fraser and Anthony Sutcliffe (eds.), *The Pursuit of Urban History* (London: Edward Arnold, 1983).

Flora Fraser, *The Unruly Queen: The Life of Queen Caroline* (London: Macmillan, 1996).

Hilary Fraser, *Beauty and Belief: Aesthetics and Religion in Victorian Literature* (New York: Cambridge University Press, 1986).

Hilary Fraser, *The Victorians and Renaissance Italy* (Oxford: Blackwell, 1994).

Sylvia Freedman, *Poor Penelope: Lady Penelope Rich, an Elizabethan Woman* (Windsor: Kensal Press, 1983).

Michael Freeman, *Edmund Burke and the Critique of Political Radicalism* (Oxford: Basil Blackwell, 1980).

Jerome Friedman, *Blasphemy, Immortality, and Anarchy: The Ranters and the English Revolution* (Athens: Ohio University Press, 1987).

Jerome Friedman, *Miracles and the Pulp Press During the English Revolution* (London: UCL Press, 1993).

Terry Friedman, *James Gibbs* (London: Yale University Press, 1984).

G. E. Fussell and K. R. Fussell, *The English Countryman* (London: Andrew Melrose, 1955).

David Gadd, *Georgian Summer: Bath in the Eighteenth Century* (Bath: Adams and Dart, 1971).

Catherine Gallagher and Thomas Laqueur (eds.), *The Making of the Modern Body: Sexuality and Society in the Nineteenth Century* (Berkeley: University of California Press, 1987).

Dorothy Gardiner, *English Girlhood at School* (Oxford: Oxford University Press, 1929).

Carl Gardner and Julia Sheppard, *Consuming*

Passion: The Rise of Retail Culture (London: Unwin Hyman, 1989).

Leon Garfield, *The House of Hanover: England in the 18th Century* (The Mirror of Britain Series, gen. ed. Kevin Crossley-Holland; London: André Deutsch, 1976).

David Garland, *Punishment and Welfare: A History of Penal Strategies* (Aldershot: Gower Publishing Co., 1985).

Martha McMackin Garland, *Cambridge before Darwin: The Ideal of a Liberal Education 1800–1860* (Cambridge: Cambridge University Press, 1980).

Clarke Garrett, 'Swedenborg and the Mystical Enlightenment in Late Eighteenth Century England', *Journal of the History of Ideas*, 45 (1984), 67–81.

Clarke Garrett, *Spirit Possession and Popular Religion: From the Camisards to the Shakers* (Baltimore: Johns Hopkins University Press, 1987).

Tom Garvin, *The Evolution of Irish Nationalist Politics* (New York: Holmes and Meier, 1982).

John Gascoigne, 'Anglican Latitudinarianism and Political Radicalism in the Late Eighteenth Century', *History*, 71 (1986), 22–38.

John Gascoigne, *Cambridge in the Age of the Enlightenment: Science, Religion and Politics from the Restoration to the French Revolution* (Cambridge: Cambridge University Press, 1989).

Norman Gash, *Pillars of Government and Other Essays on State and Society c. 1770–c. 1880* (London: Edward Arnold, 1986).

S. Martin Gaskell (ed.), *Slums* (Leicester: Leicester University Press, 1990).

Barbara T. Gates, *Victorian Suicide: Mad Crimes and Sad Histories* (Princeton: Princeton University Press, 1988).

J. Gathorne-Hardy, *The Public School Phenomenon, 597–1977* (London: Hodder and Stoughton, 1977).

V. A. C. Gatrell, *The Hanging Tree: Execution and the English People 1770–1868* (Oxford: Oxford University Press, 1994).

V. A. C. Gatrell, Bruce Lenman and Geoffrey Parker (eds.), *Crime and the Law: The Social History of Crime in Western Europe since 1500* (London: Europa, 1980).

Anne Geneva, *Astrology and the Seventeenth Century Mind: William Lilly and the Language of the Stars* (Manchester: Manchester University Press, 1995).

Lucy Gent and Nigel Llewellyn (eds.), *Renaissance Bodies: The Human Figure in English Culture c. 1540–1660* (London: Reaktion Books, 1990).

M. Dorothy George, *English Social Life in the Eighteenth Century* (London: Sheldon Press, 1923).

M. Dorothy George, *England in Johnson's Day* (London: Methuen, 1928).

M. Dorothy George, *England in Transition: Life and Work in the Eighteenth Century*, new edn. (London: Penguin, 1953).

M. Dorothy George, *English Political Caricature 1793–1832* (Oxford: Clarendon Press, 1959).

M. Dorothy George, *London Life in the Eighteenth Century* (Harmondsworth: Penguin, 1966).

M. Dorothy George, *Hogarth to Cruikshank: Social Change in Graphic Satire* (London: Allen Lane, 1967).

Jessica Gerard, *Country House Life: Family and Servants 1815–1914* (Oxford: Blackwell, 1994).

Bronislaw Geremek, *Poverty: A History* (Oxford: Blackwell, 1994).

Dorian Gerhold, *Road Transport before the Railways: Russell's London Flying Coaches* (Cambridge: Cambridge University Press, 1993).

B. J. Gibbons, *Gender in Mystical and Occult Thought: Behmenism and its Development in England* (Cambridge: Cambridge University Press, 1996).

Philip Gibbs, *England Speaks* (London: Heinemann, 1935).

Wiliam Gibson, *Church, State and Society, 1760–1850* (London: Macmillan, 1994).

A. Giddens, *The Constitution of Society: Outline of a Theory of Structuration* (Cambridge: Polity Press, 1984).

Marijke Gijswijt-Hofstra, Brian P. Levack and Roy Porter, *Witchcraft and Magic in Europe: The Eighteenth and Nineteenth Centuries* (London: Athlone, 1999).

A. D. Gilbert, *Religion and Society in Industrial England* (London: Longman, 1976).

A. D. Gilbert, *The Making of Post-Christian Britain: A History of the Secularization of Modern Society* (London: Longman, 1980).

Pamela K. Gilbert, *Disease, Desire and the Body in Victorian Women's Popular Novels* (New York and Cambridge: Cambridge University Press, 1997).

Sandra M. Gilbert and Susan Gubar, *The Madwoman in the Attic: The Woman Writer and the Nineteenth-Century Literary Imagination* (New Haven: Yale University Press, 1979).

Robin Gill, *The Myth of the Empty Church* (London: Society for Promoting Christian Knowledge, 1993).

Paula Gillett, *Worlds of Art: Painters in Victorian Society* (New Brunswick, NJ: Rutgers University Press, 1990).

Sheridan Gilley and W. J. Sheils, *A History of Religion in Britain: Practice and Belief from Pre-Roman Times to the Present* (Oxford: Blackwell, 1994).

John R. Gillis, *Youth and History: Tradition and Change in European Age Relations, 1770–Present* (New York: Academic Press, 1981).

John R. Gillis, *For Better, For Worse: British Marriages, 1600 to the Present* (Oxford: Oxford University Press, 1985).

John R. Gillis, *A World of their Own Making* (Oxford: Oxford University Press, 1997).

Ernest B. Gilman, *Iconoclasm and Poetry in the English Reformation: Down Went Dagon* (Chicago: University of Chicago Press, 1986).

Sander L. Gilman, *Difference and Pathology: Stereotypes of Sexuality, Race, and Madness* (Ithaca, NY: Cornell University Press, 1985).

Kevin Gilmartin, *Print Politics: The Press and Radical Opposition in Early Nineteenth-Century England* (Cambridge: Cambridge University Press, 1996).

Ian Gilmour, *Riot, Risings and Revolution: Governance and Violence in Eighteenth-Century England* (London: Hutchinson, 1992).

Mark Girouard, *Life in the English Country House* (New Haven: Yale University Press, 1978).

Mark Girouard, *The Return to Camelot: Chivalry and the English Gentleman* (New Haven: Yale University Press, 1981).

Mark Girouard, *The English Town* (New Haven: Yale University Press, 1990).

Clare Gittings, *Death, Burial and the Individual in Early Modern England* (London: Croom Helm, 1984; London: Routledge, 1988).

Robert Gittings and Jo Manton, *Dorothy Wordsworth* (New York: Oxford University Press, 1985).

Heather Glen, *Vision and Disenchantment: Blake's 'Songs' and Wordsworth's 'Lyrical Ballads'* (Cambridge: Cambridge University Press, 1983).

Robert Glen, *Urban Workers in the Early Industrial Revolution* (London: Croom Helm, 1984).

John Gloag, *A Social History of Furniture Design: From BC 1300 to AD 1960* (London: Cassell, 1966).

David Glover, *Vampires, Mummies, and Liberals: Bram Stoker and the Politics of Popular Fiction* (Durham, NC: Duke University Press, 1996).

Sean Glynn, *Modern Britain: An Economic and Social History* (London: Routledge, 1996).

J. M. Golby and A. W. Purdue, *The Civilization of the Crowd: Popular Culture in England, 1750–1900* (London: Batsford, 1984).

Anne Goldgar, *Impolite Learning: Conduct and Community in the Republic of Letters 1680–1750* (New Haven: Yale University Press, 1995).

Bertrand A. Goldgar, *The Curse of Party: Swift's Relations with Addison and Steele* (Lincoln: University of Nebraska Press, 1961).

Bertrand A. Goldgar, *Walpole and the Wits: The Relation of Politics to Literature, 1722–1742* (Lincoln: University of Nebraska Press, 1976).

Bette P. Goldstone, *Lessons to be Learned: A Study of Eighteenth-Century English Didactic Children's Literature* (New York: Peter Lang, 1984).

Jan Golinski, *Science as Public Culture: Chemistry and Enlightenment in Britain, 1760–1820* (Cambridge: Cambridge University Press, 1992).

Ronald K. Goodenow and William E. Marsden (eds.), *The City and Education in Four Nations* (Cambridge: Cambridge University Press, 1992).

Jordan Goodman, *Tobacco in History: The Cultures of Dependence* (London: Routledge, 1993).

Albert Goodwin, *The Friends of Liberty: The English Democratic Movement in the Age of the French Revolution* (London: Hutchinson, 1979).

Jack Goody, *The Development of the Family and Marriage in Europe* (Cambridge: Cambridge University Press, 1983).

Peter Gordon and John White, *Philosophers as Educational Reformers: The Influence of Idealism on British Educational Thought and Practice* (London: Routledge and Kegan Paul, 1979).

Alan Gore and Anne Gore, *The History of English Interiors* (Oxford: Phaidon, 1991).

Deborah Gorham, *The Victorian Girl and the Feminine Ideal* (London: Croom Helm, 1982).

Beatrice Gottlieb, *The Family in the Western World: From the Black Death to the Industrial Age* (Oxford: Oxford University Press, 1993).

Stephen Jay Gould, *Time's Arrow, Time's Cycle: Myth and Metaphor in the Discovery of Geological Time* (Cambridge, Mass.: Harvard University Press, 1987).

Tony Gould, *A Summer Plague – Polio and its Survivors* (New Haven: Yale University Press, 1995).

Todd Longstaffe Gowan, *The London Town Garden* (New Haven: Yale University Press, 2001).

Laura Gowing, *Domestic Dangers: Women, Words and Sex in Early Modern London* (Oxford: Oxford University Press, 1996).

Stephen Gradish, *The Manning of the British Navy During the Seven Years' War* (London: Royal Historical Society, 1980).

Darryll Grantley and Nina Taunton (eds.), *The Body in Late Medieval and Early Modern Culture* (Aldershot: Ashgate, 2001).

Richard Grassby, *The Business Community of Seventeenth-Century England* (Cambridge: Cambridge University Press, 1995).

M. A. R. Graves and R. H. Silcock, *Revolution, Reaction and the Triumph of Conservatism: English History 1558–1700* (London: Longman, 1984).

Richard Greaves, *Deliver Us From Evil: The Radical Underground in Britain, 1660–1663* (New York: Oxford University Press, 1986).

Richard Greaves, *Enemies Under His Feet: Radicals and Nonconformists in Britain, 1664–1677* (Stanford, Calif.: Stanford University Press, 1990).

Richard Greaves, *Secrets of the Kingdom: British Radicals from the Popish Plot to the Revolution of 1688–89* (Stanford, Calif.: Stanford University Press, 1992).

D. Green, *Great Cobbett: The Noblest Agitator* (Oxford: Oxford University Press, 1985).

David R. Green, *From Artisans to Paupers: Economic Change and Poverty in London, 1790–1870* (Aldershot: Scolar Press; Brookfield, Vt.: Ashgate, 1995).

Thomas A. Green, *Verdict According to Conscience: Perspectives on the English Criminal Trial Jury, 1200–1800* (London: University of Chicago Press, 1985).

Vivian Green, *The Madness of Kings: Personal*

Trauma and the Fate of Nations (Stroud: Alan Sutton, 1993).

Mark Greengrass, Michael Leslie and Timothy Raylor (eds.), *Samuel Hartlib and Universal Reformation: Studies in Intellectual Communication* (Cambridge: Cambridge University Press, 1995).

W. H. Greenleaf, *The British Political Tradition*, vol. 1: *The Rise of Collectivism*, vol. 2: *The Ideological Heritage* (London: Methuen, 1983); vol. 3: *A Much Governed Nation* (London: Methuen, 1987).

Germaine Greer, *The Obstacle Race* (London: Secker and Warburg, 1979).

Germaine Greer, *Slip-Shod Sibyls: Recognition, Rejection and the Woman Poet* (London: Viking, 1995).

Edward Gregg, *Queen Anne* (London: Routledge and Kegan Paul, 1980).

Derek Gregory, *Regional Transformation and Industrial Revolution: A Geography of the Yorkshire Woollen Industry* (London: Macmillan, 1982).

Ole Peter Grell, Jonathan I. Israel and Nicholas Tyacke (eds.), *From Persecution to Toleration: The Glorious Revolution and Religion in England* (Oxford: Clarendon Press, 1991).

Jukka Gronow, *The Sociology of Taste* (New York: Routledge, 1997).

Joan Grundy: *Hardy and the Sister Arts* (London: Macmillan, 1979).

David Grylls, *Guardians and Angels: Parents and Children in Nineteenth-Century Literature* (London: Faber and Faber, 1978).

W. L. Guttsman, *The British Political Elite* (London: MacGibbon and Kee, 1968).

Robin D. Gwynn, *Huguenot Heritage: The History and Contribution of the Huguenots in Britain* (London: Routledge and Kegan Paul, 1985).

Knud Haakonssen, *Enlightenment and Religion: Rational Dissent in Eighteenth-Century Britain* (Cambridge: Cambridge University Press, 1996).

H. J. Habakkuk, 'England', in Albert Goodwin (ed.), *The European Nobility in the Eighteenth Century: Studies of the Nobilities of the Major European States in the Pre-Reform Era* (London: A. & C. Black, 1953; New York: Harper and Row, 1967), 1–21.

H. J. Habakkuk, *Population Growth and Economic Development since 1750* (Leicester: Leicester University Press, 1971).

John Habakkuk, *Marriage, Debt and the Estates System: English Landownership, 1650–1950* (Oxford: Clarendon Press, 1994).

I. Hacking, *The Taming of Chance* (Cambridge: Cambridge University Press, 1990).

George E. Haggerty, *Men in Love: Masculinity and Sexuality in the Eighteenth Century* (New York: Columbia University Press, 1999).

Alan Haig, *The Victorian Clergy* (London: Croom Helm, 1984).

D. R. Hainsworth, *Stewards, Lords and People: The Estate Steward and his World in Later Stuart England* (Cambridge: Cambridge University Press, 1992).

Roger Hainsworth, *The Swordsmen in Power: War and Politics under the English Republic, 1649–1660* (Stroud: Sutton Publishing, 1997).

Elie Halévy, *A History of the English People in the Nineteenth Century*, vol. 1: *England in 1815*, 2nd edn., trans. E. I. Watkin and D. A. Barker (London: Benn, 1961).

Elie Halévy, *The Growth of Philosophic Radicalism*, trans. Mary Morris, 2 vols., new edn. (London: Faber and Faber, 1972).

Bruce Haley, *The Healthy Body and Victorian Culture* (Cambridge, Mass.: Harvard University Press, 1978).

K. H. D. Haley, *Politics in the Reign of Charles II* (Oxford: Basil Blackwell, 1985).

A. Rupert Hall, *The Revolution in Science 1500–1750* (London: Longman, 1983).

A. Rupert Hall, *Henry More: Magic, Religion and Experiment* (Oxford: Blackwell, 1990).

Catherine Hall, *White, Male and Middle Class: Explorations of Feminism in History* (Cambridge: Polity Press, 1992).

Donald E. Hall (ed.), *Muscular Christianity:*

Embodying the Victorian Age (Cambridge: Cambridge University Press, 1994).

Marie Boas Hall, *All Scientists Now: The Royal Society in the Nineteenth Century* (Cambridge: Cambridge University Press, 1984).

Lotte Hamburger and Joseph Hamburger, *Contemplating Adultery: The Secret Life of a Victorian Woman* (London: Macmillan, 1992).

Henry Hamilton, *An Economic History of Scotland in the Eighteenth Century* (Oxford: Clarendon Press, 1963).

A. James Hammerton, *Cruelty and Companionship: Conflict in Nineteenth-Century Married Life* (London: Routledge, 1992).

Brean S. Hammond, *Pope and Bolingbroke: A Study of Friendship and Influence* (Columbia: University of Missouri Press, 1984).

Brean S. Hammond, *Professional Imaginative Writing in England, 1670–1740: 'Hackney for Bread'* (Oxford: Clarendon Press, 1997).

J. L. Hammond and Barbara Hammond, *The Skilled Labourer*, ed. John Rule (London and New York: Longman, 1979).

Jean Hampton, *Hobbes and the Social Contract Tradition* (Cambridge: Cambridge University Press, 1987).

David Hancock, *Citizens of the World: London Merchants and the Integration of the British Atlantic Community* (Cambridge: Cambridge University Press, 1996).

Margaret Patterson Hannay (ed.), *Silent but for the Word: Tudor Women as Patrons, Translators, and Writers of Religious Works* (Kent, Ohio: Kent State University Press, 1985).

Nicholas Adolph Hans, *New Trends in Education in the Eighteenth Century* (London, Routledge, 1966; 1st edn. 1951).

Christopher Harding, Bill Hines, Richard Ireland and Philip Rawlings, *Imprisonment in England and Wales: A Concise History* (Beckenham: Croom Helm, 1985).

Richard Harding, *The Evolution of the Sailing Navy, 1509–1815* (London: Macmillan, 1995).

C. Hardyment, *Dream Babies: Child Care from Locke to Spock* (London: Jonathan Cape, 1983).

C. Hardyment, *From Mangle to Microwave: The Mechanization of Household Work* (Cambridge: Polity Press, 1988).

Christina Hardyment, *Home Comfort: A History of Domestic Arrangements* (London: Viking/National Trust, 1992).

Dave Harker, *Fakesong: The Manufacture of British 'Folksong' 1700 to the Present Day* (Milton Keynes: Open University Press, 1985).

Philip Harling, *The Waning of 'Old Corruption': The Politics of Economical Reform in Britain, 1779–1846* (Oxford: Oxford University Press, 1996).

Ann Harrington, *Medicine, Mind, and the Double Brain: A Study in Nineteenth-Century Thought* (Princeton: Princeton University Press, 1987).

Francis Harris, *A Passion for Government: The Life of Sarah, Duchess of Marlborough* (Oxford: Clarendon Press, 1991).

Ian Harris (ed.), *Edmund Burke: Pre-Revolutionary Writings* (Cambridge: Cambridge University Press, 1993).

John Harris, *Essays in Industry and Technology in the Eigthteenth Century: England and France* (Aldershot: Variorum, 1992).

Marvin Harris, *The Rise of Anthropological Theory* (New York: Thomas Y. Crowell, 1968).

Michael Harris, *London Newspapers in the Age of Walpole: A Study of the Origins of the Modern English Press* (Cranbury, NJ: Associated University Presses, 1987).

Michael Harris and Alan Lee (eds.), *The Press in English Society from the Seventeenth to Nineteenth Centuries* (Cranbury, NJ: Fairleigh Dickinson University Press, 1986).

R. W. Harris, *Reason and Nature in the Eighteenth Century* (London: Blandford Press, 1968).

R. W. Harris, *Romanticism and the Social Order* (London: Blandford Press, 1969).

Robert Harris, *A Patriot Press: National Politics*

and the London Press in the *1740s* (Oxford: Clarendon Press, 1993).

Tim Harris (ed.), *The French Revolution and Enlightenment in England 1789–1832* (Cambridge, Mass.: Harvard University Press, 1989).

Tim Harris, *London Crowds in the Reign of Charles II: Propaganda and Politics from the Restoration until the Exclusion Crisis* (Cambridge Studies in Early Modern British History; Cambridge: Cambridge University Press, 1990).

Tim Harris, *Politics under the Later Stuarts: Party Conflict in a Divided Society 1660–1715* (London: Longman, 1993).

Tim Harris (ed.), *Popular Culture in England, c. 1500–1850* (London: Macmillan, 1995).

Tim Harris, Paul Seaward and Mark Goldie (eds.), *The Politics of Religion in Restoration England* (Oxford: Basil Blackwell, 1990).

Jonathan Harrison, *Hume's Theory of Justice* (Oxford: Oxford University Press, 1981).

J. F. C. Harrison, *The Second Coming: Popular Millenarianism 1780–1850* (London: Routledge and Kegan Paul, 1979).

J. M. Harrison, 'The Crowd in Bristol 1790–1835' (Ph.D. thesis, University of Cambridge, 1983).

Mark Harrison, *Crowds and History: Mass Phenomena in English Towns, 1790–1835* (Cambridge: Cambridge University Press, 1988).

Peter Harrison, *'Religion' and the Religions in the English Enlightenment* (Cambridge: Cambridge University Press, 1990).

Royden Harrison (ed.), *Independent Collier: The Coal Miner as Archetypal Proletarian Reconsidered* (New York: St Martin's Press, 1979; Hassocks: Harvester Press, 1979).

James S. Hart, *Justice upon Petition: The House of Lords and the Reformation of Justice, 1621–1675* (London: HarperCollins Academic, 1991).

Vaughan Hart, *Art and Magic in the Court of the Stuarts* (London: Routledge, 1994).

Negley Harte and Roland Quinault (eds.), *Land and Society in Britain, 1770–1914: Essays*

in Honour of F. M. L. Thompson (Manchester: Manchester University Press, 1996).

Lord Hartwell, *William Camrose: Giant of Fleet Street* (London: Weidenfeld and Nicolson, 1992).

R. M. Hartwell (ed.), *The Causes of the Industrial Revolution in England* (London: Methuen, 1967).

R. M. Hartwell, *The Industrial Revolution and Economic Growth* (London: Methuen, 1971).

R. M. Hartwell, *Fontana Economic History of Europe*, vol. 3: *The Industrial Revolution*, ed. C. M. Cipolla (London: Collins/Fontana, 1973).

A. D. Harvey, *Britain in the Early Nineteenth Century* (London: Batsford, 1978).

A. D. Harvey, *Collision of Empires: Britain in Three World Wars 1793–1945* (London: Hambledon Press, 1992).

A. D. Harvey, *Sex in Georgian England: Attitudes and Prejudices from the 1720s to the 1820s* (London: Duckworth, 1994).

Andrew Hassam, *Sailing to Australia: Shipboard Diaries by Nineteenth-Century British Emigrants* (Manchester: Manchester University Press, 1994).

John Hatcher, *The History of the British Coal Industry*, vol. 1: *Before 1700* (Oxford: Oxford University Press, 1993).

Helen E. Hatton, *The Largest Amount of Good: Quaker Relief in Ireland 1654–1921* (Montreal: McGill-Queen's University Press, 1993).

Jeremy Hawthorn (ed.), *The Nineteenth-Century British Novel* (Baltimore: Edward Arnold, 1986).

Carla H. Hay, *James Burgh, Spokesman for Reform in Hanoverian England* (Washington, DC: University Press of America, 1979).

Douglas Hay et al. (eds.), *Albion's Fatal Tree: Crime and Society in Eighteenth-Century England* (London: Allen Lane, 1975).

Douglas Hay and Francis Snyder (eds.), *Policing and Prosecution in Britain 1750–1850* (Oxford: Clarendon Press, 1989).

Colin Haydon, *Anti-Catholicism in Eighteenth-Century England, c.1714–80: A Political and Social Study* (Manchester: Manchester University Press, 1994).

T. Wilson Hayes, *Winstanley the Digger: A Literary Analysis of Radical Ideas in the English Revolution* (Cambridge, Mass.: Harvard University Press, 1979).

F. Heal, 'Hospitality and Honor in Early Modern England', *Food and Foodways*, 1 (1987), 321–50.

Felicity Heal, *Hospitality in Early Modern England* (Oxford: Clarendon Press, 1990).

Felicity Heal and Clive Holmes, *The Gentry in England and Wales, 1500–1700* (Basingstoke: Macmillan, 1994).

Thomas Healy and Jonathan Sawday (eds.), *Literature and the English Civil War* (Cambridge: Cambridge University Press, 1990).

Francis Hearn, *Domination, Legitimation, and Resistance: The Incorporation of the Nineteenth-Century English Working Class* (London: Greenwood Press, 1978).

James Heath, *Torture and English Law* (London: Greenwood Press, 1982).

J. Jean Hecht, *The Domestic Servant in Eighteenth Century England* (London: Routledge and Kegan Paul, 1980).

William S. Heckscher, *Art and Literature: Studies in Relationship*, ed. Egon Verheyen (Durham, NC: Duke University Press; Baden-Baden: Verlag Valentin Koerner, 1985).

J. L. Heilbron, *Electricity in the 17th and 18th Centuries: A Study of Early Modern Physics* (London: University of California Press, 1979).

J. L. Heilbron, *Physics at the Royal Society during Newton's Presidency* (Los Angeles: William Andrews Clark Memorial Library, 1983).

Eckhart Hellmuth (ed.), *The Transformation of Political Culture: England and Germany in the Late Eighteenth Century* (Oxford: Oxford University Press, 1990).

Richard Helmstadter (ed.), *Freedom and Religion in the Nineteenth Century* (Stanford, Calif.: Stanford University Press, 1997).

Phyllis Hembry, *The English Spa 1560–1815: A Social History* (London: Athlone, 1990).

Ray Hemmings, *Liberty or Death: The Struggle for Democracy in Britain 1780–1830* (London: Lawrence and Wishart, 2000).

David Hempton, *Methodism and Politics in British Society, 1750–1850* (Stanford, Calif.: Stanford University Press, 1984).

David Hempton, *Religion and Political Culture in Britain and Ireland* (Cambridge: Cambridge University Press, 1996).

Katherine Usher Henderson and Barbara F. McManus, *Half Humankind: Contexts and Texts of the Controversy about Women in England, 1540–1640* (Urbana: University of Illinois Press, 1985).

Ursula Henriques, *Religious Toleration in England 1783–1833* (London: Routledge, 1961).

Ursula Henriques, *Before the Welfare State: Social Administration in Early Industrial Britain* (London: Longman, 1979).

A. C. Hepburn (ed.), *Documents of Modern History: The Conflict of Nationality in Modern Ireland* (London: Edward Arnold, 1980).

David Hey, *The Fiery Blades of Hallamshire: Sheffield and its Neighbourhood, 1660–1740* (Leicester: Leicester University Press, 1991).

T. W. Heyck, *The Transformation of Intellectual Life in Victorian England* (London: Croom Helm, 1982).

Caroline Hibbard, *Charles I and the Popish Plot* (London: University of North Carolina Press, 1983).

Christopher Hibbert, *The Roots of Evil: Crime and Punishment* (London: Weidenfeld and Nicolson, 1963).

Christopher Hibbert (ed.), *Louis Simond: An American in Regency England: The Journal of a Tour in 1810–1811* (London: Maxwell, 1968).

Christopher Hibbert, *The English: A Social*

History 1066–1945 (London: HarperCollins, 1987).

Alan G. Hill (ed.), *Letters of Dorothy Wordsworth: A Selection* (New York: Oxford University Press, 1985).

Brian W. Hill, *Robert Harley: Speaker, Secretary of State and Premier Minister* (New Haven: Yale University Press, 1988).

Brian Hill, *The Early Parties and Politics in Britain, 1688–1832* (London: Macmillan, 1996).

Bridget Hill, *Eighteenth-Century Women: An Anthology* (London: Allen and Unwin, 1984).

Bridget Hill, *The First English Feminist: Reflections upon Marriage and Other Writings by Mary Astell* (Aldershot: Gower, 1986).

Bridget Hill, *The Republican Virago: The Life and Times of Catharine Macaulay* (Oxford: Clarendon Press, 1992).

Bridget Hill, *Women, Work and Sexual Politics in Eighteenth-Century England* (London: UCL Press, 1994).

Bridget Hill, *Servants: English Domestics in the Eighteenth Century* (Oxford: Oxford University Press, 1996).

Christopher Hill, 'Puritans and the Poor', *Past and Present*, 2 (1952), 32–50.

Christopher Hill, *The Century of Revolution 1603–1714* (London and Edinburgh: T. Nelson, 1961).

Christopher Hill, *The Intellectual Origins of the Puritan Revolution* (Oxford: Oxford University Press, 1965).

Christopher Hill, *Puritanism and Revolution* (Harmondsworth: Penguin, 1958; repr. London: Panther, 1968).

Christopher Hill, *Reformation to Industrial Revolution* (Harmondsworth: Penguin, 1969).

Christopher Hill, *God's Englishman: Oliver Cromwell and the English Revolution* (Harmondsworth: Penguin, 1970).

Christopher Hill, *Antichrist in Seventeenth Century England* (London: Oxford University Press, 1971).

Christopher Hill, *Milton and the English Revolution* (London: Faber, 1977).

Christopher Hill, *The World Turned Upside Down: Radical Ideas During the English Revolution* (Harmondsworth: Penguin, 1972; repr. 1978).

Christopher Hill, *Some Intellectual Consequences of the English Revolution* (London: Weidenfeld and Nicolson, 1980).

Christopher Hill, *The Collected Essays of Christopher Hill*, vol. 1: *Writing and Revolution in 17th Century England*; vol. 2: *Religion and Politics in 17th Century England*; vol. 3: *People and Ideas in 17th Century England* (Brighton: Harvester Press, 1988).

Christopher Hill, *A Turbulent, Seditious and Factious People: John Bunyan and his Church 1628–1688* (Oxford: Oxford University Press, 1989).

Christopher Hill, *A Nation of Change and Novelty: Radical Politics, Religion and Literature in Seventeenth-Century England* (London: Routledge, 1990).

Christopher Hill, *The English Bible and the 17th-Century Revolution* (London: Allen Lane, 1993).

Christopher Hill, *Liberty Against the Law: Some Seventeenth-Century Controversies* (London: Penguin, 1996).

Christopher Hill, Barry Reay and William Lamont, *The World of the Muggletonians* (London: Temple Smith, 1983).

Boyd Hilton, *The Age of Atonement: The Influence of Evangelicalism on Social and Economic Thought, 1785–1865* (Oxford: Clarendon Press, 1988).

Mary Hilton, Morag Styles and Victor Watson (eds.), *Opening the Nursery Door: Reading, Writing and Childhood, 1600–1900* (London and New York: Routledge, 1997).

Gertrude Himmelfarb, *The Idea of Poverty: England in the Early Industrial Age* (London: Faber; New York: Knopf, 1984).

Gertrude Himmelfarb, *Marriage and Morals amongst the Victorians and Other Essays* (London: Faber and Faber, 1986).

Walter John Hipple, *The Beautiful, the Sublime, and the Picturesque in Eighteenth-Century Aesthetic Theory* (Carbondale: Southern Illinois University Press, 1957).

Rénee Hirschon (ed.), *Women and Property – Women as Property* (London: Croom Helm, 1984).

Derek Hirst, *Authority and Conflict: England 1603–1658* (London: Edward Arnold, 1986).

Tim V. Hitchcock *et al.* (eds.), *Stilling the Grumbling Hive: The Regulation of Social and Economic Problems in England, 1689–1750* (Stroud: Sutton; New York: St Martin's Press, 1992).

Tim Hitchcock, *English Sexualities, 1700–1800* (Basingstoke: Macmillan, 1997).

Eric Hobsbawm, *Industry and Empire: From 1750 to the Present Day* (Harmondsworth: Penguin, 1969; orig. pub. London: Weidenfeld and Nicolson, 1968).

Eric Hobsbawm, *Worlds of Labour: Further Studies in the History of Labour* (London: Weidenfeld Paperbacks, 1984).

Eric Hobsbawm and Terence Ranger (eds.), *The Invention of Tradition* (Cambridge: Cambridge University Press, 1983).

Jane Aiken Hodge, *Passion and Principle: The Loves and Lives of Regency Women* (London: John Murray, 1996).

Devon L. Hodges, *Renaissance Fictions of Anatomy* (Amherst: University of Massachussetts Press, 1985).

Edward Hodnett, *Image and Text: Studies in the Illustration of English Literature* (London: Scolar Press, 1982).

Richard Hoggart, *The Uses of Literacy* (London: Chatto and Windus, 1957).

Mike Holbrook-Jones, *Supremacy and Subordination of Labour* (London: Heinemann Educational Books, 1982).

B. A. Holderness, 'Credit in a Rural Community 1660–1800', *Midland History*, 3 (1975), 94–115.

B. A. Holderness, 'Credit in English Rural Society before the Nineteenth Century', *Agricultural History Review*, 24 (1976), 97–109.

B. A. Holderness, *Pre-Industrial England: Economy and Society 1500–1750* (London: Dent, 1976).

Robert Hole, *Pulpits, Politics and Public Order in England, 1760–1832* (Cambridge: Cambridge University Press, 1989).

Geoffrey Holmes (ed.), *Britain after the Glorious Revolution 1689–1714* (London: Macmillan, 1969).

Geoffrey Holmes, *The Trial of Doctor Sacherverell* (London: Eyre Methuen, 1973).

Geoffrey S. Holmes, *Augustan England: Professions, State and Society, 1680–1730* (London: G. Allen and Unwin, 1982).

Geoffrey S. Holmes, *Politics, Religion, and Society in England, 1679–1742* (London: Hambledon, 1986).

Geoffrey Holmes, *British Politics in the Age of Anne* (London: Hambledon, 1987).

Geoffrey Holmes, *The Making of a Great Power: Late Stuart and Early Georgian Britain, 1660–1722* (Harlow: Longman, 1993).

Geoffrey Holmes, *The Birth of Britain: A New Nation 1700–1710* (Oxford: Blackwell, 1994).

Geoffrey Holmes and Daniel Szechi, *The Age of Oligarchy: Pre-Industrial Britain, 1723–1783* (Harlow: Longman, 1993).

Richard Holmes, *Coleridge* (Oxford: Oxford University Press, 1982).

Richard Holmes, *Coleridge: Early Visions* (London: Hodder and Stoughton, 1989).

Richard Holmes, *Dr Johnson and Mr Savage: A Biographical Mystery* (London: Hodder and Stoughton, 1993).

Karl Josef Höltgen, Peter M. Daly and Wolfgang Lottes (eds.), *Word and Visual Imagination: Studies in the Interaction of English Literature and the Visual Arts* (Erlangen: Universitätsbund Erlangen-Nürnberg, 1988).

Margaret Homans, *Women Writers and Poetic Identity: Dorothy Wordsworth, Emily Brontë, and Emily Dickinson* (Princeton: Princeton University Press, 1980).

J. Ann Hone, *For the Cause of Truth: Radicalism in London, 1796–1821* (Oxford: Oxford University Press, 1982).

Katrina Honeyman, *Origins of Enterprise: Business Leadership in the Industrial Revolution* (Manchester: Manchester University Press; New York: St Martin's Press, 1982).

Hugh Honour, *The Image of the Black in Western Art*, vol. 4: *From the American Revolution to World War I* (Cambridge, Mass.: Harvard University Press, 1989).

Istvan Hont and Michael Ignatieff (eds.), *Wealth and Virtue: The Shaping of Political Economy in the Scottish Enlightenment* (Cambridge: Cambridge University Press, 1983).

H. M. Höpfl, 'From Savage to Scotsman: Conjectural History in the Scottish Enlightenment', *Journal of British Studies*, 17 (1978), 19–40.

Eric Hopkins, *Birmingham: The First Manufacturing Town in the World, 1760–1840* (London: Weidenfeld and Nicolson, 1989).

Eric Hopkins, *Childhood Transformed: Working-Class Children in Nineteenth Century England* (Manchester: Manchester University Press, 1994).

Eric Hopkins, *Working-Class Self-Help in Nineteenth-Century England: Responses to Industrialisation* (London: UCL Press, 1995).

H. Hopkins, *The Long Affray: The Poaching Wars, 1760–1914* (London: Secker and Warburg, 1985).

K. Theodore Hoppen, 'The Franchise and Electoral Politics in England and Ireland', *History*, 70 (1985), 202–17.

Julian Hoppit, 'Political Arithmetic in Eighteenth-Century England', *Economic History Review*, 49 (1996), 516–40.

Julian Hoppit, 'Financial Crises in Eighteenth Century England', *Economic History Review*, 39 (1986), 39–58.

Julian Hoppit, 'The Use and Abuse of Credit in Eighteenth Century England', in N.

McKendrick and R. B. Outhwaite (eds.), *Business Life and Public Policy: Essays in Honour of D. C. Coleman* (Cambridge: Cambridge University Press, 1986), 64–78.

Julian Hoppit, *Risk and Failure in English Business, 1700–1800* (Cambridge: Cambridge University Press, 1987).

Julian Hoppit, 'Understanding the Industrial Revolution', *Historical Journal*, 30 (1987), 211–24.

Julian Hoppit, 'Counting the Industrial Revolution', *Economic History Review*, 43 (1990), 173–93.

Julian Hoppit, 'Reforming Britain's Weights an Measures, 1600–1824', *English Historical Review*, 108 (1993).

Julian Hoppit, *A Land of Liberty? England 1689–1727* (Oxford: Oxford University Press, 2000).

Julian Hoppit and E. A. Wrigley (eds.), *The Industrial Revolution in Britain*, 2 parts (Oxford: Blackwell, 1994).

Pamela Horn, *The Rural World 1780–1850: Social Change in the English Countryside* (London: Hutchinson, 1980).

Pamela Horn, *A Georgian Parson and his Village: The Story of David Davies (1742–1819)* (Abingdon: Beacon Publications, 1981).

Pamela Horn, *Life and Labour in Rural England, 1760–1850* (Basingstoke: Macmillan, 1987).

Pamela Horn, *Children's Work and Welfare, 1780–1880s* (Basingstoke: Macmillan, 1994; Cambridge: Cambridge University Press, 1995).

Thomas A. Horne, *Property Rights and Poverty: Political Argument in Britain, 1605–1834* (Chapel Hill: University of North Carolina Press, 1990).

Ralph Houlbrooke, *The English Family, 1450–1700* (London: Longman, 1984).

Ralph Houlbrooke (ed.), *English Family Life, 1576–1716: An Anthology from Diaries* (Oxford: Basil Blackwell, 1988).

Ralph Houlbrooke (ed.), *Death, Ritual and Bereavement* (London: Routledge, 1989).

Ralph Houlbrooke, *Death, Religion and the Family in England, 1480–1750* (Oxford: Clarendon Press, 1998).

J. A. Houlding, *Fit for Service: The Training of the British Army, 1715–1795* (Oxford: Oxford University Press, 1981).

R. A. Houston, 'The Development of Literacy in Northern England, 1640–1750', *Economic History Review*, 35 (1982), 199–216.

R. A. Houston, *Scottish Literacy and the Scottish Identity: Illiteracy and Society in Scotland and Northern England, 1600–1800* (Cambridge: Cambridge University Press, 1985).

R. A. Houston, *Literacy in Early Modern Europe: Culture and Education, 1500–1800* (London: Longman, 1988).

R. A. Houston, 'Scottish Education and Literacy, 1660–1800: An International Perspective', in T. M. Devine (ed.), *Improvement and Enlightenment* (Edinburgh: John Donald, 1989), 43–61.

R. A. Houston, *The Population History of Britain and Ireland, 1500–1750* (London: Macmillan, 1992).

R. A. Houston, 'Literacy, Education and the Culture of Print in Enlightenment Edinburgh', *History*, 78 (1993).

R. A. Houston, 'Popular Politics in the Reign of George II: The Edinburgh Cordiners', *Scottish Historical Review*, 72 (1993).

R. A. Houston, *Social Change in the Age of Enlightenment: Edinburgh, 1660–1760* (Oxford: Clarendon Press, 1994).

R. A. Houston and I. D. Whyte (eds.), *Scottish Society, 1500–1800* (Cambridge: Cambridge University Press, 1989).

S. J. Houston, *James I*, 2nd edn. (London: Longman, 1995).

David Howarth (ed.), *Art and Patronage in the Caroline Courts* (Cambridge: Cambridge University Press, 1994).

Nicholas Hudson, *Samuel Johnson and Eighteenth-Century Thought* (Oxford: Clarendon Press, 1988).

Pat Hudson, *The Genesis of Industrial Capitalism: A Study of the West Riding Wool Textile Industry c. 1750–1850* (Cambridge: Cambridge University Press, 1986).

Pat Hudson, *Britain's Industrial Revolution* (London: Arnold, 1989).

Pat Hudson (ed.), *Regions and Industries: A Perspective on the Industrial Revolution in Britain* (Cambridge: Cambridge University Press, 1989).

Pat Hudson, *The Industrial Revolution* (London: Arnold, 1992).

Olwen Hufton, *The Prospect Before Her: A History of Women in Western Europe*, vol. 1: *1500–1800* (London: HarperCollins, 1995).

Suzanne W. Hull, *Women According to Men: The World of Tudor–Stuart Women* (Walnut Creek, Calif.: AltaMira Press, 1996).

Sally Humphreys, *The Family, Women and Death* (London: Routledge and Kegan Paul, 1983).

John Dixon Hunt, *Garden and Grove: The Italian Renaissance Garden in the English Imagination, 1600–1750* (Philadelphia: University of Pennsylvania Press, 1996).

Lynn Hunt (ed.), *The Invention of Pornography: Obscenity and the Origins of Modernity, 1500–1800* (New York: Zone Books, 1993).

Margaret Hunt, 'English Urban Families in Trade, 1660–1800: The Culture of Early Modern Capitalism' (Ph.D. thesis, New York University, 1986).

Margaret Hunt, 'Time-Management, Writing, and Accounting in the Eighteenth-Century English Trading Family: A Bourgeois Enlightenment?', *Business and Economic History* (2nd ser.), 18 (1989), 150–9.

Margaret Hunt, 'Wife-beating, Domesticity and Women's Independence in Eighteenth-Century London', *Gender and History*, 4 (1992), 10–33.

Margaret Hunt, 'Racism, Imperialism and the Traveler's Gaze in Eighteenth-Century England', *Journal of British Studies*, 32 (1993): 333–57.

Margaret Hunt, *The Middling Sort: Commerce, Gender, and the Family in England, 1680–1780* (Berkeley: University of California Press, 1996).

Margaret Hunt, Margaret Jacob, Phyllis Mack and Ruth Perry (eds.), *Women and the Enlightenment* (New York: Institute for Research in History and the Haworth Press, 1984).

Michael Hunter, *Science and Society in Restoration England* (Cambridge: Cambridge University Press, 1981).

Michael Hunter, *The Royal Society and its Fellows, 1680–1700: The Morphology of an Early Scientific Institution* (Chalfont St Giles: British Society for the History of Science, 1982).

Michael Hunter, *Establishing the New Science: The Experience of the Early Royal Society* (Woodbridge: Boydell and Brewer, 1989).

Michael Hunter, *Science and the Shape of Orthodoxy: Intellectual Change in Late Seventeenth-Century Britain* (Woodbridge: Boydell and Brewer, 1995).

Michael Hunter and Simon Schaffer (eds.), *Robert Hooke: New Studies* (Woodbridge: Boydell Press, 1989).

Michael Hunter and David Wootton (eds.), *Atheism from the Reformation to the Enlightenment* (Oxford: Clarendon Press, 1992).

Ronald Hutton, *The Royalist War Effort 1642–1646* (London: Longman, 1981).

Ronald Hutton, *Charles the Second, King of England, Scotland, and Ireland* (Oxford: Clarendon Press, 1989).

Ronald Hutton, *The British Republic, 1649–1660* (London: Macmillan, 1990).

Ronald Hutton, *The Restoration: A Political and Religious History of England and Wales, 1658–1667* (Oxford: Clarendon Press, 1985; 1993).

Ronald Hutton, *The Rise and Fall of Merry England: The Ritual Year, 1400–1700* (Oxford: Oxford University Press, 1994).

Ronald Hutton, *The Stations of the Sun: A History of the Ritual Year in Britain* (Oxford: Oxford University Press, 1996).

Ronald Hyam, *Empire and Sexuality* (Manchester: Manchester University Press, 1990).

Kenneth Hylson-Smith, *Evangelicals in the Church of England, 1734–1984* (Edinburgh: T. & T. Clark, 1988).

A. Hyman (ed.), *Science and Reform: Selected Works of Charles Babbage* (Cambridge: Cambridge University Press, 1989).

Brian Inglis, *Poverty and the Industrial Revolution* (London: Hodder and Stoughton, 1971).

Ulrich Im Hoff, *The Enlightenment*, trans. William E. Yuill (Oxford and Cambridge, Mass.: Blackwell, 1994).

Brian Inglis, *Natural and Supernatural: A History of the Paranormal* (London: Hodder and Stoughton, 1977).

Martin Ingram, 'Religion, Communities and Moral Discipline in Late Sixteenth- and Early Seventeenth-Century England: Case Studies', in Kaspar von Greyerz (ed.), *Religion and Society in Early Modern Europe, 1500–1800* (London: German Historical Institute, 1984), 177–93.

Martin Ingram, *Church Courts, Sex and Marriage in England, 1570–1640* (Cambridge: Cambridge University Press, 1987).

Ian Inkster, 'The Development of a Scientific Community in Sheffield, 1790–1850: A Network of People and Interests', *Transactions of the Hunter Archaeological Society*, 10 (1973), 99–131.

Ian Inkster, 'Culture, Institutions and Urbanity: The Itinerant Science Lecturer in Sheffield 1790–1850', in Sidney Pollard and Colin Holmes (eds.), *Essays in the Economic and Social History of South Yorkshire* (Barnsley: South Yorkshire County Council, 1976), 218–32.

Ian Inkster, 'Marginal Men: Aspects of the Social Role of the Medical Community in Sheffield 1790–1850', in John Woodward and David Richards (eds.), *Health Care and Popular Medicine in Nineteenth-Century*

England: Essays in the Social History of Medicine (London: Croom Helm, 1977), 128–63.

Ian Inkster, 'Science and Society in the Metropolis: A Preliminary Examination of the Social and Economic Context of the Askesian Society of London, 1796–1807', *Annals of Science*, 34 (1977), 1–32.

Ian Inkster, 'Studies in the Social History of Science in England during the Industrial Revolution' (Ph.D. thesis, University of Sheffield, 1977).

Ian Inkster, 'London Science and the Seditious Meetings Act of 1817', *British Journal of the History of Science*, 12 (1979), 192–6.

Ian Inkster, 'The Public Lecture as an Instrument of Science Education for Adults', *Paedagogica Historica*, 20 (1981), 85–112.

Ian Inkster, 'Seditious Science: A Reply to Paul Weindling', *British Journal for the History of Science*, 14 (1981), 181–7.

Ian Inkster, 'Mental Capital: Transfers of Knowledge and Technique in Eighteenth-Century Europe', *Journal of European Economic History*, 19 (1990), 403–42.

Ian Inkster, *Science and Technology in History: An Approach to Industrial Development* (Basingstoke: Macmillan, 1991).

Ian Inkster and Jack Morrell (eds.), *Metropolis and Province: Science in British Culture 1780–1850* (Philadelphia: University of Pennsylvania Press; London: Hutchinson, 1983).

J. Innes, 'The King's Bench Prison in the Later Eighteenth Century: Law, Authority and Order in a London Debtors' Prison', in John Brewer and John Styles (eds.), *An Ungovernable People: The English and their Law in the Seventeenth and Eighteenth Centuries* (London: Hutchinson, 1980), 250–98.

J. Innes, 'Jonathan Clark, Social History, and England's Ancien Régime', *Past and Present*, 115 (1987), 165–200.

J. Innes, 'Prisons for the Poor: English Bridewells, 1555–1800', in F. Snyder and D. Hay (eds.), *Labour, Law and Crime: An Historical Perspective* (London: Tavistock, 1987), 42–122.

J. Innes, 'Parliament and the Shaping of Eighteenth-Century English Social Policy', *Transactions of the Royal Historical Society*, 40 (1990), 63–92.

J. Innes and J. Styles, 'The Crime Wave: Recent Writing on Crime and Criminal Justice in Eighteenth Century England', *Journal of British Studies*, 25 (1986), 380–435.

Jonathan Israel (ed.), *The Anglo-Dutch Moment: Essays on the Glorious Revolution and its World Impact* (Cambridge: Cambridge University Press, 1991).

Malcolm R. Jack, *Corruption and Progress: The Eighteenth-Century Debate* (New York: AMS Press, 1990).

Gordon Jackson, *The British Whaling Trade* (London: A. and C. Black, 1978).

Mark Jackson, *New-Born Child Murder: Women, Illegitimacy and the Courts in Eighteenth Century England* (Manchester: University of Manchester Press, 1996).

James R. Jacob, *Henry Stubbe: Radical Protestantism and the Early Enlightenment* (Cambridge: Cambridge University Press, 1983).

Margaret C. Jacob, *The Newtonians and the English Revolution, 1689–1720* (Hassocks: Harvester Press, 1976).

Margaret C. Jacob, 'Newtonianism and the Origins of the Enlightenment', *Eighteenth-Century Studies*, 11 (1977), 1–25.

Margaret C. Jacob, *The Radical Enlightenment: Pantheists, Freemasons and Republicans* (London: Allen and Unwin, 1981).

Margaret C. Jacob, 'The Crisis of the European Mind: Hazard Revisited', in Phyllis Mack and Margaret Jacob (eds.), *Politics and Culture in Early Modern Europe* (Cambridge: Cambridge University Press, 1987), 251–71.

Margaret C. Jacob, *The Cultural Meaning of the*

Scientific Revolution (New York: A. A. Knopf, 1988).

Margaret C. Jacob, *Living the Enlightenment: Freemasonry and Politics in 18th Century Europe* (New York: Oxford University Press, 1992).

Margaret C. Jacob, 'Reflections on the Ideological Meaning of Western Science from Boyle and Newton to the Postmodernists', *History of Science*, 33 (1995), 333–57.

Margaret C. Jacob, *Scientific Culture and the Making of the Industrial West* (Oxford: Oxford University Press, 1997).

Muriel Jaeger, *Before Victoria, Changing Standards & Behaviour 1787–1837* (Harmondsworth: Penguin, 1967).

Pat Jalland, *Death in the Victorian Family* (Oxford: Oxford University Press, 1996).

Francis G. James, *Lords of the Ascendancy: The Irish House of Lords and its Members 1600–1800* (Dublin: Irish Academic Press, 1995).

Patricia James, *Population Malthus: His Life and Times* (London: Routledge and Kegan Paul, 1979).

Derek Jarrett, *Britain 1688–1815* (London: Longmans, 1965).

Derek Jarrett, *The Ingenious Mr Hogarth* (London: Joseph, 1976).

Derek Jarrett, *England in the Age of Hogarth* (London: Hart-Davis MacGibbon, 1974; New Haven: Yale University Press, 1986).

Andrew Jenkins (ed.), *Bread and the British Economy, c.* 1700–1870. (Aldershot: Scolar Press; Brookfield, Vt.: Ashgate Publishing, 1995).

Anthony Jenkins, *The Making of Victorian Drama* (New York: Cambridge University Press, 1991).

D. T. Jenkins and K. G. Ponting, *The British Wool Textile Industry, 1770–1914* (London: Heinemann Educational, 1982).

Geraint H. Jenkins, *The Foundations of Modern Wales: 1642–1780* (Oxford: Clarendon Press; Cardiff: University of Wales Press, 1987).

Philip Jenkins, *The Making of a Ruling Class: The Glamorganshire Gentry 1640–1790* (Cambridge: Cambridge University Press, 1983).

Humphrey Jennings, *Pandaemonium 1660–1886: The Coming of the Machine as Seen by Contemporary Observers*, ed. Mary-Lou Jennings and Charles Madge (London: André Deutsch, 1985).

Paul Jennings, *The Public House in Bradford, 1770–1970* (Keele: Keele University Press, 1995).

C. B. Jewson, *Jacobin City: A Portrait of Norwich in its Reaction to the French Revolution 1788–1902* (Glasgow: Blackie, 1975).

Adrian Johns, *The Nature of the Book: Print and Knowledge in the Making* (Chicago: Chicago University Press, 1998).

E. D. H. Johnson, *Paintings of the British Social Scene, from Hogarth to Sickert* (London: Weidenfeld and Nicolson, 1986).

James William Johnson, *The Formation of English Neo-Classical Thought* (Princeton: Princeton University Press, 1967).

Samuel Johnson, *A Dictionary of the English Language*, ed. Anne McDermott (Cambridge: Cambridge University Press, 1996).

Clyve Jones (ed.), *Britain in the First Age of Party, 1680–1750: Essays Presented to Geoffrey Holmes* (London: Hambledon Press, 1987).

Clyve Jones (ed.), *A Pillar of the Constitution: The House of Lords in British Politics, 1640–1784* (London: Hambledon Press, 1989).

Clyve Jones and David Lewis Jones (eds.), *Peers, Politics and Power: The House of Lords 1603–1911* (London: Hambledon Press, 1986).

Colin Jones (ed.), *Britain and Revolutionary France: Conflict, Subversion and Propaganda* (Exeter: University of Exeter Press, 1983).

Edwin Jones, *The English Nation: The Great Myth* (Stroud: Sutton, 1998).

E. L. Jones, 'English Farming before and during the Nineteenth Century', *Economic History Review*, 15 (1962–3), 145–52.

E. L. Jones (ed.), *Agriculture and Economic Growth in England, 1600–1815* (London: Methuen, 1967).

E. L. Jones, 'English and European Agricultural Development 1650–1750', in Ronald M. Hartwell (ed.), *The Industrial Revolution* (Oxford: Basil Blackwell, 1970), 42–76.

E. L. Jones, 'The Fashion Manipulators: Consumer Tastes and British Industries, 1660–1800', in L. P. Cain and P. J. Uselding (eds.), *Business Enterprise and Economic Change* (Kent, Ohio: Kent State University Press, 1973), 198–226.

E. L. Jones, *Agriculture and the Industrial Revolution* (Oxford: Basil Blackwell, 1974).

E. L. Jones and G. E. Mingay (eds.), *Land, Labour and Population in the Industrial Revolution: Essays Presented to J. D. Chambers* (London: Edward Arnold, 1967).

Gareth Elwyn Jones, *Modern Wales: A Concise History c.1485–1979* (Cambridge: Cambridge University Press, 1984).

J. R. Jones (ed.), *The Restored Monarchy, 1660–1688* (London: Macmillan, 1979).

J. R. Jones, *Britain and the World 1649–1815* (London: Fontana, 1980).

J. R. Jones, *Charles II, Royal Politician* (London: Allen and Unwin, 1987).

J. R. Jones (ed.), *Liberty Secured? Britain before and after 1688* (Stanford, Calif.: Stanford University Press, 1992).

Kathleen Jones, *A Glorious Fame: The Life of Margaret Cavendish, Duchess of Newcastle* (London: Bloomsbury Press, 1988).

R. F. Jones, *Ancients and Moderns: A Study of the Background of the Battle of the Books* (St Louis: Washington University, 1936).

Vivien Jones (ed.), *Women in the Eighteenth Century: Constructions of Femininity* (London: Routledge, 1990).

Vivien Jones, 'The Death of Mary Wollstonecraft', *British Journal for Eighteenth-Century Studies*, 20 (1997), 187–206.

Ludmilla Jordanova, *Sexual Visions: Images of* 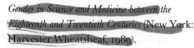 *Gender in Science and Medicine between the Eighteenth and Twentieth Centuries* (New York: Harvester Wheatsheaf, 1989).

Nicholas Jose, *Ideas of the Restoration in English Literature, 1660–71* (London: Macmillan, 1984).

Tony Joseph, *George Grossmith: Biography of a Savoyard* (Bristol: Published by the Author, 1982).

Patrick Joyce, *Work, Society and Politics* (London: Methuen, 1982).

Patrick Joyce (ed.), *The Historical Meanings of Work* (Cambridge: Cambridge University Press, 1987).

Patrick Joyce, *The Printed Image and the Transformation of Popular Culture 1790–1860* (Oxford: Clarendon Press, 1991).

Patrick Joyce, *Democratic Subjects: The Self and the Social in Nineteenth-Century England* (Cambridge: Cambridge University Press, 1994).

Margaret A. Judson, *From Tradition to Political Reality: A Study of the Ideas Set Forth in Support of the Commonwealth Government in England, 1649–1653* (Hamden, Conn.: Archon Books, for the Conference on British Studies and Wittenberg University, 1980).

Rana Kabbani, *Europe's Myths of Orient* (Bloomington: Indiana University Press, 1986).

Beth Kalikoff, *Murder and Moral Decay in Victorian Popular Literature* (Ann Arbor: UMI Research Press, 1986).

Henry Kamen, *European Society 1500–1700* (London: Hutchinson, 1984).

Penny Kane, *Victorian Families in Fact and Fiction* (New York: St Martin's Press, 1995).

Barbara Beigun Kaplan, '*Divulging of Useful Truths in Physick': The Medical Agenda of Robert Boyle* (Baltimore: Johns Hopkins University Press, 1993).

Steven L. Kaplan (ed.), *Understanding Popular Culture: Europe from the Middle Ages to the Nineteenth Century* (Berlin: Mouton, 1984).

David S. Katz, *Philo-Semitism and the*

Readmission of the Jews to England 1603–1655
(Oxford: Oxford University Press, 1982).

Harvey J. Kaye, *The British Marxist Historians: An Introductory Analysis* (New York: St Martin's Press, 1995).

Angela Keane, *Women Writers and the English Nation in the 1790s: Romantic Belongings* (Sheffield: University of Sheffield, 2001).

John Keane, *Tom Paine: A Political Life* (London: Bloomsbury, 1995).

N. H. Keeble (ed.), *The Cultural Identity of Seventeenth-Century Woman: A Reader* (London: Routledge, 1994).

Gary Kelly, *The English Jacobin Novel, 1780–1805* (Oxford: Clarendon Press, 1976).

Gary Kelly, *Revolutionary Feminism: The Mind and Career of Mary Wollstonecraft* (New York: St Martin's Press, 1992).

Gary Kelly, *Women, Writing, and Revolution, 1790–1827* (Oxford: Clarendon Press, 1993).

Gary Kelly, '(Female) Philosophy in the Bedroom: Mary Wollstonecraft and Female Sexuality', *Women's Writing*, 4 (1997), 143–54.

Paul Kennedy, *The Rise and Fall of the Great Powers: Economic Change and Military Conflict from 1500 to 2000* (London: Unwin Hyman, 1988).

John Kenyon, *The History Men: The Historical Profession in England since the Renaissance* (London: Weidenfeld and Nicolson, 1983).

John Kenyon, *The Civil Wars of England* (London: Weidenfeld and Nicolson, 1988).

John Keown, *Abortion, Doctors and the Law: Some Aspects of the Legal Regulation of Abortion in England from 1803 to 1982* (Cambridge: Cambridge University Press, 1988).

Jenny Kermode (ed.), *Woman, Crime and the Courts in Early Modern England* (London: UCL Press, 1994).

Eric Kerridge, *The Agricultural Revolution* (London: Allen and Unwin, 1967).

Eric Kerridge, *Textile Manufactures in Early Modern England* (Manchester: Manchester University Press, 1985).

Eric Kerridge, *Trade and Banking in Early Modern England* (Manchester: Manchester University Press, 1988).

Colin Kidd, *Subverting Scotland's Past* (Cambridge: Cambridge University Press, 1993).

V. G. Kiernan, *The Duel in European History: Honour and the Reign of Aristocracy* (Oxford: Oxford University Press, 1989).

V. G. Kiernan, *Tobacco: A History* (London: Hutchinson Radius, 1991).

Mark Kishlansky, *A Monarchy Transformed, Britain 1603–1714* (Penguin History of Britain; London: Allen Lane, 1996).

Khalid Kishtainy, *The Prostitute in Progressive Literature* (London: Allison and Busby, 1982).

John Van der Kiste, *George III's Children* (Stroud: Alan Sutton, 1992).

H. Gustav Klaus (ed.), *The Socialist Novel in Britain: Towards the Recovery of a Tradition* (New York: St Martin's Press, 1982).

H. Gustav Klaus, *The Literature of Labour: 200 Years of Working Class Literature* (New York: St Martin's Press, 1985).

Lawrence E. Klein, *Shaftesbury and the Culture of Politeness: Moral Discourse and Cultural Politics in Early Eighteenth-Century England* (Cambridge: Cambridge University Press, 1994).

Lawrence E. Klein, 'Gender and the Public/Private Distinction in the Eighteenth Century: Some Questions about Evidence and Analytic Procedure', *Eighteenth Century Studies*, 29 (1995), 97–110.

Charlotte Klonk, *Science and the Perception of Nature: British Landscape Art in the Late Eighteenth and Early Nineteenth Centuries* (London: Yale University Press, 1996).

David Knight, *The Age of Science: The Scientific World-View in the Nineteenth Century* (Oxford: Basil Blackwell, 1986).

Theodore Koditschek, *Class Formation and Urban Industrial Society: Bradford 1750–1850* (Cambridge: Cambridge University Press, 1990).

H. G. Koenigsberger, *Early Modern Europe 1500–1789* (London: Longman, 1987).

Stephen Koss, *The Rise and Fall of the Political Press in Britain*, vol. 1: *The Nineteenth Century* (London: Hamish Hamilton, 1981).

Elizabeth Kowaleski-Wallace, *Their Fathers' Daughters: Hannah More, Maria Edgeworth, and Patriarchal Complicity* (New York: Oxford University Press, 1991).

Elizabeth Kowaleski-Wallace, *Consuming Subjects: Women, Shopping, and Business in the Eighteenth Century* (New York: Columbia University Press, 1997).

Isaac Kramnick, *Bolingbroke and His Circle: The Politics of Nostalgia in the Age of Walpole* (Cambridge, Mass.: Harvard University Press, 1968).

Isaac Kramnick, *The Rage of Edmund Burke: Portrait of an Ambivalent Conservative* (New York: Basic Books, 1977).

Isaac Kramnick, 'Children's Literature and Bourgeois Ideology: Observations on Culture and Industrial Capitalism in the Later Eighteenth Century', *Studies in Eighteenth Century Culture*, 12 (1983), 11–44.

Isaac Kramnick, 'Eighteenth-Century Science and Radical Social Theory: The Case of Joseph Priestley's Scientific Liberalism', *Journal of British Studies*, 25 (1986), 1–30.

Isaac Kramnick, *Republicanism and Bourgeois Radicalism: Political Ideology in Late Eighteenth-Century England and America* (Ithaca, NY: Cornell University Press, 1990).

Isaac Kramnick (ed.), *The Portable Enlightenment Reader* (Harmondsworth: Penguin, 1995).

Jonathan Brody Kramnick, *Making the English Canon: Print Capitalism and the Cultural Past, 1700–1770* (Cambridge: Cambridge University Press, 1999).

Richard Kroll, Richard Ashcraft and Perez Zagorin (eds.), *Philosophy, Science and Religion in England, 1640–1740* (Cambridge: Cambridge University Press, 1992).

Bounelyn Young Kunze and Dwight D. Brautigam (eds.), *Court, Country and Culture: Essays on Early Modern British History in Honour of Perez Zagorin* (Rochester, NY: University of Rochester Press, 1992).

David Kunzle, *The Early Comic Strip: Narrative Strips and Picture Stories in the European Broadsheet from ca. 1450 to 1826* (Berkeley: University of California Press, 1973).

Tony Kushner (ed.), *The Jewish Heritage in British History* (London: Frank Cass, 1992).

Ann Kussmaul, *Servants in Husbandry in Early Modern England* (Cambridge: Cambridge University Press, 1981).

Ann Kussmaul, *A General View of the Rural Economy of England, 1538–1840* (Cambridge: Cambridge University Press, 1990).

Jonathan Lamb, *Preserving the Self in the South Seas* (Chicago: University of Chicago Press, 2001).

William M. Lamont, *Richard Baxter and the Millennium: Protestant Imperialism and the English Revolution* (Totowa, NJ: Rowman and Littlefield, 1979).

John Landers, *Death in the Metropolis* (Cambridge: Cambridge University Press, 1993).

David S. Landes, *The Unbound Prometheus: Technological Change and Industrial Development in Western Europe from 1750 to the Present* (London: Cambridge University Press, 1960; Cambridge: Cambridge University Press, 1969).

David S. Landes, *Revolution in Time: Clocks and the Making of the Modern World* (Cambridge, Mass.: Harvard University Press, 1983).

Joan Landes, *Women and the Public Sphere in the Age of the French Revolution* (Ithaca, NY: Cornell University Press, 1988).

Richard Landes, *Relics, Apocalypse and the Deceits of History* (Cambridge, Mass.: Harvard University Press, 1995).

George P. Landow (ed.), *Approaches to Victorian Autobiography* (Athens: Ohio University Press, 1979).

George P. Landow, *Victorian Types, Victorian Shadows: Biblical Typology in Victorian Literature, Art, and Thought* (Boston: Routledge and Kegan Paul, 1980).

George P. Landow, *Images of Crisis: Literary Iconology, 1750 to the Present* (Boston: Routledge and Kegan Paul, 1982).

Joan Lane, *Apprenticeship in England 1600–1914* (London: UCL Press, 1996).

Timothy Lang, *The Victorians and the Stuart Heritage: Interpretations of a Discordant Past* (Cambridge: Cambridge University Press, 1995).

Paul Langford, *A Polite and Commercial People: England 1727–1783* (Oxford: Oxford University Press, 1989).

Paul Langford, *Public Life and the Propertied Englishman 1689–1798* (Oxford: Clarendon Press, 1991).

Paul Langford, *Englishness Identified: Manners and Character 1650–1850* (Oxford: Oxford University Press, 2000).

Thomas W. Laqueur, *Making Sex: Body and Gender from the Greeks to Freud* (Cambridge, Mass.: Harvard University Press, 1990).

Vivienne Larminie, *Wealth, Kinship and Culture: The Seventeenth-Century Newdigates of Arbury and their World* (Royal Historical Society Studies in History 72; Woodbridge: Boydell, 1995).

Christina Larner, *Witchcraft and Religion: The Politics of Popular Belief* (Oxford: Basil Blackwell, 1986).

Gerald Larner and Celia Larner, *The Glasgow Style* (London: Astragal Books, 1979).

F. La Rochefoucauld, *A Frenchman in England in 1784* (London: Caliban, 1995).

Christopher Lasch, *Women and the Common Life: Love, Marriage and Feminism*, ed. Elisabeth Lasch-Quinn (London: Norton, 1997).

Peter Laslett, 'The English Revolution and Locke's *Two Treatises of Government*', *Cambridge Historical Journal*, 12 (1956), 40–55.

Peter Laslett, *Family Life and Illicit Love in Earlier Generations: Essays in Historical Sociology* (Cambridge: Cambridge University Press, 1977).

Peter Laslett, 'Studies in Social and Demographic History', in Peter Laslett, Karla Oosterveen, and Richard M. Smith (eds.), *Bastardy and its Comparative History: Studies in the History of Illegitimacy and Marital Nonconformism in Britain, France, Germany, Sweden, North America, Jamaica and Japan* (London: E. Arnold, 1980).

Peter Laslett, *The World We have Lost, Further Explored*, 3rd edn. (London: Methuen, 1983).

Peter Laslett, *A Fresh Map of Life: The Emergence of the Third Age* (London: Weidenfeld and Nicolson, 1989).

Rachel Laudan, *From Mineralogy to Geology: The Foundations of a Science, 1650–1830* (Chicago: University of Chicago Press, 1987).

Anne Laurence, *Women in England 1500–1760: A Social History* (London: Weidenfeld and Nicolson, 1994).

Anne Laurence, W. R. Owens and Stuart Sim (eds.), *John Bunyan and his England, 1628–1688* (London: Hambledon Press, 1990).

James Laver, *The Age of Illusion: Manners and Morals, 1750–1848* (London: Weidenfeld and Nicolson, 1972).

Philip Lawson, *George Grenville: A Political Life* (Oxford: Oxford University Press, 1984).

Richard Lawton and Colin G. Pooley, *Britain 1749–1950: An Historical Geography* (London: Edward Arnold, 1992).

Keith Laybourn, *The History of British Trade Unionism c. 1770–1990* (Stroud: Alan Sutton, 1992).

Douglas Leach, *Roots of Conflict: British Armed Forces and Colonial Americans, 1677–1763* (Chapel Hill: University of North Carolina Press, 1986).

C. H. Lee, *The British Economy Since 1700: A Macroeconomic Perspective* (Cambridge: Cambridge University Press, 1986).

Maurice Lee Jr., *Government by Pen: Scotland Under James VI and I* (London: University of Illinois Press, 1980).

E. S. Leedham-Green, *A Concise History of the University of Cambridge* (Cambridge: Cambridge University Press, 1996).

James Lees-Milne, *The Last Stuarts* (London: Hogarth Press, 1983).

Stanford E. Lehmberg, *Cathedrals under Siege: Cathedrals in English Society, 1600–1700* (Exeter: Exeter University Press, 1996).

Donald Leinster-Mackay, *The Rise of the English Prep School* (London: Falmer Press, 1984).

Beverly Lemire, *Fashion's Favourite: The Cotton Trade and the Consumer in Britain, 1660–1800* (Oxford: Oxford University Press, 1992).

Beverly Lemire, *Dress, Culture and Commerce: The English Clothing Trade before the Factory* (Basingstoke: Macmillan Press, 1996).

David Lemmings, *Gentlemen and Barristers: The Inns of Court and the English Bar* (Oxford: Clarendon Press, 1990).

David Lemmings, *Professors of the Law: Barristers and English Legal Culture in the Eighteenth Century* (Oxford: Oxford University Press, 2000).

Bruce Lenman, *The Jacobite Risings in Britain 1687–1746* (London: Eyre Methuen, 1980).

Bruce Lenman, *Integration, Enlightenment, and Industrialization: Scotland 1746–1832* (London: Edward Arnold, 1981).

Shirley Letwin, *The Pursuit of Certainty* (Cambridge: Cambridge University Press, 1965).

W. L. Letwin, *The Origins of Scientific Economics* (London: Methuen, 1963).

Brian P. Levack, *The Formation of the British State: England, Scotland, and the Union 1603–1707* (Oxford: Clarendon Press, 1987).

David Levine, 'Consumer Goods and Capitalist Modernization', *Journal of Interdisciplinary History*, 22 (1991), 67–77.

David Levine and Keith Wrightson, *The Making of an Industrial Society: Whickham*

1560–1765 (Oxford: Oxford University Press, 1991).

George Levine, *The Realistic Imagination: English Fiction from Frankenstein to Lady Chatterley* (Chicago: University of Chicago Press, 1981).

George Levine (ed.), *One Culture: Essays in Science and Literature* (Madison: University of Wisconsin Press, 1989).

Richard A. Levine (ed.), *The Victorian Experience: The Poets* (Athens: Ohio University Press, 1982).

Judith S. Lewis, *In the Family Way: Childbearing in the British Aristocracy 1760–1860* (New Brunswick, NJ: Rutgers University Press, 1986).

David Lieberman, *The Province of Legislation Determined: Legal Theory in Eighteenth-Century Britain* (Cambridge: Cambridge University Press, 1989).

Harry Liebersohn, *Aristocratic Encounters: European Travelers and North American Indians* (Cambridge: Cambridge University Press, 1998).

Bryant Lillywhite, *London Coffee Houses: A Reference Book of Coffee Houses of the Seventeenth, Eighteenth and Nineteenth Centuries* (London: Allen and Unwin, 1963).

Anthony Hadley Lincoln, *Some Political and Social Ideas of English Dissent, 1763–1800* (Cambridge: Cambridge University Press, 1938).

Keith Lindley, *Popular Politics and Religion in Civil War London* (London: Scolar, 1997).

Jack Lindsay, *The Monster City: Defoe's London, 1688–1730* (New York: St Martin's Press, 1978).

Peter Linebaugh, *The London Hanged: Crime and Civil Society in the Eighteenth Century* (London: Allen Lane, 1991).

Lawrence Lipking, *The Ordering of the Arts in Eighteenth Century England* (Princeton: Princeton University Press, 1970).

Louise Lippincott, *Selling Art in Georgian London: The Rise of Arthur Pond* (London:

Yale University Press for the Paul Mellon Center for Studies in British Art, 1983).

Catharina Lis and Hugo Soly, *Disordered Lives: Eighteenth-Century Families and their Unruly Relatives* (Cambridge: Polity Press, 1996).

Julian Litten, *The English Way of Death: The Common Funeral since 1450* (London: Robert Hale, 1991).

Joseph Litvak, *Strange Gourmets: Sophistication, Theory, and the Novel* (Durham, NC: Duke University Press, 1997).

Tai Liu, *Puritan London: A Study of Religion and Society in the City Parishes* (London: Associated University Presses, 1986).

Nigel Llewellyn, *The Art of Death: Visual Culture in the English Death Ritual c.1500–c.1800* (London: Victoria and Albert Museum, 1991).

David W. Lloyd, *The Making of English Towns: 2000 Years of Evolution* (London: Victor Gollancz in association with Peter Crawley, 1984).

David W. Lloyd and Paul Thomas, *Culture and the State* (New York: Routledge, 1998).

Michael Lobban, *The Common Law and English Jurisprudence, 1760–1850* (New York: Oxford University Press, 1991).

F. P. Lock, *The Politics of Gulliver's Travels* (Oxford: Oxford University Press, 1980).

F. P. Lock, *Burke's Reflections on the Revolution in France* (London: George Allen and Unwin, 1985).

Elizabeth M. R. Lomax, *Small and Special: The Development of Hospitals for Children in Victorian Britain* (London: Wellcome Institute for the History of Medicine, 1996).

Lord Longford, *A History of the House of Lords*, introd. Elizabeth Longford (London: Collins, 1988).

R. Longrigg, *The English Squire and his Sport* (London: Michael Joseph, 1977).

Roger Lonsdale (ed.), *The New Oxford Book of Eighteenth Century Verse* (Oxford: Oxford University Press, 1984).

Roger Lonsdale (ed.), *Eighteenth-Century Women Poets* (Oxford: Oxford University Press, 1989).

Irvine Loudon, *Medical Care and the General Practitioner 1750–1850* (Oxford: Oxford University Press, 1986).

Harold Love, *Scribal Publication in Seventeenth-Century England* (Oxford: Clarendon Press, 1993).

Deryck W. Lovegrove, *Established Church, Sectarian People: Itineracy and the Transformation of English Dissent, 1780–1830* (Cambridge: Cambridge University Press, 1988).

D. Lowe, *History of Bourgeois Perception* (Brighton: Harvester, 1982).

Roger D. Lund (ed.), *The Margins of Orthodoxy: Heterodox Writing and Cultural Response, 1660–1750* (Cambridge: Cambridge University Press, 1995).

Michael Lynch, *Scotland: A New History* (London: Barrie and Jenkins, 1991).

Iain McCalman, *Radical Underworld: Prophets, Revolutionaries and Pornographers in London, 1795–1840* (Cambridge: Cambridge University Press, 1988).

Seán McConville, *A History of English Prison Administration*, vol. 1: *1750–1877* (London: Routledge and Kegan Paul, 1981).

Ruth McClure, *Coram's Children: The London Foundling Hospital in the Eighteenth Century* (London: Yale University Press, 1981).

Robert McCrum, William Cran and Robert MacNeil, *The Story of English* (London: Faber and Faber, 1992).

Robert P. Maccubbin (ed.), *'Tis Nature's Fault: Unauthorized Sexuality during the Enlightenment* (Cambridge: Cambridge University Press, 1987).

Robert P. Maccubbin and Martha Hamilton-Phillips (eds.), *The Age of William III and Mary II: Power, Politics and Patronage, 1688–1702. A Reference Encylopedia and Exhibition Catalogue* (Williamsburg, Va.: William and Mary College, 1989).

Diarmaid MacCulloch, *The Later Reformation in England 1547–1603* (New York: St Martin's Press, 1990).

Michael MacDonald, *Mystical Bedlam: Madness, Anxiety, and Healing in Seventeenth-Century England* (Cambridge: Cambridge University Press, 1981).

Michael MacDonald and Terrence R. Murphy, *Sleepless Souls: Suicide in Early Modern England* (Oxford: Oxford University Press, 1990).

R. B. McDowell and D. A. Webb, *Trinity College Dublin 1592–1952: An Academic History* (Cambridge: Cambridge University Press, 1982).

D. D. MacElroy, *Scotland's Age of Improvement: A Survey of Eighteenth-Century Literary Clubs and Societies* (Pullman: Washington State University Press, 1969).

Alan Macfarlane, *The Family Life of Ralph Josselin, a Seventeenth-Century Clergyman: An Essay in Historical Anthropology* (Cambridge: Cambridge University Press, 1970).

Alan Macfarlane, *Witchcraft in Tudor and Stuart England: A Regional and Comparative Study* (London: Routledge and Kegan Paul, 1970).

Alan Macfarlane (ed.), *The Diary of Ralph Josselin 1616–1683* (Records of Social and Economic History, new ser. 3; London: Oxford University Press, 1976).

Alan Macfarlane, Book Review of Lawrence Stone, *The Family, Sex and Marriage in England, 1500–1800* (New York: Harper & Row, 1977).

Alan Macfarlane, *The Origins of English Individualism: The Family, Property and Social Transition* (Oxford: Basil Blackwell, 1978).

Alan Macfarlane, *The Justice and the Mare's Ale: Law and Disorder in Seventeenth Century England* (Oxford: Basil Blackwell, 1981).

Alan Macfarlane, *Marriage and Love in England: Modes of Reproduction, 1300–1840* (Oxford: Basil Blackwell, 1986).

Alan Macfarlane, *The Culture of Capitalism* (Oxford: Basil Blackwell, 1987).

Alan Macfarlane, *The Savage Wars of Peace: England, Japan and the Malthusian Trap,* (Oxford: Blackwell, 1997).

Anthony McFarlane, *The British in the Americas 1480–1815* (London: Longman, 1995).

Arthur Macgregor (ed.), *Sir Hans Sloane: Collector, Scientist, Antiquary* (London: British Museum Press in association with Alistair McAlpine, 1994).

Allan I. Macinnes, *Charles I and the Making of the Covenanting Movement* (Edinburgh: John Donald, 1991).

Maynard Mack, *Alexander Pope: A Life* (London: Yale University Press, 1985).

Patricia McKee, *Public and Private: Gender, Class, and the British Novel (1764–1878)* (Minneapolis: University of Minnesota Press, 1997).

Neil McKendrick, 'Josiah Wedgwood and Factory Discipline', *Historical Journal,* 4 (1961), 30–55.

Neil McKendrick, 'Wedgwood and the Factory System', *Proceedings of the Wedgwood Society,* 5 (1963), 1–29.

Neil McKendrick, 'Josiah Wedgwood and Thomas Bentley: An Inventor–Entrepreneur Partnership in the Industrial Revolution', *Transactions of the Royal Historical Society,* 14 (1964), 1–33.

Neil McKendrick, 'The Rôle of Science in the Industrial Revolution: A Study of Josiah Wedgwood as a Scientist and Industrial Chemist', in Mikuláš Teich and Robert M. Young (eds.), *Changing Perspectives in the History of Science: Essays in Honour of Joseph Needham* (London: Heinemann, 1973), 274–320.

Neil McKendrick (ed.), *Historical Perspectives: Studies in English Thought and Society in Honour of J. H. Plumb* (London: Europa, 1974).

Neil McKendrick, 'J. H. Plumb: A Valedictory Tribute', in McKendrick (ed.), *Historical Perspectives: Studies in English Thought and Society* (London: Europa, 1974), 1–18.

Neil McKendrick, ' "Gentlemen and Players" Revisited: The Gentlemanly Ideal, The Business Ideal and the Professional Ideal in English Literary Culture', in Neil McKendrick and R. B. Outhwaite (eds.), *Business Life and Public Policy* (Cambridge: Cambridge University Press, 1986).

Neil McKendrick, 'The Commercialization of Fashion', in Richard Golden (ed.), *Social History of Western Civilization* (New York, 1991), 1–24.

Neil McKendrick, John Brewer and J. H. Plumb, *The Birth of a Consumer Society: The Commercialization of Eighteenth-Century England* (London: Europa, 1982).

Charlotte MacKenzie, *Psychiatry for the Rich: A History of Ticehurst Private Asylum, 1792–1917* (New York: Routledge, 1992).

Michael McKeon, *The Origins of the English Novel, 1600–1740* (Baltimore: Johns Hopkins University Press, 1987).

Eric David Mackerness, *A Social History of English Music* (London: Routledge and Kegan Paul, 1964).

J. D. MacKillop, *The British Ethical Societies* (New York: Cambridge University Press, 1986).

Angus McLaren, *Sexuality and Social Order: The Debate over the Fertility of Women and Workers in France, 1770–1920* (New York: Holmes and Meier, 1983).

Angus McLaren, *Reproductive Rituals: The Perception of Fertility in England from the Sixeenth Century to the Nineteenth Century* (London: Methuen, 1984).

Angus McLaren, *A History of Contraception: From Antiquity to the Present Day* (Oxford: Basil Blackwell, 1990).

C. MacLeod, *Inventing the Industrial Revolution: The English Patent System, 1660–1800* (Cambridge: Cambridge University Press, 1988).

Kirsty McLeod, *Drums and Trumpets: The House of Stuart* (The Mirror of Britain Series, gen. ed. Kevin Crossley-Holland; London: André Deutsch, 1977).

Frank McLynn, *Charles Edward Stuart: A Tragedy in Many Acts* (London: Routledge, 1988).

Frank McLynn, *Crime and Punishment in Eighteenth-Century England* (London: Routledge, 1989; Oxford: Oxford University Press, 1991).

John McManners, *Death and the Enlightenment: Changing Attitudes to Death in Eighteenth-Century France* (Oxford: Oxford University Press, 1985).

Juliet McMaster and Rowland McMaster, *The Novel from Sterne to James: Essays on the Relation of Literature to Life* (Totowa, NJ: Barnes and Noble, 1981).

Maureen McNeil, *Under the Banner of Science: Erasmus Darwin and his Age* (Manchester: Manchester University Press, 1987).

Simon McVeigh, *Concert Life in London: From Mozart to Haydn* (Cambridge: Cambridge University Press, 1993).

M. Mahl and H. Koon (eds.), *The Female Spectator: English Women Writers before 1800* (Bloomington: Indiana University Press, 1977).

Howard L. Malchow, *Gothic Images of Race in Nineteenth-Century Britain* (Stanford, Calif.: Stanford University Press, 1996).

R. W. Malcolmson, *Popular Recreations in English Society 1700–1850* (Cambridge: Cambridge University Press, 1973; 1975).

R. W. Malcolmson, *Life and Labour in England, 1700–1780* (London: Hutchinson, 1981).

Gail Malmgreen, *Silk Town: Industry and Culture in Macclesfield 1750–1835* (Hull: Hull University Press; Atlantic Highlands, NJ: Humanities Press, 1985).

Gail Malmgreen (ed.), *Religion in the Lives of English Women, 1760–1930* (London: Croom Helm, 1986).

Richard D. Mandell, *Sport: A Cultural History* (New York: Columbia University Press, 1984).

Peter Mandler (ed.), *The Uses of Charity: The Poor on Relief in the Nineteenth-Century Metropolis* (Philadelphia: University of Pennsylvania Press, 1990).

Peter Mandler, *The Fall and Rise of the Stately*

Home in Britain (New Haven: Yale University Press, 1997).

Lawrence Manley, *Literature and Culture in Early Modern London* (Cambridge: Cambridge University Press, 1995).

Diana E. Manuel, *Marshall Hall (1790–1857): Science and Medicine in Early Victorian Society* (Amsterdam: Rodopi, 1996).

Frank E. Manuel, *The Eighteenth Century Confronts the Gods* (New York: Athenaeum, 1967).

Robert Markley, *Fallen Languages: Cries of Representation in Newtonian England, 1660–1740* (Ithaca, NY: Cornell University Press, 1993).

Hilary Marland and Margaret Pelling (eds.), *The Task of Healing: Medicine, Religion and Gender in England and the Netherlands: 1450–1800* (Rotterdam: Erasmus, 1996).

Gerald Mars and Valerie Mars (eds.), *Food, Culture and History*, vol. 1 (London: London Food Seminar, 1993).

D. Marshall, *The Old Poor Law 1795–1834* (London: Macmillan, 1968).

Gordon Marshall, *Presbyteries and Profits: Calvinism and the Development of Capitalism in Scotland, 1560–1707* (Oxford: Oxford University Press, 1980).

Peter Marshall (ed.), *The British Discovery of Hinduism in the Eighteenth Century* (Cambridge: Cambridge University Press, 1970).

Peter Marshall, *William Godwin: Philosopher, Novelist, Revolutionary* (London: Yale University Press, 1984).

Peter Marshall (ed.), *The Impact of the English Reformation, 1500–1640* (London: Arnold, 1997).

P. J. Marshall and Glyndwr Williams, *The Great Map of Mankind: British Perceptions of the World in the Age of Enlightenment* (London: J. M. Dent, 1982).

G. H. Martin and J. R. L. Highfield, *A History of Merton College, Oxford* (Oxford: Oxford University Press, 1997).

Lauro Martines, *Society and History in English*

Renaissance Verse (Oxford: Basil Blackwell, 1985).

Michael Mason, *The Making of Victorian Sexuality* (Oxford: Oxford University Press, 1994).

Michael Mason, *The Making of Victorian Sexual Attitudes* (Oxford: Oxford University Press, 1995).

Philip Mason, *The English Gentleman: The Rise and Fall of an Ideal* (London: André Deutsch, 1982).

Roger A. Mason (ed.), *Scotland and England, 1286–1815* (Edinburgh: John Donald, 1987).

Peter Mathias, *The Transformation of England: Essays in the Economic and Social History of England in the Eighteenth Century* (New York: Columbia University Press, 1979).

Peter Mathias and John A. Davis (eds.), *International Trade and British Economic Growth from the Eighteenth Century to the Present Day* (Oxford: Blackwell, 1997).

Trevor May, *An Economic and Social History of Britain, 1760–1970* (London: Longman, 1987).

Michael Meehan, *Liberty and Poetics in Eighteenth-Century England* (London: Croom Helm, 1986).

Ronald L. Meek, *Social Science and the Ignoble Savage* (Cambridge: Cambridge University Press, 1975).

Joseph Melling and Jonathan Barry (eds.), *Culture in History: Production, Consumption and Values in Historical Perspective* (Exeter: University of Exeter Press, 1992).

Sara Heller Mendelson, *The Mental World of Stuart Women: Three Studies* (Brighton: Harvester, 1987).

Sara Mendelson and Patricia Crawford, *Women in Early Modern England* (Oxford: Clarendon Press, 1998).

Jonathan Mendilow, *The Romantic Tradition in British Political Thought* (London: Croom Helm, 1985).

Michael Mendle, *Henry Parker and the English Civil War: The Political Thought of the Public's*

'*Privado*' (Cambridge: Cambridge University Press, 1995).

Samuel Pyeatt Menefee, *Wives for Sale: An Ethnographic Study of British Popular Divorce* (London: Blackwell, 1981).

Stephen Mennell, *All Manners of Food: Eating and Taste in England and France from the Middle Ages to the Present* (Oxford: Basil Blackwell, 1985).

Stephen Mennell, *Norbert Elias: Civilization and the Human Self-Image* (Oxford: Basil Blackwell, 1989).

Alex Mercer, *Disease, Mortality and Population in Transition* (Leicester: Leicester University Press, 1990).

Carolyn Merchant, *The Death of Nature: Women, Ecology and the Scientific Revolution* (San Francisco: Harper and Row, 1980).

J. F. Merritt (ed.), *The Political World of Thomas Wentworth, Earl of Strafford, 1621–1641* (Cambridge: Cambridge University Press, 1996).

J. F. Merritt (ed.), *Imagining Early Modern London: Perceptions and Portrayals of the City from Stow to Strype, 1598–1720* (Sheffield: University of Sheffield Press, 2001).

Helena Michie, *The Flesh Made Word: Female Figures and Women's Bodies* (New York: Oxford University Press, 1987).

Clare Midgley, *Women against Slavery: The British Campaigns 1780–1870* (London: Routledge, 1992).

Graham Midgley, *University Life in Eighteenth-Century Oxford* (New Haven: Yale University Press, 1996).

Dudley Miles, *Francis Place, 1771–1854: The Life of a Remarkable Radical* (New York: St Martin's Press, 1988).

Rosalind Miles, *Ben Jonson: His Life and Work* (London: Routledge and Kegan Paul, 1986).

Andrew H. Miller and James Eli Adams (eds.), *Sexualities in Victorian Britain* (Bloomington: Indiana University Press, 1996).

John Miller, 'The Potential for "Absolutism" in Later Stuart England', *History*, 69 (1984), 187–207.

John Miller, *Restoration England: The Reign of Charles II* (London: Longman, 1985).

John Miller, *Charles II* (London: Weidenfeld and Nicolson, 1991).

G. E. Mingay, *English Landed Society in the Eighteenth Century* (London: Routledge and Kegan Paul, 1963).

G. E. Mingay (ed.), *Arthur Young and his Times* (London: Macmillan, 1975).

G. E. Mingay (ed.), *The Agrarian History of England and Wales*, vol. 6: *1750–1858* (Cambridge: Cambridge University Press, 1989).

G. E. Mingay, *A Social History of the English Countryside* (London: Routledge, 1990).

G. E. Mingay, *Land and Society in England, 1750–1980* (London: Longman, 1994).

G. E. Mingay, *Parliamentary Enclosure in England: An Introduction to its Causes, Incidence and Impact, 1750–1850* (London: Longman, 1997).

L. G. Mitchell (ed.), *The Writings and Speeches of Edmund Burke*, vol. 8: *The French Revolution, 1790–1794* (Oxford: Clarendon Press, 1989).

L. G. Mitchell, *Charles James Fox* (Oxford: Oxford University Press, 1992).

L. G. Mitchell, *Lord Melbourne, 1779–1848* (Oxford: Oxford University Press, 1997).

Robert M. Mitchell, *Calvin's and the Puritans' View of the Protestant Ethic* (Washington, DC: University Press of America, 1979).

Rosalind Mitchison, *Lordship to Patronage: Scotland 1603–1746* (London: Edward Arnold, 1983).

Rosalind Mitchison and Leah Leneman, *Sexuality and Social Control: Scotland 1660–1780* (Oxford: Basil Blackwell, 1989).

Joel Mokyr (ed.), *The British Industrial Revolution: An Economic Perspective* (Oxford: Westview Press, 1993).

John Money, 'Public Opinion in the West Midlands, 1760–1793' (Ph.D. thesis, Cambridge University, 1967).

John Money, 'Taverns, Coffee Houses and Clubs: Local Politics and Popular Articulacy in the Birmingham Area in the Age of the American Revolution', *Historical Journal*, 14 (1971), 15–47.

John Money, *Experience and Identity: Birmingham and the West Midlands, 1760–1800* (Manchester: Manchester University Press, 1977).

Paul Kleber Monod, *Jacobitism and the English People, 1688–1788* (Cambridge: Cambridge University Press, 1989).

Massimo Montanari, *The Culture of Food* (Oxford: Blackwell, 1994).

William Monter, *Ritual, Myth and Magic in Early Modern Europe* (Brighton: Harvester Press, 1983).

Jane Moody, *Illegitimate Theatre in London, 1770–1840* (York: University of York, 2000).

Lucy Moore, *The Thieves' Opera: The Remarkable Lives and Deaths of Jonathan Wild, Thief-Taker, and Jack Sheppard, House-Breaker* (London: Penguin, 1998).

Bruce T. Moran (ed.), *Patronage and Institutions: Science, Technology and Medicine at the European Court, 1500–1750* (Woodbridge: Boydell Press, 1991).

Richard Moran, *Knowing Right from Wrong: The Insanity Defense of Daniel McNaughton* (London: Collier Macmillan, 1981).

Edmund S. Morgan, *Inventing the People: The Rise of Popular Sovereignty in England and America* (New York: Norton, 1988).

John Morgan, *Godly Learning: Puritan Attitudes Towards Reason, Learning and Education, 1560–1640* (Cambridge: Cambridge University Press, 1986).

Kenneth Morgan, *Bristol and the Atlantic Trade in the Eighteenth Century* (Cambridge: Cambridge University Press, 1993).

Marjorie Morgan, *Manners, Morals and Class in England, 1774–1858* (London: Macmillan, 1994).

John Morrill (ed.), *Reactions to the English Civil War, 1642–1649* (London: Macmillan, 1982).

John Morrill (ed.), *The Impact of the English Civil War* (London: Collins and Brown, 1991).

John Morrill (ed.), *Revolution and Restoration: England in the 1650s* (London: Collins and Brown, 1992).

John Morrill, Paul Slack and Daniel Woolf (eds.), *Public Duty and Private Conscience in Seventeenth-Century England: Essays Presented to G. E. Aylmer* (Oxford: Clarendon Press, 1993).

R. J. Morris, *Class and Class Consciousness in the Industrial Revolution, 1780–1850* (London: Macmillan, 1979).

Ornella Moscucci, *The Science of Woman: Gynaecology and Gender in England, 1800–1929* (Cambridge: Cambridge University Press, 1990).

Hoh-Cheung Mui and Lorna H. Mui, *Shops and Shopkeeping in Eighteenth-Century England*, (Kingston: McGill-Queen's University Press, 1989).

Chandra Mukerji, *From Graven Images: Patterns of Modern Materialism* (New York: Columbia University Press, 1983).

Jerry Z. Muller, *Adam Smith in his Time and Ours: Designing the Decent Society* (New York: Free Press, 1993).

Thomas Munck, *Seventeenth-Century Europe, 1598–1700* (London: Macmillan, 1990).

Roger Munting, *An Economic and Social History of Gambling* (Manchester: Manchester University Press, 1996).

Alexander Murdoch, *The People Above: Politics and Administration in Mid-Eighteenth-Century Scotland* (Edinburgh: John Donald, 1980).

David R. Murray, *Odious Commerce: Britain, Spain and the Abolition of the Cuban Slave Trade* (Cambridge: Cambridge University Press, 1981).

A. E. Musson and Eric Robinson, *Science and Technology in the Industrial Revolution* (Manchester: Manchester University Press, 1969).

Stefan Muthesius, *The English Terraced House* (London: Yale University Press, 1982).

William Myers, *Milton and Free Will: An Essay*

in Criticism and Philosophy (New York and Sydney: Croom Helm, 1987).

Tom Nairn, *The Break-up of Britain* (London: New Left Books, 1977).

Tom Nairn, *The Enchanted Glass: Britain and its Monarchy* (London: Radius, 1988).

Clark Nardinelli, *Child Labor and the Industrial Revolution* (Bloomington: University of Indiana Press, 1990).

R. S. Neale, *Bath 1680–1850: A Social History, or, A Valley of Pleasure Yet a Sink of Iniquity* (London: Routledge and Kegan Paul, 1981).

R. S. Neale, *Class in English History 1680–1850* (Oxford: Basil Blackwell; Totowa, NJ: Barnes and Noble, 1981).

R. S. Neale, *History and Class: Essential Readings in Theory and Interpretation* (Oxford: Basil Blackwell, 1983).

J. M. Neeson, *Commoners: Common Right, Enclosure and Social Change in England, 1700–1820* (Cambridge: Cambridge University Press, 1993).

Howard Nenner, *The Right to be King: The Succession to the Crown of England, 1603–1714* (Chapel Hill: University of North Carolina Press, 1995).

Victor E. Neuburg, *The Penny Histories: A Study of Chapbooks for Young Readers over Two Centuries* (London: Oxford University Press, 1968).

Victor E. Neuburg, *Popular Education in Eighteenth Century England* (London: Woburn Press, 1971).

Victor E. Neuburg, *Gone for a Soldier: A History of Life in the British Ranks from 1642* (London: Cassell, 1989).

T. R. Nevett, *Advertising in Britain: A History* (London: Heinemann, 1982).

Vincent Newey (ed.), *The Pilgrim's Progress: Critical and Historical Views* (Totowa, NJ: Barnes and Noble, 1980).

Gerald Newman, *The Rise of English Nationalism: A Cultural History, 1750–1830* (London: Weidenfeld and Nicolson, 1987).

Judith Lowder Newton, *Women, Power, and Subversion: Social Strategies in British Fiction, 1778–1800* (Athens: University of Georgia Press, 1981).

Judith L. Newton, Mary P. Ryan and Judith R. Walkowitz (eds.), *Sex and Class in Women's History* (London: Routledge and Kegan Paul, 1983).

David Nicholls, *God and Government in an 'Age of Reason'* (London: Routledge, 1995).

Phillip A. Nicholls, *Homeopathy and the Medical Profession* (London: Croom Helm, 1988).

Colin Nicholson, *Writing and the Rise of Finance: Capital Satires of the Early Eighteenth Century* (Cambridge: Cambridge University Press, 1994).

Eirwen E. C. Nicholson, 'Consumers and Spectators: The Public of the Political Print in Eighteenth-Century England', *History*, 81 (1996), 5–21.

Peter P. Nicholson, *The Political Philosophy of the British Idealists: Selected Studies* (Cambridge: Cambridge University Press, 1990).

C. D. Niven, *History of the Humane Movement* (London: Johnson, 1967).

Peter Benedict Nockles, *The Oxford Movement in Context: Anglican High Churchmanship, 1760–1857* (Cambridge: Cambridge University Press, 1994).

David Norbrook, *Writing the English Republic: Poetry, Rhetoric and Politics, 1627–1660* (Cambridge: Cambridge University Press, 1999).

Edward Norman, *Roman Catholicism in England: From the Elizabethan Settlement to the Second Vatican Council* (Oxford: Oxford University Press, 1985).

Anthony North, *Descent into Crime* (London: Allison and Busby, 2000).

Rictor Norton, *Mother Clap's Molly House: The Gay Subculture in England, 1700–1830* (London: GMP Publishers, 1992).

J. Obelkevich, 'Proverbs and Social History', in P. Burke and R. Porter (eds.), *The Social History of Language* (Cambridge: Cambridge University Press, 1987), 43–72.

James Obelkevich, Lyndal Roper and Raphael Samuel, *Disciplines of Faith: Studies in Religion, Politics and Patriarchy* (London: Routledge and Kegan Paul, 1987).

Conor Cruise O'Brien, *The Great Melody: A Thematic Biography and Commented Anthology of Edmund Burke* (London: Sinclair-Stevenson, 1992).

Patricia O'Brien, *The Promise of Punishment* (Princeton: Princeton University Press, 1982).

Patrick O'Brien, *Power with Profit: The State and the Economy, 1688–1815* (London: Institute of Historical Research, 1991).

Patrick O'Brien (ed.), *The Industrial Revolution in Europe*, 2 parts (Oxford: Blackwell, 1993 and 1994).

Patrick O'Brien and Roland Quinault (eds.), *The Industrial Revolution in British Society* (Cambridge: Cambridge University Press, 1993).

Rosemary O'Day, *The English Clergy: The Emergence and Consolidation of a Profession 1558–1642* (Leicester: Leicester University Press, 1979).

Rosemary O'Day, *Education and Society, 1500–1800: The Social Foundations of Education in Early Modern England* (London: Longman, 1982).

Rosemary O'Day, *The Debate on the English Reformation* (London: Methuen, 1986).

Rosemary O'Day, *The Family and Family Relationships, 1500–1900: England, France and the United States of America* (Basingstoke: Macmillan, 1994).

Rosemary O'Day and Felicity Heal (eds.), *Princes and Paupers in the English Church, 1500–1800* (Leicester: Leicester University Press, 1981).

D. J. Oddy, 'Food in the Nineteenth Century: Nutrition in the First Urban Society', *Proceedings of the Nutrition Society*, 29 (1970), 150–57.

D. J. Oddy, *The Making of the Modern British Diet* (London: Croom Helm, 1976).

Amy Oden, *In her own Words – Women's Writings in the History of Christian Thought* (London: SPCK, 1995).

Miles Ogborn, *Spaces of Modernity: London's Geographies, 1680–1780* (New York: Guilford Press, 1998).

Frank O'Gorman, *The Whig Party and the French Revolution* (London: Macmillan, 1967).

Frank O'Gorman, *The Rise of Party in England: The Rockingham Whigs, 1760–82* (London: Allen & Unwin, 1975).

Frank O'Gorman, *The Emergence of the British Two-party System, 1760–1832* (London: Edward Arnold, 1982).

Frank O'Gorman, *British Conservatism: Conservative Thought from Burke to Thatcher* (New York: Longman, 1986).

Frank O'Gorman, 'Recent Historiography of the Hanoverian Regime', *Historical Journal*, 29 (1986), 1005–20.

Frank O'Gorman, *Voters, Patrons, and Parties: The Unreformed Electoral System of Hanoverian England, 1734–1832* (Oxford: Clarendon Press, 1989).

Frank O'Gorman, *The Long Eighteenth Century: British Political and Social History 1688–1832* (London: Arnold, 1997).

R. C. Olby, G. N. Cantor, J. R. R. Christie and M. J. S. Hodge (eds.), *Companion to the History of Modern Science* (London: Routledge, 1990).

James Oldham, *The Mansfield Manuscripts and the Growth of English Law in the Eighteenth Century* (Chapel Hill: University of North Carolina Press, 1992).

W. H. Oliver, *Prophets and Millennialists: The Uses of Biblical Prophecy in England from the 1790s to the 1840s* (Oxford: Oxford University Press, 1979).

Richard Ollard, *The Image of the King: Charles I and Charles II* (London: Hodder and Stoughton, 1979).

Richard Ollard, *Pepys: A Biography* (Oxford: Oxford University Press, 1984).

Pat O'Mara, *The Autobiography of a Liverpool Slummy* (Liverpool: Bluecoat Press, 1995).

Janet Oppenheim, *'Shattered Nerves': Doctors, Patients and Depression in Victorian England* (Oxford: Oxford University Press, 1991).

Christopher O'Riordan, 'Popular Exploitation of Enemy Estates in the English Revolution', *History*, 78 (1993), 183–200.

Ian Ousby, *The Englishman's England: Taste, Travel and the Rise of Tourism* (Cambridge: Cambridge University Press, 1990).

R. B. Outhwaite, *Dearth, Public Policy and Social Disturbance in England 1550–1800* (London: Macmillan, 1991).

R. B. Outhwaite, *Clandestine Marriage in England, 1500–1850* (London: Hambledon Press, 1995).

Dorinda Outram, *The Enlightenment* (Cambridge: Cambridge University Press, 1995).

Mark Overton, *Agricultural Revolution in England: The Transformation of the Agrarian Economy, 1500–1850* (Cambridge: Cambridge University Press, 1996).

D. Owen, *English Philanthropy, 1660–1960* (Cambridge, Mass.: Harvard University Press, 1965).

G. W. Oxley, *Poor Relief in England and Wales 1601–1834* (Newton Abbot: David and Charles, 1974).

Steven Ozment, *When Fathers Ruled: Family Life in Reformation Europe* (Cambridge, Mass.: Harvard University Press, 1984).

Arnold Pacey, *Technology in World Civilization: A Thousand-Year History* (Oxford: Blackwell, 1990).

Arnold Pacey, *The Maze of Ingenuity: Ideas and Idealism in the Development of Technology* (Cambridge, Mass.: MIT Press, 1992).

Thomas Paine, *The Rights of Man and Common Sense*, introd. Michael Foot (London: D. Campbell, Everyman's Library, 1994).

Morton D. Paley, *The Apocalyptic Sublime* (New Haven: Yale University Press, 1986).

Colin A. Palmer, *Human Cargoes: The British Slave Trade to Spanish America, 1700–1739* (London: University of Illinois Press, 1981).

Stanley H. Palmer, *Police and Protest in England and Ireland, 1780–1850* (Cambridge: Cambridge University Press, 1988).

Panikos Panayi (ed.), *Germans in Britain since 1500* (London: Hambledon Press, 1995).

Christopher Parker (ed.), *Gender Roles and Sexuality in Victorian Literature* (London: Scolar, 1995).

Mark Parker, *Literary Magazines and British Romanticism* (Virginia: Randolph-Macon College, 2001).

Terry M. Parssinen, *Secret Passions, Secret Remedies: Narcotic Drugs in British Society, 1820–1930* (Manchester: Manchester University Press, 1983).

Graham Parry, *Hollar's England* (Salisbury: Michael Russell, 1980).

Graham Parry, *The Golden Age Restor'd: The Culture of the Stuart Court, 1603–42* (Manchester: Manchester University Press, 1981).

Sara Paston-Williams, *The Art of Dining: A History of Cooking and Eating* (London: National Trust, 1993).

C. A. Patrides and Raymond B. Waddington (eds.), *The Age of Milton: Backgrounds to Seventeenth-Century Literature* (Manchester: Manchester University Press, 1980).

Robert L. Patten, *George Cruikshank's Life, Times and Art*, vol. 1: *1792–1835* (New Brunswick, NJ: Rutgers University Press, 1992).

Annabel Patterson, *Censorship and Interpretation: The Conditions of Writing and Reading in Early Modern England* (Madison: University of Wisconsin Press, 1984).

Robert Pattison, *The Child Figure in English Literature* (Athens: University of Georgia Press, 1978).

Ronald Paulson, *Hogarth: His Life, Art and Times* (New Haven: Yale University Press, 1974).

Ronald Paulson, *Popular and Polite Art in the Age of Hogarth and Fielding* (Notre Dame: University of Notre Dame Press, 1979; 1981).

Ronald Paulson, *Book and Painting; Shakespeare, Milton, and the Bible. Literary Texts and the Emergence of English Painting* (Knoxville: University of Tennessee Press, 1982).

Ronald Paulson, *Literary Landscape: Turner and Constable* (New Haven: Yale University Press, 1982).

Ronald Paulson, *Representations of Revolution* (New Haven: Yale University Press, 1983).

Ronald Paulson, *Breaking and Remaking: Aesthetic Practice in England, 1700–1820* (New Brunswick, NJ: Rutgers University Press, 1989).

Ronald Paulson, *Hogarth*, vol. 1: *The 'Modern Moral Subject'*; vol. 2: *High Art and Low, 1732–1750*; vol. 3: *Art and Politics, 1750–1764* (Cambridge: Lutterworth, 1993).

Ronald Paulson, *The Beautiful, Novel, and Strange: Aesthetics and Heterodoxy* (Baltimore and London: Johns Hopkins University Press, 1996).

Ronald Paulson, *Don Quixote in England: The Aesthetics of Laughter* (Baltimore: Johns Hopkins University Press, 1998).

Eric Pawson, *Transport and the Economy: The Turnpike Roads of Eighteenth-Century Britain* (London: Academic Press, 1977).

Eric Pawson, *The Early Industrial Revolution: Britain in the Eighteenth Century* (London: Batsford, 1979).

Iain Pears, *The Discovery of Painting: The Growth of Interest in the Arts in England 1680–1768* (New Haven: Yale University Press, 1988).

Ronald Pearsall, *The Worm in the Bud: The World of Victorian Sexuality* (Harmondsworth: Penguin, 1971).

R. A. Pearson, *The Guardian Book of the Welfare State* (Aldershot: Wildwood House, 1988).

Linda Levy Peck, *Court Patronage and Corruption in Early Stuart England* (London: Unwin Hyman, 1990).

Linda Levy Peck (ed.), *The Mental World of the Jacobean Court* (Cambridge: Cambridge University Press, 1991).

Vincent P. Pecora, *Households of the Soul* (Baltimore: Johns Hopkins University Press, 1997).

Markku Peltonen, *Classical Humanism and Republicanism in English Political Thought, 1570–1640* (Cambridge: Cambridge University Press, 1995).

Donald Pennington and Keith Thomas (eds.), *Puritans and Revolutionaries: Essays in Seventeenth-Century History Presented to Christopher Hill* (Oxford: Oxford University Press, 1978).

Harold Perkin, *The Origins of Modern English Society 1780–1880* (Toronto: University of Toronto Press, 1967; London: Routledge and Kegan Paul, 1969).

Harold Perkin, *The Structured Crowd: Essays in English Social History* (Brighton: Harvester Press, 1981).

Joan Perkin, *Women and Marriage in Nineteenth-Century England* (London: Routledge, 1988; Chicago: Lyceum Books, 1989).

Philippe Perrot, *Fashioning the Bourgeoisie: A History of Clothing in the Nineteenth Century* (Princeton: Princeton University Press, 1994).

Ruth Perry, *The Celebrated Mary Astell: An Early English Feminist* (Chicago: University of Chicago Press, 1986).

Karl Gunnar Persson, *Grain Markets in Europe, 1500–1900: Integration and Deregulation* (Cambridge: Cambridge University Press, 1999).

Marie Peters, *Pitt and Popularity: The Patriot Minister and London Opinion during the Seven Years' War* (Oxford: Oxford University Press, 1981).

Marie Peters, *The Elder Pitt* (London: Longman, 1998).

William Petersen, *Malthus* (Cambridge, Mass.: Harvard University Press, 1979).

Nikolaus Pevsner, *The Englishness of English Art* (Harmondsworth: Penguin, 1976; orig. pub. London: Architectural Press, 1956).

Naomi Pfeffer, *The Stork and the Syringe: A Political History of Reproductive Medicine* (Cambridge: Polity Press, 1993).

John A. Phillips, *Electoral Behaviour in Unreformed England: Plumpers, Splitters and Straights* (Guildford: Princeton University Press, 1982).

Roderick Phillips, *Putting Asunder: A History of Divorce in Western Society* (Cambridge: Cambridge University Press, 1988).

Nicholas Phillipson, 'Towards a Definition of the Scottish Enlightenment', in Paul Fritz and David Williams (eds.), *City & Society in the 18th Century* (Toronto: A. M. Hakkert, 1973), 125–47.

Nicholas Phillipson, 'The Scottish Enlightenment', in Roy Porter and Mikuláš Teich (eds.), *Enlightenment in National Context* (Cambridge: Cambridge University Press, 1981), 19–40.

Nicholas Phillipson, *Hume* (London: Weidenfeld and Nicolson, 1989).

Nicholas Phillipson and Rosalind Mitchison (eds.), *Scotland in the Age of Improvement: Essays in Scottish History in the Eighteenth Century* (Edinburgh: Edinburgh University Press, 1970).

Charles Phythian-Adams (ed.), *Societies, Cultures and Kinship, 1580–1850: Cultural Provinces and English Local History* (Leicester: Leicester University Press, 1993).

S. F. Pickering Jr., *John Locke and Children's Books in Eighteenth-Century England* (Knoxville: University of Tennessee Press, 1981).

E. R. Pike, *Human Documents of the Industrial Revolution* (London: Allen and Unwin, 1966).

E. R. Pike, *Human Documents of Adam Smith's Time* (London: Allen and Unwin, 1974).

John Alfred Ralph Pimlott, *The Englishman's Holiday: A Social History* (London: Faber and Faber, 1947).

Ivy Pinchbeck, *Women Workers and the Industrial Revolution, 1750–1850*, 3rd edn. (London: Virago, 1981).

Ivy Pinchbeck and Margaret Hewitt, *Children in English Society*, 2 vols. (London: Routledge and Kegan Paul, 1969–73).

Steven Pincus, *Protestantism and Patriotism: Ideologies and the Making of English Foreign Policy, 1650–1668* (Cambridge: Cambridge University Press, 1996).

Philip Pinkus, *Grub St. Stripped Bare: The Scandalous Lives and Pornographic Works of the Original Grub St. Writers, Together With the Battle Songs Which Led to Their Drunkenness, the Shameless Pamphleteering Which Led Them to Prison, & the Continual Pandering to Public Taste Which Put Them Among the First Almost to Earn a Fitful Living From Their Writing Alone* (Hamden, Conn.: Archon Books, 1968).

Murray G. H. Pittock, *The Invention of Scotland: The Stuart Myth and the Scottish Identity: 1638 to the Present* (London: Routledge, 1991).

Andrejs Plakans, *Kinship in the Past: An Anthropology of European Family Life 1500–1900* (New York: Basil Blackwell, 1984).

Marjorie Plant, *The English Book Trade: An Economic History of the Making and Sale of Books* (London: Allen and Unwin, 1965).

J. H. Plumb, *England in the Eighteenth Century, 1714–1815* (Harmondsworth: Penguin, 1950).

J. H. Plumb, *The First Four Georges* (London: Batsford, 1956).

J. H. Plumb, *Men and Places* (Harmondsworth: Pelican, 1966).

J. H. Plumb, *The Growth of Political Stability in England, 1675–1725* (London: Macmillan, 1967).

J. H. Plumb, *In the Light of History* (London: Allen Lane, 1972).

J. H. Plumb, 'The Public, Literature and the Arts in the Eighteenth Century', in P. Fritz and D. Williams (eds.), *The Triumph of Culture* (Toronto: A. M. Hakkert, 1972), 27–48.

J. H. Plumb, *The Commercialisation of Leisure in Eighteenth-Century England* (Reading: University of Reading, 1973).

J. H. Plumb, 'The New World of the Children in Eighteenth-Century England', *Past and Present*, 67 (1975), 64–95.

J. H. Plumb, *Sir Robert Walpole*, 2 vols. (London: Allen Lane, 1976).

J. H. Plumb, *The Pursuit of Happiness* (New Haven: Yale University Press, 1977).

J. H. Plumb, *The Death of the Past* (London: Macmillan, 1978).

J. H. Plumb, *Georgian Delights* (London: Weidenfeld and Nicolson, 1980).

J. G. A. Pocock, *Politics, Language and Time: Essays in Political Thought and History* (London: Methuen, 1972).

J. G. A. Pocock (ed.), *Three British Revolutions: 1641, 1688, 1776* (Princeton: Princeton University Press, for the Folger Shakespeare Library, 1980).

J. G. A. Pocock, *Virtue, Commerce and History: Essays on Political Thought and History, Chiefly in the Eighteenth Century* (Cambridge: Cambridge University Press, 1985).

Colin Podmore, *The Moravian Church in England, 1728–1760* (Oxford: Clarendon Press, 1998).

Marcia Pointon, *Hanging the Head: Portraiture and Social Formation in Eighteenth-Century England* (New Haven: Yale University Press, 1993).

Sidney Pollard, *The Idea of Progress: History and Society* (London: Watts and Co., 1968).

Sidney Pollard and David W. Crossley, *The Wealth of Britain, 1085–1966* (London: Batsford, 1968).

Harold Pollins, *Economic History of the Jews in England* (London: Associated University Presses, 1983).

Linda A. Pollock, *Forgotten Children: Parent–Child Relations from 1500 to 1900* (Cambridge: Cambridge University Press, 1983).

Linda A. Pollock, *A Lasting Relationship: Parents and Children over Three Centuries* (London: Fourth Estate, 1987).

Clive Ponting, *World History: A New Perspective* (London: Chatto and Windus, 2000).

Robert Poole, ' "Give us our Eleven Days!": Calendar Reform in Eighteenth-Century England', *Past and Present*, 149 (1995), 95–139.

Dorothy Porter and Roy Porter, *Patient's Progress: Doctors and Doctoring in Eighteenth-Century England* (Cambridge: Polity Press, 1989).

Roy Porter, *English Society in the Eighteenth Century* (London: Allen Lane, 1982).

Roy Porter (ed.), *Patients and Practitioners: Lay Perceptions of Medicine in Pre-Industrial Society* (Cambridge: Cambridge University Press, 1985).

Roy Porter, *Edward Gibbon: Making History* (London: Weidenfeld and Nicolson, 1988).

Roy Porter, *Health for Sale: Quackery in England 1660–1850* (Manchester: Manchester University Press, 1989).

Roy Porter (ed.), *Myths of the English* (Cambridge: Polity Press, 1992).

Roy Porter, *London: A Social History* (London: Hamish Hamilton, 1994).

Roy Porter (ed.), *Rewriting the Self* (London: Routledge, 1996).

Roy Porter, *Quacks: Fakers and Charlatans in English Medicine* (Stroud: Tempus, 2000).

Roy Porter and Lesley Hall, *The Facts of Life: The Creation of Sexual Knowledge in Britain 1650–1950* (New Haven: Yale University Press, 1995).

Roy Porter and Marie Mulvey Roberts (eds.), *Pleasure in the Eighteenth Century* (London: Macmillan, 1996).

John D. Post, *Food Shortage, Climatic Variability and Epidemic Disease in Preindustrial Europe: The Mortality Peak in the Early 1740s* (London: Cornell University Press, 1985).

Harry Potter, *Hanging in Judgment: Religion and the Death Penalty from the Bloody Code to Abolition* (London: SCM Press, 1993).

Wilfrid Prest (ed.), *The Professions in Early Modern England* (Beckenham: Croom Helm, 1987).

Martin Price, *Forms of Life: Character and Moral Imagination in the Novel* (New Haven: Yale University Press, 1983).

Richard Price, *Labour in British Society: An*

Interpretative History (London: Croom Helm, 1986).

Mary Prior (ed.), *Women in English Society, 1500–1800* (London: Methuen, 1985).

F. K. Prochaska, *Women and Philanthropy in Nineteenth-Century England* (Oxford: Clarendon Press, 1980).

Kathy Alexis Psomiades, *Beauty's Body: Femininity and Representation in British Aestheticism* (Stanford, Calif.: Stanford University Press, 1997).

S. Pugh (ed.), *Reading Landscape: Country-City-Capital* (Manchester: Manchester University Press, 1990).

Diane Purkiss, *The Witch in History: Early Modern and Twentieth Century Representations* (London: Routledge, 1996).

Diane Purkiss, *Troublesome Things: A History of Fairies and Fairy Stories* (London: Allen Lane, The Penguin Press, 2000).

G. R. Quaife, *Wanton Wenches and Wayward Wives* (London: Croom Helm, 1979).

Peter Quennell, *The Pursuit of Happiness* (London: Constable, 1988).

Michael C. Questier, *Conversion, Politics and Religion in England, 1580–1685* (Cambridge: Cambridge University Press, 1996).

Claude Quétel, *History of Syphilis*, trans. Judith Braddock and Brian Pike (Oxford: Polity Press, 1990).

Maurice Quinlan, *Victorian Prelude: A History of English Manners, 1700–1830* (London: Cass, 1941).

M. Quinlan, *William Cowper* (Minneapolis: University of Minnesota Press, 1953).

M. Quinlan, *Samuel Johnson: A Layman's Religion* (Madison: University of Wisconsin Press, 1964).

Anthony Quinton, *The Politics of Imperfection: The Religious and Secular Traditions of Conservative Thought in England from Hooker to Oakeshott* (London: Faber and Faber, 1978).

Henry Rack, *Reasonable Enthusiast: John Wesley and the Rise of Methodism* (London: Epworth, 1989).

Leon Radzinowicz and Roger Hood, *A History of English Criminal Law and its Administration from 1750*, vol. 5: *The Emergence of Penal Policy* (London: Stevens and Sons, 1986).

Deirdre Raftery, *Women and Learning in English Writing, 1600–1900* (Dublin: Four Courts Press, 1997).

Michael Ragussis, *Figures of Conversion: 'The Jewish Question' and English National Identity* (Durham, NC: Duke University Press, 1995).

Arthur Raistrick, *Quakers in Science and Industry; Being an Account of the Quaker Contributions to Science and Industry During the 17th and 18th Centuries* (London: Bannisdale Press, 1950).

James Raven, *Judging New Wealth: Popular Publishing and Responses to Commerce in England 1750–1800* (Oxford: Clarendon Press, 1992).

James Raven, Helen Small and Naomi Tadmor (eds.), *The Practice and Representation of Reading in England* (Cambridge: Cambridge University Press, 1996).

Philip Rawlings (ed.), *Drunks, Whores and Idle Apprentices: Criminal Biographies of the Eighteenth Century* (London: Routledge, 1992).

C. Rawson, *Gulliver and the Gentle Reader: Studies in Swift and our Time* (London: Routledge and Kegan Paul, 1973).

Claude Rawson, *Satire and Sentiment 1660–1830* (Cambridge: Cambridge University Press, 1994).

Joad Raymond (ed.), *Making the News: An Anthology of the Newsbooks of Revolutionary England, 1641–1660* (Moreton-in-Marsh: Windrush Press, 1993).

Peter Razzell, *Essays in English Population History* (London: Caliban, 1994).

Donald Read, *The English Provinces c. 1760–1960: A Study in Influence* (London: Edward Arnold, 1964).

W. J. Reader, *At Duty's Call: A Study in Obsolete*

Patriotism (Manchester: Manchester University Press, 1988).

Barry Reay (ed.), *Popular Culture in Seventeenth-Century England* (London: Croom Helm, 1985).

Barry Reay, *The Quakers and the English Revolution* (London: Temple Smith, 1985).

Barry Reay, *The Last Rising of the Agricultural Labourers: Rural Life and Protest in Nineteenth-Century England* (Oxford: Clarendon Press, 1990).

Barry Reay, *Popular Cultures in England 1550–1750* (London: Longman, 1998).

John Redwood, *Reason, Ridicule and Religion: The Age of Enlightenment in England, 1660–1750* (London: Thames and Hudson, 1976; repr. 1996).

Michael Reed, *The Age of Exuberance 1550–1700* (London: Routledge and Kegan Paul, 1986).

Michael Reed, *The Landscape of Britain: From the Beginnings to 1914* (London: Routledge, 1990).

Michael Reed and Roger Wells (eds.), *Class Conflict and Protest in the English Countryside, 1700–1880* (Savage, Md.: Frank Cass, 1990).

Philip F. Rehbock, *The Philosophical Naturalists: Themes in Early Nineteenth-Century British Biology* (Madison: University of Wisconsin Press, 1983).

John Phillip Reid, *The Concept of Liberty in the Age of the American Revolution* (Chicago: University of Chicago Press, 1988).

Robin Reilly, *Josiah Wedgwood* (London: Macmillan, 1992).

Jane Rendall (ed.), *The Origins of the Scottish Enlightenment 1707–1776* (London: Macmillan, 1978).

Jane Rendall, *The Origins of Modern Feminism: Women in Britain, France, and the United States, 1780–1860* (London: Macmillan, 1985).

Jane Rendall, *Sexuality and Subordination* (London: Routledge, 1989).

Jane Rendall, *Women in an Industrializing Society: England 1750–1880* (Oxford: Basil Blackwell, 1990).

Myra Reynolds, *The Learned Lady in England 1650–1760* (Boston: Houghton Mifflin, 1920).

Aileen Ribeiro, *Dress in Eighteenth-Century Europe, 1715–1789* (New York: Holmes and Meier, 1985).

Aileen Ribeiro, *The Art of Dress: Fashion in England and France, 1750–1820* (New Haven: Yale University Press, 1995).

Robert J. Richards, *Darwin and the Emergence of Evolutionary Theories of Mind and Behaviour* (Chicago: University of Chicago Press, 1987).

R. C. Richardson (ed.), *Town and Countryside in the English Revolution* (Manchester: Manchester University Press, 1993).

R. C. Richardson and T. B. James (eds.), *The Urban Experience: A Sourcebook. English, Scottish and Welsh Towns, 1450–1700* (Manchester: Manchester University Press, 1983).

Ruth Richardson, *Death, Dissection and the Destitute* (London: Routledge and Kegan Paul, 1987).

P. W. J. Riley, *King William and the Scottish Politicians* (Edinburgh: John Donald, 1979).

P. W. J. Riley, *The Union of England and Scotland: A Study in Anglo-Scottish Politics of the Eighteenth Century* (Manchester: Manchester University Press, 1979).

Guenter B. Risse, *Hospital Life in Enlightenment Scotland: Care and Teaching at the Royal Infirmary of Edinburgh* (Cambridge: Cambridge University Press, 1986).

Harriet Ritvo, *The Animal Estate: The English and Other Creatures in the Victorian Age* (Cambridge, Mass.: Harvard University Press, 1987).

Isabel Rivers (ed.), *Books and their Readers in Eighteenth-Century England* (Leicester: Leicester University Press; New York: St Martin's Press, 1982).

Isabel Rivers, *Reason, Grace, and Sentiment: A Study of the Language of Religion and Ethics in*

England, 1660–1780, vol. 1: *Whichcote to Wesley* (Cambridge: Cambridge University Press, 1991).

J. Roach, *Social Reform in England, 1780–1880* (London: Batsford, 1978).

Clayton Roberts, *Schemes & Undertakings: A Study of English Politics in the Seventeenth Century* (Columbus: Ohio State University Press, 1985).

David Roberts, *The Ladies: Female Patronage of Restoration Drama* (Oxford: Clarendon Press, 1991).

J. M. Roberts, *The Penguin History of Europe* (Harmondsworth: Penguin, 1996).

Marie Mulvey Roberts and Roy Porter (eds.), *Literature and Medicine during the Eighteenth Century* (London: Routledge, 1993).

Nicholas K. Robinson, *Edmund Burke: A Life in Caricature* (New Haven: Yale University Press, 1996).

Betsy Rodgers, *Cloak of Charity: Studies in Eighteenth-century Philanthropy* (London: Methuen, 1949).

N. A. M. Rodger, *The Wooden World: An Anatomy of the Georgian Navy* (Annapolis, Md.: Naval Institute Press; London: Collins, 1986).

N. A. M. Rodger, *The Insatiable Earl: A Life of John Montagu, Fourth Earl of Sandwich, 1718–1792* (London: HarperCollins, 1993).

Richard Rodger, *Housing in Urban Britain 1780–1914: Class, Capitalism and Construction* (Basingstoke: Macmillan Education, 1989; Cambridge: Cambridge University Press, 1995).

Peter Roebuck, *Yorkshire Baronets 1640–1760: Families, Estates and Fortunes* (Oxford: Oxford University Press for the University of Hull, 1980).

H. C. B. Rogers, *The British Army of the Eighteenth Century* (London: Allen and Unwin, 1977).

Katharine M. Rogers, *Feminism in Eighteenth-Century England* (Urbana: University of Illinois Press, c1982).

Katharine M. Rogers, *The Troublesome*

Helpmate (Seattle: University of Wisconsin Press, 1968).

Nicholas Rogers, 'Resistance to Oligarchy: The City Opposition to Walpole and his Successors, 1725–47', in J. Stevenson (ed.), *London in the Age of Reform* (Oxford: Basil Blackwell, 1977), 1–29.

Nicholas Rogers, 'Popular Protest in Early Hanoverian London', *Past and Present*, 79 (1978), 70–100.

Nicholas Rogers, 'Money, Land and Lineage: The Big Bourgeoisie of Hanoverian London', *Social History*, 4 (1979), 437–54.

Nicholas Rogers, *Whigs and Cities: Popular Politics in the Age of Walpole and Pitt* (Oxford: Clarendon Press, 1989).

Nicholas Rogers, 'Making the English Middle Class, ca 1700–1850', *Journal of British Studies*, 32 (1993).

Nicholas Rogers, *Crowds, Culture and Politics in Georgian Britain* (Oxford: Clarendon Press, 1998).

Pat Rogers, *Grub Street: Studies in a Subculture* (London: Methuen, 1972).

Pat Rogers, *The Augustan Vision* (London: Weidenfeld & Nicolson, 1974).

Pat Rogers (ed.), *The Context of English Literature: The Eighteenth Century* (London: Methuen 1978).

Pat Rogers, 'Gulliver's Glasses', in Clive T. Probyn (ed.), *The Art of Jonathan Swift* (London: Vision Press, 1978), 179–88.

Pat Rogers, *Hacks and Dunces: Pope, Swift and Grub Street* (London: Methuen, 1980).

Pat Rogers, 'Tristram's Polite Conversation', *Essays in Criticism*, 32 (1982).

Pat Rogers, *Eighteenth-Century Encounters: Studies in Literature and Society in the Age of Walpole* (Brighton: Harvester Press; Totowa, NJ: Barnes and Noble, 1985).

Pat Rogers, *Literature and Popular Culture in Eighteenth-Century England* (Brighton: Harvester Press; Totowa, NJ: Barnes and Noble, 1985).

Pat Rogers, *Samuel Johnson* (Oxford: Oxford University Press, 1993).

Pat Rogers, *Johnson and Boswell: The Transit of Caledonia* (Oxford: Clarendon Press, 1995).

Erich Roll, *A History of Economic Thought* (London: Faber, 1938).

David Rollison, *The Local Origins of Modern Society: Gloucestershire 1500–1800* (London: Routledge, 1992).

Derek Roper, *Reviewing before the Edinburgh: 1788–1802* (London: Methuen, 1978).

H. Rosaveare, *The Treasury, 1660–1870: The Foundations of Control* (London: Allen and Unwin, 1973).

M. E. Rose, *The English Poor Law 1760–1830* (Newton Abbot: David and Charles, 1971).

Mary B. Rose, *The Gregs of Quarry Bank Mill: The Rise and Decline of a Family Firm, 1750–1914* (New York: Cambridge University Press, 1986).

Mary B. Rose (ed.), *The Lancashire Cotton Industry: A History since 1700* (Preston: Lancashire County Books, 1996).

Sonya O. Rose, *Limited Livelihoods: Gender and Class in Nineteenth-Century England* (Berkeley: University of California Press, 1992).

Charles E. Rosenberg, *Explaining Epidemics and Other Studies in the History of Medicine* (Cambridge: Cambridge University Press, 1992).

Doreen M. Rosman, *Evangelicals and Culture* (London: Croom Helm, 1984).

Robert I. Rotberg and Theodore K. Rabb (eds.), *Population and Economy: Population and History from the Traditional to the Modern World* (New York: Cambridge University Press, 1986).

Eric Rothstein and Frances M. Kavenik, *The Designs of Carolean Comedy* (Carbondale: Southern Illinois University Press, 1988).

G. S. Rousseau and Roy Porter (eds.), *Sexual Underworlds of the Enlightenment* (Manchester: Manchester University Press, 1988).

Nick Rowling, *Commodities: How the World was Taken to Market* (London: Free Association Books, 1987).

A. L. Rowse, *Reflections on the Puritan Revolution* (London: Methuen, 1986).

A. L. Rowse, *The Regicides and the Puritan Revolution* (London: Duckworth, 1994).

Edward Royle, *Radical Politics 1790–1900: Religion and Unbelief* (Harlow: Longman, 1971).

Edward Royle, *Victorian Infidels: The Origins of the British Secularist Movement, 1791–1848* (Manchester: Manchester University Press, 1974).

Edward Royle, *Modern Britain: A Social History, 1750–1985* (London: Edward Arnold, 1987).

E. Royle and J. Walvin, *English Radicals and Reformers 1760–1848* (Brighton: Harvester, 1982).

G. R. Rubin and David Sugarman (eds.), *Law, Economy and Society, 1750–1914: Essays in the History of English Law* (Abingdon: Professional Books, 1984).

W. D. Rubinstein, 'The End of "Old Corruption" in Britain 1780–1860', *Past and Present*, 101 (1983), 55–86.

W. D. Rubinstein, *Elites and the Wealthy in Modern British History: Essays in Social and Economic History* (Brighton: Harvester, 1987).

W. D. Rubinstein, *Capitalism, Culture and Economic Decline in Britain, 1750–1990* (London: Routledge, 1993).

George Rudé, *Wilkes and Liberty: A Social Study of 1763–1774* (Oxford: Clarendon Press, 1962).

George Rudé, *The Crowd in History* (New York: John Wiley, 1964).

G. Rudé, *Paris and London in the Eighteenth Century: Studies in Popular Protest* (London: Collins, 1970).

George Rudé, *Hanoverian London, 1714–1808* (London: Secker and Warburg, 1971).

George Rudé, *Ideology and Popular Protest* (London: Lawrence and Wishart, 1980).

George Rudé, *Criminal and Victim: Crime and Society in Early Nineteenth-Century England* (Oxford: Clarendon Press, 1985).

Richard Rudgely, *The Alchemy of Culture: Intoxicants in Society* (London: British Museum Press, 1993).

J. Rule, *The Experience of Labour in Eighteenth Century Industry* (London: Croom Helm, 1981).

J. Rule, *The Labouring Classes in Early Industrial England 1750–1850* (London: Longman, 1986).

J. Rule, *British Trade Unionism, 1750–1850: The Formative Years* (London: Longman, 1988).

John Rule, *Albion's People: English Society, 1714–1815* (London: Longman, 1992).

John Rule, *The Vital Century: England's Developing Economy 1714–1815* (London: Longman, 1992).

John Rule and Robert Malcolmson (eds.), *Protest and Survival: The Historical Experience. Essays for E. P. Thompson* (London: Merlin Press, 1993).

John Rule and Roger Wells, *Crime, Protest and Popular Politics in Southern England, 1740–1850* (London: Hambledon Press, 1997).

Gordon Rupp, *Religion in England 1688–1791* (Oxford: Clarendon Press, 1986).

Anthony Russell, *The Clerical Profession* (London: SPCK, 1980).

Colin Russell (ed.), *Science and Religious Belief: A Selection of Recent Historical Studies* (London: University of London Press, 1973).

Colin Russell, *Science and Social Change in Britain and Europe, 1700–1900* (London: Macmillan, 1983).

Colin A. Russell, *Cross-currents: Intersections between Society and Faith* (Leicester: Intervarsity, 1984).

Colin Russell, N. G. Coley and G. K. Roberts, *Chemists by Profession: The Origins and Rise of the Royal Institute of Chemistry* (Milton Keynes: Open University, 1977).

Conrad Russell, *The Causes of the English Civil War* (Oxford: Clarendon Press, 1990).

Conrad Russell, *The Fall of the British Monarchies 1637–42* (Oxford: Clarendon Press, 1991).

Gillian Russell, *The Theatres of War: Performance, Politics, and Society, 1793–1815* (Oxford: Clarendon Press, 1995).

W. Rybczynski, *Home: A Short History of an Idea* (London: Heinemann, 1988).

James J. Sack, *From Jacobite to Conservative: Reaction and Orthodoxy in Britain, c.1760–1832* (Cambridge: Cambridge University Press, 1993).

David Harris Sacks, *The Widening Gate: Bristol and the Atlantic Economy, 1450–1700* (Berkeley: University of California Press, 1991).

Edward W. Said, *Culture and Imperialism* (New York: Alfred A. Knopf, 1993).

Andrew St George, *The Descent of Manners: Etiquette, Rules & the Victorians* (London: Chatto & Windus, 1993).

Roger Sales, *English Literature in History, 1780–1830: Pastoral and Politics* (London: Hutchinson, 1983).

P. Salzman, *English Prose Fiction 1558–1700: A Critical History* (Oxford: Oxford University Press, 1985).

Pamela Sambrook, *Country House Brewing in England 1500–1900* (London: Hambledon Press, 1996).

Anthony Sampson, *The Essential Anatomy of Britain: Democracy in Crisis* (London: Hodder and Stoughton, 1992).

H. Sampson, *A History of Advertising* (London: Chatto and Windus, 1974).

Raphael Samuel (ed.), *People's History and Socialist Theory* (London: Routledge and Kegan Paul, 1981), 227–40.

Raphael Samuel (ed.), *Patriotism. The Making and Unmaking of British National Identity*, 3 vols. (London: Routledge, 1989).

Raphael Samuel, *Island Stories: Unravelling Britain. Theatres of Memory*, vol. 1: *History and Politics*; vol. 2: *Minorities and Outsiders*; vol. 3: *National Fictions* (London: Verso, 1998).

Raphael Samuel and G. Stedman Jones (eds.), *Culture, Ideology and Politics* (London: Routledge and Kegan Paul, 1982).

Raphael Samuel and Paul Thompson (eds.),

The Myths we Live By (London: Routledge, 1990).

Elizabeth C. Sanderson, *Women and Work in Eighteenth-Century Edinburgh* (London: Macmillan, 1996).

John Sanderson, *'But the People's Creatures': The Philosophical Basis of the English Civil War* (Manchester: Manchester University Press, 1989).

Mollie Sands, *Robson of the Olympic* (London: Society for Theatre Research, 1979).

Rose-Mary Sargent, *The Diffident Naturalist: Robert Boyle and the Philosophy of Experiment* (Chicago: University of Chicago Press, 1995).

J. W. Saunders, *The Profession of English Letters* (London: Routledge and Kegan Paul, 1964).

Lyndel Saunders King, *The Industrialization of Taste: Victorian England and the Art Union of London* (Ann Arbor: UMI Research Press, 1985).

Jonathan Sawday, *The Body Emblazoned: Dissection and the Human Body in Renaissance Culture* (London: Routledge, 1995).

Simon Schaffer, 'Natural Philosophy', in G. S. Rousseau and R. Porter (eds.), *The Ferment of Knowledge: Studies in the Historiography of Eighteeenth-Century Science* (Cambridge: Cambridge University Press, 1980), 55–91.

Simon Schaffer, 'Natural Philosophy and Public Spectacle in the Eighteenth Century', *History of Science*, 21 (1983), 1–43.

Simon Schaffer, 'Priestley's Questions', *History of Science*, 22 (1984), 151–83.

Simon Schaffer, 'Newton's Comets and the Transformation of Astrology', in P. Curry (ed.), *Astrology, Science and Society* (Woodbridge, Suffolk: Boydell Press, 1987), 219–43.

Simon Schaffer, 'Defoe's Natural Philosophy and the Worlds of Credit', in John Christie and Sally Shuttleworth (eds.), *Nature Transfigured: Science and Literature,*

1700–1900 (Manchester: Manchester University Press, 1989), 13–44.

Simon Schaffer, 'Genius in Romantic Natural Philosophy', in A. Cunningham and N. Jardine (eds.), *Romanticism and the Sciences* (Cambridge: Cambridge University Press, 1990), 82–98.

Simon Schaffer, 'States of Mind: Enlightenment and Natural Philosophy', in G. S. Rousseau (ed.), *The Languages of Psyche: Mind and Body in Enlightenment Thought* (Berkeley: University of California Press, 1990), 233–90.

Simon Schaffer, 'Visions of Empire: Afterword', in David Philip Miller and Peter Hanns Reill (eds.), *Visions of Empire: Voyages, Botany, and Representations of Nature* (Cambridge: Cambridge University Press, 1996), 335–52.

Simon Schama, *The Embarrassment of Riches: An Interpretation of Dutch Culture in the Golden Age* (London: Fontana, 1988).

Simon Schama, *Landscape and Memory* (London: HarperCollins, 1995).

Bernard M. Schilling, *Conservative England and the Case against Voltaire* (New York: Columbia University Press, 1950).

Cannon Schmitt, *Alien Nation: Nineteenth-Century Gothic Fictions and English Nationality* (Philadelphia: University of Pennsylvania Press, 1997).

Robert E. Schofield, 'John Wesley and Science in Eighteenth-Century England', *Isis*, 44 (1953), 331–40.

Robert E. Schofield, 'Josiah Wedgwood, Industrial Chemist', *Chymia*, 5 (1959), 180–92.

Robert E. Schofield, *The Lunar Society of Birmingham: A Social History of Provincial Science and Industry in Eighteenth-Century England* (Oxford: Clarendon Press, 1963).

Robert E. Schofield, 'Joseph Priestley, the Theory of Oxidation and the Nature of Matter', *Journal of the History of Ideas*, 25 (1964), 285–94.

Robert E. Schofield (ed.), *A Scientific*

Autobiography of Joseph Priestley (1733–1804): Selected Correspondence (Cambridge, Mass., MIT Press, 1966).

Robert E. Schofield, 'Joseph Priestley, Natural Philosopher', *Ambix*, 14 (1967), 1–15.

Robert E. Schofield, 'The Lunar Society and the Industrial Revolution', *University of Birmingham Historical Journal*, 11 (1967–8), 94–111.

Robert E. Schofield, *Mechanism and Materialism: British Natural Philosophy in an Age of Reason* (Princeton: Princeton University Press, 1970).

Robert E. Schofield, 'The Industrial Orientation of Science in the Lunar Society of Birmingham', in A. E. Musson (ed.), *Science, Technology and Economic Growth in the Eighteenth Century* (London: Methuen, 1972), 136–47.

Robert E. Schofield, 'Joseph Priestley: Theology, Physics and Metaphysic' *Enlightenment and Dissent*, 2 (1983), 69–81.

Robert E. Schofield, *The Enlightenment of Joseph Priestley: A Study of his Life and Work from 1733 to 1773* (Philadelphia: Pennsylvania State University Press, 1997).

R. S. Schofield, 'Dimensions of Illiteracy, 1750–1850', *Explorations in Economic History*, 10 (1972–3), 436–54.

R. S. Schofield, *The Population History of England 1541–1971: A Reconstruction* (London: Edward Arnold, 1981).

R. S. Schofield, 'Population Growth and the Century after 1750: The Role of Mortality Decline', in T. Bengtsson *et al.* (eds.), *Pre-Industrial Population Change* (Stockholm: Almqvist & Wiskell, 1984).

Esther Schor, *Bearing the Dead: The British Culture of Mourning from the Enlightenment to Victoria* (Princeton: Princeton University Press, 1994).

Max F. Schub, *Paradise Preserved: Recreations of Eden in Eighteenth- and Nineteenth-Century England* (New York: Cambridge University Press, 1986).

Wayne Schumaker, *English Autobiography* (Berkeley: University of California Press, 1954).

Hillel Schwartz, *The French Prophets: The History of a Millenarian Group in Eighteenth-Century England* (London: University of California Press, 1980).

Bill Schwarz (ed.), *The Expansion of England: Race, Ethnicity and Cultural History* (London: Routledge, 1996).

L. D. Schwarz, *London in the Age of Industrialisation: Entrepreneurs, Labour Force and Living Conditions, 1700–1850* (Cambridge: Cambridge University Press, 1992).

Lois Schwoerer, *Lady Rachel Russell* (Baltimore: Johns Hopkins University Press, 1988).

Lois Schwoerer (ed.), *The Revolution of 1688–1689: Changing Perspectives* (Cambridge: Cambridge University Press, 1992).

Roger Scola, *Feeding the Victorian City: The Food Supply of Manchester, 1770–1870* (Manchester: Manchester University Press, 1992).

J. Scott, *Gender and the Politics of History* (New York: Columbia University Press, 1988).

Jonathan Scott, *England's Troubles: Seventeenth-Century Political Stability in European Context* (Cambridge: Cambridge University Press, 2000).

I. Scoutland (ed.), *Huguenots in Britain and their French Background, 1550–1800* (Basingstoke: Macmillan, 1987).

Andrew Scull (ed.), *Madhouses, Mad-Doctors, and Madmen* (Philadelphia: University of Pennsylvania Press, 1981).

Andrew Scull, *The Most Solitary of Afflictions: Madness and Society in Britain, 1700–1900* (New Haven: Yale University Press, 1993).

Andrew Scull, *Masters of Bedlam: The Transformation of the Mad-Doctoring Trade* (Princeton: Princeton University Press, 1996).

L. C. B. Seaman, *A New History of England*

410–1975 (Brighton: Harvester Press, 1981).

Peter Searby, *A History of the University of Cambridge*, vol. 3: *1750–1870* (Cambridge: Cambridge University Press, 1997).

Paul S. Seaver, *Wallington's World: A Puritan Artisan in Seventeenth-Century London* (London: Methuen, 1985).

Paul Seaward, *The Cavalier Parliament and the Reconstruction of the Old Regime, 1661–1667* (Cambridge: Cambridge University Press, 1989).

Paul Seaward, *The Restoration, 1660–1668* (New York: St Martin's Press, 1991).

Wally Seccombe, *Weathering the Storm: Working-Class Families from the Industrial Revolution to the Fertility Decline* (London: Verso, 1993).

John Sekora, *Luxury: The Concept in Western Thought, Eden to Smollett* (Baltimore: Johns Hopkins University Press, 1977).

Janet Semple, *Bentham's Prison: A Study of the Panopticon Penitentiary* (Oxford: Clarendon Press, 1993).

Richard Sennett (ed.), *Classic Essays on the Culture of Cities* (Englewood Cliffs, NJ: Prentice-Hall, 1969).

Richard Sennett, *The Fall of Public Man* (Cambridge: Cambridge University Press, 1976; London: Faber, 1986).

Richard Sennett, *Flesh and Stones: The Body and the City in Western Civilisation* (London: Faber and Faber, 1994).

Richard Sennett, *The Uses of Disorder: Personal Identity & City Life* (London: Faber and Faber, 1996).

Carole Shammas, 'The Domestic Environment in Early Modern England and America', *Journal of Social History*, 14 (1980), 1–24.

C. Shammas, 'Food Expenditure and Well-being in Early Modern England', *Journal of Economic History*, 43 (1983), 89–100.

C. Shammas, 'The Eighteenth-Century English Diet and Economic Change', *Explorations in Economic History*, 21 (1984), 254–69.

Carole Shammas, *The Pre-Industrial Consumer in England and America* (Oxford: Clarendon Press, 1990).

Steven Shapin, *A Social History of Truth: Civility and Science in Seventeenth-Century England* (Chicago: University of Chicago Press, 1994).

Steven Shapin, *The Scientific Revolution* (Chicago: University of Chicago Press, 1996).

Steven Shapin and Simon Schaffer, *Leviathan and the Air-Pump: Hobbes, Boyle, and the Experimental Life* (Guildford: Princeton University Press, 1985).

Barbara J. Shapiro, *Probability and Certainty in Seventeenth-Century England: A Study of the Relationships between Natural Science, Religion, History, Law, and Literature* (Guildford: Princeton University Press, 1983).

Barbara Shapiro and Robert G. Frank Jr., *English Scientific Virtuosi in the 16th and 17th Centuries* (Los Angeles: University of California Press, 1979).

Susan C. Shapiro, 'A Seventeenth-Century Hermaphrodite', *Seventeenth-Century News*, 45 (1987).

Buchanan Sharp, *In Contempt of All Authority: Rural Artisans and Riot in the West of England, 1586–1660* (London: University of California Press, 1980).

J. A. Sharpe, *Defamation and Sexual Slander in Early Modern England: The Church Courts at York* (York: University of York, Borthwick Institute of Historical Research, 1980).

J. A. Sharpe, 'Domestic Homicide in Early Modern England', *Historical Journal*, 24 (1981), 29–48.

J. A. Sharpe, *Crime in Seventeenth-Century England: A County Study* (Cambridge: Cambridge University Press, 1983).

J. A. Sharpe, *Crime in Early Modern England 1550–1750* (London: Longman, 1984).

J. A. Sharpe, 'Last Dying Speeches: Religion, Ideology and Public Execution in Seventeenth-Century England', *Past and Present*, 107 (1985), 144–67.

J. A. Sharpe, 'Plebeian Marriage in Stuart England', *Transactions of the Royal Historical Society*, 36 (1986), 69–90.

J. A. Sharpe, *Early Modern England: A Social History 1550–1760* (London: Edward Arnold, 1987).

J. A. Sharpe, *Judicial Punishment in England* (London: Faber, 1990).

James Sharpe, 'History from Below', in Peter Burke (ed.), *New Perspectives on Historical Writing* (Cambridge: Polity Press, 1991), 24–41.

James Sharpe, *Instruments of Darkness: Witchcraft in England 1550–1750* (London: Hamish Hamilton, 1996).

Kevin Sharpe and Steven N. Zwicker (eds.), *Politics of Discourse: The Literature and History of Seventeenth-Century England* (Berkeley: University of California Press, 1987).

W. Sheils (ed.), *The Church and Healing* (Oxford: Basil Blackwell, 1982).

Richard Sher, *Church and University in the Scottish Enlightenment: The Moderate Literati of Edinburgh* (Princeton: Princeton University Press, 1985; Edinburgh: Edinburgh University Press, 1990).

Richard Sher and Jeffrey Smitten, *Scotland and America in the Age of the Enlightenment* (Edinburgh: Edinburgh University Press, 1990).

William H. Sherman, *John Dee: The Politics of Reading and Writing in the English Renaissance* (Amherst: University of Massachusetts Press, 1995).

Kathryn Shevelow, *Women and Print Culture: The Construction of Femininity in the Early Periodical* (London: Routledge, 1989).

Robert B. Shoemaker, *Prosecution and Punishment: Petty Crime and the Law in London and Rural Middlesex, c.1660–1725* (Cambridge: Cambridge University Press, 1991).

Robert B. Shoemaker, *Gender in English Society 1650–1850: The Emergence of Separate Spheres?* (London: Longman, 1998).

Jack Simmons and Gordon Biddle (eds.), *The Oxford Companion to British Railway History* (Oxford: Oxford University Press, 1997).

David Sinclair, *Two Georges: The Making of the Modern Monarchy* (London: Hodder and Stoughton, 1988).

Rob Sindall, *Street Violence in the Nineteenth Century* (Leicester: Leicester University Press, 1990).

Alan Sinfield, *Literature in Protestant England, 1560–1660* (Totowa, NJ: Barnes and Noble, 1983).

Andrew S. Skinner, *A System of Social Science: Papers Relating to Adam Smith* (Oxford: Oxford University Press, 1979).

Vieda Skultans, *English Madness: Ideas on Insanity 1580–1890* (London: Routledge and Kegan Paul, 1979).

Paul Slack, 'Vagrants and Vagrancy in England 1598–1664', *Economic History Review*, 27 (1974), 369–70.

Paul Slack (ed.), *Rebellion, Popular Protest and Social Change in Early Modern England* (Cambridge: Cambridge University Press, 1984).

Paul Slack, *The Impact of Plague in Tudor and Stuart England* (London: Routledge and Kegan Paul, 1985).

Paul Slack, 'Responses to Plague in Early Modern Europe: The Implications of Public Health', *Social Research*, 55 (1988), 433–53.

Paul Slack, *The English Poor Law, 1531–1782* (Cambridge: Cambridge University Press, 1995).

Miriam Slater, *Family Life in the Seventeenth Century: The Verneys of Claydon House* (London: Routledge and Kegan Paul, 1984).

A. W. Sloan, *English Medicine in the Seventeenth Century* (Durham: Durham Academic Press, 1996).

John Small, *The Origins of Middle-Class Culture: Halifax, Yorkshire, 1660–1780* (Ithaca, NY: Cornell University Press, 1994).

Sam Smiles, *The Image of Antiquity: Ancient*

Britain and the Romantic Imagination (New Haven: Yale University Press, 1994).

B. Smith, *European Vision and the South Pacific, 1768–1850: A Study in the History of Art and Ideas* (Oxford: Clarendon Press, 1960).

Bruce R. Smith, *Homosexual Desire in Shakespeare's England: A Cultural Poetics* (Chicago: University of Chicago Press, 1991).

David Smith (ed.), *A People and a Proletariat: Essays in the History of Wales, 1780–1980* (London: Pluto Press, in association with Llafur, the Society for the Study of Welsh Labour History, 1980).

David L. Smith, *A History of the Modern British Isles 1603–1707: The Double Crown* (Oxford: Blackwell, 1998).

Nigel Smith (ed.), *A Collection of Ranter Writings from the 17th Century* (London: Junction Books, 1983).

Nigel Smith, *Perfection Proclaimed: Language and Literature in English Radical Religion, 1640–1660* (Oxford: Clarendon Press, 1989).

Nigel Smith, *Literature and Revolution in England, 1640–1660* (New Haven: Yale University Press, 1994).

Robert A. Smith, *A Social History of the Bicycle: Its Early Life and Times in America* (New York: American Heritage, 1972).

Robert A. Smith, *Late Georgian and Regency England, 1760–1837* (Cambridge: Cambridge University Press, for the Conference on British Studies, 1984).

Robert A. Smith (ed.), *The House of Lords: A Thousand Years of British Tradition* (London: Smith's Peerage, 1994).

Roger Smith, *Trial by Medicine: Insanity and Responsibility in Victorian Trials* (Edinburgh: Edinburgh University Press, 1981).

Ruth Smith, *Handel's Oratorios and Eighteenth-Century Thought* (Cambridge: Cambridge University Press, 1995).

T. C. Smout, *A History of the Scottish People, 1560–1830* (London: Collins, 1969; 1970).

T. C. Smout, *Nature Contested: Environmental History in Scotland and Northern England since*

1600 (Edinburgh: Edinburgh University Press, 2000).

Hannah Snell, *The Secret Life of a Female Marine 1723–1792* (London: Ship Street Press, 1997).

Keith D. M. Snell, *Annals of the Labouring Poor: Social Change and Agrarian England, 1660–1900* (Cambridge: Cambridge University Press, 1985).

David Snodin, *A Mighty Ferment: Britain in the Age of Revolution, 1750–1850* (The Mirror of Britain Series, gen. ed. Kevin Crossley-Holland; London: André Deutsch, 1978).

Graeme Snooks (ed.), *Was the Industrial Revolution Necessary?* (London: Routledge, 1994).

David H. Solkin, *Painting for Money: The Visual Arts and the Public Sphere in Eighteenth-Century England* (New Haven: Yale University Press, 1983).

Leo F. Solt, *Church and State in Early Modern England, 1509–1640* (Oxford: Oxford University Press, 1990).

C. John Somerville, *The Discovery of Childhood in Puritan England* (Athens: University of Georgia Press, 1992).

C. John Somerville, *The Secularization of Early Modern England: From Religious Culture to Religious Faith* (Oxford: Oxford University Press, 1992).

C. John Sommerville, 'The Secularization Puzzle', *History Today*, 44 (1994), 14–19.

C. John Sommerville, *The News Revolution in England* (Oxford: Clarendon Press, 1997).

Johann P. Sommerville, *Thomas Hobbes: Political Ideas in Historical Context* (Basingstoke: Macmillan, 1992).

Margaret R. Sommerville, *Sex and Subjection: Attitudes to Women in Early Modern Society* (London: Edward Arnold, 1995).

Thomas Somerville, *My Own Life and Times 1741–1814* (Bristol: Thoemmes Press, 1995).

Tom Sorell, *Hobbes* (London: Routledge and Kegan Paul, 1986).

David Spadafora, *The Idea of Progress in*

Eighteenth-Century Britain (New Haven: Yale University Press, 1990).

W. A. Speck, *The Divided Society: Parties and Politics in England, 1694–1716* (London: Edward Arnold, 1967).

W. A. Speck, *Tory and Whig: The Struggle in the Constituencies 1701–1715* (London: Macmillan, 1970).

W. A. Speck, *Stability and Strife: England, 1714–1760* (London: Edward Arnold, 1977).

W. A. Speck, *Society and Literature in England, 1700–1760* (Dublin: Gill and Macmillan, 1983).

W. A. Speck, 'English Politics and Society in the Eighteenth Century', *Historian*, 12 (1986), 13–16.

W. A. Speck, *Reluctant Revolutionaries: Englishmen and the Revolution of 1688* (Oxford: Oxford University Press, 1988).

W. A. Speck, *A Concise History of Britain, 1707–1975* (Cambridge: Cambridge University Press, 1993).

W. A. Speck, *The Birth of Britain: A New Nation 1700–1710* (Oxford: Blackwell, 1994).

W. M. Spellman, *John Locke* (London: Macmillan, 1997).

Peter Spence, *The Birth of Romantic Radicalism: War, Popular Politics and English Radical Reformation, 1800–1815* (London: Scolar Press, 1996).

Jane Spencer, *The Rise of the Woman Novelist: from Aphra Behn to Jane Austen* (Oxford: Blackwell, 1986).

Dale Spender, *Women of Ideas and What Men Have Done to Them: From Aphra Behn to Adrienne Rich* (London: Routledge and Kegan Paul, 1982).

Dale Spender (ed.), *Feminist Theorists: Three Centuries of Women's Intellectual Traditions* (London: Women's Press, 1983).

Dale Spender, *Mothers of the Novel: 100 Good Women Writers before Jane Austen* (London: Pandora, 1986).

Pieter Spierenburg, *The Spectacle of Suffering: Executions and the Evolution of Repression. From a Preindustrial Metropolis to the European*

Experience (Cambridge: Cambridge University Press, 1984).

Pieter Spierenburg, *The Broken Spell: A Cultural and Anthropological History of Preindustrial Europe* (London: Macmillan; New Brunswick, NJ: Rutgers University Press, 1991).

Pieter Spierenburg, *The Prison Experience: Disciplinary Institutions and their Inmates in Early Modern Europe* (New Brunswick, NJ: Rutgers University Press, 1991).

Edward M. Spiers, *The Army and Society 1815–1914* (London: Longman, 1980).

Edward M. Spiers, *Haldane: An Army Reformer* (Edinburgh: Edinburgh University Press, 1980).

Lucio Sponza, *Italian Immigrants in Nineteenth-Century Britain: Realities and Images* (Leicester: Leicester University Press, 1988).

Margaret Spufford, *Contrasting Communities: English Villagers in the Sixteenth and Seventeenth Centuries* (London: Cambridge University Press, 1974).

Margaret Spufford, 'First Steps in Literacy: The Reading and Writing Experiences of the Humblest Seventeenth-Century Spiritual Autobiographers', *Social History*, 4 (1979), 407–37.

Margaret Spufford, *Small Books and Pleasant Histories: Popular Fiction and its Readership in Seventeenth-Century England* (Athens: University of Georgia Press, 1981; London: Methuen, 1981).

Margaret Spufford, *The Great Reclothing of Rural England* (London: Hambledon Press, 1984).

M. Spufford, 'The Pedlar, the Historian and the Folklorist: 17th Century', *Folklore*, 105 (1994), 13–24.

Margaret Spufford (ed.), *The World of Rural Dissenters, 1520–1725* (Cambridge: Cambridge University Press, 1995).

Margaret Spufford, *Figures in the Landscape: Rural Society in England, 1500–1700* (Aldershot: Ashgate, 2000).

Frank Staff, *The Penny Post 1680–1918* (Cambridge: Lutterworth Press, 1992).

William Stafford, *Socialism, Radicalism, and Nostalgia: Social Criticism in Britain 1775–1830* (Cambridge: Cambridge University Press, 1987).

Daniel Statt, *Foreigners and Englishmen: The Controversy over Immigration and Population, 1660–1760* (Newark: University of Delaware Press, 1995).

Susan Staves, *'Our Fortunes are in Your Possession': Married Women's Separate Property 1660–1830* (Cambridge, Mass.: Harvard University Press, 1990).

Carolyn Steedman, *Strange Dislocations: Childhood and the Idea of Human Interiority, 1780–1930* (London: Virago, 1995).

John Steegman, *The Rule of Taste from George I to George IV* (London: Macmillan, 1936).

David A. Steel, *A Lincolnshire Village: The Parish of Corby Glen in its Historical Context* (London: Longman, 1979).

Don Steel and Lawrence Taylor (eds.), *Family History in Focus* (Cambridge: Lutterworth Press, 1984).

Ian K. Steele, *The English Atlantic, 1675–1740: An Exploration of Communication and Community* (New York: Oxford University Press, 1986).

Peter Stein, *Legal Evolution: The Story of an Idea* (Cambridge: Cambridge University Press, 1980).

Leslie Stephen, *Selected Writings in British Intellectual History*, ed. Noel Annan (London: University of Chicago Press, 1979).

John Stevenson, *Popular Disturbances in England, 1700–1870* (London: Longman, 1979).

A. T. Q. Stewart, *The Narrow Ground: Aspects of Ulster, 1609–1969* (London: Faber and Faber, 1977).

Garrett Stewart, *Death Sentences: Styles of Dying in British Fiction* (Cambridge, Mass.: Harvard University Press, 1984).

Garrett Stewart, *Dear Reader: The Conscripted Audience in Nineteenth-Century British Fiction* (Baltimore: Johns Hopkins University Press, 1996).

Larry Stewart, *The Rise of Public Science: Rhetoric, Technology, and Natural Philosophy in Newtonian Britain, 1660–1750* (Cambridge: Cambridge University Press, 1992).

Larry Stewart, *Industry and Enterprise in Britain: From the Scientific to the Industrial Revolution 1640–1790* (London: Athlone Press, 1995).

Robert Stewart, *Henry Brougham, 1778–1868: His Public Career* (London: Bodley Head, 1985).

E. Stokes, *The English Utilitarians and India* (Oxford: Clarendon Press, 1959).

Lawrence Stone, 'The Educational Revolution in England, 1560–1640', *Past and Present*, 28 (1964), 41–80.

Lawrence Stone, *The Crisis of the Aristocracy 1558–1641* (London: Oxford University Press, 1965).

Lawrence Stone, 'Social Mobility in England, 1500–1700', *Past and Present*, 33 (1966), 16–73.

Lawrence Stone, 'Literacy and Education in England 1640–1900', *Past and Present*, 42 (1969), 67–139.

Lawrence Stone, *Family and Fortune: Studies in Aristocratic Finance in the Sixteenth and Seventeenth Centuries* (Oxford: Clarendon Press, 1973).

Lawrence Stone (ed.), *The University in Society*, 2 vols. (Princeton: Princeton University Press, 1975).

Lawrence Stone, *The Family, Sex and Marriage in England, 1500–1800* (London: Weidenfeld and Nicolson, 1977).

Lawrence Stone, 'The Residential Development of the West End of London in the Seventeenth Century', in Barbara C. Malament (ed.), *After the Reformation: Essays in Honor of J. H. Hexter* (Manchester: Manchester University Press, 1980; orig. pub. Philadelphia: University of Philadelphia Press, 1979), 167–212.

Lawrence Stone, 'The New Eighteenth

Century', *New York Review of Books*, 31 (1984), 42–8.

Lawrence Stone, *The Past and Present Revisited*, 2nd edn. (London: Routledge, 1987).

Lawrence Stone, *The Road to Divorce, England 1530–1987* (Oxford: Oxford University Press, 1990).

Lawrence Stone, 'History and Post-modernism', *Past and Present*, 131 (1991), 217–18; 133 (1991), 204–13.

Lawrence Stone, *Uncertain Unions: Marriage in England 1660–1753* (Oxford: Oxford University Press, 1992).

Lawrence Stone, *Broken Lives: Separation and Divorce in England 1660–1857* (Oxford: Oxford University Press, 1993).

Lawrence Stone (ed.), *An Imperial State at War: Britain from 1689 to 1815* (London and New York: Routledge, 1994).

Lawrence Stone and Jeanne C. Fawtier Stone, *An Open Elite? England 1540–1880* (Oxford: Clarendon Press, 1984).

Robert D. Storch (ed.), *Popular Culture and Custom in Nineteenth-Century England* (London: Croom Helm, 1982).

Kristina Straub, *Divided Fictions: Fanny Burney and Feminine Strategy* (Lexington: University of Kentucky Press, 1987).

Roland N. Stromberg, *Religious Liberalism in Eighteenth-Century England* (London: Oxford University Press, 1954).

Roy C. Strong, *Splendour at Court: Renaissance Spectacle and Illusion* (London: Weidenfeld and Nicolson, 1973).

Roy Strong, *The Artist and the Garden* (New Haven: Yale University Press, 2000).

D. Stuart (ed.), *A Social History of Yoxall in the Sixteenth and Seventeenth Centuries* (Keele: Department of Adult Education, Keele University, 1990).

Keith Sturgess, *Jacobean Private Theatre* (London: Routledge and Kegan Paul, 1987).

Geoffrey Summerfield, *Fantasy and Reason: Children's Literature in the Eighteenth Century* (London: Methuen, 1984).

Ronald M. Sunter, *Patronage and Politics in Scotland, 1707–1832* (Edinburgh: John Donald, 1986).

Anthony Sutcliffe (ed.), *British Town Planning: The Formative Years* (Leicester: Leicester University Press; New York: St Martin's Press, 1981).

Anthony Sutcliffe, *Towards the Planned City: Germany, Britain, the United States and France, 1780–1914* (New York: St Martin's Press; Oxford: Blackwell, 1981).

James Sutherland, *The Restoration Newspaper and its Development* (Cambridge: Cambridge University Press, 1986).

Lucy Sutherland, 'Sampson Gideon, 18th c. Jewish Financier', *Transactions of the Jewish Historical Society*, 17 (1951–2), 79–90.

Lucy Sutherland, *The East India Company in Eighteenth-Century Politics* (Oxford: Clarendon Press, 1952).

Lucy Sutherland, 'The City of London in Eighteenth-Century Politics', in A. J. P. Taylor and Richard Pares (eds.), *Essays Presented to Sir Lewis Namier* (London: Macmillan, 1956), 49–74.

Lucy Sutherland, *The City of London and the Opposition to Government 1768–74* (Creighton Lecture in History, 1958; London: Athlone Press, 1959).

Lucy Sutherland, 'The City of London and the Devonshire–Pitt Administration 1756–7', *Proceedings of the Royal Academy*, 46 (1960), 147–93.

Lucy Sutherland, 'Edmund Burke and the Relations between Members of Parliament and their Constituents', *Studies in Burke and his Time*, 10 (1968), 1005–21.

Lucy Sutherland, *Politics and Finance in the Eighteenth Century*, ed. Aubrey Newman (London: Hambledon Press, 1984).

Lucy Sutherland and L. G. Mitchell (eds.), *The History of the University of Oxford*, vol. 5, *The Eighteenth Century* (Oxford: Clarendon Press, 1986).

N. Sykes, *Edmund Gibson, Bishop of London, 1669–1748: A Study in Politics and Religion in the Eighteenth Century* (London: Oxford University Press, 1926).

N. Sykes, *Church and State in England in the Eighteenth Century* (Cambridge: Cambridge University Press, 1934).

Daniel Szechi, *Jacobitism and Tory Politics, 1710–1714* (Edinburgh: John Donald, 1984).

Daniel Szechi, *The Jacobites: Britain and Europe 1688–1788* (Manchester: Manchester University Press, 1994).

Naomi Tadmor, *Family and Friends in Eighteenth-Century England: Household, Kinship and Patronage* (Cambridge: Cambridge University Press, 2001).

Frank Tallett and Nicholas Atkin (eds.), *Catholicism in Britian and France since 1789* (London: Hambledon Press, 1996).

Nathan Tarcov, *Locke's Education for Liberty* (Chicago: University of Chicago Press, 1984).

Richard Tawney, *Religion and the Rise of Capitalism* (New York: Harcourt, Brace and Co., 1926).

A. J. Taylor (ed.), *The Standard of Living in Britain in the Industrial Revolution* (London: Methuen, 1975).

Arthur Taylor, *Laissez-Faire and State Intervention in Nineteenth-Century Britain* (London: Macmillan, 1972).

David Taylor, *The New Police in Nineteenth-Century England: Crime, Conflict and Control* (Manchester: Manchester University Press, 1997).

Geoffrey Taylor, *The Problem of Poverty, 1660–1834* (Harlow: Longmans, 1969).

George Taylor, *Players and Performances in the Victorian Theatre* (Manchester: Manchester University Press, 1989).

Gordon Rattray Taylor, *The Angel Makers: A Study in the Psychological Origins of Historical Change 1750–1850* (London: Secker and Warburg, 1958).

Melanie Tebbutt, *Making Ends Meet: Pawnbroking and Working-Class Credit* (London: Methuen, 1984).

Michael S. Teitelbaum, *The British Fertility Decline: Demographic Transition in the Crucible of the Industrial Revolution* (Princeton: Princeton University Press, 1984).

Pat Thane (ed.), *The Origins of British Social Policy* (London: Croom Helm, 1978).

Pat Thane, *Old Age in English History: Past Experiences, Present Issues* (Oxford: Oxford University Press, 2000).

Margaret Olofson Thickstun, *Fictions of the Feminine Puritan Doctrine and the Representation of Women* (Ithaca, NY: Cornell University Press, 1988).

Joan Thirsk, *Economic Policy and Projects: The Development of a Consumer Society in Early Modern England* (Oxford: Clarendon Press, 1978).

Joan Thirsk (ed.), *The Agrarian History of England and Wales* vol. 5: *1640–1750*, part I: *Regional Farming Systems*, part II: *Agrarian Change* (London and New York: Cambridge University Press, 1984–5).

Joan Thirsk, *Agricultural Regions and Agrarian History in England, 1500–1750* (Basingstoke: Macmillan, 1987).

Joan Thirsk, *Alternative Agriculture: A History. From the Black Death to the Present Day* (Oxford: Oxford University Press, 1997).

Keith Thomas, 'The Double Standard', *Journal of the History of Ideas*, 20 (1959), 195–216.

Keith Thomas, 'Work and Leisure in Pre-industrial Society', *Past and Present*, 29 (1964), 50–66.

Keith Thomas, 'An Anthropology of Religion and Magic', *Journal of Interdisciplinary History*, 6 (1975), 91–110.

Keith Thomas, 'Age and Authority in Early Modern Britain', *Proceedings of the Royal Academy*, 62 (1976; 1977).

Keith Thomas, *Religion and the Decline of Magic: Studies in Popular Beliefs in Sixteenth and Seventeenth Century England* (London: Weidenfeld & Nicolson, 1971; Harmondsworth: Penguin, 1973; repr., Harmondsworth: Penguin, 1978;

London: Weidenfeld and Nicolson, 1981).

Keith Thomas, *Man and the Natural World: Changing Attitudes in England 1500–1800* (London: Allen Lane; Harmondsworth: Penguin, 1983).

Keith Thomas, 'Numeracy in Early Modern England', *Transactions of the Royal Historical Society*, 37 (1987), 103–32.

Peter D. G. Thomas, 'George III and the American Revolution', *History*, 70 (1985), 16–31.

Peter D. G. Thomas, *Politics in Eighteenth-Century Wales* (Cardiff: University of Wales Press, 1998).

Malcolm Thomis, *The Town Labourer and the Industrial Revolution* (London: Batsford, 1974).

Malcolm Thomis, *Responses to Industrialization* (Newton Abbot: David and Charles, 1976).

Malcolm Thomis and Peter Holt, *Threats of Revolution in Britain 1789–1848* (London: Macmillan, 1977).

Dorothy Thompson, *Outsiders: Class, Gender and Nation* (London: Verso, 1993).

E. P. Thompson (ed.), *The Railway: An Adventure in Construction* (London: British Yugoslav Association, 1948).

E. P. Thompson, *The Struggle for a Free Press* (London: People's Press Printing Society, 1952).

E. P. Thompson (ed.), *Out of Apathy* (London: Stevens and Sons, 1960).

E. P. Thompson, 'Time, Work-Discipline and Industrial Capitalism', *Past and Present*, 38 (1967), 56–97.

E. P. Thompson, *The Making of the English Working Class* (Harmondsworth: Penguin, 1968).

E. P. Thompson, 'The Moral Economy of the English Crowd in the Eighteenth Century', *Past and Present*, 50 (1971), 76–136.

E. P. Thompson, 'Anthropology and the Discipline of Historical Context', *Midland History*, 1 (1972), 41–55.

E. P. Thompson, 'Rough Music', *Annales ESC*, 27 (1972), 285–310.

E. P. Thompson, 'Patrician Society, Plebeian Culture', *Journal of Social History*, 7 (1973–4), 382–405.

E. P. Thompson, *Whigs and Hunters: The Origin of the Black Act* (London: Allen Lane, 1975).

E. P. Thompson, 'The Grid of Inheritance: A Comment', in Jack Goody, Joan Thirsk and E. P. Thompson (eds.), *Family and Inheritance: Rural Society in Western Europe, 1200–1800* (Cambridge: Cambridge University Press, 1976), 328–60.

E. P. Thompson, *Folklore, Anthropology and Social History* (Brighton: Noyce, 1979).

E. P. Thompson, 'Eighteenth Century English Society: Class Struggle without Class?', *Social History*, (1978), 133–65.

E. P. Thompson, *The Poverty of Theory and Other Essays* (London: Merlin, 1978).

E. P. Thompson, *Writing by Candlelight* (London: Merlin, 1980).

E. P. Thompson, *Società patrizia, cultura plebea: Otto saggi di antropologia storica sull' inghilterra del settecento* (2nd edn.; Torino: Einaudi, 1982).

E. P. Thompson, *Customs in Common* (London: Merlin Press, 1991).

E. P. Thompson, *Witness Against the Beast: William Blake and the Moral Law* (Cambridge: Cambridge University Press, 1993).

F. M. L. Thompson, *English Landed Society in the Nineteenth Century* (London: Routledge and Kegan Paul; Toronto: University of Toronto Press, 1963).

F. M. L. Thompson, *Hampstead: Building a Borough, 1650–1964* (London: Routledge and Kegan Paul, 1974).

F. M. L. Thompson (ed.), *The Cambridge Social History of Britain 1750–1950*. vol. 1: *Regions and Communities*; vol. 2: *People and their Environment*; vol. 3: *Social Agencies and Institutions* (Cambridge: Cambridge University Press, 1990).

F. M. L. Thompson (ed.), *Landowners,*

Capitalists and Entrepreneurs: Essays for Sir John Habakkuk (Oxford: Clarendon Press, 1994).

F. M. L. Thompson, *Gentrification and the Enterprise Culture: Britain 1780–1980* (Oxford: Oxford University Press, 2001).

Roger Thompson, *Women in Stuart England and America: A Comparative Study* (London: Routledge and Kegan Paul, 1974).

Roger Thompson, *Unfit for Modest Ears: A Study of Pornographic, Obscene and Bawdy Works Written or Published in England in the Second Half of the 17th Century* (London: Macmillan, 1979).

Norman J. W. Thrower (ed.), *The Compleat Plattmaker: Essays on Chart, Map and Globe Making in England in the Seventeenth and Eighteenth Centuries* (London: University of California Press, 1978).

Kathryn Tidrick, *Empire and the English Character* (London: J. B. Tauris, 1992).

Stella Tillyard, *Aristocrats: Caroline, Emily, Louisa and Sarah Lennox* (London: Chatto and Windus, 1994).

Stella Tillyard, *Citizen Lord: Edward Fitzgerald 1763–1798* (London: Chatto and Windus, 1997).

J. J. Tobias, *Crime and Police in England 1700–1900* (Dublin: Gill and Macmillan, 1979).

Beth Fowkes Tobin, *Superintending the Poor: Charitable Ladies and Paternal Landlords in British Fiction, 1770–1860* (New Haven: Yale University Press, 1993).

Dennis Todd, *Imagining Monsters: Miscreations of the Self in Eighteenth-Century England* (Chicago: University of Chicago Press, 1995).

Janet Todd, *Women's Friendship in Literature* (New York: Columbia University Press, 1980).

Janet Todd, *Men by Women* (New York: Holmes and Meier, 1981).

Janet Todd, *Sensibility: An Introduction* (London: Methuen, 1986).

Janet Todd, *The Sign of Angellica: Women,*

Writing and Fiction, 1660–1800 (London: Virago, 1989).

Janet Todd (ed.), *A Wollstonecraft Anthology* (Cambridge: Polity Press, 1989).

Janet Todd and Marilyn Butler (eds.), *The Works of Mary Wollstonecraft*, 7 vols. (London: Pickering and Chatto, 1989).

Claire Tomalin, *The Life and Death of Mary Wollstonecraft* (London: Weidenfeld and Nicolson, 1974).

James D. Tracy, *Europe's Reformations 1450–1650* (Totowa, NJ: Rowman and Littlefield, 2000).

N. L. Tranter, *Population and Society 1750–1940* (London: Longman, 1985).

Neil Tranter, *Sport, Economy and Society in Britain 1750–1914* (Cambridge: Cambridge University Press, 1998).

John F. Travis, *The Rise of the Devon Seaside Resorts, 1750–1900* (Exeter: Exeter University Press, 1993).

Geoffrey Trease, *Portrait of a Cavalier: William Cavendish, First Duke of Newcastle* (London: Macmillan, 1979).

G. R. R. Treasure, *The Making of Modern Europe 1648–1780* (London and New York: Methuen, 1985).

H. R. Trevor-Roper, *Catholics, Anglicans and Puritans: Seventeenth Century Essays* (London: Secker and Warburg, 1987).

Barrie Trinder, *The Making of the Industrial Landscape* (London: Dent, 1982).

Randolph Trumbach, *The Rise of the Egalitarian Family: Aristocratic Kinship and Domestic Relations in Eighteenth-Century England* (New York: Academic Press, 1978).

Randolph Trumbach, 'Sodomitical Assaults, Gender Identity and Individual Development in Eighteenth Century London', in K. Gerard and G. Hekma (eds.), *The Pursuit of Sodomy: Male Homosexuality in Renaissance and Enlightenment Europe* (New York: Harington Park Press, 1987), 407–29.

Randolph Trumbach, *Sex and the Gender Revolution*, vol. 1: *Heterosexuality and the Third*

Gender in Enlightenment London (Chicago: Chicago University Press, 1998).

Richard Tuck, *Natural Rights Theories: Their Origin and Development* (Cambridge: Cambridge University Press, 1979).

James Tully, *A Discourse on Property: John Locke and his Adversaries* (Cambridge: Cambridge University Press, 1980).

David Turley, *The Culture of English Anti-slavery, 1780–1860* (London: Routledge, 1991).

James Grantham Turner, *One Flesh: Paradisal Marriage and Sexual Relations in the Age of Milton* (Oxford: Clarendon Press, 1987).

J. Turner, *Reckoning with the Beast: Animals, Pain, and Humanity in the Victorian Mind* (Baltimore: Johns Hopkins University Press, 1980).

Michael Turner, *Enclosures in Britain 1750–1830* (London: Macmillan, 1984).

Jon Turney, *Frankenstein's Footsteps* (New Haven: Yale University Press, 1998).

John Twigg, *The University of Cambridge and the English Revolution, 1625–1688* (Woodbridge: Boydell/Cambridge University Library, 1990).

Nicholas Tyacke, *Anti-Calvinists: The Rise of English Arminianism, c.1590–1640s* (Oxford: Oxford University Press, 1987).

Jenny Uglow, *William Hogarth: A Life and a World* (London: Faber and Faber, 1997).

David Underdown, *Revel, Riot and Rebellion: Popular Politics and Culture in England 1603–1660* (Oxford: Oxford University Press, 1985).

David Underdown, *Fire from Heaven: The Life of an English Town in the Seventeenth Century* (London: HarperCollins, 1992).

David Underdown, *A Freeborn People: Politics and the Nation in Seventeenth-Century England* (Oxford: Clarendon Press, 1996).

Albion M. Urdank, *Religion and Society in a Cotswold Vale: Nailsworth, Gloucestershire, 1780–1865* (Berkeley: University of California Press, 1990).

John Ure, *Trespassers on the Amazon* (London: Constable, 1986).

Deborah M. Valenze, *Prophetic Sons and Daughters: Female Preaching and Popular Religion in Industrial England* (Princeton: Princeton University Press, 1985).

Frederick Valletta, *Witchcraft, Magic and Superstition in England, 1640–70* (Aldershot: Ashgate, 2000).

W. Vamplew, *The Turf: A Social and Economic History of Horse Racing* (London: Allen Lane, 1976).

John A. Vance, *Samuel Johnson and the Sense of History* (Athens: University of Georgia Press, 1984).

W. Van Lennep *et al.* (eds.), *Index to the London Stage, 1660–1800* (Carbondale: Southern Illinois University Press, 1979).

V. Van Muyden (trans. and ed.), *A Foreign View of England in 1725–1729: The Letters of M. César de Saussure to his Family* (London: Caliban: 1995).

Linda Van Norden, *The Black Feet of the Peacock: The Color-Concept 'Black' from the Greeks through the Renaissance*, ed. John Pollock (Lanham, Md.: University Press of America, 1985).

Ann Jessie Van Sant, *Eighteenth-Century Sensibility and the Novel: The Senses in Social Context* (Cambridge: Cambridge University Press, 1993).

Karen Iversen Vaughn, *John Locke: Economist and Social Scientist* (London: Athlone Press, 1980).

Amanda Vickery, 'Golden Age to Separate Spheres?: A Review of the Categories and Chronology of English Women's History', *Historical Journal*, 36/2 (1993).

Amanda Vickery, *The Gentleman's Daughter: Women's Lives in Georgian England* (New Haven: Yale University Press, 1998).

Andrew Vincent and Raymond Plant, *Philosophy, Politics and Citizenship: The Life and Thought of the British Idealists* (Oxford: Blackwell, 1984).

David Vincent (ed.), *Testaments of Radicalism* (London: Europa Publications, 1977).

David Vincent, *Bread, Knowledge and Freedom:*

A Study of Nineteenth-Century Working Class Autobiography (London: Routledge, 1982).

D. Vincent, *Literacy and Popular Culture: England 1750–1914* (Cambridge: Cambridge University Press, 1989).

J. Viner, *The Role of Providence in the Social Order: An Essay in Intellectual History* (Philadelphia: American Philosophical Society, 1972).

Peter Virgin, *The Church in an Age of Negligence: Ecclesiastical Structure and Problems of Church Reform, 1700–1840* (Cambridge: Peter Clarke and Co., 1900).

Rozina Visram, *Ayahs, Lascars and Princes: The Story of Indians in Britain 1700–1947* (London: Pluto Press, 1986).

Ivan Waddington, *The Medical Profession in the Industrial Revolution* (Dublin: Gill and Macmillan, 1984).

Peter Wagner, *Eros Revived: Erotica in the Age of Enlightenment* (London: Secker and Warburg, 1986).

Peter Wagner, *Reading Iconotexts: From Swift to the French Revolution* (London: Reaktion Books, 1995).

Dror Wahrman, *Imagining the Middle Class: The Political Representation of Class in Britain, c. 1780–1840* (Cambridge: Cambridge University Press, 1995).

D. P. Walker, *Spiritual and Demonic Magic from Ficino to Campanella* (London: Warburg Institute, 1958).

D. P. Walker, *The Decline of Hell: Seventeenth-Century Discussions of Eternal Torment* (London: Routledge and Kegan Paul, 1964).

D. P. Walker, *Unclean Spirits* (London: Scolar Press, 1980).

Maureen Waller, *1700: Scenes from London Life* (London: Hodder, 2000).

Immanuel Maurice Wallerstein, *The Modern World-System: Capitalist Agriculture and the Origins of the European World-Economy in the Sixteenth Century* (New York: Academic Press, 1974).

John Walsh, Colin Haydon and Stephen Taylor (eds.), *The Church of England*

c.1689–c.1833: From Toleration to Tractarianism (Cambridge: Cambridge University Press, 1993).

Alexandra Walsham, *Church Papists: Catholicism, Conformity and Confessional Polemic in Early Modern England* (Woodbridge: Boydell Press/Royal Historical Society, 1993).

John K. Walton, 'The Social Development of Blackpool 1788–1914' (Ph.D. thesis, Lancaster University, 1974).

John K. Walton, *The English Seaside Resort: A Social History 1750–1914* (Leicester: Leicester University Press; New York: St Martin's Press, 1983).

John K. Walton, *Lancashire: A Social History, 1558–1939* (Manchester: Manchester University Press, 1988).

John K. Walton and James Walvin (eds.), *Leisure in Britain, 1780–1939* (Manchester: Manchester University Press, 1983).

J. Walvin, *The Black Presence: A Documentary History of the Negro in Britain* (London: Orbach and Chambers, 1971; New York: Schocken Books, 1972).

James Walvin, *Black and White: The Negro and English Society, 1555–1945* (London: Allen Lane, 1973).

James Walvin, *Slavery and British Society, 1776–1848* (London: Macmillan; Baton Rouge: Louisiana State University Press, 1982).

James Walvin, *Slavery and the Slave Trade: A Short Illustrated History* (London: Macmillan, 1983).

James Walvin, *English Urban Life, 1776–1851* (London: Hutchinson, 1984).

James Walvin, *Passage to Britain: Immigration in History and Politics* (Harmondsworth: Penguin, in association with Belitha Press, 1984).

James Walvin, *England, Slaves and Freedom, 1776–1838* (London: Macmillan, 1987).

James Walvin, *Black Ivory: A History of British Slavery* (London: HarperCollins, 1992).

James Walvin, *Slaves and Slavery: The British*

Colonial Experience (Manchester: Manchester University Press, 1992).

James Walvin, *Questioning Slavery* (London: Routledge, 1996).

James Walvin, *The Quakers: Money and Morals* (London: John Murray, 1997).

James Walvin, *The Life and Times of Olaudah Equiano: An African's Life, 1745–1797* (London: Cassell Academic, 1998).

James Walvin, M. Craton and D. Wright (eds.), *Slavery, Abolition and Emancipation: Black Slaves and the British Empire* (London: Longman, 1976).

James Walvin and Paul Edwards, *Black Personalities in the Era of Slavery* (London: Macmillan; Baton Rouge: Louisiana State University Press, 1983).

James Walvin and D. Eltis (eds.), *Abolition of the Atlantic Slave Trade* (Madison: University of Wisconsin Press, 1981).

James Walvin and C. Emsley (eds.), *Artisans, Peasants and Proletarians: Essays Presented to Gwyn A. Williams* (London: Croom Helm, 1985).

James Walvin and E. Royle, *English Radicals and Reformers, 1776–1848* (Brighton: Harvester Press; Lexington: University of Kentucky Press, 1982).

J. T. Ward, *The Factory System*, 2 vols. (Newton Abbot: David and Charles, 1970).

J. T. Ward and W. Hamish Fraser (eds.), *Workers and Employers: Documents on Trade Unions and Industrial Relations in Britian Since the Eighteenth Century* (London: Macmillan, 1980).

W. Peter Ward, *Birth Weight and Economic Growth: Women's Living Standards in the Industrializing West* (Chicago: University of Chicago Press, 1993).

W. R. Ward, *Religion and Society in England, 1790–1850* (London: Batsford, 1972).

W. R. Ward, *The Protestant Evangelical Awakening* (Cambridge: Cambridge University Press, 1992).

W. R. Ward, *Faith and Faction* (London: Epworth Press, 1993).

John Wardroper, *Lovers, Rakes and Rogues: Amatory, Merry and Bawdy Verse from 1580 to 1830* (London: Shelfmark Books, 1995).

M. Warner, *Alone of All her Sex: The Myth and the Cult of the Virgin Mary* (London: Weidenfeld and Nicolson; New York: Alfred A. Knopf, Inc., 1976; Pan Books, 1985).

Marina Warner, *From the Beast to the Blonde: On Fairy Tales and their Tellers* (London: Chatto and Windus, 1994).

Marina Warner, *No Go the Bogeyman: Scaring, Lulling and Making Mock* (London: Chatto and Windus, 1998).

A. M. C. Waterman, *Revolution, Economics and Religion: Christian Political Economy, 1793–1833* (Cambridge: Cambridge University Press, 1991).

Merlin Waterson, *The Servants' Hall: A Domestic History of Erddig* (London: Routledge and Kegan Paul, 1980).

Ian Watson, *Song and Democratic Culture in Britain: An Approach to Popular Culture in Social Movements* (London: Croom Helm, 1983).

J. P. N. Watson, *Captain-General and Rebel Chief: The Life of James, Duke of Monmouth* (London: George Allen and Unwin, 1979).

Michael R. Watts, *The Dissenters*, vol. 1: *From the Reformation to the French Revolution* (Oxford: Clarendon Press, 1978).

Michael R. Watts, *The Dissenters*, vol. 2: *The Expansion of Evangelical Nonconformity* (Oxford: Clarendon Press, 1995).

Sheldon J. Watts, *A Social History of Western Europe 1450–1720: Tensions and Solidarities among Rural People* (London: Hutchinson, 1984).

Andrew Wear (ed.), *Medicine in Society: Historical Essays* (Cambridge: Cambridge University Press, 1992).

L. Weatherill, *The Pottery Trade and North Staffordshire, 1660–1760* (Manchester: Manchester University Press, 1971).

Lorna Weatherill, 'Consumer Behaviour and Social Status in England', *Continuity and Change*, 2 (1986), 191–216.

Lorna Weatherill, 'A Possession of One's Own: Women and Consumer Behaviour in England, 1660–1740', *Journal of British Studies*, 25 (1986), 131–56.

Lorna Weatherill, *Consumer Behaviour and Material Culture, 1660–1760* (London: Routledge, 1988).

Lorna Weatherill (ed.), *The Account Book of Richard Latham* (Oxford: Oxford University Press, 1990).

R. K. Webb, *Modern England: From the Eighteenth Century to the Present* (London: Routledge, 1969, 1980).

Stephen Saunders Webb, *The Governors-General: The English Army and the Definition of the Empire, 1569–1681* (Chapel Hill: University of North Carolina Press for the Institute of Early American History and Culture, Williamsburg, Va., 1979).

Harold W. Weber, *Paper Bullets: Print and Kingship under Charles II* (Lexington: University Press of Kentucky, 1996).

Max Weber, *The Protestant Ethic and the Spirit of Capitalism* (London: Allen and Unwin, 1930).

William Weber, *The Rise of Musical Classics in Eighteenth-Century England: A Study in Canon, Ritual, and Ideology* (New York: Oxford University Press, 1992).

Barbara Wedgwood and Hensleigh Wedgwood, *The Wedgwood Circle 1730–1897: Four Generations of a Family and their Friends* (London: Studio Vista, 1980).

Jeffrey Weeks, *Sex, Politics and Society: The Regulation of Sexuality Since 1800* (London: Longman, 1981).

R. William Weisberger, *Speculative Freemasonry and the Enlightenment: A Study of the Craft in London, Paris, Prague and Vienna* (Boulder, Colo.: East European Monographs, 1993).

Michael R. Weisser, *Crime and Punishment in Early Modern Europe* (Hassocks: Harvester Press, 1979).

Roger Wells, *Insurrection: The British Experience, 1795–1803* (Stroud: Alan Sutton, 1983).

Roger Wells, *Wretched Faces: Famine in Wartime England, 1793–1801* (Stroud: Alan Sutton, 1988).

Corinne C. Weston and Janelle R. Greenberg, *Subjects and Sovereigns: The Grand Controversy over Legal Sovereignty in Stuart England* (Cambridge: Cambridge University Press, 1981).

Joyce Whalley, *Cobwebs to Catch Flies: Illustrated Books for the Nursery and Schoolroom, 1700–1800* (Berkeley: University of California Press, 1975).

Lois Whitney, *Primitivism and the Idea of Progress, English Popular Literature in the Eighteenth Century* (Baltimore: Johns Hopkins University Press, 1934).

Ian D. Whyte, *Migration and Society in Britain, 1550–1830* (Basingstoke: Macmillan, 2000).

Chris Wiesenthal, *Figuring Madness in Nineteenth-Century Fiction* (London: Macmillan; New York: St Martin's Press, 1997).

Roy McKeen Wiles, *Serial Publication in England before 1750* (Cambridge: Cambridge University Press, 1957).

Roy McKeen Wiles, *Freshest Advices: Early Provincial Newspapers in England* (Columbus: Ohio State University Press, 1965).

Roy McKeen Wiles, 'The Relish for Reading in Provincial England Two Centuries Ago', in Paul J. Korshin (ed.), *The Widening Circle: Essays on the Circulation of Literature in Eighteenth-Century Europe* (Philadelphia: University of Pennsylvania Press, 1976), 85–115.

Tom Wilkinson, *Polite Landscapes: Gardens and Society in Eighteenth-Century England* (Baltimore: Johns Hopkins University Press, 1995).

Basil Willey, *The Eighteenth Century Background: Studies on the Idea of Nature in the Thought of the Period* (Harmondsworth: Penguin, 1962).

A. Susan Williams, *The Rich Man and the Diseased Poor in Early Victorian Literature* (Atlantic Highlands, NJ: Humanities Press, 1987).

Carolyn Williams, 'The Genteel Art of Resuscitation', *Transactions of the International Congress of Enlightenment*, 8 (1982), 1887–90.

Carolyn D. Williams, *Pope, Homer and Manliness: Some Aspects of Eighteenth-Century Classical Learning* (London: Routledge, 1993).

E. N. Williams, *Powder and Paint* (London: Longmans, 1957).

E. N. Williams (ed.), *The Eighteenth-Century Constitution 1688–1815* (Cambridge: Cambridge University Press, 1960).

E. N. Williams, *Life in Georgian England* (London: Batsford, 1962).

Glyn Williams and John Ramsden, *Ruling Britannia: Political History of Britain, 1688–1988* (London: Longman, 1990).

Gwyn Williams, 'Romanticism in Wales', in Roy Porter and Mikuláš Teich (eds.), *Romanticism in National Context* (Cambridge: Cambridge University Press, 1988), 1–8.

J. Gwynn Williams, *The University Movement in Wales* (Cardiff: University of Wales Press, 1993).

Karel Williams, *From Pauperism to Poverty* (London and Boston: Routledge and Kegan Paul, 1981).

Raymond Williams, *The Country and the City* (London: Chatto and Windus, 1973).

Jeffrey C. Williamson, *Did British Capitalism Breed Inequality?* (Boston: Allen and Unwin, 1985).

Frances Willmoth, *Sir Jonas Moore: Practical Mathematics and Restoration Science* (Woodbridge: Boydell Press, 1993).

S. Wilmot, *'The Business of Improvement': Agriculture and Scientific Culture in Britain, c.1770–c.1870* (Historical Geography Research Group Series, no. 24, n.p. 1990).

Adrian Wilson (ed.), *Rethinking Social History: English Society 1570–1920 and its Interpretation* (Manchester: Manchester University Press, 1993).

Adrian Wilson, *The Making of Man-Midwifery:*

Childbirth in England, 1660–1770 (London: University College London Press, 1995).

C. Anne Wilson (ed.), *'Banquetting Stuffe': The Fare and Social Background of the Tudor and Stuart Banquet* (Edinburgh: Edinburgh University Press, 1991).

C. Anne Wilson (ed.), *The Appetite and the Eye* (Edinburgh: Edinburgh University Press, 1991).

Charles Wilson, *England's Apprenticeship, 1603–1763*, 2nd edn. (London: Longman, 1984).

Charles Wilson, *First with the News: The History of W. H. Smith 1792–1972* (London: Cape, 1985).

David A. Wilson, *Paine and Cobbett: The Transatlantic Connection* (Kingston: McGill-Queen's University Press, 1988).

Francesca M. Wilson, *Strange Island: Britain through Foreign Eyes* (London: Longman Green, 1955).

Katharina M. Wilson (ed.), *Women Writers of the Renaissance and Reformation* (Athens: University of Georgia Press, 1987).

Kathleen Wilson, 'The Rejection of Deference: Urban Provincial Culture in England, 1715–1785' (Ph.D. thesis, Yale University, 1985).

Kathleen Wilson, 'Empire, Trade and Popular Politics in Mid-Hanoverian Britain', *Past and Present*, 121 (1988), 74–109.

Kathleen Wilson, 'Citizenship, Empire and Modernity in the English Provinces, c. 1720–1790', *Eighteenth Century Studies*, 29 (1995), 69–96.

Kathleen Wilson, *The Sense of the People: Politics, Culture and Imperialism in England, 1715–1785* (Cambridge: Cambridge University Press, 1995).

Donald Winch, *Adam Smith's Politics: An Essay in Historiographic Revision* (Cambridge: Cambridge University Press, 1978).

Donald Winch, 'Science and the Legislator: Adam Smith and After', *Economic Journal*, 93 (1982), 501–29.

Donald Winch, *Malthus* (New York: Oxford University Press, 1987).

Donald Winch, *Riches and Poverty: An Intellectual History of Political Economy in Britain, 1750–1834* (Cambridge: Cambridge University Press, 1996).

Anthony S. Wohl, *Endangered Lives: Public Health in Victorian Britain* (London: J. M. Dent, 1983).

John Wolffe (ed.), *Evangelical Faith and Public Zeal: Evangelicals and Society in Britain, 1780–1980* (London: SPCK, 1995)

Sybil Wolfram, *In-Laws and Outlaws: Kinship and Marriage in England* (New York: St Martin's Press, 1987).

Florence Wood and Kenneth Wood (eds.), *A Lancashire Gentleman: The Letters and Journals of Richard Hodgkinson 1763–1847* (Stroud: Sutton, 1992).

Linda Woodbridge, *Women and the English Renaissance: Literature and the Nature of Womenkind, 1540–1620* (Urbana: University of Illinois Press, 1984).

S. R. J. Woodell (ed.), *The English Landscape: Past, Present and Future* (Oxford: Oxford University Press, 1985).

Robert Woods and John Woodward (eds.), *Urban Disease and Mortality in Nineteenth-Century England* (London: Batsford Academic and Educational; New York: St Martin's Press, 1984).

Donald Woodward, *Men at Work: Labourers and Building Craftsmen in the Towns of Northern England, 1450–1750* (Cambridge: Cambridge University Press, 1995).

Austin Woolrych, *Commonwealth to Protectorate* (Oxford: Oxford University Press, 1982).

Blair Worden (ed.), *Stuart England* (Oxford: Phaidon Press, 1980).

J. R. Wordie, *Estate Management in Eighteenth-Century England: The Building of the Leveson–Gower Fortune* (London: Royal Historical Society, 1982).

Jenny Wormald, 'James VI and I: Two Kings or One?', *History*, 68 (1983).

D. G. Wright, *Popular Radicalism: The Working Class Experience, 1770–1880* (London: Longman, 1988).

K. Wrightson, *English Society, 1580–1680* (New Brunswick, NJ: Rutgers University Press; London: Hutchinson, 1982).

Keith Wrightson, 'The Social Order of Early Modern England: Three Approaches', in Lloyd Bonfield *et al.* (eds.), *The World We Have Gained: Histories of Population and Social Structure. Essays Presented to Peter Laslett on his Seventieth Birthday* (New York: Basil Blackwell, 1986), 177–202.

Keith Wrightson, 'The Enclosure of English Social History', *Rural History*, 1 (1990), 73–81.

Keith Wrightson and David Levine, *Poverty and Piety in an English Village* (New York: Academic Press, 1979).

E. A. Wrigley (ed.), *An Introduction to English Historial Demography from the Sixteenth to the Nineteenth Century* (London: Weidenfeld and Nicolson, 1966).

E. A. Wrigley, 'A Simple Model of London's Importance in Changing English Society and Economy, 1650–1750', *Past and Present*, 37 (1967), 44–70.

E. A. Wrigley, *Population and History* (London: Weidenfeld and Nicolson, 1969).

E. A. Wrigley, 'The Growth of Population in Eighteenth Century England: A Conundrum Resolved', *Past and Present*, 98 (1983), 121–50.

E. A. Wrigley, *Reproducing Families: The Political Economy of English Population History* (Cambridge: Cambridge University Press, 1984).

E. A. Wrigley, 'No Death without Birth: The Implications of English Mortality in the Early Modern Period', in R. Porter and A. Wear (eds.), *Problems and Methods in the History of Medicine* (London: Croom Helm, 1987), 133–50.

E. A. Wrigley, *People, Cities and Wealth: The Transformation of Traditional Society* (Oxford: Basil Blackwell, 1987).

E. A. Wrigley, *The Character of the Industrial*

Revolution in England (Cambridge: Cambridge University Press, 1988).

E. A. Wrigley, 'The Limits to Growth: Malthus and the Classical Economists', in Michael S. Teitelbaum and Jay M. Winter (eds.), *Population and Resources in Western Intellectual Traditions* (Cambridge: Cambridge University Press, 1989), 30–48.

E. A. Wrigley, R. S. Davies, J. E. Oeppen and R. S. Schofield, *English Population History from Family Reconstitution 1580–1837* (Cambridge: Cambridge University Press, 1997).

J. A. Yelling, *Common Fields and Enclosure in England 1450–1850* (London: Macmillan, 1977).

Eileen Janes Yeo, *The Contest for Social Science: Relations and Representations of Gender and Class* (London: Rivers Oram Press, 1996).

Eileen Janes Yeo (ed.), *Mary Wollstonecraft and 200 Years of Feminism* (London: Rivers Oram Press, 1997).

Eileen Janes Yeo and Stephen Yeo (eds.), *Popular Culture and Class Conflict, 1590–1914: Explorations in the History of Labour and Leisure* (Brighton, Sussex: Harvester Press; Atlantic Highlands NJ: Humanities Press, 1981).

Richard Yeo, *Defining Science: William Whewell, Natural Knowledge, and Public Debate in Early Victorian Britain* (Cambridge: Cambridge University Press, 1992).

D. Valenze York, *The First Industrial Women* (Oxford: Oxford University Press, 1995).

James D. Young, *The Rousing of the Scottish Working Class* (London: Croom Helm, 1979).

James D. Young, *Women and Popular Struggles: A History of Scottish and English Working-Class Women 1500–1984* (Edinburgh: Mainstream Publishing; Atlantic Highlands, NJ: Humanities Press International, 1985).

A. J. Youngson, *The Scientific Revolution in Victorian Medicine* (London: Croom Helm, 1979).

William Zachs, *Without Regard to Good Manners: A Biography of Gilbert Stuart 1743–1786* (Edinburgh: Edinburgh University Press, 1992).

Perez Zagorin (ed.), *Culture and Politics from Puritanism to the Enlightenment* (London: University of California Press, 1980).

Perez Zagorin, *Rebels and Rulers, 1500–1660*, vol. 1: *Society, States and Early Modern Revolution, Agrarian and Urban Rebellions*; vol. 2: *Provincial Rebellion, Revolutionary Civil Wars, 1560–1660* (Cambridge: Cambridge University Press, 1982).

Perez Zagorin, *Ways of Lying: Dissimulation, Persecution, and Conformity in Early Modern Europe* (Cambridge, Mass.: Harvard University Press, 1990).

Perez Zagorin, *Milton: Aristocrat and Rebel. The Poet and his Politics* (New York: Brewer, 1992).

Linda Gertner Zatlin, *The Nineteenth-Century Anglo-Jewish Novel* (Boston: G. K. Hall and Co., 1981).

John P. Zomchick, *Family and Law in Eighteenth-Century Fiction* (Cambridge: Cambridge University Press, 1993).

Steven Zwicker, *Lines of Authority: Politics and English Literary Culture, 1649–1689* (Ithaca, NY: Cornell University Press, 1992).

INDEX

Figures in **bold** indicates a definition or an explanation. Figures followed by a lower case 'n' refer to footnotes.